IMMUNOPHARMACOLOGY REVIEWS VOLUME 2

IMMUNOPHARMACOLOGY REVIEWS VOLUME 2

Edited by

John W. Hadden
and
Andor Szentivanyi

University of South Florida
College of Medicine
Tampa, Florida

PLENUM PRESS • NEW YORK AND LONDON

Library of Congress Cataloging-in-Publication Data

ISBN-13: 978-1-4613-8010-8 e-ISBN: 978-1-4613-0349-7
DOI: 10.1007/978-1-4613-0349-7

Softcover reprint of the hardcover 1st edition 1996
A Division of Plenum Publishing Corporation
233 Spring Street, New York, N. Y. 10013

10 9 8 7 6 5 4 3 2 1

CONTRIBUTORS

CHRISTINE M. ABARCA • Department of Internal Medicine, University of South Florida Colleges of Medicine and Public Health, Tampa, Florida 33612

DENNIS J. BEER • Pulmonary Medicine, Newton–Wellesley Hospital, Newton, Massachusetts 02162

STUART M. BROOKS • Department of Environmental and Occupational Health, University of South Florida Colleges of Medicine and Public Health, Tampa, Florida 33612

RONALD G. COFFEY • Department of Pharmacology, University of South Florida College of Medicine, Tampa, Florida 33612

JOHN J. COSTA • Departments of Pathology and Medicine, Beth Israel Hospital and Harvard Medical School, and Division of Experimental Pathology, Beth Israel Hospital, Boston, Massachusetts 02215

SANDRA DANIEL • Department of Microbiology, College of Veterinary Medicine, University of Tennessee, Knoxville, Tennessee 37916

M. JANE EHRKE • Grace Cancer Drug Center, Roswell Park Cancer Institute, Buffalo, New York 14263

NICOLA FABRIS • Immunology Center, Gerontological Research Department, INRCA, 60100 Ancona, and Institute of Haematology, Medical Faculty, University of Pavia, 27100 Pavia, Italy

STEPHEN J. GALLI • Department of Pathology, Beth Israel Hospital and Harvard Medical School, and Division of Experimental Pathology, Beth Israel Hospital, Boston, Massachusetts 02215

JOHN W. HADDEN • Department of Internal Medicine, Division of Immunopharmacology, University of South Florida College of Medicine, Tampa, Florida 33612

DAVID W. HOROHOV • Department of Microbiology, College of Veterinary Medicine, Louisiana State University, Baton Rouge, Louisiana 70803

TAMMIE L. KEADLE • Department of Ophthalmology, Washington University School of Medicine, St. Louis, Missouri 63130

RICHARD F. LOCKEY • Departments of Internal Medicine, Neurology, Pharmacology, and Environmental and Occupational Health, University of South Florida Colleges of Medicine and Public Health, Tampa, Florida 33612

K. NOEL MASIHI • Robert Koch Institute, Federal Institute for Infectious and Non-Communicable Diseases, D-13353 Berlin, Germany

ENRICO MIHICH • Grace Cancer Drug Center, Roswell Park Cancer Institute, Buffalo, New York 14263

LEON D. PROCKOP • Department of Neurology, University of South Florida Colleges of Medicine and Public Health, Tampa, Florida 33612

ROSS E. ROCKLIN • Clinical Research, Astra USA, Inc., Westborough, Massachusetts 01581

BARRY T. ROUSE • Department of Microbiology, College of Veterinary Medicine, University of Tennessee, Knoxville, Tennessee 37916

VIBEKE STRAND • Division of Immunology, Stanford University, Stanford, California 94305

ANDOR SZENTIVANYI • Departments of Internal Medicine, Neurology, Pharmacology, and Environmental and Occupational Health, University of South Florida Colleges of Medicine and Public Health, Tampa, Florida 33612

NORMAN TALAL • Clinical Immunology Section, Audie L. Murphy Memorial Veterans Hospital, and Department of Medicine, The University of Texas Health Science Center at San Antonio, San Antonio, Texas 78284

JAMES E. TALMADGE • University of Nebraska Medical Center, Omaha, Nebraska 68198

CONTENTS

PART I. INTRODUCTION

CHAPTER 4

IMMUNOPHARMACOLOGY OF ANTICANCER AGENTS

M. Jane Ehrke and Enrico Mihich

PART III. MICROBIAL IMMUNOPHARMACOLOGY

CHAPTER 5

VIRUS-INDUCED IMMUNOSUPPRESSION

TAMMIE L. KEADLE, SANDRA DANIEL, BARRY T. ROUSE, AND DAVID W. HOROHOV

Chapter 6

Immunotherapy of Microbial Diseases

K. Noel Masihi

Part IV. Allergy Immunopharmacology

Chapter 7

Basophils and Mast Cells: Basic Biology and Clinical Significance

John J. Costa and Stephen J. Galli

CHAPTER 8

HISTAMINE

ROSS E. ROCKLIN AND DENNIS J. BEER

Part V. Autoimmunity

Chapter 9

Biologic Interventions in Autoimmune Diseases

Vibeke Strand and Norman Talal

Part VI. Neuroimmunomodulation

Chapter 10

Neuroendocrine–Immune Interactions

Nicola Fabris

Chapter 11

Thymic Endocrinology and Prospects for Treating Thymic Involution

John W. Hadden

Chapter 12

Some Evolutionary, Morphoregulatory, and Functional Aspects of the Immune–Neuroendocrine Circuitry

Andor Szentivanyi, Christine M. Abarca, Stuart M. Brooks, Richard F. Lockey, and Leon D. Prockop

IMMUNOPHARMACOLOGY REVIEWS VOLUME 2

PART I

INTRODUCTION

CHAPTER 1

IMMUNOMODULATORS

JOHN W. HADDEN

Immunomodulators are agents that are intended to modify immune response in an attempt to restore immunity and/or to direct it toward tumor or pathogen in the treatment of human diseases. These agents are also termed *biological response modifiers* (BRMs). The agents currently used include drugs, microbial products, and proteins derived from the immune system. These proteins include cytokines and antibodies. The cytokines (referred to as *lymphokines* and *interleukins*) are generally produced by recombinant genetic techniques in various vectors and the antibodies by monoclonal antibody-producing cell cultures. Several of these agents have direct anticancer activity. The growth of this area of immunopharmacology in recent years and the extensive development of these agents in the United States and abroad indicate that many of these agents have and will enter clinical use in the years to come.

1. BACKGROUND

Various cellular populations of the immune system are targets of immunomodulators. The immune system is composed of many different cell populations having distinct functional roles in defending the host against tumor or pathogen. The cell populations are linked in a complex network by many different low-molecular-weight mediators and protein cytokines. While complex and difficult to understand, the immune system is amenable to manipulation not only through vaccination or immunization but also by immunomodulation.

Developmentally, the immune system is derived as an offshoot of the hematopoietic system. Its specialized cells called *lymphocytes* consist of two main classes,

JOHN W. HADDEN • Department of Internal Medicine, Division of Immunopharmacology, University of South Florida College of Medicine, Tampa, Florida 33612.

Immunopharmacology Reviews, Volume 2, edited by John W. Hadden and Andor Szentivanyi. Plenum Press, New York, 1996.

bone marrow-derived antibody-producing "B" lymphocytes and thymus-derived lymphokine-producing "T" lymphocytes. B lymphocytes develop early in life and are distributed to the spleen and peripheral lymphoid tissues such as lymph nodes, tonsils, and Peyer's patches of the intestine where they form follicles. These follicles trap antigen and process it with the help of macrophages. The precommitted reactive B lymphocytes are stimulated by antigen to proliferate and mature to antibody-producing cells. This process is delicately regulated by the sequential actions of various interleukins (especially IL-1, 4, 5, 6, and 10) produced by B and T lymphocytes and macrophages. Once these B lymphocytes have matured into "antibody factories" called plasma cells, they produce large quantities of antibodies which circulate in the blood and coat mucosal surfaces. Acting alone and in concert with the complement cascade, these antibodies offer a strong neutralizing defense against invading pathogens. These antibodies bind to the surfaces of phagocytic cells like polymorphonuclear granulocytes and macrophages and assist them in opsonizing and ingesting various pathogens. The five different classes of antibody (IgA, M, G, D, and E) confer a spectrum of different defense capacities. In general, the B-cell system confers humoral immunity and, therefore, resistance to high-grade pyogenic pathogens, particularly bacteria; thus, the primary manifestations of B-cell deficiency as occurs in agamma globulinemia are respiratory tract infections (sinusitis, otitis, bronchitis, and pneumonia) and gastrointestinal tract infections (particularly with enteroviruses). Most viral infections are dealt with normally by these patients, although hepatitis and enterovirus infections can prove fatal. The B-cell system develops soon after birth and remains remarkably stable throughout life. The system is relatively resistant to suppression by cancer chemotherapy and immunosuppressive drugs and is much more resistant to environmental toxicants and aging than is the T-cell system. Primary hypogammaglobulinemia and antibody deficiency syndromes are relatively rare; more often, dysfunction of the system is observed in autoimmune diseases and in leukemias and lymphomas. The B-cell system has, for decades, been therapeutically manipulated through immunization and as a result, diseases such as diphtheria, tetanus, measles, mumps, and polio have been markedly reduced or eradicated in certain areas. The function of the B-cell system has been substantially replaced in deficient individuals through the immunoprophylactic use of gamma globulin and both intramuscular and intravenous preparations are available. Hyperimmune globulin and fresh frozen plasma have been used in the treatment of active infections of various types in these deficient individuals.

A recent discovery is that antibody-producing B lymphocytes can be fused in culture to produce immortalized B cells that generate monospecific antibodies. The monoclonal antibodies produced by these clones of B cells can be generated in large quantities and in a high degree of purity and are being used extensively in clinical trials as potential diagnostic and therapeutic agents.

T lymphocytes develop in the thymus. This process is delicately regulated by the sequential action of various interleukins (especially IL-1, 2, 4, 6, 7, 8, and 12). T lymphocytes distribute only in small part to the peripheral lymphoid organs where they play a major role in the regulation of antibody production by B lymphocytes via the two major subpopulations of helper and suppressor T cells. The major population circulates in the blood (approximately 80% of blood lymphocytes are T cells), percolates through the tissues, and returns to the circulation via lymphatics and the thoracic duct. The T-cell system confronts pathogen or tumor directly and is thus called the *cellular immune system* in contrast to the *humoral immune B-cell system*. The T-cell system responds to antigenic challenge by the clonal expansion of precommitted sensitized T cells, the direct cytotoxic action of killer T cells, and the synthesis and secretion of a myriad of lymphokines. In addition to helper, suppressor, and growth-regulating factors for B lymphocytes, the major lymphokines include (1) IL-2 whose major function is in concert with macrophage-produced IL-1 to regulate both the ontogeny of T and natural killer (NK) cells and the clonal proliferation of T cells in response to antigen, (2) macrophage regulatory lymphokines including macrophage chemotactic factor, migration inhibitory factor, activating factors, growth and colony-stimulating factors (CSFs), and a fusion factor, (3) IFN-γ which participates in antiviral defense and activates macrophages and NK cells for enhanced microbicidal and tumoricidal capacity, and (4) lymphotoxin (also called *tumor necrosis factor* β) which is directly tumoricidal. A number of other interleukins modulate the movement and/or secretion of granulocytic populations (Table I). The various interleukins are, in general, produced by both $CD4^+$ and $CD8^+$ subclasses of T lymphocytes and interact with each other and with cytokines from both monocytes and B cells in a highly synergistic manner (i.e., the combined action exceeds the sum of individual actions). The major form of expression of the T-cell system is variously termed *delayed-type hypersensitivity* (DTH) or *cell-mediated immunity* (CMI). Its hallmarks are a slow development (24–48 hr to peak) and its mixed cellular expression. The two principal cellular components are activated T cells as a minor population and monocyte-derived macrophages in various stages of activation, as the major population. The cellular immune system is responsible for defending the host against a broad spectrum of invasive bacteria, fungi, viruses, and parasites and against spontaneous malignancies; thus, cellular immune deficiency is characterized by a high incidence of systemic infections with mycobacteria (e.g., tuberculosis), fungi (e.g., candidiasis), and parasites (e.g., pneumocystis, toxoplasma) and of malignancies such as lymphomas and Kaposi's sarcoma. Primary deficiencies of CMI are rare; however, secondary deficiencies are common in cancer, human immunodeficiency virus (HIV) infection and other viral infections, and malnutrition and parasitosis. The T-cell system is very sensitive to suppression by cancer chemotherapy and immunosuppressive drugs and is much more sensitive than the B-cell system to environmental toxicants and to aging. Replacement of the functions of the T-cell system has been attempted in primary deficiency through the use of bone marrow and fetal thymus transplants. Only recently have T-cell products been used as replacement therapy. A number of T-cell-produced lymphokines have been produced by genetic engineering and many interleukins, IFN-γ, and CSFs are being used in clinical trials. At the present time, the expansion of tumor-infiltrating lymphocytes (TIL) in culture is in vogue as an

TABLE I
Interleukins

	Source				
	T cell	NK cell	Macrophage/ monocyte	Other	Action
IL-1B	±	+	+	+	Augmentation of IL-2 and IFN-γ on T cells ↑ NK, proinflammatory
IL-2	+	+			T-cell proliferation, cytotoxicity
IL-3	+		+		Stem cell proliferation, augmentation of mast cell and basophil
IL-4	+ (TH_2)				Induction of IgG_1 and IgE Downregulation of TH_2
IL-5	+				Activation of eosinophils IgE promotion
IL-6			+	+	T-cell differentiation Acute-phase proteins
IL-7			+	+ (BM & TEC)	Pre-B and early T-cell growth
IL-8	+		+	+	Chemotaxis of neutrophils
IL-9	+				Stem cell growth and development
IL-10	+		+		B-cell growth and development
IL-11				+ (BM)	
IL-12	+		+		Promotes $TH_0 \rightarrow TH_1$, ↑ NK and LAK
IL-13	+				Cell differentiation
GM-CSF	+		+	+	BM stem cell growth
IFN-γ	+ (TH_1)	+	+		Macrophage activation, upregulation of TH_1, ↑ CMI
TNF-α			+		Proinflammatory, cachexis

anticancer treatment. Nonspecific augmentation of the T-cell system has been attempted with thymomimetic drugs (i.e., drugs that mimic the action of the thymus) and with biologicals such as hormones extracted from the thymus. Specific augmentation has been attempted with factors like transfer factor derived from T cells and through immunization with live organisms such as bacille Calmette–Guérin (BCG).

As detailed, phagocytic cells like granulocytes and macrophages are important companion populations in the expression of both cellular and humoral immunity. These populations of cells produce a number of important mediators and cytokines. Of particular note from an immunopharmacologic standpoint are (1) the colony-stimulating factors for granulocytes (CSF-G), monocytes (CSF-M or CSF1) and for both populations (CSF-GM), (2) tumor necrosis factor α and (3) IL-1β. These cytokines have been genetically cloned and are under development for replacement therapy.

In addition, NK cells form a unique group of presumed pre-T cells which participate in a relatively primitive defense mechanism against both pathogens and tumor cells. This population of cells when activated by IL-2 and IFN-γ can kill a number of tumor cell types particularly those of hematopoietic origin. When cloned *in vitro* in the presence of IL-2, they are thought to form a population called *lymphokine-activated killer* (LAK) cells which then show a broad spectrum of antitumor activity. The *in vitro* expansion of autologous LAK cells with subsequent infusion of high doses of IL-2 has provided the basis for a novel form of anticancer therapy used experimentally in renal cell cancer and malignant melanoma.

These cell populations (Fig. 1) form the targets for immunotherapy with various immunomodulators. Their products as antibodies or recombinant cytokines also have provided immunomodulating biologicals for therapy. In addition, natural regulatory hormones (e.g., thymic hormones) and immunomodulatory products derived from bacteria complete the repertoire of our current armamentarium.

Before discussing the basic immunopharmacology of the agents, it is important

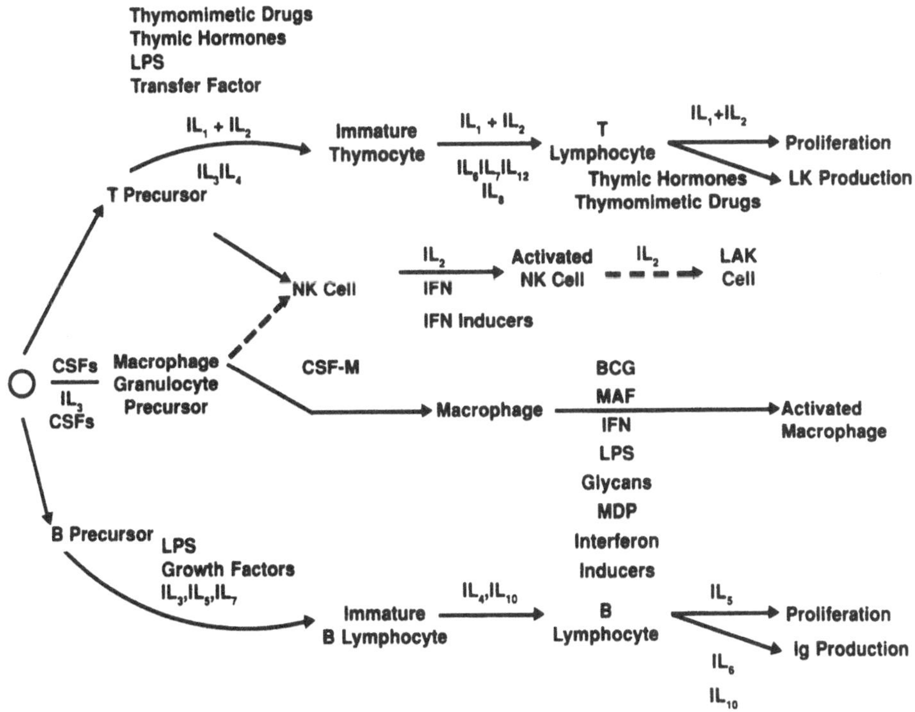

Figure 1. Immune development schematic.

to note that therapy development in this area is in its early experimental phases. Development initially stressed nonspecific immunomodulation with drugs and bacterial products in cancer but has advanced to include the extensive use of recombinant biologicals in cancer and HIV infection [acquired immunodeficiency syndrome (AIDS) and AIDS-related complex (ARC)] and the use of drugs and biologicals in the treatment of rheumatoid arthritis and in the treatment or prophylaxis for various other infectious illnesses. It has been demonstrated that thymus involution and T-cell deficiencies are central issues in immune senescence and contribute to mortality and morbidity through increased incidence of cancer, infection, and autoimmunity. Immunoprophylactic treatments to restore cellular immunity to ensure longevity and to reduce morbidity are a logical future projection. Only now is the immunopharmacology of these clinical efforts coming into clear focus; the present portends the emergence of an important new therapeutic science.

2. BASIC IMMUNOPHARMACOLOGY: HOST-MODIFYING AGENTS

Immunomodulator effectiveness is related to the cellular targets of action. The agents to be discussed can be divided into two partially overlapping groups, the host modifying agents and the direct-acting anticancer agents. The host modifying agents can be further divided as to their primary cellular targets; however, it is important to remember that the molecular and cellular networks that constitute the immune system dictate that an agent acting primarily on one cell target generally influences secondarily other cell populations.

2.1. Thymomimetic Biologicals and Drugs

The central role of the thymus in evolving T cells and its early involution has naturally led to the search for drugs and biologicals that will mimic the role of the thymus in inducing or promoting the development and function of T lymphocytes. These agents are collectively called *thymomimetic biologicals* and *drugs*. Despite a midlife thymic "menopause," the thymus can rejuvenate to repopulate the system following radiation injury or other T-cell-removing influences. The key regulatory influences acting to populate the system initially and to repopulate it after depletion are only now under study.

A number of peptides have been derived from the thymus and developed for clinical use in an attempt to replace the involuted thymus. Mixtures of peptides from bovine thymus include thymosin fraction 5 and thymostimulin. Purified peptides include thymopoietin, thymulin, thymosin α_1, and thymic humoral factor (Fig. 2). These agents have been shown to induce T-cell surface markers on prothymocytes and to modulate the display of these receptors on mature T cells. In addition, they modulate a number of responses of T cells including proliferation, interleukin production, cytotoxicity, and helper and suppressor function. Interestingly, a role for them in

THYMOSIN

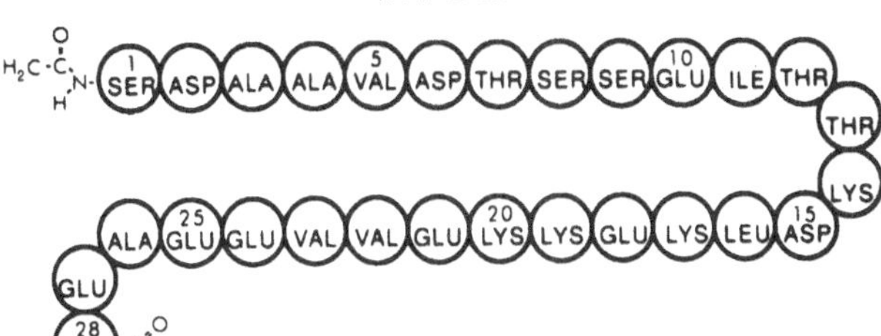

THYMIC HUMORAL FACTOR

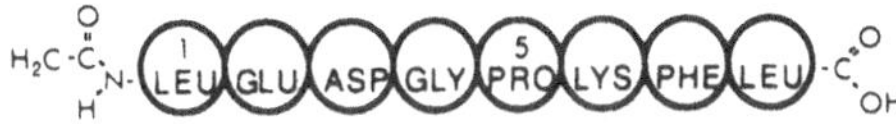

THYMOPOIETIN

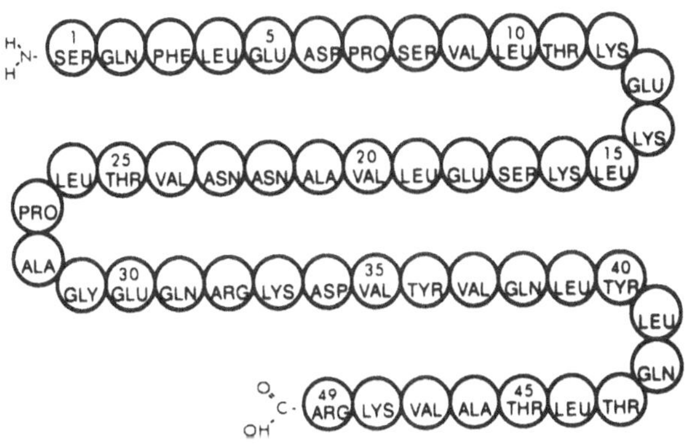

THYMULIN

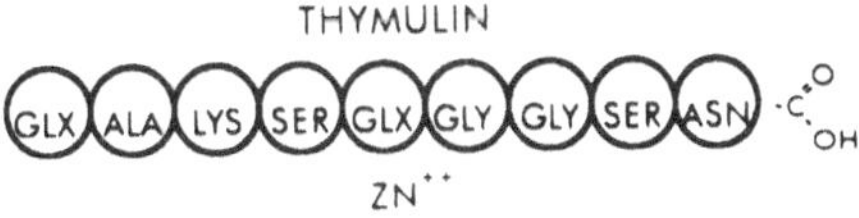

Figure 2. Sequence analysis of purified thymic hormones.

intrathymic evolution of T cells has not emerged suggesting that these peptides commit T cells to the lineage but other signals govern the timing of T-cell maturation and seeding into the periphery.

In experimental animals, they have shown activity to modulate T-cell markers and function and to increase cell-mediated immunity and resistance in infection, cancer, autoimmunity, and aging models. In humans, a number of these effects have been confirmed. These studies have provided the rationale for their use as immunorestorative agents in human diseases. This effort, however, has been complicated by several problems. All agents require injection with the use of the mixtures from bovine thymus, and allergic responses to bovine proteins have been observed. The smaller defined peptides, while not immunogenic, show short half-lives in the circulation, requiring frequent administration of relatively large amounts. Finally, insufficient knowledge about the differential actions of the individual peptides makes it unclear whether one is more appropriate for a specific condition or whether multiple hormones should be given to achieve reconstitution. Despite these drawbacks, physician acceptance and patient tolerance for these agents have been demonstrated by widespread clinical use in Europe, particularly Italy and Germany. Efficacy and appropriate clinical indications by U.S. standards remain to be determined.

The two main classes of compounds having thymomimetic action by the minimum criteria that, directly or indirectly via induced factors, they are active in the differentiation of prothymocytes and in the modulation of mature T-cell receptors and functions, are represented by the drugs isoprinosine and levamisole (Fig. 3).

The effect of isoprinosine to induce T-cell maturation and to promote T-cell function can be directly demonstrated *in vitro* while a similar effect of levamisole can only be demonstrated to occur *in vivo* and apparently results from the induction in the serum of a thymic hormone-like factor putatively derived from liver. Each class is also represented by structurally similar chemical compounds which insofar as has been examined, share similar immunopharmacologies [e.g., diethyldithiocarbamate (DTC) for levamisole and methyl IMP for isoprinosine]. Representatives of both classes of agents augment cell-mediated immune responses as measured both *in vitro* and *in vivo*.

For the purpose of simplicity, in the remaining discussion, only the immunopharmacologies of levamisole and isoprinosine will be considered. The reader is referred to other sources for expanded discussion and references on the immunopharmacologies of these two compounds and their structurally related compounds.

Not all of the activities of the two compounds can be regarded as thymomimetic. Additional features of levamisole's *in vitro* actions that are not strictly thymomimetic include: augmentation of lymphokine-induced macrophage phagocytosis and activation, augmentation of macrophage and granulocyte motility, and induction of interferon.

Additional features of isoprinosine's *in vitro* action that are not strictly thymomimetic include: induction of B-cell differentiation, increase in NK cell activity, increased monocyte phagocytosis, potentiation of lymphokine-induced macrophage proliferation and activation, and increased antibody-dependent cytotoxicity by eosinophils.

Both levamisole and isoprinosine have received extensive *in vivo* immunopharmacologic testing in animals and humans. Many of the immune functions shown to be affected by levamisole, isoprinosine, and the thymic hormones *in vitro* have been confirmed *in vivo* following administration to experimental animals and to human subjects (Table II). Table II makes the general point that, to the extent tested, levamisole and isoprinosine share the immunopharmacologic actions of the thymic

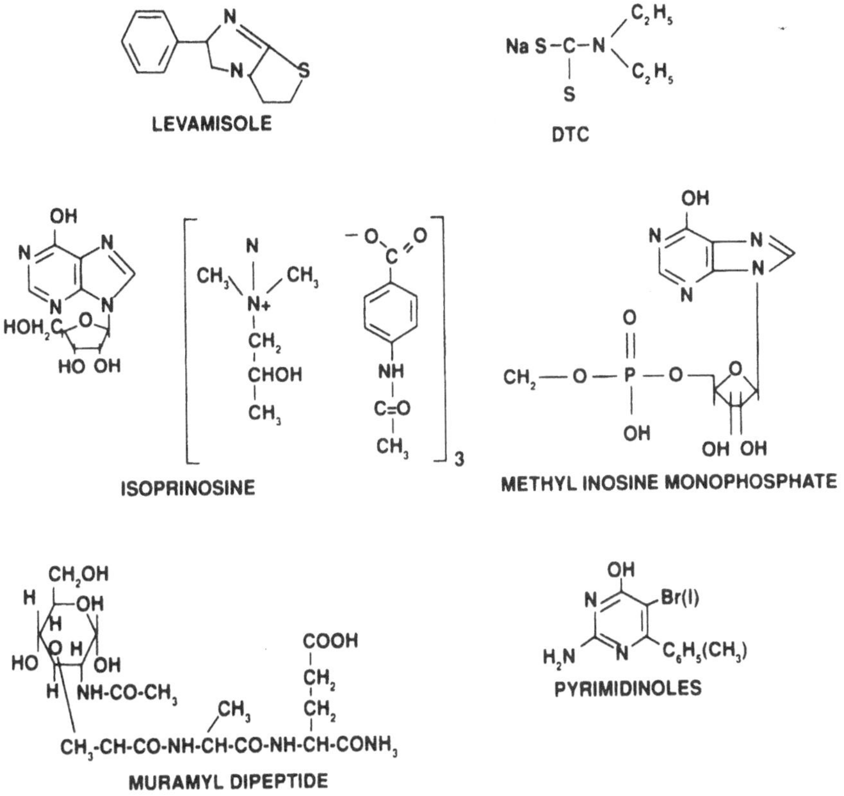

LEVAMISOLE

DTC

ISOPRINOSINE

METHYL INOSINE MONOPHOSPHATE

MURAMYL DIPEPTIDE

PYRIMIDINOLES

Figure 3. Chemical immunomodulators.

hormones as assessed by *in vitro* parameters, DTH, and resistance to viral infection, cancer, and autoimmunity.

While both levamisole and isoprinosine are orally active, both have limitations in their therapeutic usefulness. Both are relatively mild in their action. Levamisole often takes weeks to months to achieve effects and nonresponder animals and humans exist in any particular disease category without immunopharmacologic explanation. Its side effects (particularly agranulocytosis) are significant. Apparently some of the other sulfur-containing compounds, e.g., DTC, are less toxic and may be more potent and, therefore, offer significant potential for improving on the immunotherapeutic efficacy of levamisole. Isoprinosine, generally, requires relatively high doses but is somewhat more consistent in its action than levamisole and it is nontoxic. Other 9-substituted hypoxanthines, in particular methyl IMP, are more potent on a weight basis and have more prolonged actions. Isoprinosine has been extensively analyzed in viral infection in humans and animals.

Both levamisole and isoprinosine have demonstrated activity in infectious and

TABLE II
In Vivo Effects of Levamisole, Isoprinosine, and Thymic Hormones on Immune Function of Experimental Animals and Humans

Immune function	Levamisole	Isoprinosine	Thymic hormones
Experimental animals			
T-cell marker induction in athymic or thymectomized mice	+	+	+
T-cell mitogen responses	+	+	+
Lymphokine production	+	+	+
Cytotoxicity of T cells	+	+	+
Cell-mediated immunity			
DTH or graft rejection	+	+	+
T-dependent antibody production	+	+	+
Resistance to tumor recurrence			
Following cytoreductive therapy	+	NT	+
Without cytoreductive therapy	0	0	0
Reduction of autoimmunity	+	+	+
Reversal of effects of aging on IR	+	+	+
Humans			
Active rosettes of T cell	+	+	+
T-cell mitogen response	±	+	+
Lymphocyte counts	±	±	±
DNCB or skin tests	+	+	+
Resistance to cancer	+	NT	+
Resistance to viral infection	+	+	+
Decreased autoimmunity	+	+	+

autoimmune models. Both have reversed the immunodepression of aging in animals in association with decreased tumor incidence and/or increased survival. These activities parallel those reported for the thymic hormones. Therefore, the clinical indications for use are and will be predictably similar.

In addition to the thymomimetic drugs and biologicals, a number of other agents have actions on T cells and can be used either in a thymomimetic way or in a T-cell adjuvant mode.

IL-2 (formerly *T-cell growth factor*) promotes mature T-cell proliferation by acting as a second signal in the mitogen-signal sequence and both the induction of markers and proliferation of prothymocytes and early T cells. It has been postulated to constitute one of several "signals from the periphery" to promote T-cell development and exodus from the thymus. As such it can act to promote development of T cells and expand antigen-stimulated T cells in an adjuvant mode. It also can enhance and expand tumoricidal NK and LAK cells. Enhancement of NK cell activity, while not a potent direct antitumor mechanism, appears to relate to the inhibition of metastases. Activation of LAK cells, particularly by *ex vivo* means, does appear to be active against progressive tumor growth (see the discussion on adoptive cell therapy).

Administration of recombinant IL-2 (rIL-2) to animals has demonstrated antitumor activity by a T-cell adjuvant mechanism at low doses and activation of LAK cells at high doses. The half-life of rIL-2 is rather short following intravenous administration; however, more sustained levels follow intramuscular or intraperitoneal administration. More impressive immunopharmacologic effects have been shown by its regional administration by the intralymphatic or perilymphatic route.

IL-1 (formerly *T-cell activating factor*) is a monokine produced by activated monocyte/macrophages. It is active on many different cell populations contributing to inflammatory responses; however, its primary immunopharmacologic action at low levels appears to lie in its T-cell-activating characteristics. It also acts synergistically with IL-2 to induce proliferation and development of prothymocytes and immature T cells. It induces IL-2 and high-affinity IL-2 receptors and promotes T-cell clonal proliferation. Important issues for preclinical immunopharmacologic studies as well as clinical indications remain to be determined; however, the synergy of IL-1 with IL-2 on T-cell development and function suggests thymomimetic actions and indications.

One class of compounds that has seen extensive clinical application over several decades is the transfer factor/dialyzed leukocyte extract (DLE) group of substances. The essence of the phenomena is that T cells are the source of small peptides that nonspecifically stimulate T-cell function and, in some cases, can transfer cell-mediated immunity from a sensitized to a nonsensitized human. The basis for the specific transfer (e.g., hapten, a peptide complementary to hapten, or a derepressor molecule) has not been determined; however, nonspecific immunostimulation has been variously attributed to the inosine in transfer factor (giving it actions like isoprinosine) or to the Tyr-Gly-Gly or Tyr-Gly sequences present in Imreg 1 and 2. Evidence suggests that transfer factor induces T-cell differentiation and thus may have thymomimetic actions on both T-cell development and function. Its development in this context is awaited.

2.2. Macrophage-Activating Agents

Macrophage-activating agents have been extensively employed to enhance tumor immunity and resistance to pathogen challenge, particularly to facultative intracellular pathogens, and to increase antibody production as adjuvants. Initially, complex microbial products like BCG and *Corynebacterium parvum* were used to nonspecifically enhance tumor immunity in animals and more recently in humans. Parallel immunopharmacologic studies defined their actions as being primarily mediated by activated macrophages. Their antigenicity and the capacity of mixed bacterial vaccines to induce the symptoms of infection and in the case of BCG actual infection made them ambivalent agents. The results of the preclinical and clinical studies were neither consistent nor predictable. Considerable effort has been invested in finding less toxic and more reliable microbe-derived agents. While the search continues, several have emerged as clinically active.

Part of the macrophage activity of mixed bacterial and other microbial agents can be ascribed to polysaccharide components of their cell walls. Several reasonably pure polysaccharide preparations of varying molecular weight have been prepared from fungi. Examples include lentinan, krestin, glucan, schizophyllan, and levan. The immunopharmacologies of these glycans are quite similar and the activity appears to depend on the presence of 1,3 rather than 1,4 or 1,6 glycosidic linkages. All apparently activate macrophages. *In vivo*, particularly in high-molecular-weight forms, they expand the reticuloendothelial system and produce hepatosplenomegaly. Symptoms are generally fever and a "flulike" syndrome presumed to be mediated by monokines such as IL-1 and CSF, and prostaglandins. In preclinical models they have shown effects to enhance resistance to pathogen challenge prophylactically but not therapeutically. Effects have been observed in cancers in animal models particularly when treatment is combined with cytoreductive therapy.

Part of the macrophage activity particularly of the mycobacterial preparations appears to reside in the presence of the muramyl dipeptides resident therein. Synthetic muramyl dipeptides (MDPs) of many types have been produced and patented and are under development. MDP and its derivatives activate macrophages directly and promote proliferation, secretion of monokines including CSF and TNF, and both microbicidal and tumoricidal function. In the latter regard, MDPs have potent synergy with IFN-γ and lipopolysaccharide (LPS) endotoxin (particularly in liposomes) in inducing tumoricidal macrophages. MDP with endotoxin can elicit the tumor necrosis phenomena *in vivo*. Projected clinical applications focus on adjuvant use and antitumor immunotherapy. The requirement for preadministration for antiinfective use presently limits their usefulness in this area.

Still another component of bacteria having macrophage activation potential lies in the LPS endotoxin component. This component has a spectrum of immunopharmacologic features by both direct and indirect means. While profoundly active, the most important features appear to be direct macrophage activation for secretion, microbicidal and tumoricidal activity, and polyclonal B-cell activation. These characteristics make LPS, like MDP, potently active as an adjuvant and an enhancer of resistance for both tumor and pathogen challenge. LPS, unfortunately, is very toxic, producing shock in addition to fever and other symptoms. The toxic activity and certainly a large part of the immunopharmacologic actions of LPS reside in its lipid A moiety. The removal of a phosphate by acid hydrolysis to yield a monophosphoryl lipid A yields an active but less toxic LPS. Synthetic derivatives of lipid A also show greater antitumor activity with reduced toxicity.

Other active components of bacterial cell walls (e.g., lipoteichoic acids, lysopeptides, trehalose dimycolate, and cell wall skeleton) are under study and the future surely will see an effective harnessing of these potent microbial immunomodulators for clinical use.

Another approach to macrophage activation has been the development of cytokines that act as macrophage activators for microbicidal and tumoricidal capacity. These include IFN-α, -β, and -γ and CSF1. These cytokines, now available in recombinant form, have been demonstrated to activate macrophages for various functions *in vitro* and *in vivo*. The most extensive experience preclinically and clinically has been with rIFN-α of which there exist 20 genetically different types. There is also the possibility of using hybrid forms in the future.

It is important to note that many of the macrophage-activating compounds induce fever mediated by prostaglandin synthesis. The adjuvant and protective effects of these compounds are not reduced by concurrent administration of a nonsteroidal antiinflammatory agent to block prostaglandin synthesis. While fever is an unwanted side effect of the compound, it may contribute to an immunotherapeutic result, particularly in cancer.

2.3. Interferons and Inducers as NK Cell Activators

Another large class of immunotherapeutic agents involves the interferons and their inducers as NK cell activators.

NK cells are central to the resistance to low levels of pathogen and tumor challenge. They exist as part of natural surveillance mechanisms and are nonspecific in their responses. They do not expand with antigen challenge; however, they can be expanded by persistent exposure to relatively high doses of IL-2. IFN-α, -β, and -γ are all activators of NK cells. This action is part of the rationale for their clinical application in human cancer. The interferons, particularly IFN-α and -β, are antiproliferative for lymphocytes as well as tumor cells and thus their *in vivo* use at high doses results in suppressed lymphoproliferative responses and suppressed humoral and cellular immunity. At lower doses CMI has been observed to be augmented. Interferons are protective against a variety of viral challenges when given prophylactically. IFN-γ is more immunostimulating. So far most of the clinical experience has been obtained with IFN-α in cancer. IFN-α is more stable and distributes better than IFN-β following intramuscular administration; however, their pharmacokinetics are similar when administration is by the intravenous route. Both forms produce fever and "flulike" symptoms which are dose dependent. At low doses, NK cell activity and other immune parameters are increased; at higher doses, most responses are suppressed, including NK cell activity, and both lymphopenia and anemia occur. The interferons remain important components of the immunomodulator repertoire and clearly have both immunostimulating and immunosuppressive effects depending on the dose and the response measured. With the heavy emphasis on the maximum tolerated doses used in cancer, the optimalization of the immunopharmacologic effects of the interferons alone and in conjunction with other agents has been neglected. Interferons have been observed experimentally to synergize with other agents (Table III) and the use of lower doses of IFN in combinations should maximize the immunopharmacologic effects as well as lessen its toxicity for use in cancer, AIDS, and chronic viral and bacterial infectious diseases.

A number of IFN inducers have been studied including various viruses, viral components, and polynucleotides and other polymers. In general, they share the effects and toxicities of IFN. It was noted, however, that the inducers produce a refractory state for IFN induction lasting up to 1 week and they are thought to be

TABLE III
Interferon Synergistic Interactions

IFN-α + IFN-β; IFN-α + IFN-γ
IFN + chemotherapy
IFN + immunomodulators (e.g., isoprinosine, cimetidine)
IFN + IL-2
IFN + TNF
IFN + MDP/LPS/liposomes
IFN + monoclonal antibody (imaging)

inferior to exogenous IFN administration in the levels of IFN achieved and the persistence of effects. Pyran copolymers (maleic anhydride-divinyl ether) and poly I:C LC have proved more toxic and less active than IFN-α. The mismatched double-stranded polymer ampligen (poly I:poly C with interspersed uracil) appears to have less immunosuppressive and other side effects and is under study in HIV infection. The pyrimidinoles (AIBP and AIPP) are the only IFN inducers that appear to be orally active and nontoxic. Their persistent positive effects in tumor and infectious challenge models following weekly administration indicate that IFN induction does not have to be great to produce positive challenge results.

These three major categories allow an effective grouping of most host-modifying immunomodulators (see Fig. 1). It perhaps underestimates the extent to which growth factors for all lineages of cells will be useful to enhance resistance. It neglects, for lack of classification, agents with mixed or poorly characterized actions.

2.4. Anticancer Agents Derived from the Immune System

The interferons (α and β) whose immunopharmacologies are discussed in the previous section were the first biologicals to be explored for effects as anticancer agents. Their inhibition of the growth of many malignant cell types was envisioned to be a direct anticancer effect. In addition, IFNs enhance cell surface receptor expression for a number of markers indicating a differentiation-inducing effect which might translate into enhanced tumor immunogenicity. The most clear-cut antitumor effects in animal models were those that concerned virally induced tumors; spontaneous tumors as occur in humans were in general poorly responsive. In a number of models, high doses were no more effective than low doses; nevertheless, human trials were designed with the assumption that maximum tolerated doses would be tumoricidal and maximally immunotherapeutic as well. These assumptions have proven false and a need exists to reevaluate the immunopharmacology of IFN treatment of cancer to determine the extent to which IFNs are directly anticancer and indirectly so through immunopharmacologic mechanisms. Synergistic combinations of IFNs with other therapies could then be better exploited.

Tumor necrosis factors α and β have been genetically engineered and demonstrated to inhibit the growth of a number of tumor cell types *in vitro* particularly when combined with an antimetabolite. The tumor necrosis phenomenon *in vivo* appears to result from endothelial–granulocyte interactions leading to ischemic necrosis of the tumor. Toxicity of rTNFs are currently under study. Much information is needed before we can harness the activity of TNF.

Monoclonal antibody-producing clones have been developed from mice immunized with human tumors and a number of unique tumor epitopes have been defined that are sufficiently distinct from host antigens to allow the use of these antibodies to target human tumors *in vivo*. In the presence of complement, certain monoclonal antibodies will lyse tumor cells *in vitro*, suggesting tumoricidal potential. Non-complement-fixing antibodies are envisioned to need to be armed with cytotoxic agents such as radionuclides or toxins such as ricin A chain. A number of problems are associated with monoclonal antibody therapy. Mouse monoclonal antibodies are antigenic in humans, leading to allergic responses and rapid clearing. Use of human–mouse hybrids and eventually human–human hybrids will hopefully obviate this problem. Many antibodies yield poor localization because of poor entry. This may be overcome with enhancers (e.g., IFN-α) or use of antigen-binding fragments of multiple antibodies identifying different tumor epitopes. Monoclonal antibodies are also being explored for use in diagnostic tumor imaging using various isotope conjugates.

2.5. Adoptive Cell Therapy

The use of autologous tumoricidal cell population expanded *in vitro* has recently gained interest for cancer therapy. It was observed in mice that IL-2 could at very high doses invoke destruction of a number of tumor types by activating LAK cells, in part from NK cell precursors. In humans, it was evident that such doses of IL-2 could not be tolerated because of a greater sensitivity to the toxicity of IL-2. This led to a protocol involving *in vitro* expansion of LAK cells from buffy coat cells obtained from patients using IL-2. The activated LAK cells are then reinfused with high doses of IL-2. The toxicities are extreme in terms of vascular leak; however, tumor responses have obtained that were not seen with IL-2 alone. Recent data in cancer patients indicate that less toxic protocols using lower doses of IL-2 without LAK cells may produce better results when combined with low-dose cyclophosphamide to inhibit suppressor T cells, indomethacin to inhibit suppressor macrophages, and/or administration with tumor vaccines.

Many animal tumors have been noted to contain infiltrating T lymphocytes (TILs). It has recently been observed experimentally that these T lymphocytes can be activated and expanded *in vitro* using IL-2. When these cells are readministered with IL-2 and cyclophosphamide, tumor responses in mice occur. Recently, human tumors have been confirmed to contain such TIL cells and initial efforts to expand these populations for reinfusion have begun.

3. PRECLINICAL IMMUNOPHARMACOLOGIC CONSIDERATIONS

Before discussing the clinical applications of immunotherapeutic agents, it is important to review some basic principles of immunopharmacology, particularly those that appear to be distinct from conventional pharmacology.

Dose–response characteristics in immunopharmacology are often unique in that a rather low dose of an agent may stimulate an immune function while a higher dose is inactive or even immunosuppressive. Thus, the maximum effective dose is generally lower than the maximum tolerated dose. This difference is important when considering cancer therapy since cancer chemotherapy generally stresses the maximum tolerated dose.

The pharmacokinetics of immunotherapeutic agents generally diverge from their pharmacodynamics (Fig. 4). In general, the pharmacokinetics of immunotherapeutic drugs are similar to other drugs. For the biologicals, small peptides may have very short half-lives in the circulation, yet others like immunoglobulins may persist. In any case, the effects of an agent often outlive its presence in the patient. These persisting effects often have undulating patterns typical of "waves in a pool," indicating the complex reverberating circuitry of the immune system. In other cases, a period of refractoriness may occur. For example, for several days following the administration of an interferon inducer a second treatment will fail to induce further interferon. Despite this refractoriness to a second induction, an interferon-mediated state of resistance to viral challenge will persist. For these reasons, immunotherapeutic agents are often administered intermittently, e.g., several times per week rather than several times per day. With immunorestorative treatments the response depends on the

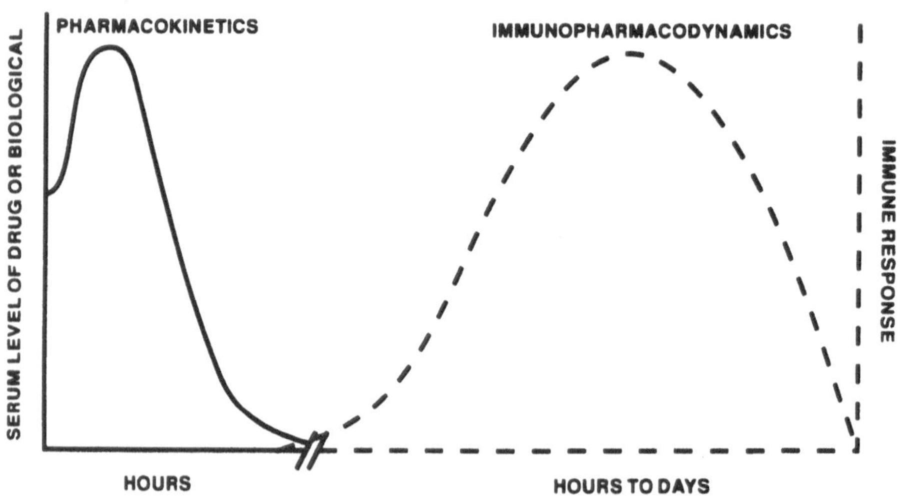

Figure 4. Dissociation of pharmacokinetics and immunopharmacodynamics.

integrity and functional status of the patient's immune system at the time of treatment. A normal immune system may respond little. A hyperactive system may be downregulated. A hyporeactive immune system may be upregulated but the degree may depend on the extent of dysfunction. If the destruction or dysfunction of the system is extreme, no response may result. For example, AIDS in its late stages is associated with profound pan-T lymphocytopenia and thymic involution and in such a condition immunorestorative attempts have not been effective.

In cancer, the immune system has been demonstrated to be impaired, particularly the T-cell system. This cellular immune deficiency is progressive with the stage of the cancer and is compounded by poor nutrition and immunosuppressive cancer chemotherapeutic agents. The degree of secondary immunodeficiency correlates inversely with prognosis in cancer patients as measured by mean survival time and response to cytoreductive therapy. Most patients will die of infection secondary to these causes. Stimulating the cellular immune system in cancer is oriented toward improving the general state of resistance and toward reducing the cancer. The latter objective is only observed clinically when cytoreductive therapy is nearly complete and the immune system can effectively eradicate the minimal residual tumor. This concept of immunotherapy is referred to as "remission stabilization" (Fig. 5). For this reason, this type of therapy is usually administered in an adjuvant manner, e.g., as chemoimmunotherapy. Immunotherapy is not given concurrently *with* the anticancer therapy since it is not

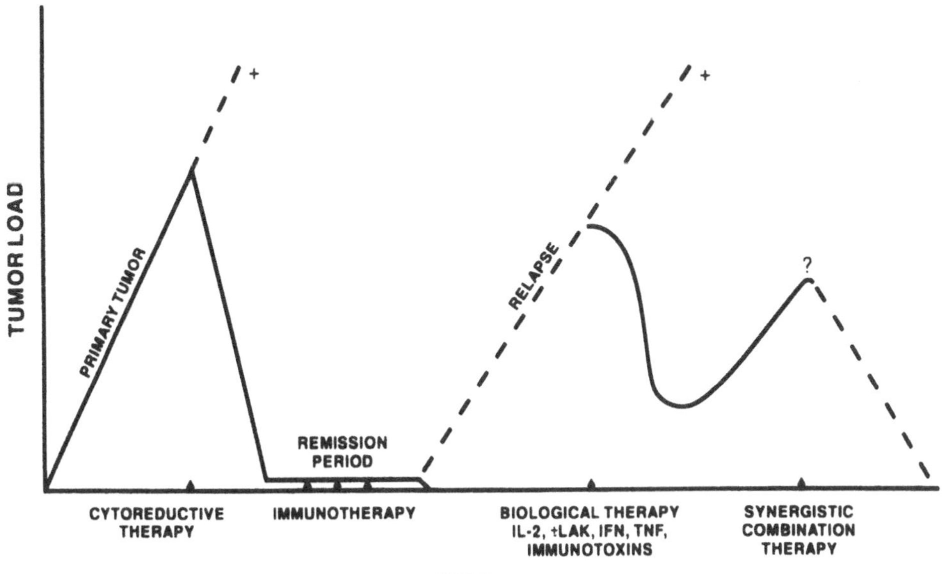

Figure 5. Immunotherapy models.

effective and even enhances the immunosuppressive side effects of the anticancer theapy.

In general, stimulation of the immune system is not associated with effect on active progressive disease and once recurrence appears the ultimate outcome is little affected.

The use of immunologic agents that act directly to kill the tumor can have an impact on active progressive disease (Fig. 6). Examples are interferons, tumor necrosis factors, monoclonal antibodies, immunotoxins, and IL-2 in conjunction with LAK cells or TIL. Tumor cell vaccines using autologous tumor or tumor-associated antigens are increasingly being used with various adjuvant techniques to immunize the patient to his tumor. Finally, immunosuppression in the tumor-bearing patient may result from tumor-derived immunosuppressive factors and from immune system-derived suppressive factors. Cancer chemotherapy, even low doses, may relieve immune suppression and enhance response. Antisuppressor cell therapy with low-dose cyclophosphamide or cimetidine to block T-suppressor cells or with indomethacin to block prostaglandin-produced macrophage suppressors has been effective in animals and is increasingly being used experimentally in human patients.

As with multiagent cancer chemotherapy, multiagent immunotherapy is emerging and the future success of immunotherapy of cancer will predictably depend on selection of the appropriate combinations (see Fig. 6).

In the treatment of infectious disorders, immunotherapeutic agents have a number of demonstrated actions that should make them important adjuncts to antimicrobial therapy where available and as bolsterers of host defense where unavail-

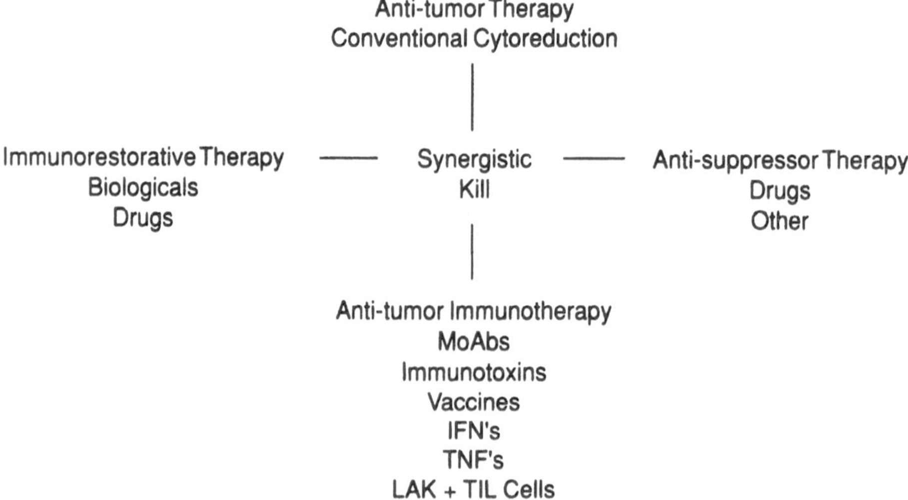

Figure 6. Synergistic combination therapy in cancer.

able. The classic use of immunotherapeutics is in vaccines. The combination of adjuvants with a killed or attenuated microbe or with microbial antigens is well known to produce long-standing protection against infection. New vaccines in the future will derive from the attachment of potent immunoadjuvants (e.g., the muramyl peptides) to genetically engineered or synthetic protein epitopes. These vaccines will be specifically geared toward the relevant defense mechanism, i.e., cellular or humoral immunity or both.

Immunorestorative agents will be used to prevent infections in patients known to be at risk. For example, T-cell stimulants and marrow-stimulating growth factors have been demonstrated experimentally to hasten recovery and reduce susceptibility to pathogen challenge in animals treated with immunosuppressive cancer chemotherapy. Pretreatment with various agents (Table IV) has been shown to protect against subsequent pathogen challenge, e.g., interferons protect against viral challenge and MDPs protect against bacterial challenge. This type of therapy is termed *immunoprophylaxis*. Other agents have been employed experimentally to enhance resistance in the treatment of infection. This type of therapy can be expected to shorten the duration of the infection, protect against dissemination, or to prevent secondary infection. It is important to note that most viruses have been demonstrated to be immunosuppressive and a high incidence of secondary bacterial infection currently requires extensive antibiotic use. "Prohost" therapy in microbial infections may be an important use of immunotherapeutic agents in the future. Immunotherapeutic agents have been demonstrated to have beneficial effects in situations involving immunodeviation as occurs in autoimmune disease. Treatment with thymic hormones or thymomimetic drugs has modified the course of experimental autoimmune diseases in animals and clinical studies are in progress to determine whether this offers adjuncts or alternatives to antiinflammatory or immunosuppressive therapy.

Finally, tolerance induction with selectively suppresssive immune adjuvants can be envisioned to impact on the future treatment of allergies and allograft immunity.

Importantly, effective immunotherapeutics in the future will depend on a knowledge of the specific immune defects related to a particular disease and contributing to

TABLE IV
Agents with Activity
in Animal Models of Bacterial,
Viral, and Fungal Challenge

Immunoprophylactic	Immunotherapeutic
Interferon	Interferon
Interferon inducers	Thymic hormones
MDP and analogues	Levamisole
RES expanders—glycans	Isoprinosine

its pathogenesis. More precise immunodiagnostics in the clinic are necessary to this development. With the appropriate diagnosis of the nature of the immunodeficiency, the more selective agents or combinations of agents can be employed to reverse the defect and yield a beneficial therapeutic outcome.

4. CLINICAL PHARMACOLOGY

4.1. Cancer

The most extensive use of immunotherapy in humans has been in cancer. The longest experience with any agent in human cancer has been with BCG. It has been demonstrated to consistently induce clearance of injected malignant melanoma but not uninjected nodules. It is licensed by the U.S. Food and Drug Administration (FDA) for use in bladder cancer when given by the intravesicular route with chemotherapy. The interferons, initially as mixed lymphokine preparation and more recently in recombinant forms (particularly IFN-α preparations), have been used in a wide range of human cancers. Side effects include a "flulike syndrome" and at high doses marrow and immune suppression. Approximately one-third of cancer patients will show a significant palliative response but rarely a curative response. The most and least responsive cancers are listed in Table V. The success of IFN-α is comparable to single-agent cancer chemotherapy. Combination therapy using interferon with chemotherapy or with other immunotherapy will likely improve the results in the future. IFN-α is licensed by the FDA as a treatment of choice in hairy cell leukemia, venereal papillomas, Kaposi's sarcoma and is likely to be approved soon for other tumors.

Intensive efforts have been employed to evaluate IL-2 and LAK therapy in human cancer. The treatment has had significant palliative effects in approximately 20% of patients with disseminated malignant melanoma and renal cell carcinoma. The side effects of this therapy, in addition to the "flulike" syndrome seen with interferon, include fluid accumulation and transudation leading to vascular collapse, respiratory distress, and even death. Efforts are in progress to alleviate the toxicity of this therapy and to obviate the cumbersome *ex vivo* phase involving the LAK cell

TABLE V
Interferon Treatment of Human Cancers

Very responsive	Moderately responsive	Unresponsive
Hairy cell leukemia	Myeloma	Colon cancer
Nodular lymphoma	Kaposi's sarcoma	Breast cancer
Mycosis fungoides	Renal cell cancer	Lung cancer
Chronic myeloid leukemia	Melanoma	Large solid tumors
Laryngeal and venereal papillomas	Carcinoid tumors	

propagation. IL-2 alone is currently licensed by the FDA for renal cell cancer. In disseminated malignant melanoma, preliminary data suggest that IL-2 without LAK cells but with low-dose cyclophosphamide and indomethacin may be more effective in inducing objective responses.

Monoclonal antibodies to human tumor-associated antigens have been tested successfully in patients with leukemia, colorectal cancer, malignant melanoma, and ovarian cancer. Phase II and III trials are in progress with several of these immunotoxins in leukemia, malignant melanoma, ovarian and colon cancer. Similar progress is occurring using monoclonal antibody–isotope conjugates for diagnostic imaging of human cancers. Side effects have been minimal but include allergic reactions to mouse immunoglobulins.

The glycans, krestin and lentinan, are already licensed in Japan for use in gastric cancer following surgery and one MDP derivative (MDP-Lys L18) is licensed in Japan for bone marrow recovery following cancer chemotherapy.

Levamisole has seen extensive testing in various cancers using combined chemoimmuno protocols. While mild effects to induce "remission stabilizations" were observed in the majority of studies, side effects and inconsistent effects have delayed regulatory approval. Levamisole is licensed only for Duke's "C" colon cancer in combined use with 5-fluorouracil.

4.2. Infectious Diseases

Many studies in AIDS and the AIDS-related complex (ARC) have employed IL-2, thymic hormones, and the thymomimetic drugs and transfer factor/Imreg. To date, no significant immunorestorative responses have been observed in patients with AIDS; however, effects to modify immune responses have been observed in ARC patients with decreased progression from ARC to AIDS. The development and licensing of azidothymidine (AZT) as an effective anti-human immunodeficiency virus (HIV) agent has allowed combined trials of AZT with various immunorestorative agents to proceed; their results are awaited. Vaccine prospects for HIV are also under intensive evaluation.

IFN-α, which has been used effectively for Kaposi's sarcoma in AIDS, has not, as yet, proven to modify the underlying HIV-mediated immunodeficiency disease. It has proven effective and is licensed for the treatment of venereal and laryngeal warts by local injection. IFN-α is licensed for chronic granulomatous disease of childhood.

Isoprinosine has been licensed in 80 countries outside the United States in the treatment of a number of viral infections. In this country, efficacy has been documented in recurrent herpes, early HIV infection, and subacute sclerosing panencephalitis; however, licensing by the FDA has not been forthcoming. Levamisole has been used experimentally in a large number of different infections with a corresponding long list of successful treatment reports; however, toxicity and inconsistent effects have apparently prevented its licensing for infections.

4.3. Other Diseases

Levamisole, DTC, isoprinosine, thymulin, and thymopentin have all been reported to be active in experimental autoimmune disease and in rheumatoid arthritis. None is approved by the FDA. The muramyl peptides are being considered for synthetic vaccine use.

As a closing thought I would like to put forth the following: Conventional pharmacological and therapeutic principles dictate that a failing organ system should be treated to prevent the development of more serious disease and death. Thus, we treat hypertension and coronary artery disease to prevent subsequent vascular accidents. The only recent development of our understanding of the immune system and its apparently staggering complexity have made it difficult for physicians and others to recognize that it too is a system deserving of treatment, when failing, to prevent the sequelae of infection, cancer, and autoimmunity. Further development of the field of basic immunopharmacology along its present lines and increased clinical experience will ensure the emergence of a successful clinical immunopharmacology.

BIBLIOGRAPHY

General References

Dale, M., and Foreman, J. E., eds., 1984, *Textbook of Immunopharmacology*, Blackwell Scientific, Oxford.

Fenichel, R. L., and Chirigos, M. A., eds., 1984, *Immune Modulation Agents and Their Mechanisms*, Dekker, New York.

Girdlestone, D., 1993, Immunopharmacology, *Trends Pharmacol.* Sci. **14**:137.

Hadden, J. W., and Spreafico, F., eds., 1985 and 1986, *Springer Seminars in Immunopathology: New Perspectives in Immunotherapy I & II*, Springer-Verlag, Berlin.

Hadden, J. W., and Szentivanyi, A., eds., 1992, *Immunopharmacology Reviews*, Plenum Press, New York.

Hadden, J. W., Coffey, R. G., and Spreafico, F., eds., 1977, *Immunopharmacology*, Plenum Press, New York.

Hadden, J. W., *et al.*, 1981, 1983, 1988, 1991, and 1994, *Advances in Immunopharmacology I–V*, Pergamon Press, New York.

Hersh, E. M., Chirigos, M. A., and Mastrangelo, M. J., eds., 1981, *Augmenting Agents in Cancer*, Raven Press, New York.

Specific References

Goldstein, A. L., ed., 1984, *Thymic Hormones and Lymphokines*, Plenum Press, New York.

Majde, J. A., ed., 1987, *Immunopharmacology of Infectious Diseases*, Liss, New York.

Miescher, P. A., Bolis, L., and Ghione, M., eds., 1985, *Immunopharmacology*, Raven Press, New York.

Mihich, E., and Fefer, A., eds., 1983, *Biological Response Modifiers Subcommittee Report*, National Cancer Institute Monograph 63, U.S. Government Printing Office, Washington, DC.

CHAPTER 2

DRUGS FOR THE TREATMENT OF INFLAMMATORY AND AUTOIMMUNE DISEASE

JOHN W. HADDEN and RONALD G. COFFEY

1. INTRODUCTION

Drugs that are used to treat acute and chronic inflammatory disorders suppress natural processes that contribute to the signs and symptoms of inflammation. Drugs that are used to treat simple forms of arthritis such as gout and osteoarthritis relieve pain and swelling and improve mobility. These agents are often referred to as *nonsteroidal antiinflammatory drugs* (NSAIDs). In the absence of known infection, chronic inflammation with strong immune components is termed *autoimmune*. Drugs that are used to treat autoimmune arthritides such as rheumatoid arthritis and the reactive arthritides (psoriatic arthritis and Reiter's syndrome) act not only to suppress inflammation but also to modify the disease process by impairing the expression of the immune components of the inflammation. These latter drugs are often referred to as *disease-modifying antirheumatic drugs* (DMARDs). DMARDs can act as immunomodulators or as immunosuppressive agents. Autoimmune disorders without attendant inflammation are generally treated with immunosuppressive drugs alone. Antiinflammatory and immunosuppressive drugs are listed in Table I.

JOHN W. HADDEN • Department of Internal Medicine, Division of Immunopharmacology, University of South Florida College of Medicine, Tampa, Florida 33612. RONALD G. COFFEY • Department of Pharmacology, University of South Florida College of Medicine, Tampa, Florida 33612.

Immunopharmacology Reviews, Volume 2, edited by John W. Hadden and Andor Szentivanyi. Plenum Press, New York, 1996.

TABLE I
Antiinflammatory and Immunosuppressive Drugs

Nonsteroidal antiinflammatory agents	
Aspirin	Ketoprofen
Diflunisal	Meclofenamate
Fenoprofen	Naproxen
Ibuprofen	Phenylbutazone
Indomethacin	Piroxicam
Sulindac	Tolmetin
Glucocorticosteroids, antigout drugs	
Colchicine	Probenecid
Allopurinol	Sulfinpyrazone
Immunomodulators	
Chloroquine	Aurothioglucose
Hydroxychloroquine	Gold sodium thiomalate
Auranofin	Penicillamine
Immunosuppressive drugs	
Azathioprine	Cyclophosphamide
Methotrexate	Cyclosporin A

2. BACKGROUND

Inflammatory mediator release and action are the targets of antiinflammatory drug action. Celsus (30 B.C.–38 A.D.) described the basic features of inflammation as heat ("color"), redness ("rubor"), swelling ("tumor"), and pain ("dolor"). More recent physicians have emphasized loss of motion or function. Local inflammation, e.g., joints or soft tissues, may be associated with generalized inflammation including vasculitis and nephritis and with constitutional symptoms of fever and malaise. The clinical decision to treat inflammation depends on the cause and the degree of distress.

Inflammation can be classified in many different ways. Figure 1 shows one paradigm based on the antigenicity of the inciting agent and whether the process is acute or chronic. Examples of acute, nonantigenic, nonspecific inflammation are trauma or acute gout. Examples of acute, antigenic immune inflammation are acute rheumatic fever or septic arthritis. Examples of chronic, nonspecific, nonantigenic inflammation are osteoarthritis, gout, or foreign body granuloma. Examples of such inflammation in the immune form are rheumatoid arthritis and other autoimmune or reactive disorders (where the cause is unknown) or tuberculosis or leprosy (where the cause is known).

Simple acute trauma generally requires little more than immobilization, emotional support, and mild analgesics such as aspirin. Acute septic inflammation necessitates specific antimicrobial therapy. When the inflammation is chronic and debilitating, therapy specifically designed to suppress the inflammation is warranted.

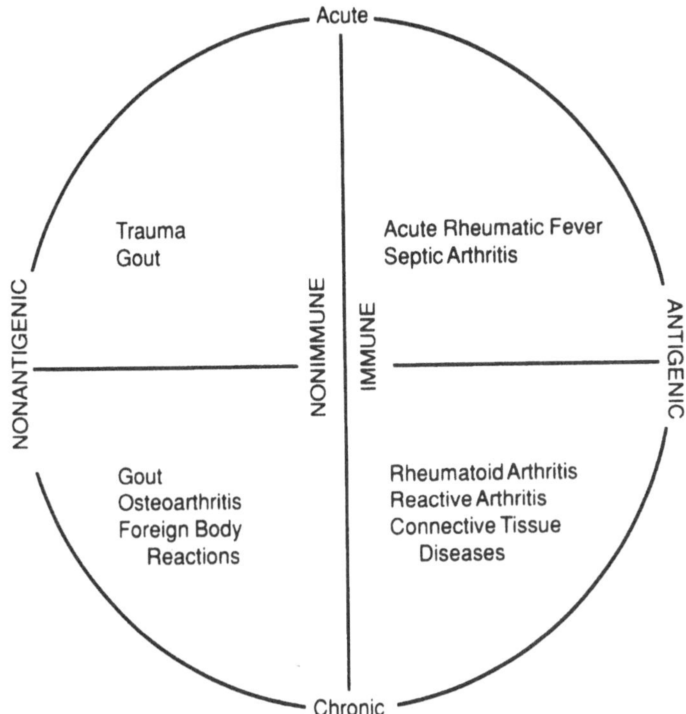

Figure 1. Model of inflammation.

Given the many causes of inflammation and their complexities, this chapter will emphasize two diseases, gouty arthritis and rheumatoid arthritis, as examples of simple inflammation and immune inflammation, respectively. The basic mechanisms of pathogenesis and concepts of treatment can be generalized to other inflammatory conditions on the one hand and to other autoimmune diseases on the other hand.

For the purposes of this discussion the term *autoimmune* is used to refer to disorders involving antigens that are associated with host cells and induce both humoral and cellular forms of immunity. The nature of these antigens are not known, i.e., whether they are typical host antigens or altered host antigens. If they are typical host antigens, the reactive antibody-producing B cells are presumed to lack appropriate suppressor T-cell regulation to keep them unreactive and are, therefore, called *hidden clones.*

While obvious viral and bacterial pathogens have been ruled out in the tissues of patients with these diseases, latent and retroviruses have not been excluded. The attendant signs of altered cellular immunity in these diseases have led many immunologists and rheumatologists to believe that in fact they represent "hidden pathogen" diseases resulting from primary or secondary immunodeficiency in genetically predisposed individuals. Despite this belief and because the human suffering is great, the treatment is oriented toward symptom relief rather than removal of the primary cause. Only with the elucidation of causative agents can future therapies be oriented toward cure.

The early signs of acute inflammation, whether immune or not, are indistinguishable and are characterized by dilatation and fenestration of the microvasculature, leakage of blood and/or serum into the interstitium (leading to fluid accumulation), and the movement of blood cells, particularly granulocytes, into the affected tissue. This process is mediated by a number of inflammatory mediators derived from cells in the damaged tissue (fibroblasts, mast cells, nerves, and endothelial cells) and from the infiltrating inflammatory cells (neutrophils, monocytes, basophils, eosinophils, platelets, and lymphocytes).

As the exudate progressively accumulates, the initial mediators observed are histamine and serotonin (5-hydroxytryptamine) derived from mast cells and platelets; these decline and are followed by bradykinin and complement fragments generated from serum components (Fig. 2). A third wave of mediators involves the products of arachidonic acid derived via metabolism through the cyclooxygenase and the lipoxygenase pathways (Fig. 3). The release of arachidonic acid from the membrane lipids of mast cells, platelets, granulocytes, monocytes, and endothelial cells results from the activation of phospholipases in the plasma membranes of these cells while different cells contribute different metabolites of arachidonic acid and the molecular scenario is not entirely worked out. The pharmacologic approach to these events reveals the basic processes that are most critical and that can be effectively modulated to reduce the inflammation. For example, if antihistamines, antiserotonin, or antikinin agents are given, little beneficial effect results presumably from the rapid, transient nature of the effects of these mediators. If granulocytes are removed from the circulation using a drug causing neutropenia or if the serum is decomplemented with an agent such as cobra venom, the reactions are markedly inhibited. Thus, both cellular and complement-dependent phases are important in generating the inflammatory exudate. These procedures are compromising to host defenses and are, therefore, not used clinically. If agents that inhibit arachidonic acid release or its metabolism to eicosanoids like prostaglandins, thromboxanes, and leukotrienes are used, the resulting inflammatory signs and symptoms of pain, vasodilatation, and swelling are attenuated. These agents, in general, do not compromise host resistance and, therefore, constitute the first line of therapeutic defense against inflammation, whatever the cause.

For simple inflammation, aspirin in various forms is the single best agent for analgesia and reduction of inflammation. In the case of gout, the removal of offending urate crystals through diet adjustment and treatment with uricosuric and other agents, is complementary to analgesia and inflammation reduction. In the case of rheumatoid arthritis, immunomodulating and immunosuppressive agents, in addition to anti-inflammatory agents, are often necessary to quell the inflammation.

In the case of gout, removal of urate cyrstals can reverse the arthritic process; however, in the case of rheumatoid arthritis a chronic arthritic process supervenes

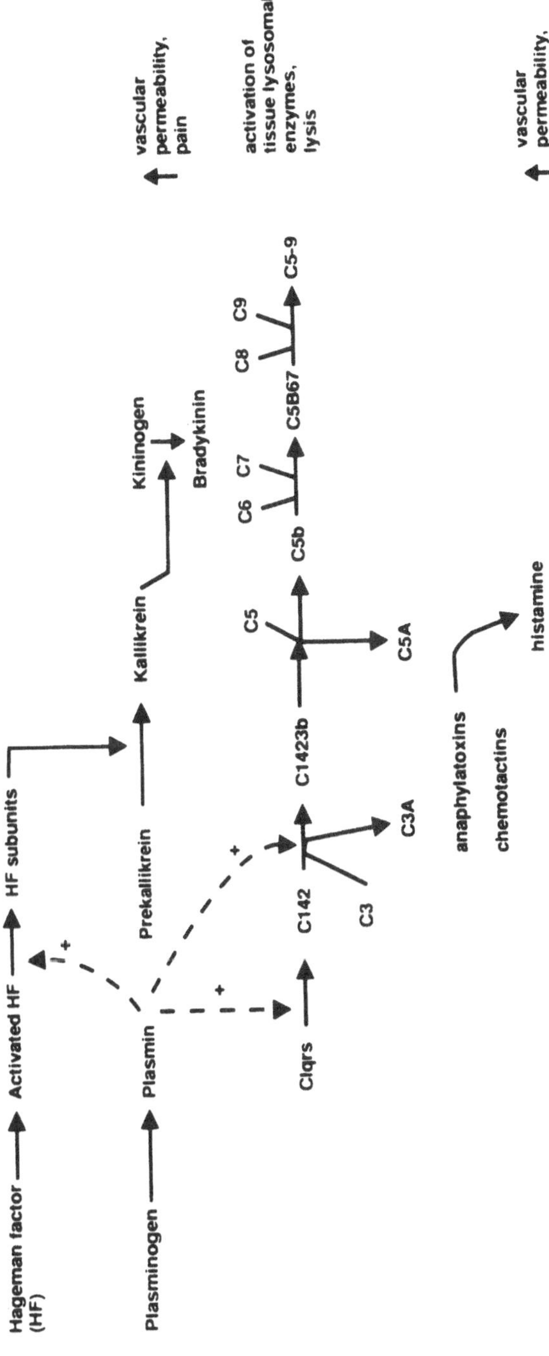

Figure 2. Inflammatory mediators.

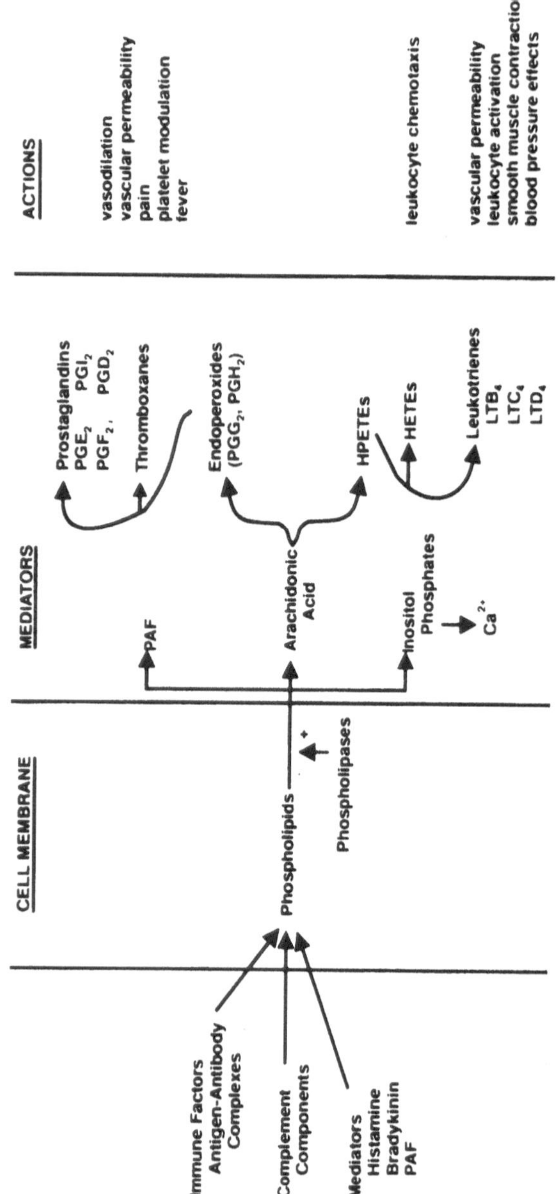

Figure 3. Lipid mediators.

which has signs of immune perpetuation. The initial cellular infiltrate progressively shifts from a granulocyte-based population to one of macrophages (monocyte-derived) and lymphocytes. These form dense cellular aggregates in the periarticular tissues, particularly the fingerlike projections (pannus) which form from these tissues and penetrate into the joint. Both thymus-dependent T lymphocytes and bone marrow-derived B lymphocytes are present and both populations are activated as indicated by the presence of activation markers [e.g., interleukin 2 (IL-2) receptor for T cells or intracytoplasmic immunoglobulin (Ig) for B cells] and of the secretion of cellular products (lymphokines from T cells and IgG, IgM, and IgG–IgM rheumatoid factor from B cells). Also evident is the action of the products on their target cells [macrophage activation, interleukin 1 (IL-1) production, arachidonic acid metabolites, etc. for lymphokines from T cells and complement fixation for antibody from B cells].

The activation of granulocytes and macrophages by interleukins (particularly IL-1, IL-6, and CSFs), antigen–antibody complex, and complement components all contribute to the formation and release of tissue-damaging oxygen metabolites and exocytosed lysosomal enzymes. These are thought to be the final common pathway leading to joint destruction through articular cartilage erosion and bone digestion. Healing, when it occurs, is characterized by intense fibrosis which results in further restriction of the joint. Thus, the normal mobile joint with its delicate, lubricated sliding surfaces becomes fused and immobile. In the case of gout, failure to reverse the urate deposition can lead to a similar, yet less extensive, end-stage process of joint ankylosis.

During the active phase of rheumatoid arthritis, extra-articular manifestations may be present and fever and malaise may be debilitating. Serum reflects disturbances of acute-phase reactants (e.g., β_2 microglobulin, C-reactive protein), hyperfibrinogenemia leading to an enhanced erythrocyte sedimentation rate (ESR), modification of trace metal levels, hyperglobulinemia, the presence of rheumatoid factor (an IgG–IgM complex), and altered complement levels reflecting complement consumption. Other attendant findings include evidence of altered T-cell-mediated immunity (decreased mitogen responses, increased helper/suppressor cell ratio, decreased skin test reactivity).

The therapeutic strategies that are employed to combat the more severe forms of autoimmune-based inflammation, as seen in rheumatoid arthritis, are based on a tiered approach in which the intensity and severity of the inflammatory process determine the intensity and risk of the therapy.

3. BASIC PHARMACOLOGY OF NSAIDs

All NSAIDs act, in part, by inhibiting cyclooxygenase activity, thereby preventing the formation of the cycloendoperoxide precursors of prostaglandins (PGs) and thromboxanes (TXs). Aspirin covalently acetylates cyclooxygenase and inhibits it irreversibly; the other NSAIDs inhibit the enzyme in a reversible way. PGs and TXs are derived from arachidonic acid, cleaved from phosphatidylcholine and other lipids by the reactions shown in Fig. 3. In addition to these reactions, which occur in nearly all eukaryotic cells, arachidonic acid is metabolized in leukocytes and certain other cells by the lipoxygenase pathway to form the leukotrienes (LTs), hydroxy and hydroperoxy eicosatetraenoic acids (HETEs and HPETEs), and lipoxins, all of which have potent biological effects. NSAIDs do not inhibit the formation of these substances. The release of arachidonate is the rate-limiting step for the biosynthesis of all cyclooxygenase and lipoxygenase products, collectively termed *eicosanoids*. Another important lipid mediator, 2-acetyl-1-ether-glycero-phosphocholine [also known as platelet-activating factor (PAF)], is formed by activated phagocytic cells and certain other cells. Release occurs in response to a host of hormones, cytokines, drugs, tissue injury, and inflammatory conditions. To understand the mechanism of NSAID actions, it is necessary to briefly review the physiological actions of the prostaglandins and the related eicosanoids.

The formation of the eicosanoids is highly tissue-specific. For example, TXA_2 is the principal cyclooxygenase product in platelets, PGD_2 is synthesized chiefly in mast cells, while prostacyclin (PGI_2) is the major arachidonate metabolite of the vascular endothelium. PGE_2, generally the major PG formed at inflammatory sites, acts on afferent nerve endings to cause pain. It also has hyperalgesic effects, enhancing the pain caused by other agents such as bradykinin or histamine. PGE_2 has a direct effect to cause headache. It also causes fever by acting on the hypothalamus to increase the temperature set point. Endogenous pyrogen, or IL-1 (secreted by activated monocytes, macrophages, and a few other cell types), is thought to cause fever by stimulating increases in hypothalamic PGE_2. PGI_2 often has effects similar to PGE_2.

Both PGE_2 and PGI_2 exert their effects, to a large degree, by stimulating production of intracellular cyclic AMP. $PGF_{2\alpha}$ may have similar actions as PGE_2 in a few instances, but in most cases it acts in a way that opposes PGE_2. For example, PGE_2 and PGI_2 cause vasodilatation, while $PGF_{2\alpha}$ causes vasoconstriction. TXA_2, LTC_4, LTD_4, and PAF are also potent vasoconstrictors. Vascular permeability (extravasation of plasma) is enhanced by the prostaglandins, LTB_4, LTC_4, LTD_4, and PAF. Thus, different products of lipid metabolism may have opposing or similar effects, and the overall effect of mobilization of these lipids depends on the nature of the stimulus as well as the responding tissue.

There are several functions of the prostaglandins that are considered normal and beneficial for the host, and the interruption of these functions by NSAIDs can have serious consequences. Important effects of PGE_2 and PGI_2 include the enhancement of both cardiac and renal blood flow and renal diuresis. PGD_2 and, to a lesser extent, $PGF_{2\alpha}$ also increase salt and water excretion. Inhibition of cyclooxygenase does not alter renal or cardiac perfusion under normal circumstances. However, in both the heart and kidney, stress caused by anoxia or reduced blood flow results in enhanced release of the vasodilatory PGs, which help to maintain regional blood flow. NSAIDs should be used with caution in patients receiving diuretics or in those with impaired renal function. Antihypertensive agents including diuretics, β-adrenoceptor antagonists, and angiotensin-converting enzyme inhibitors are antagonized by certain NSAIDs. Increases in blood pressure have been observed on administration of NSAIDs to patients receiving such therapy. PGs are involved in uterine contractions and may be used as abortifacients, especially in the second trimester of pregnancy. The inappropriate use of NSAIDs can prevent normal delivery. The effects of PGE_2 to inhibit gastric acid secretion and to stimulate the production of a protective gastric mucus are other important physiological roles of this substance; therefore, NSAIDs should be used with great caution by subjects with peptic ulcers. Thromboxanes are synthesized in platelets in response to thrombin and stimulate platelet aggregation, while PGI_2 is synthesized by the vascular endothelium and inhibits platelet aggregation. Cyclooxygenase inhibition can, therefore, have important effects on blood clotting.

The inhibition of cyclooxygenase by NSAIDs may be associated with enhancement of the formation of products of the lipoxygenase pathway. One of the consequences of the lipoxygenase products LTC_4, LTD_4, and LTE_4 [collectively known as *slow-reacting substance of anaphylaxis* (SRS-A)] is the contraction of airway smooth muscle. In patients with NSAID-evoked asthma, this response may be greatly exaggerated by cyclooxygenase inhibition and for these patients NSAIDs are contraindicated.

PGs inhibit most functions of mature blood cells, including lymphocyte activation, immunoglobulin and lymphokine release, phagocyte activation and release of monokines, superoxide, and hydrolytic enzymes. One function of macrophages that is promoted by PGE_2 is the release of collagenase. Inhibition of this release by NSAIDs may account for a portion of their antiinflammatory effects. NSAIDs at high doses inhibit migration and adherence of neutrophils, thus decreasing local accumulation of neutrophils and therefore the production of leukotrienes and PAF as well as PGs. NSAIDS are used for control of pain, fever, and inflammation.

NSAIDs do not affect ongoing pain *per se*, but by preventing PG synthesis, they reduce pain and hyperalgesia caused by PGs. NSAIDs are only effective against pain of low to moderate intensity, having much less effects than opioids; however, the NSAIDs do not cause dependence and do not have many other of the unwanted side effects of opioids on the central nervous system. NSAIDs are particularly useful for the pain associated with inflammation. They are, of course, the mainstay for treatment of most simple headaches, but are not very good for migraine. Oral NSAIDs are quite useful for toothaches; however, NSAIDs are not useful for pain associated with the viscera. Postoperative pain, related to inflammation, is particularly well controlled by the aspirinlike drugs.

NSAIDs reduce the fever caused by PGs. Since PGs only augment the hypothalamic set point, NSAIDs do not lower normal body temperature. NSAIDs are widely used for their antiinflammatory activity in the treatment of rheumatoid arthritis, osteoarthritis, ankylosing spondylitis, juvenile arthritis, acute gouty arthritis, and Reiter's syndrome (see Section 8). The drugs provide only symptomatic relief, and do not arrest the progression or injury to the tissue. The choice of the drug to use depends on several factors. If antipyretic or analgesic action is desired, the choice is seldom a problem. If antiinflammatory properties are required, the choice is more complex and very high, sustained levels are needed. In this case, severe side effects and cost become important considerations.

3.1. Salicylates

The bark of the common white willow has been known for centuries to have medicinal properties. The active ingredient, the glycoside salicin, was purified in 1829 by Leroux, who discovered its antipyretic activity. Sodium salicylate was first used to treat rheumatic fever in 1875. Bayer patented the synthetic acetylsalicylic acid or aspirin in 1899, and it has been used for its antiinflammatory, analgesic, and antipyretic properties ever since (see Fig. 4). It was not until 1971 that Vane and others found that aspirin inhibits the formation of PGs. The mode of inhibition of PG synthesis is not well understood. Although aspirin acetylates and thereby inhibits cyclooxygenase *in vitro*, most of ingested aspirin is quickly converted to salicylate *in vivo*. Salicylates are not potent inhibitors of cyclooxygenase *in vitro*; however, *in vivo*, they are just as potent as aspirin in preventing PG synthesis.

The action of salicylates to inhibit PG synthesis is most consistently manifest by their action to reduce pain and fever. Their use is extensive in this regard. Acute rheumatic fever is one example of such a medical indication. Another prominent physiological effect is the inhibition of platelet aggregation. Aspirin and other salicylates have not been found useful to inhibit thrombosis in acute myocardial infarction, but they do protect to some extent individuals with incipient coronary thrombosis and unstable angina. Salicylic acid is used topically as a keratolytic agent to remove warts and corns. Methyl salicylate is commonly used topically for painful muscles or joints.

Diflunisal is a derivative of salicylic acid, containing fluorine. It is more potent than aspirin in antiinflammatory tests, but is not useful in controlling fever. Diflunisal has been used chiefly as an analgesic in treatment of simple arthritis and muscle strains. It has no auditory side effects, and the gastrointestinal side effects are less than those of aspirin.

Adverse effects of salicylates apply to almost all of the NSAIDs to one degree or another. Important exceptions will be mentioned later.

PGE_2 and PGI_2 normally inhibit gastric acid secretion and also promote the secretion of cell protective mucus in the intestine. Aspirin and similar drugs prevent these effects, thus promoting acid secretion; they also cause local irritation, which is more severe if the drugs persist for a long time undissolved. High doses of salicylates can cause nausea and vomiting, gastric ulceration and hemorrhage, and exacerbation of peptic ulcer. These side effects rarely occur with low doses, and the salicylate-induced gastric bleeding usually involves minimal blood loss, is painless, and pre-

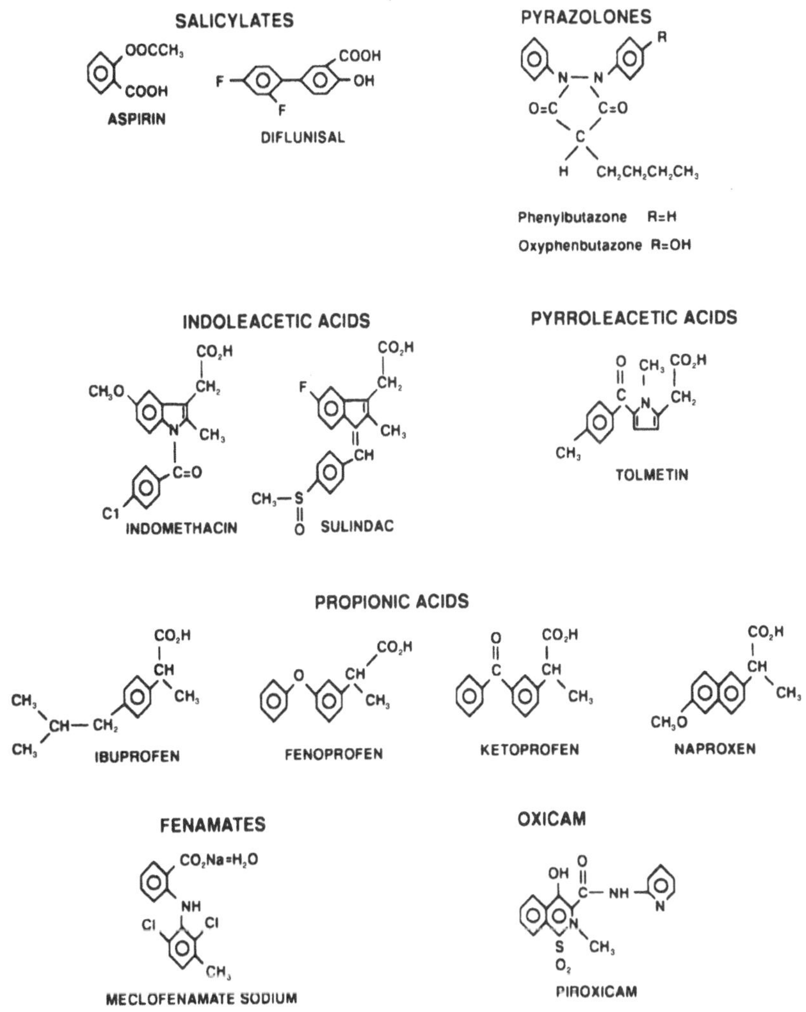

Figure 4. Nonsteroidal antiinflammatory drugs.

sents no problem. Rare individuals experience extreme blood loss and iron deficiency anemia caused by salicylates, and they must avoid the drugs.

Two tablets of aspirin approximately double the mean bleeding time as a result of the effect on platelet aggregation. Since platelets cannot regenerate cyclooxygenase after it has been irreversibly inhibited by aspirin, this persists until new platelets are formed (up to 7 days). Obvious contraindications for aspirin include patients with thrombocytopenia, hypoprothrombinemia, vitamin K deficiency, or hemophilia. Also, aspirin and most other NSAIDs should be discontinued 1 week before surgery. These drugs are contraindicated for patients receiving anticoagulants, except in certain cases, when NSAIDs and anticoagulants are deliberately combined for the prophylaxis of coronary or cerebral arterial thrombosis.

Some patients are aspirin intolerant; the symptoms range from rhinitis and urticaria to bronchoconstriction, shock, and vasomotor collapse. This reaction resembles anaphylaxis, but apparently is not immunologic in nature. It may be related to increased formation of PAF or lipoxygenase metabolites. It occurs very rarely, but when it does, a cross-reactivity with all of the other NSAIDs has been observed and none of them should be used.

Over 10,000 cases of salicylate intoxication occur in the United States each year; many of them are children. Children with fever and dehydration are particularly vulnerable to small doses of salicylates. Early symptoms are thirst, tinnitus, and hearing loss (reversible in 2–3 days). Dangerous levels of salicylates cause confusion, dizziness, and delirium. The occurrence of hyperthermia, sweating, diarrhea, and vomiting leads to dehydration. Stimulation of respiration is accompanied by increased oxygen uptake and CO_2 release. This respiratory alkalosis is followed by metabolic acidosis (salicylic acid and organic acids). Treatment of a toxic overdose involves several maneuvers including first of all removal by gastric lavage followed by treatment of the hyperthemia, dehydration, and metabolic acidosis.

Finally, Reye's syndrome is a neurological disorder usually occurring in children who have recently had a viral infection, particularly chicken pox or influenza, and were treated with NSAIDs. NSAIDs, especially salicylates, are also thought to cause the hepatic injury seen in this syndrome.

3.2. Pyrazolones

Phenylbutazone was introduced in 1949 for rheumatoid arthritis. Its analgesic activity is inferior to salicylates, but it is a very effective antiinflammatory agent. Toxic effects occur in nearly half of all patients. Phenylbutazone causes water and electrolyte retention, ulcers, hemorrhage, nephritis, and gastric problems; the other effects of salicylates are common. The most serious side effects are leukopenia, aplastic anemia, and agranulocytosis. Several deaths have also occurred. Its serious toxicity, therefore, limits its use to short-term therapy. It is recommended for control of acute exacerbations of rheumatoid arthritis or related conditions, and not for trivial uses such as musculoskeletal disorders. It should only be tried if other NSAIDs have failed, and it is not advisable for the elderly.

Oxyphenbutazone is a metabolite of phenylbutazone; it shares the same activities and toxicities.

3.3. Pyrrole Acetic Acids

Indomethacin was introduced in 1963 for the treatment of rheumatoid arthritis and related disorders. In this respect, it is equal in potency to phenylbutazone and is more potent than aspirin. Indomethacin is a very potent inhibitor of cyclooxygenase activity, but its capacity to inhibit cyclic nucleotide phosphodiesterase and to interfere directly with the migration of leukocytes may further contribute to its antiinflammatory effect. Indomethacin also has antipyretic and analgesic properties. It is usually not used for long periods of time because of severe side effects. Toxic effects include the usual gastrointestinal complaints including ulcers, blood loss, and diarrhea. Serious hepatic and renal effects are rare, but liver and kidney function should be monitored in patients. Several effects on the CNS are common, especially severe frontal headache, dizziness, vertigo, and depression. Neutropenia and other blood problems occur rarely. Hypersensitivity reactions such as rashes and asthma have been reported.

Sulindac and tolmetin are similar in action and use to indomethacin. Sulindac lacks significant effects on the kidney, which converts it back to the inactive prodrug. It, therefore, does not inhibit PGI_2 synthesis and usually can be safely used in cases of mild renal impairment. Tolmetin can be used with warfarin, causing no displacement from binding sites. This is an unusual feature of a NSAID which is shared with ibuprofen. Also, tolmetin does not change prothrombin time.

3.4. Propionic Acid Derivatives

There are eight or more of these in use in the world, but only four are presently in use in the United States (ibuprofen, ketoprofen, naproxen, and fenoprofen; benoxaprofen, a very potent drug with lipoxygenase inhibitory actions, has been withdrawn). Ibuprofen was the first of these compounds to come into use in the United States (1974). All of these drugs are effective antiinflammatory agents, and all have analgesic and antipyretic properties. They are more effective than aspirin in the relief of pain from dysmenorrhea. This was one reason for ibuprofen's release in 1984 for nonprescription use. These compounds would undoubtedly be used more if they were less expensive.

All of the propionic acid derivatives are well tolerated by patients, but they can cause gastrointestinal side effects. These are usually much less severe than those of aspirin or indomethacin. Ibuprofen has been used in patients with ulcers.

All of the propionic acid drugs inhibit platelets and one of them (naproxen) is notable for its ability to inhibit leukocyte migration. This group of NSAIDs does not interact with other drugs significantly despite the high degree of protein binding. Although they will displace other binding drugs from binding sites, they may, with caution, be used by patients receiving oral anticoagulants and hypoglycemics. They are metabolized in the kidney and excreted in the urine. They are, therefore, contraindicated in kidney disease, but can often be safely used with diuretics, while aspirin and indomethacin cannot.

3.5. Fenamates

Fenamates are anthranilic acid derivatives. At least five of these agents are in use; two are commonly prescribed in the United States: meclofenamate and mefenamic acid. In addition to inhibition of PG synthesis, the drugs compete for binding sites at PG receptors. Their antiinflammatory actions are good, and comparable to those of aspirin or indomethacin, as are their analgesic and antipyretic activities. These drugs were discovered in the 1950s, but have not gained wide acceptance. Frequent side effects, dyspepsia and diarrhea in particular, are severe.

3.6. Piroxicam

Piroxicam is the newest NSAID to be introduced into clinical use in the United States (1982). It is the most potent antiinflammatory NSAID on a weight basis and also has good analgesic and antipyretic activities. It is tolerated better than aspirin or indomethacin and less than 5% of patients discontinue the drug because of its NSAID side effects.

4. STEROIDAL ANTIINFLAMMATORY AGENTS

Glucocorticoids are potent antiinflammatory agents (Fig. 5). Like the NSAIDs, they are only palliative and do not arrest the progress of arthritis. The basic pharmacology of adrenocortical steroids and related drugs is presented elsewhere and will be alluded to only briefly here. In 1950, the Nobel prize in medicine was awarded to Kendall, Reichstein, and Hench for the basic chemical research and clinical use of the glucocorticoids in rheumatoid arthritis.

Cortisol and synthetic analogues (prednisone, prednisolone, betamethasone, dexamethasone, triamcinolone, and others) rapidly suppress inflammatory signs and symptoms. The goal of treatment with steroids is to attain reasonable control of symptoms, not complete relief. Intraarticular injection of glucocorticoids is often employed for control of acute episodes of arthritis.

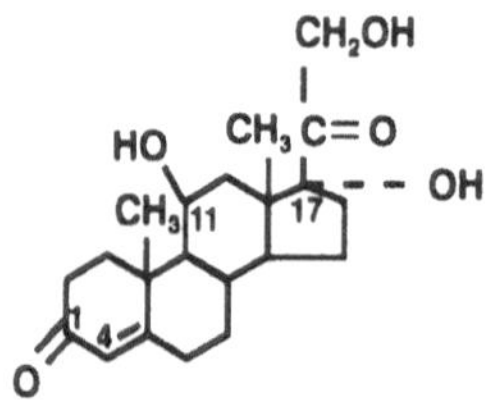

Slight structural modifications yield more potent derivatives:

Prednisolone:	**1,2-dehydro**
Prednisone:	**1,2-dehydro, 11-keto**
Dexamethasone:	**1,2-dehydro, 9-a-fluoro, 16-a-methyl**
Triamcinolone:	**1,2-dehydro, 9-a-fluoro, 16-a-hydroxyl**

Figure 5. Steroid structures.

Glucocorticoids alter leukocyte circulation; however, their antiinflammatory effects are mediated largely by the ability of glucocorticoids to inhibit the adherence of phagocytes, and therefore the recruitment of neutrophils and monocytes/macrophages into the affected area. They also inhibit the cells' responses to phagocytic and lymphokine signals.

Very specific effects of glucocorticoids to inhibit the production of IL-1 by monocytes and macrophages, and the synthesis of IL-2 and other lymphokines by lymphocytes, account in part for the profound inhibitory effects of these agents on the immune response.

The mechanism of action of glucocorticoid antiinflammatory effects involves enhancing transcription of a specific mRNA for the synthesis of macrocortin (lipocortin, lipomodulin), a peptide with profound antiinflammatory effects. It specifically inhibits phospholipases that break down membrane lipids (Fig. 3), and therefore inhibits the production of both cyclooxygenase products (PGs and TXs) and lipoxygenase products (HETEs, leukotrienes, and lipoxins). Glucocorticoids also enhance, by a rapid membrane effect, the production of cyclic AMP by leukocytes responding to other stimulants. Cyclic AMP is involved in the inhibition of nearly all lymphocyte and phagocyte functions.

Adverse effects of glucocorticoids are not usually severe if therapy is restricted to a few days, but limit their use for long-term therapy. In addition to the profound immunosuppression discussed above, the drugs cause osteoporosis, arrest of growth, electrolyte and fluid imbalances, increased risk of ulcers, myopathy, and Cushing's syndrome with behavioral disturbances. The administration of glucocorticoids inhibits the endogenous production of both ACTH and hydrocortisone. Since the glucocorticoids are synthesized at rates proportional to secretion, glucocorticoid therapy is followed by a period of very low endogenous hydrocortisone levels.

5. ANTIGOUT THERAPY

Gouty arthritis is unique in the nature of the inflammatory stimulus, sodium urate crystals. Uric acid is the end product of purine metabolism and when plasma levels become excessive sodium urate crystals are deposited in the kidney and joint tissue.

Regardless of the cause of excessive urate, the crystals cause infiltration of neutrophils to the site of deposition. The consequent phagocytosis of sodium urate crystals results in neutrophil disruption and release of lysosomal enzymes and other inflammatory mediators. The kallikrein and complement systems are also activated. The resultant inflammatory symptoms and erosion of articular tissue proceed as described for other types of arthritic inflammation.

The three approaches to treat gout that are distinctive from those used to treat other arthritides include the use of colchicine as an antiinflammatory agent, of allopurinol to inhibit uric acid synthesis, and of probenecid or sulfinpyrazone to enhance uric acid secretion (see Fig. 6).

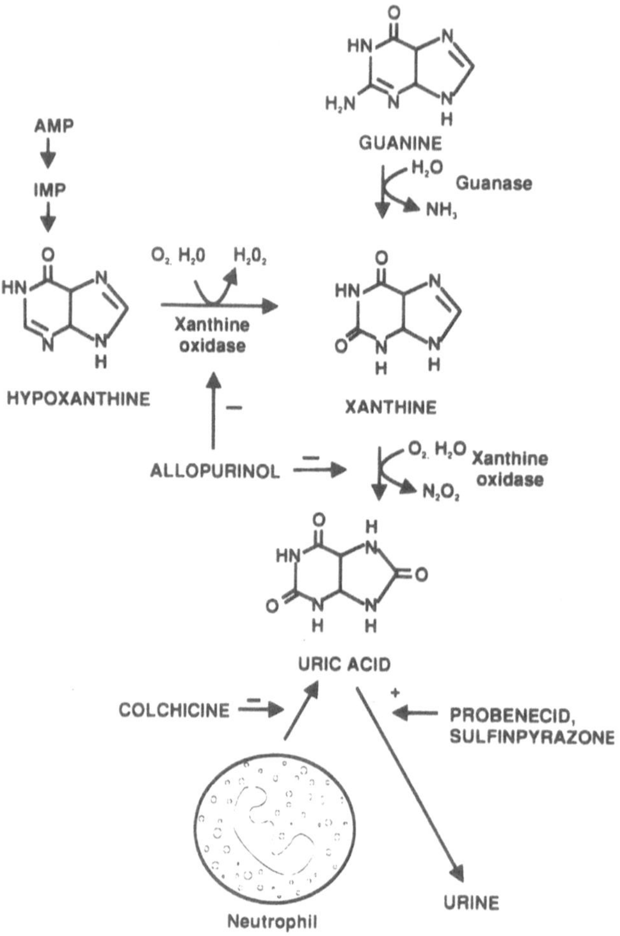

Figure 6. Gout model.

Colchicine is used prophylactically to prevent attacks of gout and it also affords relief from ongoing attacks (Fig. 7). It is an alkaloid of the autumn crocus of Colchis in Asia Minor. Its antiinflammatory effect is specific for gouty arthritis for which it has been used for 200 years. It binds to microtubular proteins, causing depolymerization and disappearance of the microtubular structures of the mitotic spindle at high doses. Since motile cells such as neutrophils depend on microtubule structures for movement, it has long been accepted that colchicine acts beneficially in gout by inhibiting movement of neutrophils into synovial spaces. Colchicine inhibits mast cell degranulation, and therefore prevents the release of neutrophil chemotaxins from mast cells. A more direct and dramatic effect of colchicine has been uncovered recently. On

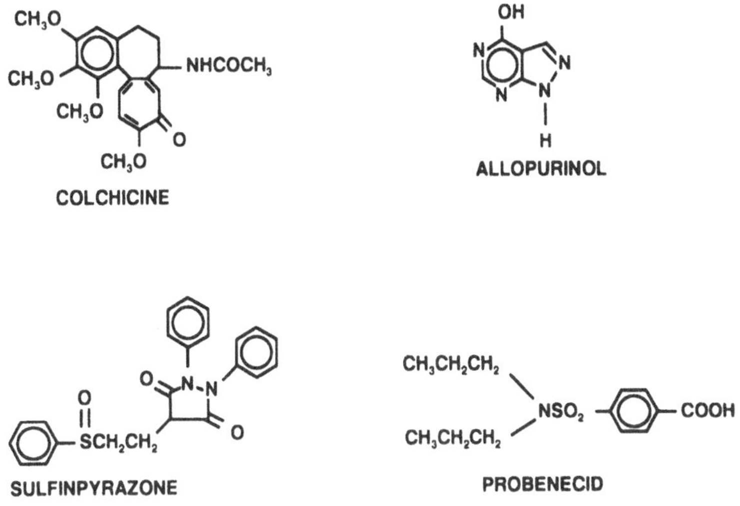

Figure 7. Drugs used in gout.

ingestion of urate crystals, neutrophils produce a glycoprotein that, when injected into joints, produces a profound arthritis histologically identical to that caused by urate crystals. Colchicine has a dramatic effect to specifically prevent the formation and release of this protein.

Most adverse effects of colchicine are gastrointestinal (nausea, vomiting, abdominal pain, and diarrhea). These are considerably reduced if the drug is given intravenously. Colchicine affects the proliferating cells of the bone marrow and chronic administration may result in agranulocytosis and aplastic anemia. Symptoms of acute poisoning are hemorrhagic gastroenteritis, nephrotoxicity, an ascending paralysis of the CNS, and disseminated intravascular coagulation. Colchicine should be used with caution by older patients and those with renal, hepatic, gastrointestinal, or cardiac disease.

Allopurinol decreases the production of uric acid. This analogue of hypoxanthine inhibits xanthine oxidase, the enzyme that catalyzes the conversion of hypoxanthine to xanthine and xanthine to uric acid. In addition, it reduces *de novo* purine synthesis through a feedback mechanism involving hypoxanthine-quanine phosphoribosyl transferase. Allopurinol is converted by xanthine oxidase to alloxanthine (oxypurinol), which also inhibits xanthine oxidase.

Allopurinol is the preferred drug for treatment of chronic gout and other conditions such as leukemia associated with excessive uric acid production. By inhibiting uric acid formation, allopurinol reduces serum and urine levels, permitting solubilization of the urate crystals and, eventually, dissolution of gouty tophi.

Allopurinol is well tolerated by most patients. Renal insufficiency and hepatic dysfunction have been reported. Adverse reactions (headache, drowsiness, nausea, vomiting, vertigo, diarrhea) are usually minor. Certain drug interactions may be of major importance. Clearance of theophylline is reduced and a metabolite, 1-methyltheophylline, appears in elevated levels. Allopurinol delays the excretion of probenecid and increases its concentration in plasma, while probenecid, in turn, increases the urinary excretion of allopurinol. These interactions are common because combination therapy with the two agents is frequently employed for gout. Other examples of negative interactions include thiazide diuretics and 6-mercaptopurine (6-MP) or azathioprine. Since allopurinol prevents enzymatic inactivation of 6-MP, it increases by three- to fourfold the bone marrow toxicity of 6-MP. Allopurinol also increases the bone marrow toxicity of unrelated cytotoxic agents such as cyclophosphamide.

Probenecid and sulfinpyrazone are organic acids that enhance uric acid excretion by acting on the anionic transport sites of the renal tubule to inhibit uric acid reabsorption. As the urinary excretion of uric acid increases, the formation of uric acid stones is favored; therefore, urine volume should be maintained at a high level and the pH kept high (> 6) with sodium bicarbonate therapy. Uricosuric agents may lower plasma levels only slowly since turnover of urate from tissue deposits is necessary before plasma levels decline. Both agents can induce gastrointestinal irritation, allergic dermatitis, and, rarely, aplastic anemia.

6. DISEASE-MODIFYING AGENTS

6.1. Antimalarial Drugs

The 4-aminoquinoline compounds, chloroquine and hydroxychloroquine, are orally active antiinflammatory agents used in second-line therapy in rheumatoid arthritis and in related inflammatory connective tissue diseases (Fig. 8). The mechanisms of their actions from an immunopharmacologic standpoint are unclear. The accumulated evidence indicates these drugs act both *in vitro* and *in vivo* to suppress leukocyte responses including leukotaxis, IL-1 production by macrophages, lymphoproliferative responses of T lymphocytes, and cytotoxic responses of T lymphocytes and NK cells. While these agents inhibit RNA and DNA synthesis at high doses, the therapeutic effects appear to result from an attenuation of activation events of leukocytes, perhaps through the inhibition of sulfhydryl systems or membrane phospholipases.

At therapeutic levels these agents are not clinically immunosuppressive and are relatively nontoxic (mild gastrointestinal and CNS effects). Their use is complicated by long half-life in the circulation (> 6 days), tissue concentration, and thus slow turnover and excretion. Their capacity to accumulate in pigmentated tissues such as the retina can occasionally lead to a sometimes irreversible, "doughnut" retinopathy and care must be taken to avoid exceeding recommended doses and to monitor the fundi for degenerative changes.

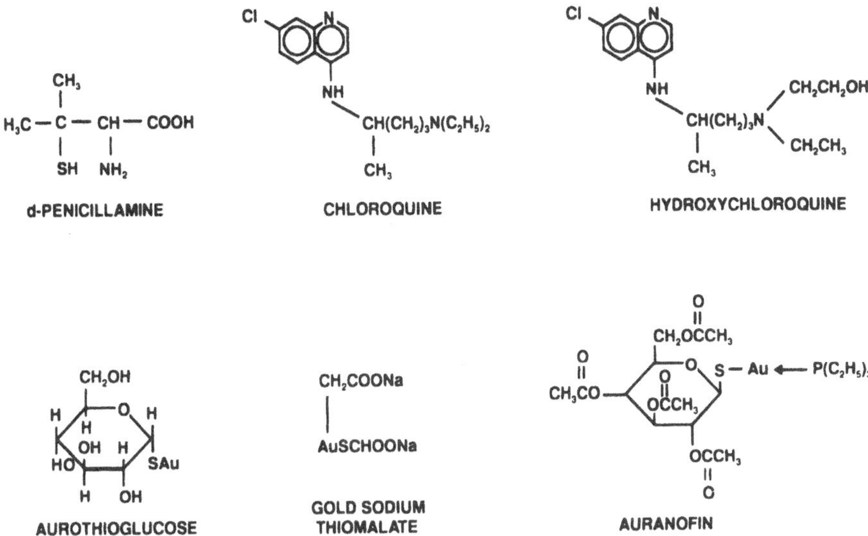

Figure 8. Drugs used in rheumatoid arthritis.

6.2. Gold Preparations

Gold has traditionally been used to treat palmar pruritis ("itching palms"); however, its use in juvenile and adult rheumatoid arthritis is more recent. Two parenteral gold salt preparations, aurothioglucose and gold sodium thiomalate, and an oral form, auranofin, are effective remission inducers (15%) in the more active and severe forms of rheumatoid arthritis. The mechanism of this latter action is not well understood. While not generally immunosuppressive, gold salts modulate a spectrum of immune and inflammatory responses and reduce adjuvant-type arthritides in animals. The primary cellular targets appear to be phagocytic cell populations. Following administration, gold is taken up in "aurosomes" of these cells in the synovium and elsewhere in the reticuloendothelial system (liver, spleen, bone marrow, and lymph nodes). A decrease in leukotactic and phagocytic activity results and, while the cells are capable of degranulating, the activities of various lysosomal enzymes are reduced. Reduced lymphoproliferative responses likely result in great part from impaired accessory macrophage function and perhaps cytokine release. In addition, complement activation is directly impaired by gold salts.

The molecular bases of these many actions are inferred to involve binding of sulfur by gold and an interference in sulfhydryl (SH-SS) exchange. Possibly other antiinflammatory or antimicrobial actions may be involved.

Because of a high degree of binding of gold salts to serum proteins, particularly albumin, and deposition in cellular storage sites, the turnover of gold is slow, allowing infrequent administration but favoring cumulative toxicity. The mechanism of toxicity, seen as limiting in at least one-third of the patients, is not clear. The most common problems involve skin lesions (erosive dermatitis) and mucous membrane lesions (stomatitis, enteritis); gastrointestinal disturbances progressing to diarrhea are also common. Nephrosis with proteinuria, hematologic and allergic reactions, and hepatitis also limit therapy. Immunosuppressive effects and secondary infections are not a problem; however, the frequency and severity of side effects restrict gold therapy to those who are generally healthy and preclude its use with other toxic agents (phenylbutazone, steroids, and cytotoxic agents).

6.3. D-Penicillamine

D-Penicillamine is a dimethyl analogue of D-cysteine which is used as a second-line agent in juvenile and adult rheumatoid arthritis. The best characterized action of D-penicillamine is its action to chelate trace metals such as copper, lead, and mercury, which provides the rationale for its clinical use in Wilson's disease and heavy metal poisoning. The basis for its activity in rheumatoid arthritis from an immunopharmacologic standpoint is far from clear. It is neither overtly antiinflammatory nor immunosuppressive. Two types of actions have been focused on. The first relates to a direct action to dissociate rheumatoid factor and Ag–Ab complexes *in vitro*. This action is associated with decreased immune complexes in serum and synovia; yet in many patients increased deposition occurs in kidney glomeruli with associated nephropathy. The second action relates to modulation of T-lymphocyte proliferative and helper and/or suppressor cell function. These actions are favored to explain decreased autoimmune phenomena rather than alternative actions on macrophage function. A variety of studies indicate a complex immunomodulatory effect of D-penicillamine alone and in conjunction with metal chelates. The major toxicities of D-penicillamine related to its mechanism of action are the nephropathy with proteinuria (20%) which may progress to nephrotic syndrome and be associated with other autoimmune phenomena. Skin rash, gastrointestinal symptoms, and abnormal hematologic findings are also seen with regularity. The pharmacokinetics of D-penicillamine, unlike the antimalarials and gold salts, are similar to other drugs with a relatively short serum half-life (2 hr); nevertheless, it is given on a daily basis.

6.4. New Agents

Two orally active immunomodulators, levamisole and diethyldithiocarbamate (DTC), have shown efficacy in rheumatoid arthritis. Neither drug is directly anti-inflammatory in its actions and both are classified as "thymomimetic" in their actions in that they promote T-lymphocyte functions, particularly in impaired individuals. Like D-penicillamine, both contain sulfur. In addition, DTC, like D-penicillamine, is a chelator of metals. The basis of their activity in rheumatoid arthritis is not clear, yet the primary immunoregulatory actions of these agents suggest that correction of

T-cell-related immunodeficiency or restoration of suppressor cell functions is involved. DTC is relatively nontoxic while levamisole induces a reversible agranulocytosis, particularly in HLA B27-bearing individuals. Both drugs are slow in onset and occasionally remission-inducing. Neither is approved by the U.S. Food and Drug Administration (FDA).

The two thymic hormone preparations thymopentin and thymulin have shown activity in initial clinical trials in patients with rheumatoid arthritis. These parenterally administered peptides modulate the functions of T cells. The basis of their activity in rheumatoid arthritis is not clear, but like the immunomodulators, they presumably correct T-cell deficiency or restore suppressor T-cell function. Both are nontoxic. Neither is approved by the FDA.

Increasing emphasis on finding new immunomodulators that can act as disease-modifying agents in rheumatoid arthritis has focused on agents that regulate the activity of T lymphocytes. Other examples are bucillamine and lobenzarit. Agents that inhibit arachidonic acid release and metabolism to eicosanoids via the lipoxygenase pathway (e.g., CI949 and 959) are also of interest.

7. IMMUNOSUPPRESSIVE AGENTS

Cytotoxic, immunosuppressive drugs have been employed in severe, recalcitrant rheumatoid arthritis as well as other severe forms of autoimmunity. The agents used include cyclophosphamide, azathioprine, methotrexate, and cyclosporine A (see Table II). These agents are not generally considered to be directly antiinflammatory and their actions in rheumatoid arthritis can be attributed to effects to reduce the number and function of both T and B lymphocytes and of phagocytic populations. While reversible in their actions, their toxicities are considerable and include secondary infections and increased incidence of malignancy. The appropriateness of their use depends on the severity of the underlying disease and its consequences.

Special mention should be made about low-dose methotrexate use in rheumatoid arthritis. Clinical studies indicate that low-dose methotrexate may have antiinflammatory effects independent of its immunosuppressive actions. The fact that intraarticular injection is ineffective suggests these antiinflammatory actions are indirect; however, their mechanisms remain obscure at present. At low doses the side effects of methotrexate are minimal.

8. CLINICAL PHARMACOLOGY

Symptom relief for nonperpetuating inflammation as occurs with simple trauma relies on restriction of movement and mild analgesia (it remains to be decided whether hot or cold compresses are initially useful). For more severe and chronic forms of

TABLE II
Immunosuppressive Drugs Used in Autoimmune Diseases

	Disease indication[a]	Cell targets: T cell	Cell targets: B cell	Myelosuppression	Other toxic effects
Cyclophosphamide	RA SLE Autoimmune blood dyscrasias	+	+	+	Alopecia, GI sympotoms, cystitis, infertility
Azathioprine	RA SLE Polymyositis Collagen diseases	+	+	+	GI symptoms, hepatotoxicity
Methotrexate	Psoriatic arthritis Dermatomyositis Polymyositis	+	+	+	Ulcerative stomatitis, pulmonary fibrosis
Cyclosporin A	Experimental in RA and SLE Type I diabetes Psoriasis Uveitis	+	0	0	Hepatotoxic, renotoxic, neurotoxic, hypertoxic
Glucocorticoids	RA SLE Autoimmunity	+	0	0	Cushing's syndrome, ulcers

[a]RA, rheumatoid arthritis; SLE, systemic lupus erythematosus.

inflammation as occurs in the connective tissue diseases such as rheumatoid arthritis, a tiered or stepwise approach is taken. In each case the intensity of therapy is dictated by the intensity of the disease.

8.1. Rheumatoid Arthritis

The initial approaches to the treatment of rheumatoid arthritis (Fig. 9) emphasize patient education and physical therapy. Aspirin remains the drug of choice for initiating antiinflammatory therapy partly because of its low cost. The amounts of aspirin required for antiinflammatory treatment are far in excess of those used for analgesia and approach the maximum tolerated doses. The side effect of nausea or tinnitus which generally occurs at serum levels above 300 μg/ml is sometimes used as an index of having reached therapeutic levels (200–300 μg/ml). When therapeutic levels are achieved and the side effects described (e.g., increased bleeding tendency, gastrointestinal upset, intolerence) do not supervene to curtail therapy, responses can be expected to occur within 3 months and maximum effect can be realized by 6 months. Generally, responses are measured in rheumatoid arthritis in terms of scales

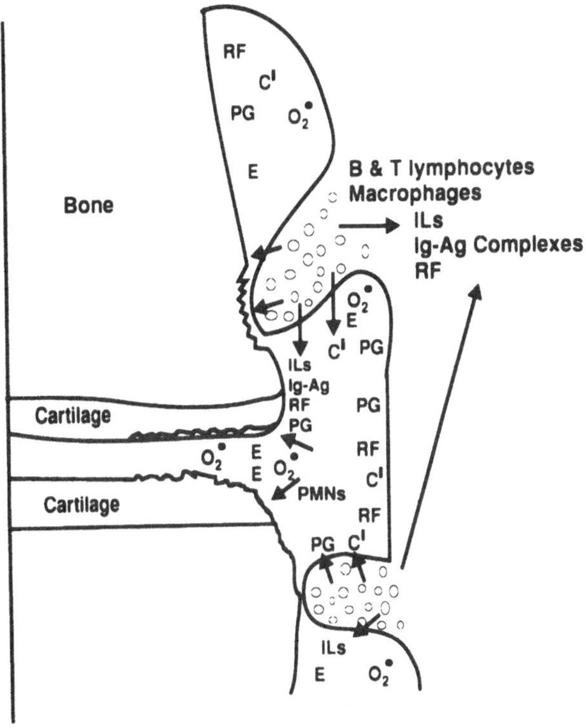

Figure 9. Process of joint inflammation and destruction in rheumatoid arthritis. PMN, polymorphonuclear neutrophils; Ig-Ag, antigen-antibody complexes; RF, rheumatoid factor; C^I, complement factors; PG, prostaglandins; E, hydrolytic enzymes; $O_2^{\bullet}$ oxygen radicals; ILs, interleukins.

such as the Ritchie or the Landsbury indices which take into account laboratory parameters of inflammation (erythrocyte sedimentation rate and/or C-reactive protein) and both objective and subjective parameters of joint involvement (e.g., number of joints involved, duration of morning stiffness, pain score, and grip strength).

Generally, glucocorticoids are avoided in the routine treatment of rheumatoid arthritis; however, when the disease is acute and systemic symptoms are present, they are useful in obtaining a prompt reduction of inflammatory symptoms. They also may be used in low doses, often intermittently, to complement other DMARDs. Intraarticular use of steroids is effective particularly when few large joints are involved. Injectable gold salts are generally the first choice in managing acute, progressive disease unresponsive to NSAIDs. In this setting, responses are obtained in two-thirds of the patients with a 15% overall remission rate. The responses occur slowly (3–6 months) and are characterized by progressive declines of rheumatoid factor, sedimentation rate, immunoglobulin levels, and joint inflammation (Ritchie index). The comparative efficacy of oral gold is somewhat less. Response is associated with reduced progression of joint destruction by radiologic criteria. One-third of the patients will suffer significant toxicity and in one-half of these discontinuance will be necessary. Gastrointestinal and skin reactions and proteinuria are the most common limiting side effects; however, they also occur in untreated patients. Side effects may be aggravated by other illnesses (e.g., renal or hepatic disease). The range of toxicity precludes concurrent therapy with other agents besides NSAIDs and requires careful monitoring to minimize the impact. Steroid therapy and gold chelation may be useful to treat severe toxicity. Gold salts are less useful in late-stage destructive disease and are not used to treat other autoimmune or inflammatory diseases.

The antimalarial compounds offer a complementary therapy with NSAIDs in patients who need more intense therapy. Approximately two-thirds of patients with rheumatoid arthritis will respond slowly to these agents (3–12 months) and only 5% will not tolerate the therapy as a result of toxicity (including retinopathy). Those who benefit show progressive declines in rheumatoid factor, sedimentation rate, and other objective inflammatory signs and symptoms and some remissions occur. Long-term effects to reverse joint destruction in those with progressive disease have not, however, been documented. Antimalarials are also reported to be effective in juvenile arthritis, lupus erythematosis, and other inflammatory connective tissue diseases; however, they are generally avoided in psoriatic arthritis because of a high incidence of dermatitis.

D-Penicillamine, like gold salts and antimalarials, is useful in patients with active, severe disease unresponsive to NSAIDs. Approximately two-thirds of patients respond and some remissions are observed. Also, like the other agents, the action is slow to develop (> 3 months) and toxicity restricts their use to combination with NSAIDs and/or glucocorticoids. Because approximately 20% of patients will suffer some toxicity involving blood dyscrasias (anemia/thrombocytopenia) or nephropathy, regular blood counts with platelet counts and urinalyses are necessary. Skin rashes and gastrointestinal effects are also limiting. In responders, progressive falls in rheumatoid factor and Ig levels are observed with diminished signs and symptoms of inflammation and with retardation of joint destruction. D-Penicillamine is not used in other connective tissue diseases.

At present, low-dose methotrexate is increasingly being employed as a second-line antiinflammatory DMARD. At levels of 7.5–25 mg/week, responses are generally prompt (within 2–3 weeks) and side effects are minimal.

In patients unresponsive or poorly responsive to the second-line DMARDs, a third line of immunosuppressive agents is considered. In addition to their own individual toxicities, they share the side effects of bone marrow suppression (except cyclosporine A), increased incidence of infection, and increased incidence of late-occurring malignancies, particularly leukemias and lymphomas. The use of this type of therapy should be restricted to those with special training in rheumatology or clinical immunology.

Azathioprine, particularly in combination with glucocorticosteroids, has seen a wide use in bone marrow transplantation and in systemic lupus erythematosus with nephritis and/or vasculitis. Its use in rheumatoid arthritis to reduce the use of steroids or to decrease disease activity directly is considered experimental.

Cyclophosphamide given orally in severe rheumatoid arthritis and intravenously with glucocorticoids in acute lupus nephritis has demonstrated efficacy; however, its use in these and other arthropathies is experimental.

Cyclosporine A has demonstrated initial activity in several autoimmune disorders; however, initial reports in rheumatoid arthritis suggest that, although active, its renal and hepatic toxicity may preclude wide use.

Methotrexate use in low doses in rheumatoid arthritis has been discussed. The use of similar doses has also been reported to be effective in recalcitrant psoriatic arthritis and Reiter's syndrome. Antineoplastic doses of methotrexate are not accepted for use in autoimmune diseases.

A variety of new agents are under study in rheumatoid arthritis. Thymomimetic drugs and the thymic hormones offer insights into ways to modify the disease processes through modulation of the immune system rather than the inflammatory process itself; however, the efficacy of these agents so far does not appear to differ markedly from the other DMARDs. Their ultimate approval will, therefore, depend on their comparative toxicities. Another approach to increase efficacy while limiting toxicity has been the combined use of low doses of DMARDs of both the antiinflammatory and immunosuppressive type. At the present time, azathioprine is being tested with cyclophosphamide or antimalarials. More effective approaches will probably depend on the better elucidation of etiologic factors or agents.

8.2. Gout

The therapy of acute gout is based on four strategies: (1) antiinflammatory therapy with glucocorticoids and/or symptomatic relief with NSAIDs, especially indomethacin, but also phenylbutazone, fenoprofen, ibuprofen, naproxen, and sulindac; (2) inhibition of neutrophil mobility (with colchicine); (3) inhibition of uric acid synthesis (with allopurinol); and (4) augmentation of uric acid excretion with probenecid or sulfinpyrazone.

The first two approaches have been described. Colchicine is given orally or intravenously to prevent and to abort attacks of gout. Pain and inflammation begin to subside within 6–12 hr after intravenous administration or 24–48 hr after oral therapy. The drug is discontinued when the pain disappears or gastrointestinal symptoms develop. Treatment should not be resumed for at least 3 days to avoid cumulative toxicity. Allopurinol is not useful during an acute attack of gouty arthritis. In fact, it may increase the frequency of gouty arthritis attacks in the early stages of treatment. Treatment is, therefore, initiated during remissions of chronic gouty arthritis or in secondary hyperuricemia. Probenecid or sulfinpyrazone are often used concurrently with allopurinol to enhance secretion of uric acid. A large volume of alkaline urine should be maintained to reduce the possibility of urate stone formation. Colchicine is often concurrently administered in small doses between attacks until all urate deposits (gouty tophi) have dissolved. Control with allopurinol may take several months.

As with rheumatoid arthritis, salicylates are preferred initial agents for the treatment of ankylosing spondylitis and the reactive arthritides (Reiter's syndrome and psoriatic arthritis).

When toxicity supervenes or clinical response is deemed inadequate in each of these diseases, a decision to try other NSAIDs is made. Often several will be tried since patient tolerance and response appear to have unique individual components. If remission occurs, maintenance therapy is not generally employed. With the persistance of active, progressive disease, the second-line agents or DMARDs are considered.

BIBLIOGRAPHY

General References

Bonta, I. L., Bray, M. A., and Parnham, M. J., eds., 1985, *Handbook of Inflammation*, Elsevier, Amsterdam. A useful source on the mechanisms of inflammation.

Drug Evaluations, 6th ed., 1986, American Medical Association, Chicago. A useful general source on the treatments of inflammation.

Espinosa, L., ed., 1988, *Infections in the Rheumatic Diseases*, Grune & Stratton, New York. A text on the role of infection in rheumatoid arthritis and the reactive arthritides.

McCarthy, D. J., ed., 1985, *Arthritis*, Lea & Febiger, Philadelphia. A classic reference for the rheumatologist.

Roth, S. M., ed., 1985, *Rheumatic Therapeutics*, McGraw–Hill, New York. A useful general source on the treatment of rheumatic disease.

Specific References

Dunn, M., and Weissman, G., eds., 1987, Arachidonic acid metabolism and inflammation: Therapeutic implications, *Drugs* **33**, Suppl. 1:1. A collection of seven reviews of arachidonic acid metabolites and NSAIDs in physiologic and pathologic processes.

Hench, P. S., Kendall, E. D., Slocumb, C. H., and Polley, H. F., 1949, The effect of a hormone of the adrenal cortex (17-hydroxy-11-dehydrocorticosterone; compound E) and of pituitary adrenocorticotropic hormone on rheumatoid arthritis, *Proc. Staff Meet. Mayo Clin.* **24**:181. Classic paper describing effects of ACTH and glucocorticoids on arthritis symptoms.

Lipsky, P. E., 1983, Immunopharmacology of remission-inducing drugs in rheumatoid arthritis, in: *Advances in Immunopharmacology 2* (J. W. Hadden, L. Chedid, P. Dukor, F. Spreafico, and D. Willoughby, eds.), Pergamon Press, Elmsford, NY, pp. 345–350. A review of new approaches to the treatment of rheumatoid arthritis.

Oates, J. A., Fitzgerald, G. A., Branch, R. A., Jackson, E. K., Knapp, H. R., and Roberts, L. J., II, 1988, Clinical implications of prostaglandin and thromboxane formation, *N. Engl. J. Med.* **319**:689–761. A review of the physiological actions of eicosanoids and effects of NSAIDs.

Talal, N., and Hadden, J. W., 1985, Hormones, immunomodulating drugs and autoimmunity, in: *Handbook of Inflammation*, Volume 5 (I. L. Bonta, M. A. Bray, and M. J. Parnham, eds.), Elsevier, Amsterdam, p. 335–345. A review of new antirheumatic agents.

Vane, J., 1971, Inhibition of prostaglandin synthesis as a mechanism of action for aspirin-like drugs, *Nature New Biol.* **231**:232–235. Classic paper describing aspirin inhibition of cyclooxygenase.

PART II

CANCER IMMUNOPHARMACOLOGY

CHAPTER 3

IMMUNOPHARMACOLOGY AND IMMUNOTHERAPY OF HUMAN CANCER

JAMES E. TALMADGE

1. INTRODUCTION

Immunoregulatory and hematoaugmenting cytokines have come into their own as novel therapeutic compounds for diverse indications including oncology and infectious, iatrogenic, and congenital diseases. Immunopharmacologic analyses of structure–activity relationships, toxicology, pharmacokinetics, and immunopharmacodynamics have yielded information contributing to the more effective use of these agents in disease models, as well as in the clinic. Current strategies for cytokine therapy suggest that the ultimate use of these drugs will be as adjuvants in combination with other therapeutics for immunodeficiencies, myeloid aplasia, cancer, and infectious diseases. This chapter briefly reviews the cytokines relevant to these indications, discusses the prioritization of these compounds for clinical entry, and emphasizes the recombinant biologics that are currently either licensed or in active clinical trials in the United States, Europe, and Asia. In addition to providing a compendium of immunologically active agents we have addressed some of the strategies used for the development of these pharmacophores as well as the difficulties and scientific–clinical challenges for their development.

The primary emphasis in this chapter is on the use of adjuvant immune-mediated therapy for the treatment of neoplasia. However, immunotherapy appears to be primarily active in a minimal residual disease setting and to date has not shown reproducible efficacy against bulky, clinically apparent disease. Thus, the current

---

JAMES E. TALMADGE • University of Nebraska Medical Center, Omaha, Nebraska 68198.

Immunopharmacology Reviews, Volume 2, edited by John W. Hadden and Andor Szentivanyi. Plenum Press, New York, 1996.

strategy is to use immunotherapy as an adjuvant strategy in patients with minimal residual disease and/or following chemotherapy. Remarkable progress has been made in the treatment of primary human cancer by cytotoxic therapy in past decades. Increasing the intensity of cytoreductive therapy has a therapeutic advantage for the treatment of cancer; however, toxicity to normal tissue limits the possible dose escalation. Typically, the tissue that limits dose escalation is the bone marrow (BM). The use of high doses of chemo/radiotherapy can (and often does) lead to myelotoxicity, failure of the BM, aplasia, infection, and death. To circumvent these complications, BM transplantation (BMT) or peripheral blood stem cell (PSC) transplantation (PSCT) have been used to reinstate stem cells that were not exposed to the cytotoxic events. In this approach, BM or PSC are first removed from the patient before high-dose therapy (HDT) and the patient "rescued" from the myelotoxic effects of the therapy by the subsequent administration of the harvested stem cells.

The use of HDT is critical, as shown in a retrospective analysis by Hryniuk and Levine who concluded that dose intensity rather than the cumulative dose of planned chemotherapy (Hryniuk and Levine, 1986) correlated with response rate in neoplasia. This hypothesis was confirmed and extended by Tannock and colleagues, who undertook a prospectively randomized trial of two dose levels of cyclophosphamide, methotrexate, and 5-fluorouracil chemotherapy (CMF) for patients with metastatic breast cancer (Tannock *et al.*, 1988). In this prospectively randomized clinical trial, they demonstrated that patients who received higher doses of CMF chemotherapy had a longer survival than those receiving the lower dose. However, the effectiveness of chemotherapy is confounded by drug resistance, particularly for tumors at relapse, and the toxicity of chemotherapy drugs to normal tissues. Thus, tumor cell resistance can be overcome to some extent by increased dose intensity but only at the expense of increased toxicity. PSCT and BMT, therefore, provide a strategy to limit the myelotoxicity associated with HDT and rescue the patient from the risk of iatrogenic infectious disease.

Despite the success of HDT and the high frequency of complete responses (CR) following HDT and stem cell transplantation, the duration of the response is often short. However, the reduction in tumor burden, although not of long duration, provides an ideal situation for adjuvant therapy. At present, one of the more intriguing forms of adjuvant therapy (other than a second cycle of HDT and stem cell rescue) is the use of immunotherapy. Indeed, with appropriate manipulation, the stem cell product itself may also provide a basis for immunotherapy (Vose *et al.*, 1993). These developing forms of adjuvant treatment include monoclonal antibodies with and without radioisotopes or toxins (not discussed in this review), adoptive cellular therapy, and cytokine therapy to augment immune function posttransplantation. In theory, the combination of immune augmentation strategies and tumor reduction by HDT and stem cell rescue should result in a longer response duration following HDT if not a "cure." The concept that induction therapy and stem cell transplantation are not the final stage in the treatment of metastatic disease, versus being the first step in multiple cycles of primary and adjuvant therapy, is "novel" and the source of ongoing preclinical and clinical research. This review discusses many of the concepts and strategies involved in the use of adjuvant immunotherapy.

2. RECOMBINANT PROTEINS

Cytokines and growth factors are relatively low-molecular-weight proteins that are secreted in minute quantities and act in either an autocrine or paracrine manner. The isolation of cDNA clones for cytokines and growth factors has permitted their production in large and reproducible quantities, which in turn has accelerated the preclinical and clinical study of their function and therapeutic attributes. The ability to cut and rejoin DNA at any desired site or to introduce point mutations at directed sites has resulted in the development and clinical use of mutant as well as chimeric therapeutic proteins. Thus, we can now utilize proteins that are either exact or mutated forms of the naturally occurring ones, or design proteins that are composed of various polypeptide structures derived from different sequences, e.g., the humanized monoclonal antibodies. The use of various point mutations has resulted in drugs with decreased toxicity, better production capabilities, or higher expression levels such as the mutant IL-2, IL-3, or CSF-G molecules (Kuga *et al.*, 1989; Rosenberg *et al.*, 1984; Lu *et al.*, 1989; Krown *et al.*, 1992), where, for example, serines are substituted for cysteines to reduce the development of aberrant tertiary structures. Furthermore, there is the development of chimeric cytokines expressing properties associated with multiple parent structures such as PIXY-321, which is a single biologically active drug comprised of IL-3 and CSF-GM (Williams *et al.*, 1990; Bruno *et al.*, 1992; Bhalla *et al.*, 1992) or an IL-3 and EPO fusion protein (Welch *et al.*, 1993).

There are a large and expanding number of cytokines and growth factors that are currently in preclinical and clinical studies. Cytokines and growth factors are defined as proteins that modulate cell growth, induce differentiation, and/or augment function and often have a limited cellular specificity. For instance, many cytokines influence cellular proliferation with individual cytokines having distinct lineage specificities. Cytokines also have activities based on the induction of differentiated functions which may be lineage specific. For example: the cytokines capable of the modulation of eosinophils, mast cells, or lymphokine-activated killer (LAK) cells appear to be restricted (IL-5, -3, and -2, respectively). In contrast, some cytokines appear to have a much broader spectrum of action, including IL-6, -1, and TNF which have activities on immune, hematopoietic, mesenchymal, and epithelial cells. The cytokines and growth factors shown in Table I have been limited to those that at present appear to have therapeutic efficacy for myelosuppression, infectious disease, and/or neoplasia, i.e., the cells of the immune and hematopoietic system. It does not include cytokines and growth factors with activities on other cell types including ones of neural and epithelial origin.

There are several examples of cytokines that share similar functions overall yet bind to different receptors and have no sequence or structural homology. In contrast,

TABLE I
Cytokines[a]

	MHC class I/II	B-cell activation	B-cell proliferation	B-cell differentiation	Ig isotype selection	T-cell activation
IFN-αs	I/II		yes	yes		
IFN-β	I/II		yes			
IFN-γ	I/II	yes	yes	yes	IgG2a	
TNF		yes	yes/no	yes/no		
LT			yes	yes		
IL-1α	no	yes	yes	yes		yes
IL-1β	no	yes	yes	yes		yes
IL-2			yes	yes		yes
IL-3	II		yes	yes		
IL-4	II	yes	yes	yes	IgE IgG1	yes
IL-5		yes	yes/no	yes/no	IgA	
IL-6				yes		yes
IL-7			yes	yes		yes
Chemokines α						yes
Chemokines β						
IL-9						
IL-10	II			yes	yes	
IL-11						
IL-12					IgE	
IL-13	II	yes	yes	yes	IgG4	
IL-14		yes	yes			
IL-15						yes
G-CSF						
M-CSF						
GM-CSF						
SCF		yes	yes			
Flk-2/Flt-3						
TPO						
TGF-α						
TGF-β	II		yes	yes	IgA	yes
IL-IRa			yes/no			

[a]Abbreviations: IFN, interferon; TNF, tumor necrosis factor; LT, lymphotoxin; IL, interleukin; CSF, colony-stimulating factor; G-CSF, granulocyte CSF; M-CSF, macrophage CSF; GM-CSF, granulocyte–macrophage CSF; SCF, stem cell factor; TPO, thrombopoietin; TGF, tumor growth factor; IL-1Ra, IL-1 receptor antagonist; Flk-2/Flt-3, fetal liver kinase.

there are also cytokines that have disparate functionality, no structural homology, and yet share receptors with similar components. This occurs most often with the beta subunit of the heterodimeric receptor, the classic example being that of IL-3, -5, and GM-CSF (Takai *et al.*, 1994; Sato *et al.*, 1993; Miyajima *et al.*, 1993). Similarly, a common receptor subunit is shared between IL-6, -11, leukemia inhibitor factor, oncostatin-M and ciliary neurotropic factor which share the signal transducer GP-130 (Kishimoto *et al.*, 1994; Miyajima *et al.*, 1992; Davis *et al.*, 1993; Gearing *et al.*, 1992). However, it is

TABLE I
(Continued)

T-cell proliferation	T-cell differentiation	Chemotaxis	Hemato-poiesis	Molecular weight	Chromosome	Receptor MW
yes		yes		16–27	9q	95–110
				20	9q	95–110
no		yes		20–24	12q	90,95
yes		yes	yes	3×17	6p	75,55
			yes	20–25	6p	75,55
yes		yes	yes	17.5	2q	80,60
yes		yes	yes	17.5	2q	80,60
yes	yes	yes		15–20	4q	50,64,75
		yes	yes	14–30	5q	120
yes	yes	yes	yes	15–19	5q	120
		yes		2×21.5	5q	60,130
yes	yes		yes	21–28	7q	80/130
yes	yes			25	8q	70
		yes	yes	8–10	4q	67,59
		yes	yes	8–10	17q	
yes			yes	32–39	5	64
yes		yes		1	1	
			yes	23		151
yes			yes	35,40		
			no	12	5q	?,130
				53	14q	
yes	yes			14		?,64,?
			yes	18–22	17q	140
		yes	yes	45–70	5q or 1p	
yes		yes/no	yes	22	5q	80/150
			yes	37–42×2		
			yes	53		160/130
			yes	38	7?	
				5–6	2	170
yes	yes	yes/no		12.5×2	19q,14q	1–53
yes/no				17–25		

(continued)

not clear whether this duplication of cytokine function represents a significant biologic redundancy. In other instances such as with the chemokines (e.g., IL-8), there are significant levels of ligand structural homology and concomitant receptor promiscuity whereby multiple receptors are able to bind and complete for multiple ligands (Stein and Dalgleish, 1994; Sozzani *et al.*, 1994). In like fashion, IL-15 (Grabstein *et al.*, 1994; Burton *et al.*, 1994; Bamford *et al.*, 1994), which has no sequence homology to IL-2, has substantial three-dimensional similarity to IL-2 consisting of a four-helix

TABLE I
(*Continued*)

	Cross species reactivity	Mito-genesis	Cytostasis/toxicity	Macro-phages	Granulo-cytes	Eosino-phils	NK	LAK
IFN-αs	no		yes	yes		no	yes	yes
IFN-β	no		yes	yes	yes		yes	yes
IFN-γ	no	yes	yes	yes	yes		yes/no	yes
TNF	P	yes	yes	yes	yes	yes	no	yes/no
LT	P	yes	yes		yes			
IL-1α	yes	yes	yes		yes	yes	yes	
IL-1β	yes	yes	yes		yes	yes	yes	
IL-2	yes	yes		yes		no	yes	yes
IL-3	no	yes				yes	yes	yes
IL-4	no	yes	yes	yes		yes	yes	yes/no
IL-5		yes			yes/no	yes		
IL-6	no	yes	yes				yes	no
IL-7		yes		yes			yes	yes
Chemokines α	yes	yes		yes	yes			
Chemokines β		yes		yes				
IL-9	P	yes						
IL-10		yes		yes				yes
IL-11		yes						
IL-12	P	yes					yes	yes
IL-13	no			yes				
IL-14								
IL-15								
G-CSF		yes			yes	no		
M-CSF			yes		yes		no	
GM-CSF	no	yes		yes	yes	yes		
SCF		yes			yes			
Flk-2/Flt-3	yes	yes						
TPO	yes	yes						
TGF-α		yes						
TGF-β	yes	yes	yes/no				yes	no
IL-IRa	yes	yes/no		yes/no				

bundle. In preliminary data, it appears that IL-15 shares the IL-2 β receptor but has a disparate γ receptor necessary for its high-affinity binding. Interestingly, the γ receptor for IL-2 is also shared by other cytokines including IL-4 and -7 (Kondo *et al.*, 1993; Noguchi *et al.*, 1993; Russell *et al.*, 1993). Gene knock-out mice for the γ receptor (Voss *et al.*, 1994; Rosenberg *et al.*, 1993) are profoundly immunosuppressed, resulting in severe combined immunodeficiency (SCID). However, the loss of IL-2 in gene knock-out mice has minimal effects which suggests a functional redundancy for IL-2, -7, and -4.

Cytokine action is influenced by a number of factors. The response of a cell or tissue to an individual cytokine *in vitro* or *in vivo* depends on the context in which it receives the signal. The level of differentiation, nutrition, presence of pathogens, and cellular damage will also affect the response. Equally, and potentially more important is the influence of other cytokines, hormones, neurotransmitters, and the like that may be present in the microenvironment. The response of a cell to a cytokine is limited to those cells that express the appropriate receptor(s) and such expression may be restricted *in vivo*. In addition, individual cytokines may be produced by a limited number of cell types. Further, stringent control of cytokine production occurs at multiple levels including DNA methylation and *trans*-acting repressors of DNA transcription. However, there appears to be an overlap in signal transduction pathways between individual cytokines, both in terms of postreceptor signal transduction and activation of similar transcription factors. Thus, structurally unrelated cytokines may have evolved similar actions for distinct physiological or pathological situations. In addition, there is a clear need for multiple and, in some instances, sequential cytokine interactions in the differentiation–maturation of hematopoietic and lymphopoietic cells. Perhaps the group of cytokines with the greatest overlap in function which have been isolated to date are those that play a role in B-cell maturation and differentiation. These include not only IL-1, -4, -6, and -10, which have become associated with B-cell maturation and differentiation, but also IL-13 and -14 (Ambrus *et al.*, 1991, 1993). Understanding the cytokine network (Burke *et al.*, 1993) requires numerous technologies including gene knock-out mice, and mice transgenic for reporter gene constructs particularly in studies under conditions of stress such as acute or chronic infections, autoimmune processes, or neoplasia. *In situ* studies of RNA and cytokine protein or receptors in development, tissue repair, infection, inflammation, and neoplasia also contribute to our knowledge of cytokine function. While *in vitro* activities of cytokines can provide useful indications of *in vivo* action, some of the *in vivo* behaviors of cytokines cannot be predicted by the *in vitro* studies.

Therapeutic proteins, including the cytokines and growth factors, have emerged as a new and important class of drugs for the treatment of cancer, immunodepression, myeloid dysplasia, and infectious disease (Oldham, 1982). However, their development has been slowed by our limited understanding of their pharmacology and mechanism of action. To facilitate the development of these immunoregulatory proteins, additional information is needed on their pharmacology (Talmadge and Herberman, 1986; Mihich, 1986). One approach to the development of these proteins is to identify a clinical hypothesis based on preclinical therapeutic surrogate (Ellenberg, 1993; Holden, 1993). A surrogate for clinical efficacy may be a phenotypic biochemical, enzymatic, functional (immunologic, molecular, or hematologic), or quality of life measurement which is believed to be associated with therapeutic activity. Phase I clinical trials can then be designed to identify the optimal and maximum tolerated dose (MTD) and treatment schedule for protein administration which maximizes the augmentation of the surrogate end point(s). Subsequent Phase II/III trials can then be established to determine if the changes in the surrogate levels correlate with therapeutic activity. Table II lists the immunologically and hematologically active cytokines and growth factors that are approved for general use in the United States, while the proteins that are currently in clinical trials are listed in Table III along with the indications under investigation.

In contrast to strategies based on the identification of surrogates for therapeutic efficacy, many protocols for recombinant proteins have been predicated on practices developed for conventional low-molecular-weight drugs and may not be advantageous for the development of proteins. This is because of the unique pharmacologic attributes of proteins which require selective or targeted delivery to the desired site [i.e., the bone marrow, spleen, or tumor (Tomlinson, 1989, 1991)]. To optimally administer proteins as drugs and ensure their targeting is the primary challenge for their development. One additional difficulty in the development of a recombinant protein is that in many instances there is little relationship between the dose administered and biologic effect. Indeed, in some instances there is a nonlinear dose relationship that has been described as bell-shaped (Talmadge *et al.*, 1987a). This dose–response relationship, or lack thereof, may be the result of the nonlinear manner in which the drug is dispersed in the body; a poor ability to enter into a saturable receptor-mediated transport process; chemical instability; sequence of administration with other agents or an incorrect time of administration; and/or an inappropriate location and response of the target cells. Further, a "bell-shaped" dose–response curve could be associated with the tachyphylaxis of receptor expression or a signal transduction mechanism whereby the cells become refractory to subsequent receptor-mediated augmentation. Because the regulation of biological control can and likely will lead to numerous physiologically untoward events, it is important that both the

TABLE II
Approved Biotechnology Drugs

Product type	Abbreviated indication	U.S. status
Interferon gamma-1b	Chronic granulomatous disease	Dec. 1990
Interferon alpha-n3	Genital warts	Oct. 1989
Epoetin alpha	Anemia of chronic renal failure	June 1989
	Anemia of chronic renal failure	Dec. 1990
Inteferon alpha-2b	Hairy cell leukemia	June 1986
	Genital warts	June 1986
	AIDS-related Kaposi's sarcoma	Nov. 1988
	Non-A, non-B hepatitis	Feb. 1991
Sargramostim (CSF-GM)	Autologous bone marrow transplantation	Mar. 1991
Filgrastim (CSF-G)	Chemotherapy-induced neutropenia	Feb. 1991
Inteferon alpha-2a	Hairy cell leukemia	June 1986
	AIDS-related Kaposi's sarcoma	Nov. 1988
Aldesleukin (IL-2)	Renal cell carcinoma	May 1992
Interferon beta	Multiple sclerosis	1993–1994

TABLE III
Biotechnology Drugs in Development

Product type	Abbreviated indication	U.S. status
Colony-stimulating factors		
CSF-GM	Adjuvant to chemotherapy	Phase I/II
	Low blood cell counts	Submitted
Sargramostim (CSF-GM)	Allogeneic bone marrow transplantations, chemotherapy adjuvant	Phase III
	Adjuvant to AIDS therapy	Phase II
CSF-M	Cancer, fungal disease	Phase I
CSF-M	Cancer, hematologic neoplasms, bone marrow transplantations	Phase I
Filgrastim (R-CSF-G)	AIDS, leukemia, aplastic anemia	Submitted
Sargramostim (CSF-GM)	Neutropenia to secondary chemotherapy	Phase III
PiXy	Neutropenia	Phase I/II
Stem Cell Factor (SCF)	Neutropenia/thrombocytopenia	Phase I
Erythropoietins		
Epoetin beta	Anemia secondary to kidney disease	Submitted
	Autologous transfusion	Phase II/III
Epoetin alpha	Anemia of cancer and chemotherapy	Submitted
	Anemia of surgical blood loss, autologous transfusion	Phase III
Interferons		
Interferon gamma-1b	Small-cell lung cancer, atopic dermatitis	Phase III
	Trauma-related infections, renal cell carcinoma, asthma, and allergies	Phase II
Interferon alpha-n3	ARC, AIDS	Phase I/II
Interferon beta	Cancer	Phase I/II
Interferon gamma	Rheumatoid arthritis	Phase II/III
	Venereal warts	Phase II
Interferon consensus	Cancer, infectious disease	Phase II/III
Interferon gamma	Cancer, infectious disease	Phase II
Interferon alpha-2b	Superficial bladder cancer, basal cell carcinoma, chronic hepatitis B, delta hepatitis	Submitted
	Acute hepatitis B, delta hepatitis, acute chronic myelogenous leukemia	Phase III
	HIV (with Retrovir)	Phase I
Interferon beta	Unresponsive malignant diseases	Phase I
Interferon alpha-2a	Colorectal cancer (with 5-fluorouracil); chronic, acute hepatitis B; non-A, non-B hepatitis; chronic myelogenous leukemia; HIV positive, ARC, AIDS (with Retrovir)	Phase II
Interleukins		
PEG IL-2	AIDS (with Retrovir)	Phase I
Aldesleukin (IL-2)	Cancer	Phase II/III
	Kaposi's sarcoma (with Retrovir)	Phase I
Human IL-1 α	Bone marrow suppression (chemo-, radiotherapy)	Phase I/II

(continued)

TABLE III
(*Continued*)

Product type	Abbreviated indication	U.S. status
Human IL-1 β	Bone marrow suppression, melanoma, immunotherapy	
	Wound healing	Phase II
Human IL-2	Cancer immunotherapy	Phase III
	Cancer immunotherapy (with Roferon-A)	In clinical trials
Human IL-3	Bone marrow failure, platelet deficiencies, autologous marrow transplant, chemotherapy adjuvant	Phase II/III
	Peripheral stem cell transplant	Phase II
Human IL-4	Immunodeficient disease, cancer therapy, vaccine adjuvant, immunization	Phase I/II
	Cancer immunomodulator	Phase II
Human IL-6	Platelet deficiencies	Phase II
Human IL-9	Thrombocytopenia	Phase I/II
Human IL-11	Thrombocytopenia	Phase II
Tumor necrosis factor		
TNF	Cancer	Phase II
Others		
Anakinra (IL-1 receptor antagonist)	AML, CML, inflammatory bowel disease, rheumatoid arthritis, sepsis, septic shock	Phase II
TNF-B	Cancer	Phase II

physicochemical structure and the mechanism of administration of recombinant proteins be developed to ensure that the required physiological activity occurred.

3. IFN-α: IMMUNOMODULATORY AND THERAPEUTIC PROPERTIES

The initial clinical studies with IFN-α were the subject of much enthusiasm when these nonrandomized studies suggested therapeutic activity against malignant melanoma, osteosarcoma, and various lymphomas (Misset *et al.*, 1982; Foon *et al.*, 1985; Golomb *et al.*, 1988; Quesada *et al.*, 1984; Bunn *et al.*, 1984; Muss, 1987; O'Connell *et al.*, 1986). However, subsequent randomized trials with IFN-α demonstrated significant therapeutic activity only against less common tumor histiotypes including hairy cell leukemia and chronic myelogenous leukemia (CML) (Misset *et al.*, 1982; Foon *et al.*, 1985), a few types of lymphoma (Golomb *et al.*, 1988), including low-grade non-Hodgkin's lymphoma (O'Connell *et al.*, 1986) and cutaneous T-cell lymphoma (Burton *et al.*, 1994). Recently, the list of responding indications has been expanded to include renal cell carcinoma (Muss, 1987; Quesada *et al.*, 1985), AIDS and Kaposi's sarcoma (Lane *et al.*, 1988; Bhalla *et al.*, 1989; Rios *et al.*, 1985;

Groopman *et al.*, 1984), and hepatitis and bladder papillomatosis (Torti *et al.*, 1988). It is now agreed that most patients with hairy cell lymphoma respond to low doses of chronically administered IFN-α. However, it is clear that despite IFN-α activity against specific leukemias and lymphomas, it has limited activity against solid tumors.

Thus, it has taken almost three decades to translate the concept of IFN-α as an antiviral to its routine utility in clinical oncology. Despite extensive clinical studies, the development of IFN-α is still in its early stages, and such basic parameters as optimal dose and therapeutic schedule remain to be determined (Golomb *et al.*, 1988; Quesada *et al.*, 1984; Moormeier *et al.*, 1988; Jones and Itri, 1986). The mechanism of activity is also controversial since IFN-α has been shown to have dose-dependent antitumor activities *in vitro*, yet be active at low doses for hairy cell leukemia (Golomb *et al.*, 1988; Quesada *et al.*, 1984; Moormeier *et al.*, 1988; Jones and Itri, 1986). Immunomodulation as the mechanism of the therapeutic activity with IFN-α is perhaps best supported by its action against hairy cell leukemia. Treatment with IFN-α is associated with a 90–95% response rate; however, this is not fully achieved until the patients have been on protocol for a year and it appears that low doses of IFN-α are as active as higher doses, i.e., $0.3–0.4 \times 10^6$ U/meter$(M)^2$ versus the MTD of $5–20 \times 10^6$ U/M^2 (Moormeier *et al.*, 1988; Jones and Itri, 1986; Teichmann *et al.*, 1988). The toxicity of IFN-α is both dose and possibly peak level dependent (Crum and Kaplan, 1991). In contrast to the clinical results, IFN-α is most active *in vitro* when added to tumor cells as a continuous low-dose exposure (Cantell and Hirvonen, 1977). Phase II clinical trials have shown that significant objective results can be achieved with IFN-α following continuous infusion of low doses of IFN-α over a 28-day period (Quesada *et al.*, 1984). In contrast, chronic administration of high doses of IFN-α does not appear to augment immune reactivity, and may reduce stem cell and NK cell activity (Teichmann *et al.*, 1988; Maluish *et al.*, 1983).

Initial dose finding studies by Quesada and colleagues determined that a dose of 12×10^6 U/M^2 of r-IFN-α was not tolerable in patients with hairy cell leukemia (Quesada *et al.*, 1984; Smalley *et al.*, 1991). Subsequently, they demonstrated that a dose of 2×10^6 U/M^2 was both well tolerated and effective when administered three times per week (Lim *et al.*, 1992). In a recent report by Smalley *et al.* (1991), highly purified natural IFN-α at a dose of 2×10^6 U/M^2 when administered for 28 days was well tolerated in most patients with hairy cell leukemia but it was suggested that this dose might be myelosuppressive in some patients as well as neurotoxic or cardiotoxic in other patients. In their studies, a lower dose of 2×10^5 U/M^2 was also administered for 28 days and it was found that this dose was better tolerated and also induced improvements in peripheral neutrophil and platelet counts as rapidly as the standard dose. In this trial, substantial clinical improvement, primarily in terms of increased platelet or neutrophil count, was observed within the first 4 to 8 weeks of treatment in patients receiving the low dose of IFN-α. This gain was obtained with an improved quality of life, and decreased cardiac and neurologic toxicity, flulike syndrome, myelosuppression, need for platelet transfusion, and incidence of bacterial infections.

They suggested that once such an improvement has been obtained at 2×10^5 U/M^2, and patients have become tolerant to the acute toxicity associated with IFN-α, the dose could then be increased to the standard 2×10^6 U/M^2 to obtain the significantly greater antileukemia effect of the higher dose. In their study, Smalley *et al.* escalated the dose following 6 months of low-dose treatment. However, they suggested that this dosage escalation could occur earlier, perhaps 3 months after induction therapy. Their results confirmed previous reports (Golomb *et al.*, 1988) which demonstrated a low-dose effect of IFN-α on platelet and neutrophil counts. It appears that significant improvement in thrombocytopenia and neutropenia can be rapidly induced in the majority of patients when low and minimally toxic doses of IFN-α are used. However, there is also a therapeutic dose–response effect, whereby higher doses of IFN-α will induce a quantitatively greater antileukemic response than that observed with low doses of IFN-α. It should be noted that the mechanism of action of IFN-α remains obscure. It may act as an antiproliferative, immunoaugmenting, or differentiation induction agent. Alternatively, it may function via multiple mechanisms; however, it is clear that it continues to have potential not only as a single agent but also in synergy with other biologics.

4. IFN-γ: IMMUNOMODULATORY AND THERAPEUTIC PROPERTIES

Preclinical studies have revealed that murine r-IFN-γ has significant therapeutic activity in animal models of experimental and spontaneous metastasis which occurs with a reproducible bell-shaped dose–response curve (Talmadge *et al.*, 1987a). Further, studies of macrophage activation in normal animals have revealed that the same bell-shaped dose–response curve occurs for the augmentation of macrophage tumoricidal activity. Studies by Black *et al.* (1993) identified the mechanism of action of r-Mu-IFN-γ in tumor-bearing animals. They treated mice with r-Mu-IFN-γ and at various times thereafter monitored levels of effector cell activity. Optimal therapeutic activity was observed with the three time per week administration (i.v.) of r-Mu-IFN-γ for the treatment of experimental and spontaneous melanoma metastasis. The dosage optimum was 30–50,000 units per animal with significantly less therapeutic activity observed at lower and higher doses. In these studies they noted a significant and inverse correlation between macrophage augmentation in the lungs of the pulmonary metastasis-bearing mice and therapeutic efficacy (Black *et al.*, 1993). The results suggested that immunological augmentation provides an indirect mechanism for the therapeutic effect of r-Mu-IFN-γ and supports the hypothesis that treatment with the MTD of 4-Mu-IFN-γ may not be optimal in an adjuvant setting.

The preclinical hypothesis of a bell-shaped dose–response curve for r-IFN-γ has been confirmed in numerous clinical studies of the immunoregulatory effects of r-IFN-γ and defined an optimal immunomodulatory dose (OID) (Maluish *et al.*, 1988; Jaffe and Herberman, 1988). In general, the OID for r-IFN-γ has been found to be between 0.1 and 0.3 mg/M^2 following i.v. or i.m. injection. In contrast, the MTD for r-IFN-γ may range from 3 to 10 mg/M^2 depending on the source of the r-IFN-γ and/or the clinical center. The identification of an OID for r-IFN-γ in patients with minimal tumor burden has resulted in the development of clinical trials to test the hypothesis that the immunological enhancement induced by r-IFN-γ will result in prolongation of the disease-free and overall survival of patients in an adjuvant setting (Jaffe and Herberman, 1988). However, it should be noted that r-IFN-γ was found on an empirical basis to have therapeutic activity in chronic granulomatous disease (CGD) (Lane *et al.*, 1988; Bhalla *et al.*, 1989) and it was for this indication that the FDA approved r-IFN-γ. Thus, despite the use of a rational developmental strategy, r-IFN-γ was initially licensed predicated on an empirical developmental strategy. The studies in CGD suggested that the mechanism of therapeutic activity for IFN-γ was associated with enhanced phagocytic oxidase activity and increased superoxide production by neutrophils. However, more recent data suggest that the majority of CGD patients obtained clinical benefit by prolonging IFN-γ therapy, and the mechanism of action may not be related to enhanced neutrophil oxidase activity but rather may be related to the correction of a respiratory burst deficiency in a subset of monocytes (Talpaz *et al.*, 1986; Woodman *et al.*, 1991).

IFN-γ has a relatively mild toxicity profile compared to other cytokines such as IL-2, tumor necrosis factor (TNF), or IL-1 (all discussed later). The MTD appears to be about 8×10^6 U/M^2, a dose at which almost all patients experience fever greater than 40°C, elevated SGOT levels greater than six times normal, and reversible hypotension. In addition, patients at this dose typically experience severe chills and confusion. The clinical toxicity suggests a dose relationship with fever normally beginning 1–2 hr after initial injection, peaking at 4–6 hr, and resolving by 24 hr. Tachyphylaxis to fever usually develops within a week's time. In addition to the fever; fatigue, myalgia, and influenzalike syndrome occur frequently and are considered to be the primary chronic toxicity for most patients. On discontinuation of IFN-γ, such side effects are reversed. In addition, cardiovascular toxicity is observed with hypotension occurring in approximately 50 to 60% of patients. Peak hypotension occurs 3–8 hr after initial dosing and often precedes the fever peak. IFN-γ also has hematopoietic toxicity with the induction of granulocytopenia and occasionally thrombocytopenia.

5. IL-2: STUDIES OF PHARMACOKINETICS, IMMUNOMODULATORY ACTIVITY, AND TOXICITY

IL-2 is a T-cell proliferative agent; however, it is also a potent NK cell augmenting agent and can activate lymphokine-activated killer (LAK) cells *in vitro* or *in vivo* following chronic (72 hr) interaction with lymphoid cells. As such, IL-2 is important to all facets of T-cell as well as NK cell augmentation and proliferation. In addition, IL-2 can augment monocyte–macrophage function. IL-2 has been approved for use as a single agent for the treatment of renal cell carcinoma although it is also administered in conjunction with LAK or T-cell infiltrating lymphocytes (TILs) in adoptive cellular therapy protocols. However, it has been questioned whether the adoptive transfer of LAK cells is necessary or adds to the clinical efficacy of r-IL-2. Indeed, there has been little indication of an improved therapeutic effect by r-IL-2 plus LAK cells versus IL-2 alone (Rosenberg *et al.*, 1993; West *et al.*, 1987; Oldham *et al.*, 1989; Gore *et al.*, 1994). When the clinical trials with IL-2 are rigorously examined, neither strategy has impressive (as opposed to significant) therapeutic activity (Rosenberg *et al.*, 1993; West *et al.*, 1987; Oldham *et al.*, 1989; Gore *et al.*, 1994). The overall response rate with r-IL-2 is 7–14% which is also associated with considerable toxicity (Lotze *et al.*, 1986). One unanticipated clinical observation (Ghosh *et al.*, 1989) posttreatment with r-IL-2 was a rapid depletion of peripheral blood lymphocytes with a subsequent rebound at 4–7 days (Ghosh *et al.*, 1989; Sosman *et al.*, 1988; Sano *et al.*, 1988; Creekmore *et al.*, 1989; Sondel *et al.*, 1988). The rebound results in a 2-fold increase in peripheral blood lymphocytes, increased numbers of r-IL-2 receptor positive (CD25) lymphocytes (4- to 15-fold increase), and an increase in NK-like (anti-K-562) and LAK-like (anti-Daudi cell) tumoricidal activity. In the initial clinical study (Ghosh *et al.*, 1989), partial responses were observed in 4 of 31 patients. Interestingly, these partial responders did not correspond to the patients with increased LAK or NK cell activity. However, the partial response could be related to an antitumor effect mediated by *in situ* LAK cells that are not represented in the peripheral population. The functional differences between LAK cells and TILs are not clear since LAK cells are present among TILs as shown in several studies using both functional and phenotypic criteria (West *et al.*, 1987; Lotze *et al.*, 1986; Ghosh *et al.*, 1989). The antitumor effect of both of these cell types could be the result of either a direct activity or secondary to the generation of other cytokine mediators acting in concert with the immune effector cells and/or on the tumor cells. The latter is suggested by the observation that r-IL-2-stimulated lymphocytes produce IFN-γ and TNF as well as other cytokines and that the therapeutic activity of r-IL-2 may be synergistic with either of these cytokines (Heslop *et al.*, 1989).

The r-IL-2-augmented activity *in vivo*, be it NK or LAK cell, is transient and dependent on recent exposure to IL-2. This is consistent with the requirement for continuous exposure to IL-2 to augment NK cells in culture (Talmadge *et al.*, 1987b). The *in vitro* augmentation of maximal NK cell cytotoxicity, by IL-2, requires receptor occupancy for 16 to 24 hr at approximately 100 U/ml (Talmadge *et al.*, 1987b). To achieve these parameters clinically, either a continuous IL-2 infusion, or multiple daily injections of high IL-2 doses by push administration are required (Moertel, 1986). Clinical trials have demonstrated that i.v. bolus injections of r-IL-2 at doses sufficient to achieve a continuous low serum level result in appreciable toxicity (Sano *et al.*, 1988). It appears that the pharmacologically appropriate route of administration is continuous infusion and that significantly less protein per M^2 is required (Crum and Kaplan, 1991; Lim *et al.*, 1992; Oldham *et al.*, 1989; Sano *et al.*, 1988; Thompson *et al.*, 1988; Herberman, 1989a,b; Stevenson *et al.*, 1990; Alper, 1988; Konrad *et al.*, 1990; Lu *et al.*, 1989; Jujjwara *et al.*, 1990; Vlasveld *et al.*, 1992; Clark *et al.*, 1990; Thompson *et al.*, 1992; Bush, 1984), although this remains somewhat controversial (Alper, 1988). The route of r-IL-2 administration is important because of its influence on the bioavailability and serum half-life of the r-IL-2. The preclinical observations of therapeutic activity at low doses by continuous infusion (Talmadge *et al.*, 1987b) suggest that r-IL-2 might be therapeutically effective using this less toxic protocol

(Oldham *et al.*, 1989; Sano *et al.*, 1988; Creekmore *et al.*, 1989; Sondel *et al.*, 1988; Thompson *et al.*, 1988; Herberman, 1989a,b; Stevenson *et al.*, 1990; Alper, 1988). Indeed, the lymphoid hyperplasia and therapeutic activity that are observed with continuous administration of r-IL-2 suggest that *ex vivo* LAK cell induction, cultivation, and infusion technology may be unnecessary (Thompson *et al.*, 1988; Konrad *et al.*, 1990; Lu *et al.*, 1989). Similar therapeutic and immunomodulatory activity have been shown preclinically with low doses of r-IL-2 when it was delivered chronically by solid phase (Crum and Kaplan, 1991) or minipellet administration (Jujjwara *et al.*, 1990).

The hypothesis that moderate doses of r-IL-2 when administered by continuous infusion will have decreased toxicity with the retention of therapeutic activity has been examined in the clinic. There are some indications that continuous infusion may be associated with lower toxicity than i.v. bolus administration and yet have comparable immunoregulatory activity *in vivo* (Lim *et al.*, 1992; Creekmore *et al.*, 1989; Lu *et al.*, 1989; Vlasveld *et al.*, 1992, 1993; Caligiuri *et al.*, 1993). The observation of decreased toxicity with a similar response rate has also been reported with continuous infusion versus i.v. bolus studies with r-IL-2 in combination with LAK cell therapy (Lim *et al.*, 1992; West *et al.*, 1987; Vlasveld *et al.*, 1992; Clark *et al.*, 1990). In a report by West *et al.* (1987), responses were found in 9 of 16 evaluable melanoma patients (West *et al.*, 1987), and it has been suggested that maintenance administration of r-IL-2 by continuous infusion for 1 week each month following two cycles of r-IL-2 and LAK therapy may prolong the response as compared to two or three cycles of r-IL-2 and LAK. Because the acute toxicity of r-IL-2 is rapidly reversed following cessation of treatment, continuous infusion provides a safer way of regulating dosage and avoiding the hypotension that usually terminates treatment when r-IL-2 is given by an intensive push schedule (q 8 hr). Indeed, using continuous infusion only 6 of the 40 patients of West *et al.* could not be managed on an ordinary ward. Toxicity is further diminished with a regular temporal interruption of infusion (Sosman *et al.*, 1988). Additional Phase I–II clinical trials with this protocol using r-IL-2 alone have reported response rates similar to r-IL-2 and LAK protocols (Sano *et al.*, 1988; Moertel, 1986; Thompson *et al.*, 1988). Several studies in the United States and in Europe have revealed that immune parameters are significantly enhanced by repetition(s) of r-IL-2 cycles beyond the first week of therapy and that bolus r-IL-2 has less immunostimulatory activity than continuous r-IL-2 administration. It appears that the toxicity by r-IL-2 is dose dependent and immunomodulation is maximal by continuous infusion compared with 2- or 8-hr infusion, or t.i.d. push injections (Woodman *et al.*, 1992). In addition, r-IL-2 induces a rebound lymphocytosis that is directly related to dose following continuous infusion. In such studies, continuous infusion of r-IL-2 initially produces leukopenia, but later results in lymphoid hyperplasia and increased LAK cell activity in the peripheral blood as determined *ex vivo*.

Many of the trials of continuous i.v. infusion of IL-2 with or without LAK cell therapy in metastatic renal cell carcinoma have used an MTD of IL-2 (i.e., $3–6 \times 10^6$ U/M^2 per day). A recent study by Fefer and colleagues (Thompson *et al.*, 1992) compared maintenance IL-2 therapy at the MTD of 6×10^6 U/M^2 per day to 2×10^6 U/M^2 per day. They found that it was possible to maintain the patients for a median of 4 days at 6×10^6 U/M^2 per day but in the presence of severe hypotension and capillary leak syndrome. In the lower dose protocol, none of the patients experienced severe hypotension or capillary leak syndrome and the median duration of maintenance IL-2 therapy was 9 days. In the lower dose protocol, there was a response rate of 41%. This was in contrast to the higher dose protocol (with a shorter duration of administration) which had a 22% response rate. These investigators suggest that it is unlikely that a dose–response relationship exists between continuous i.v. infusion of IL-2 and LAK cells and antitumor activity and that there may be an improved therapeutic activity associated with a longer maintenance protocol at lower doses which is associated with significantly less toxicity. In a number of clinical studies IL-2 has shown a very significant toxicity profile. Typically at doses of 3×10^5 U/M^2 per day the clinical toxicity profile is relatively mild and rarely requiring pharmacologic intervention. Nonetheless, even at this low dose IL-2 may have toxicities including hypotension, weight gain, and mild azotemia. Higher doses of IL-2 (3×10^6 U/M^2 per day) induce a more severe toxicity profile with flulike symptoms consisting of fevers, chills, and myalgias that increase in severity over a course of infusion resolving within 72 hr of discontinuation of administration. In most cases a combination of acetaminophen, diphenhydramine, and meperidine can alleviate the symptoms. In higher dose groups there are also severe hemodynamic effects including marked fluid retention, prerenal azotemia, and oliguria. These symptoms typically require clinical support including i.v. fluids, low-dose dopamine and albumin. In addition, anorexia, nausea, and vomiting are not unusual over the first few days of the course of therapy. A transient confusion is also observed although at a lesser frequency and does not normally require medication or psychiatric intervention. Eosinophilia is observed in most treatment groups perhaps related to the upregulation of IL-5 by L-2 administration. Combination therapy with IL-2 and LAK cells is also associated with significant cardiorespiratory effects including what is termed a *leaky capillary syndrome*. The most significant toxicities includes severe peripheral edema and ascites or plural effusions. Severe respiratory distress is also experienced and in some instances requires intubation. Cardiovascular effects include tachycardia and hypotension requiring vasopressor and i.v. fluid administration. Arrhythmias that are observed are primarily supraventricular and, in a limited percentage of patients, angina or an ischemic change is noted. In addition, myocardial infarctions have been observed at an incidence of approximately 1%.

6. TNF AND IL-1: EXAMPLES OF PRECLINICAL PROMISE AND CLINICAL TOXICITY

6.1. TNF-α

The ability of TNF to induce hemorrhagic necrosis of intradermal tumors in experimental animals has not translated into clinical efficacy. Indeed, not only does TNF appear to have minimal systemic antitumor activity, but it is also very toxic, having potent effects on the vascular endothelium resulting in localized coagulation and thrombosis, hypotension and shock (Schiller *et al.*, 1991). At its MTD, TNF-associated toxicities include hypotension, transient elevation of transaminase levels, neurological dysfunction, and thrombocytopenia. Serum concentrations of TNF attained in patients (peak levels 137 ng/ml after a 5 mg/M^2 short infusion, <0.2 ng/ml after 80 μg/m^2 per day by i.v. continuous infusion) seem to be substantially less than the levels that are required for antitumor activity *in vitro* or in animal models (Rudolph *et al.*, 1989). TNF also has effects on tumor cells, tumor vasculature, and the host immune response. *In vitro*, TNF has demonstrated direct cytotoxic or cytostatic effects on a variety of cell lines (Sugarman *et al.*, 1985; Salmon *et al.*, 1987) and antitumor activity has been observed against both murine tumors and human tumor xenografts *in vivo* (Asher *et al.*, 1987; Balkwill *et al.*, 1986). The mechanisms responsible for TNF's activity *in vivo* are not completely understood, although TNF has been shown to induce rapid hemorrhagic necrosis in subcutaneously implanted tumors, presumably caused by direct or indirect effects on the tumor vasculature. Large tumors at visceral sites can also be responsive to TNF treatment, although the role of hemorrhagic necrosis in these tumors is not clear. Development of tumor hemorrhagic necrosis has been observed in both immunogenic and nonimmunogenic tumors implanted in wild-type or nude mice. However, sustained reduction of tumor size and cures are usually noted only in hosts with intact immune systems bearing immunogenic tumors.

Clinical experience with TNF in combination with chemotherapy has been primarily limited to etoposide and dactinomycin (Orr *et al.*, 1989; Sherman *et al.*, 1992). Preliminary clinical experience indicates that TNF enhances etoposide-induced myelosuppression; however, efficacy and pharmacokinetic data have not been reported. A recent study administered TNF at high doses (2 to 4 mg) by isolated limb perfusion in combination with IFN-γ, melphalan (38 to 120 mg), and hyperthermia (Lienard *et al.*, 1992). All patients had recurrent extremity melanoma or sarcoma and 21 of 23 (89%) achieved a complete response lasting 3 to 29 months, with 12 responses ongoing from 5+ to 23+ months. The contribution of each of the components to the efficacy of therapy is unknown; however, the data suggest that potent antitumor activity can be observed with high doses of TNF in combination with chemotherapy. Agents that reduce the systemic toxicity (hypotension) of TNF are in development. If the toxic and beneficial biological effects of TNF can be separated, future trials of high-dose TNF administered systemically with chemotherapy may be possible. At present, there are few clinical studies attempting to exploit the biological effects of TNF. The future use of TNF-α will likely be limited to low-dose schedules involving the coadministration of other cytokines such as IL-2.

6.2. IL-1

Two distinct IL-1 genes, and their corresponding proteins, α and β (approximately 25% homology), have been identified. However, both IL-1 species act through the same receptors and appear to have similar biological properties (Dinarello, 1991).

The immunoregulatory activities of IL-1 include effects on B, T, and NK cells and the induction of many inflammatory and hematopoietic responses, including neutrophilia. The extent to which these effects are directly mediated is unclear, as IL-1 is able to induce many other cytokines, including TNF, IL-2, -4, and -6. Although IL-1 has direct antiproliferative effects against a number of cultured human tumor cell lines, including melanoma (Hirose *et al.*, 1993), and ovarian (Kilian *et al.*, 1991) cell lines, direct tumor cell inhibition is the exception rather than the rule (Hanauske *et al.*, 1992). A number of murine tumors have been found to regress *in vivo* in response to IL-1 (North *et al.*, 1988; Neville *et al.*, 1990) but this probably occurs indirectly through the induction of other cytokine effectors. At high doses, IL-1 is able to induce hemorrhagic necrosis of some murine tumors in a TNF-independent manner (Johnson *et al.*, 1992). The relevance of this observation to the treatment of human cancer is uncertain as such high doses would not be tolerated. Synergy has been shown to occur between IL-1 and various cytotoxic drugs in murine tumor models (Braunschweiger *et al.*, 1991), but a similar synergy between IL-1 and cytotoxic drugs has not yet been shown to be applicable to human cancer. In addition to its effects on tumors, IL-1 is able to protect mice against the lethal effects of radiation injury and some cytotoxic drugs (Neta *et al.*, 1992; Castelli *et al.*, 1988; Damia *et al.*, 1992a). The mechanisms are complex and apparently include protection of the stem cell compartment from lethal injury.

Phase I trials of both IL-1α (Dainippon Pharmaceutical Co.) (Smith *et al.*, 1992) and IL-1β (Immunex) (Crown *et al.*, 1993) in patients with advanced cancer have been reported. In both studies, r-Hu-IL-1 was administered by short i.v. infusion, once daily, for either 7 (IL-1α) or 2 (IL-1β) consecutive days. The MTDs were 0.3 μg/kg for IL-1α and 0.1 μg/kg for IL-1β. The dose-limiting toxicities were similar to those reported for TNF-α and IL-2, i.e., prominent hypotension and evidence of vascular leak syndrome with fevers, chills, emesis, and malaise. IL-1 and TNF induce the synthesis of nitric oxide, a potent physiological vasodilator, by direct action on vascular smooth muscle (Busse and Mulsch, 1990; Kilbourn *et al.*, 1992). This mechanism may represent a common pathway for the hypotension associated with both exogenous and endogenous cytokines. The hypotensive effects of IL-1 in anesthetized dogs have been reported to be rapidly reversed by the administration of nitric oxide synthesis inhibitors, which has obvious therapeutic implications.

The principal hematological effects of IL-1 are a rise in neutrophil counts and a late rise in platelet counts (Smith *et al.*, 1992, 1993; Crown *et al.*, 1993; Dennis *et al.*, 1992; Vadhan-Raj *et al.*, 1994; Nemunaitis *et al.*, 1994). Several studies suggest that IL-1 may ameliorate chemotherapy-induced myelosuppression, particularly thrombocytopenia (Crown *et al.*, 1993; Smith *et al.*, 1993; Vadhan-Raj *et al.*, 1994; Nemunaitis *et al.*, 1994). However, in a small study, no beneficial effects were noted on hematological indices in four patients with refractory aplastic anemia (Walsh *et al.*, 1992). In another limited study in patients with advanced urological malignancies, IL-2-induced *in vitro* LAK cell generation was enhanced following daily s.c. injection of IL-1β suggesting a possible role for combination therapy with these agents (Marumo *et al.*, 1992). The infusion of IL-1α has also been shown to have multiple effects on monocytes in clinical trials. r-Hu-IL-1α therapy has been shown to enhance monocyte functions in ovarian cancer patients when they received the IL-1 prior to chemotherapy. After 4 days of continuous infusion there was a significant increase in the number and function of monocytes. Overall, there was a 6-fold increase in the number of monocytes compared to preinfusion levels. These monocytes also had a significantly increased ability to produce superoxide ion in response to stimulation. They also had an increased ability to secrete IL-1α and IL-1β but not TNF-α (Lee *et al.*, 1993). In other studies using 30-min infusions of r-Hu-IL-1β in metastatic melanoma patients for 5 consecutive days, an upregulation of circulating IL-1 receptor antagonist and soluble TNF binding proteins has been observed. There was an 86-fold increase in IL-1Ra, a 78-fold increase for TNF-R-55-bp, and a 2- to 3-fold increase in TNF-R-75-bp seen at 2–4, 1, and 4 hr, respectively, after the 30-min IL-1β infusion (Bargetzi *et al.*, 1993).

In other studies, r-Hu-IL-1β was administered to patients undergoing autologous BMT for acute myelogenous leukemia. In this study, r-Hu-IL-1β was administered at 0.01, 0.02, or 0.05 μg/kg by 30-min i.v. infusion once a day beginning on the day of cell infusion and continuing for 5 days thereafter. Dose escalation was discontinued at the 0.05 μg/kg dose level and all patients experienced fever and chills within 30 min after initiation of IL-1β administration. In addition, hypertension was observed in the majority of patients 5–8 hr following infusion. In these studies, the number of days required to achieve an ANC $> 500/\text{mm}^3$ was significantly improved (25 versus 34, p=0.02) compared to patients not receiving cytokines. This correlated with the reduced incidence of infection between day 0 and 28 following BM infusion (12 versus 23%, p=0.049). In addition, there was a significant increase in the survival of patients who received r-Hu-IL-1β compared to historical patients (30 versus 20%, p=0.04). However, there was a significant toxicity associated with the administration of r-Hu-IL-1β which appeared to be higher than that associated with the administration of GM- or G-CSF although this remains to be demonstrated in a randomized trial (Nemunaitis *et al.*, 1994).

7. BIOLOGY AND PHARMACOLOGY OF IL-4

Native IL-4 has properties that exemplify many of the characteristics of immune recognition-induced lymphokines (Dean *et al.*, 1992). It is produced principally, although not exclusively, by activated ($CD4^+$) T lymphocytes (Ben-Sasson *et al.*, 1990) and exerts much of its pharmacological action locally between target cells and IL-4-producing cells. As with most molecules whose biologic functions were initially detected by *in vitro* assays, a question still remains as to the major physiological action of IL-4, although it is now recognized that it has a wide range of biological functions (Paul, 1988). It is clear that IL-4 does express at least one critical *in vivo* function and in the mouse it is principally responsible for the production of IgE in response to a variety of stimuli that elicit Ig class switching (Finkelman *et al.*, 1990). *In vitro* analysis has indicated functions of IL-4 on B cells, T cells, macrophages, hematopoietic precursors, and stromal cells, although the biological relevance of some of these findings *in vivo* has not yet been determined. IL-4 was described initially because of its ability to enhance DNA synthesis by resting B lymphocytes stimulated with anti-IgM antibodies and was thus designated B-cell growth factor (BCGF). This was superseded by the name IL-4, which was proposed at the time of the derivation of cDNA clones and because of the recognition of its action on non-B-cell targets. It also enhances hematopoiesis and is synergistic with G-CSF and EPO via the release of other CSFs. IL-4 also induces differentiation of BM pre-B cells, stimulates the clonal proliferation of resting B cells increases immunoglobulin production *in vitro*, and regulates the expression of the CD23 receptor.

It is known that resting human T cells do not respond directly to the addition of r-Hu-IL-4, but do so if they have been previously activated with mitogen (PHA or Con A) or selective stimuli (anti-CD3 or PMA) (Mitchell *et al.*, 1989). IL-4 also enhances antigen-specific T-cell-mediated cytotoxicity (Finkelman *et al.*, 1990) and may augment the growth of TILs in the presence of IL-2 (Kawakami *et al.*, 1988). However, it does inhibit antigen-unrestricted LAK-cell production. Because of its potential to enhance several functions of the immune system thought to be relevant for preventing neoplasia, it is being tested for the treatment of refractory cancer.

The cells of the immune system communicate, at least in part, via a network of interacting cytokines. In the mouse, and in humans, T-helper (TH) cells have been divided into two major subsets (TH-1 and TH-2) based on distinct cytokine secretion patterns (Mosmann *et al.*, 1986). TH-1 cells produce IL-2, IFN-γ, and lymphotoxin whereas TH-2 cells predominately secrete IL-4, -5, -10, and -13 (Mosmann *et al.*, 1986; Mosmann and Moore, 1991). Because in most instances, immunization with a strong immunogen activates not only TH-1 but also Th-2 cells, the question has arisen as to whether these cells may be reciprocally regulated by their respective cytokines. IL-10, which is produced by TH-2 cells and which was originally known as cytokine synthesis inhibitory factor, has been shown to inhibit the synthesis of most cytokines produced by TH-1 cells (Florentin *et al.*, 1989). Similarly, IL-4, which is also a TH-2 product, can negatively regulate delayed-type hypersensitivity (DTH) and inhibit other models of contact hypersensitivity (Subhash *et al.*, 1992). IL-4 can also partially block the efferent phase of hapten-specific contact sensitization, but has no effect on the afferent phase of the response. It also appears that IL-4 inhibits the expression of TNF-β and IP-10 messenger RNA in macrophages treated with culture supernatants from immune lymph node cells. Thus, IL-4 exhibits antiinflammatory activity which may act by inhibiting cytokine secretion by mononuclear cells. Similarly, IL-4 has been shown to inhibit IL-1α-induced GM-CSF expression in murine B-lymphocyte cell lines via the downregulation of RNA (Akahane and Pluznik, 1992). In other studies (Nishioka *et al.*, 1991), it has been shown that IL-4 could downregulate not only cytokine production but also the activation of human alveolar macrophages to the tumoricidal state.

Recent studies have also shown that IL-4 can upregulate the immune response to a tumor vaccine. In studies from several laboratories (Golumbek *et al.*, 1991; Tepper *et al.*, 1989), it has been demonstrated that genetically engineered renal carcinoma cells which secrete IL-4 have a significant increase in adjuvancy and subsequent protection against tumor challenge. Studies by Tepper *et al.* (1989) suggested that IL-4 exhibits antitumor activity *in vivo*. They demonstrated that tumor cells transfected with cDNA for IL-4 were less tumorigenic than the parental line and that this inhibitory effect could be blocked by the coadministration of an antibody to IL-1. In preliminary studies, r-Hu-IL-4 has been shown to have a direct antiproliferative effect on tumor cells, including specimens from most B-cell chronic lymphocytic leukemia (CLL) and 50% of the specimens from adult T-cell leukemia. Likewise, r-Hu-IL-4 can inhibit the proliferation of melanoma and lymphoma tumor specimens.

The immunoregulatory properties of IL-4 on cytotoxic cells are highly variable and dependent on their phenotype and state of activation (Atkins *et al.*, 1992). IL-4 inhibits the induction of cytotoxic T cells from resting cells if added before alloantigen, antagonizes the ability of IL-2 to induce NK cells to develop LAK activity (Horohov *et al.*, 1988; Kawakami *et al.*, 1989; Spits *et al.*, 1988), and inhibits the antiproliferative effects of monocytes on melanoma cells *in vitro* (Te Velde *et al.*, 1988). On the other hand, IL-4 accounts for most of the non-IL-2 cytotoxicity inducing factor activity present in T-cell culture supernatant (Garman and Fan, 1983), acts with IL-2 to augment the proliferation and cytolytic activity of alloantigen-specific cytotoxic T lymphocytes or TILs derived from melanoma (Kawakami *et al.*, 1988; Widmer *et al.*, 1987), and has therapeutic activity perhaps related to the stimulation of antigen-specific cytotoxic T lymphocytes which may contribute to tumor regression *in vivo*. In addition to its effects on cytolytic cells, IL-4 has been shown to strongly inhibit the induction of both IL-1 and TNF synthesis by a variety of stimuli (Essner *et al.*, 1989; Te Velde *et al.*, 1990; Kotik and Mier, 1992). Because these two pyrogenic cytokines are felt to be responsible for many of the side effects observed with high-dose cytokine therapy, there is the potential that IL-4 may activate cytotoxic cells without inducing the release of these "negative" cytokines.

Recombinant human IL-4 is available in both a glycosylated (Sterling, U.K.) and a nonglycosylated (Schering-Plough, Bury St. Edmonds, U.K.) form. Phase I trials of both i.v. and s.c. administration have been reported (Atkins *et al.*, 1992; Gilleece *et al.*, 1992; Freimann *et al.*, 1991; Davis *et al.*, 1991). The major adverse effects reported are fatigue, headache, emesis, diarrhea, and nasal congestion. Gastrointestinal ulceration, predominantly of the gastric antrum, was reported in 9 of 44 patients in one series, most of whom were treated daily with 30 or 60 μg/kg i.v. IL-4 (Davis *et al.*, 1991). Hypotension, fever, and edema (with features of the capillary leak syndrome), although recorded, were not prominent in these studies. It is interesting to note that circulating levels of TNF-α and IL-1β did not increase in patients treated with IL-4 (in contrast to those receiving IL-2), whereas C reactive protein concentrations in serum increased slightly and IL-1Ra levels in plasma increased markedly. Patients receiving once daily s.c. nonglycosylated IL-4 (Gilleece *et al.*, 1992) show a spectrum of toxicities similar to those receiving the higher-dose i.v. therapy although, in this study, nasal stuffiness was not reported. Phenotypic analysis of the PBL from these studies demonstrated a decrease in the frequency of circulating CD16- and CD14-positive cells. In the initial Phase I trials, no significant tumor responses were observed although one might not expect this to occur in a preliminary study. It appears, based on these preliminary results, that 15 μg/kg of IL-4 is the MTD using this protocol of administration. Several of the Phase I studies indicate encouraging signs of clinical activity, but only one convincing response (in a case of Hodgkin's disease) has been reported (Davis *et al.*, 1991). Phase II studies are in progress with IL-4 being administered both alone and in combination with IL-2.

8. IL-6: A PLEOTROPIC CYTOKINE

IL-6 is best known for its ability to stimulate the production of acute-phase reaction proteins. It is also able to promote the growth of B and T cells, to act as a differentiation factor for cytotoxic lymphocytes, and to enhance NK cell, LAK cell, and TIL activity (Kishimoto *et al.*, 1992). Its actions overlap with those of IL-1 and TNF-α, both of which are stimulators of IL-6 production *in vivo*. IL-6 has been reported to induce regression of small tumors from a weakly immunogenic murine transplantable tumor, but is ineffective against more advanced tumors and in nonimmunogenic tumor models (Mule *et al.*, 1992). IL-6 also demonstrates significant synergy with other antitumor cytokines and chemotherapy agents in mediating regression of established tumors in mice (Mule *et al.*, 1990, 1992). Experiments using tumor cells transduced with the IL-6 gene have demonstrated that local, high levels of IL-6 can augment tumor immunity and induce complete protection against a challenge with a lethal number of tumor cells (Porgador *et al.*, 1992; Mullen *et al.*, 1992). When IL-6 was complexed with a collagen matrix to result in a slow release or was mixed with tumor cells and inoculated subcutaneously in mice, tumors were generated whose TILs were more therapeutic than similar lymphocytes derived from untreated tumors (Marcus *et al.*, 1994). IL-6 has also shown an antiproliferative effect on tumor cells *in vitro*, and to decrease the growth of carcinoma lines passaged in nude mice (Chen *et al.*, 1988; Mayer *et al.*, 1992). Radiation-induced leukemia in mice is also inhibited by IL-6 treatment and a conversion of leukemic bone marrow cells to more differentiated precursors has been reported (Miyaura *et al.*, 1988; Chiu and Lee, 1989; Givon *et al.*, 1992).

A Phase I trial of daily s.c. IL-6 for 7 days has been reported in which all of the patients developed fever, chills, and fatigue. A number of immunological effects, including rises in C-reactive protein levels and platelet count and increased expression of the IL-2 receptor on lymphocytes, were observed at a daily dose of 10 μg/kg. At a dose of 30 μg/kg, hepatotoxicity and cardiac dysrhythmias were also observed (Weber *et al.*, 1993). In contrast, little toxicity has been observed in mice, even with extremely high doses (Mule *et al.*, 1990). In a Phase I clinical trial of r-Hu-IL-6, 20 patients with advanced cancer received daily s.c. injections of r-Hu-IL-6 over 7 days followed by a 2-week observation period and another 4 weeks of daily 4-Hu-IL-6 injections (Scheid *et al.*, 1994). Doses varied between 0.5 and 20 μg/kg and immune functions were monitored throughout. At all dose levels, IL-6 administration led to a marked increase in serum levels of C-reactive protein and an increase in complement factor C3. The proportions of $CD4^+$, $CD8^+$, or $HLA\text{-}Dr^+$ lymphocytes in peripheral blood did not alter with r-Hu-IL-6 administration nor did the *in vitro* proliferation of peripheral blood mononuclear cells supported by T-cell mitogens. However, NK and LAK cell activity and proliferation induced by *in vitro* culture with IL-2 were suppressed at doses of IL-6 exceeding 2.5 μg/kg. Serum IgE levels were consistently elevated over the r-Hu-IL-6 dose range but IgM, IgG, and IgA levels were unaffected. In summary, there appears to be a dose-dependent induction of acute-phase proteins by *in vivo* r-Hu-IL-6 treatment. At higher r-Hu-IL-6 doses there is a suppressive effect on NK and LAK activity as measured *in vitro*. r-Hu-IL-6 may thus be useful in combination with cytokine therapies that seek to suppress LAK and increase cytotoxic T-lymphocyte responses. Regardless, it should be noted that in some hematological malignancies (particularly myeloma) and Kaposi's sarcoma, IL-6 has been implicated as a growth factor for malignancy proliferation.

IL-6 is also produced by a variety of cells after inflammatory stimulation, such as occurs with infection, trauma, or immunological challenge. IL-6 has a protective role in the lipopolysaccharide (LPS)-galactosamine septic shock model in mice (Barton and Jackson, 1993). It also suppresses the acute neutrophil exudation caused by an intratracheal instillation of endotoxin in rats (Ulich *et al.*, 1991). TNF-α levels measured in the bronchoalveolar fluid of these animals were also significantly reduced. Earlier studies showed that IL-6 inhibits LPS-induced TNF-α and IL-1β production in cultured human monocytes, U937 cells, and in mice *in vivo* (Schnidler *et al.*, 1990; Aderka *et al.*, 1989). Together, these data suggest that IL-6 also possesses antiinflammatory properties.

Naturally occurring TNF antagonists have been identified in the urine of patients with febrile conditions (Seckinger *et al.*, 1988; Engelmann *et al.*, 1989). These inhibitors were subsequently shown to represent the extracellular part of the two known TNF receptors (p55 and p75) and have therefore been designated soluble TNF receptors p55 and p75 (TNFsRp55 and TNFsRp75) (Schall *et al.*, 1990; Lotscher *et al.*, 1990; Kohno *et al.*, 1990; Nophar *et al.*, 1990). Soluble forms of both TNF receptors block LPS-mediated lethality in animal models, particularly when administered as IgG fusion proteins (Ashkenazi *et al.*, 1991; Mohler *et al.*, 1991). In a Phase I clinical trial (Tilg *et al.*, 1994b), the effect of IL-6 on the induction of IL-1 and TNF antagonist was studied. Serial plasma samples were obtained from cancer patients participating in clinical trials of r-IL-6 administered as a 120-hr continuous i.v. infusion. Plasma IL-1Ra and TNFsRp75 levels were measured by radioimmunoassays (RIAs). RIA levels increased rapidly peaking within 2–4 hr of IL-6 infusion. Thereafter, levels declined reaching baseline within 1 day despite continuous infusion of IL-6. TNFsRp55 plasma levels increased to detectable levels within 48 hr after the initiation of infusion and progressively increased throughout the remaining infusion. IL-1β and TNF-α plasma levels, however, did not increase to detectable levels. This study suggests that the infusion of IL-6 has antiinflammatory properties which may be due in part to the induction of IL-1Ra synthesis and the release of soluble TNF receptors. In addition, it was suggested that tissue macrophages may provide an important source of IL-6-induced IL-1Ra.

9. IL-1 RECEPTOR ANTAGONIST

IL-1 receptor antagonist (IL-1Ra) is a member of the IL-1 family that antagonizes the effects of both IL-1α and IL-1β by blocking the binding of IL-1 to cell surface receptors (Dinarello and Thompson, 1991; Arend, 1991). IL-1Ra has protective effects against several IL-1-mediated pathological processes in preclinical models, including septic shock and inflammatory bowel disease (Dinarello and Thompson, 1991; Arend, 1991). Several cytokines have been demonstrated to induce IL-1Ra synthesis, including IL-1, IL-2, IL-4, IL-6, IFN-α, IFN-γ, GM-CSF, and transforming growth factor-β (TGF-β) (Vannier *et al.*, 1992; Atkins *et al.*, 1992; Tilg *et al.*, 1993, 1994a; Poutsiaka *et al.*, 1991; Turner *et al.*, 1991). Two structural variants of IL-1 receptor antagonists exist: S-IL-1Ra, a secretory molecule produced by monocytes, macrophages, neutrophils, fibroblasts, and other cells; and IC-IL-1Ra, an intracellular molecule produced by keratinocytes and other epithelial cells, macrophages, and fibroblasts. IL-1Ra production by monocytes, macrophages, and neutrophils may be regulated differently than IL-1β. Human IL-1Ra binds to both human IL-1R1 and IL-2R2 on cell surfaces, although with a 100-fold greater avidity to IL-1R1. IL-1Ra may bind preferentially to soluble IL-1R1 and not at all to soluble IL-1R2's. Il-1Ra competitively inhibits the binding of both IL-1α and IL-1β to cell surface receptors without inducing any intracellular responses. All three forms of IL-1 may bind to IL-1 receptors, although IL-1Ra may lack the secondary interactions necessary to trigger signal transduction. Hundredfold or greater excess of IL-1Ra over IL-1 appears to be necessary to inhibit biological responses to IL-1 both *in vitro* and *in vivo*. The roles of S-IL-1Ra and IC-IL-1Ra in normal physiologic defense mechanisms remain unclear. IL-1Ra has activity in animal models of inflammation and preliminary results of clinical trials in humans indicate its possible efficacy in septic shock, rheumatoid arthritis, and GVHD. However, the preliminary suggestion of efficacy by IL-1Ra in septic shock required a retrospective analysis of patient subset data. Subsequent appropriately randomized trials have suggested that in the specific subset of patients, those with more extensive shock symptoms did not confirm the earlier suggestion of efficacy (Arend, 1993) and further clinical development of IL-1Ra has been halted as a therapy for shock (Editorial, 1994).

10. CYTOKINES WITH SIGNIFICANT POTENTIAL FOR CLINICAL EFFICACY: IL-7 AND IL-12

IL-7 and IL-12 act as T-cell growth factors and are available as recombinant proteins. To date neither has reached clinical trials, but preclinical tests indicate a potential role for IL-7 in immunotherapy while IL-12 has promising potential to induce *in vitro* cytotoxicity against tumor cells as well as *in vivo* therapeutic efficacy. IL-7 is a 25-kDa glycoprotein, which was originally isolated from bone marrow and thymic stromal cells. It acts as a growth factor for immature B and T cells and for mature T cells, both *in vitro* (Londei *et al.*, 1990) and *in vivo* (Samaridis *et al.*, 1991). IL-7 induces LAK activity in PBMC (Naume and Espevik, 1991) and generates tumor-specific CTLs from both murine tumor-draining lymph node lymphocytes (Lynch *et al.*, 1991) and human TIL (Ditonno *et al.*, 1992; Lynch and Miller, 1994). IL-7 also synergizes with IL-2 for human lymphocyte proliferation. In addition, murine IL-7-generated antitumor CTLs are effective in adoptive immunotherapy protocols (Jicha *et al.*, 1991). Studies on the effects of IL-7 *in vivo* have also been initiated. One report on IL-7 transgenic mice demonstrated increased numbers of pre-B cells, mature B cells, thymocytes, and T cells (Samaridis *et al.*, 1991) while another report demonstrated cutaneous lymphoproliferation and lymphomas (Rich *et al.*, 1993). The administration of recombinant murine IL-7 to normal mice results in a reversible increase in B-lineage and T-cell numbers and accelerates lymphocyte repopulation in cyclophosphamide-induced lymphopenic mice (Morrissey *et al.*, 1991a). The treatment of normal mice with r-Hu-IL-7 results in a three- to five-fold increase in PBLs (Damia *et al.*, 1992b), a 90% decrease in myeloid progenitors in the bone marrow, and a fivefold increase in progenitors in the spleen as a result of exportation from the bone marrow to the spleen (Grzegorzewski *et al.*, 1994). More recently, it has been shown that adoptively transferred, IL-7-generated CTLs can specifically reduce the number of early syngeneic pulmonary metastases (Jicha *et al.*, 1991) or subsequently injected highly immunogenic fibrosarcomas (Lynch *et al.*, 1991) in mice. Further, primary mouse plasmacytomas or murine glioma cells that had been transfected with the mouse IL-7 gene are rejected by a $CD4^+$ or $CD8^+$ T-lymphocyte-dependent mechanism, respectively (Hock *et al.*, 1991; Aoki *et al.*, 1992). *In vivo*, IL-7 also has demonstrated antiviral effects in the Friend virus leukemia model (Lu *et al.*, 1992). The administration of r-Hu-IL-7 to normal mice caused a pronounced leukocytosis (three- to fivefold increase over background) in the spleen and lymph nodes, with B-lineage and T cells, NK cells, and macrophages all being increased. $CD8^+$ T cells increased disproportionately, such that the CD4:CD8 cell ratio decreased dramatically (Koschlies *et al.*, 1994). The IL-7-induced effects were dose-dependent, increased with the duration of treatment, and were reversible after cessation of r-Hu-IL-7 administration. The increase in the number of cells after IL-7 treatment was primarily a result of the expansion of the peripheral T-cell population. Importantly, splenocytes from IL-7-treated mice have enhanced proliferative responses to various T-cell stimuli *in vitro* and are able to potentiate an allogeneic CTL response *in vivo*. The IL-7-induced changes in T-cell number and the CD4:CD8 ratio were also observed in mice bearing early Renca (renal adenocarcinoma) pulmonary metastases, and these changes coincided with up to a 75% reduction in pulmonary metastases.

IL-12, initially termed natural killer cell stimulatory factor (NKSF) and cytotoxic lymphocyte maturation factor (CLMF) (Kobayashi *et al.*, 1989; Stern *et al.*, 1990), was cloned on the basis of two distinct activities: induction of IFN-γ from T and NK cells, and enhancement of T-cell activity (Wolf *et al.*, 1991; Gubler *et al.*, 1991). IL-12 is a structurally unique cytokine composed of two unrelated glycoproteins of approximately 40 kDa (p40) and 35 kDa (p35). The two are covalently linked by a single disulfide bond to form an active heterodimeric molecule of approximately 70 kDa. The *in vitro* biological activities of IL-12 include activities on both mature T and NK cells, and the promotion of TH-1 cell differentiation. In addition to its activity on immune development, IL-12 has been found to synergize with stem cell factor and IL-3 to promote the development of multilineage hematopoietic colony formation *in vitro* from BM progenitor cells (Hirayama *et al.*, 1994; Jacobsen *et al.*, 1993), suggesting that it may play a role in hematopoiesis.

Differential activity of IL-12 on helper T cells extends to the TH-1 T-cell subset. This subset of T cells was first recognized in mice (Mosmann *et al.*, 1986) but has recently been observed in humans as well (Del Prete *et al.*, 1991). IL-12 has also been shown to suppress TH-2 development. T-cell lines and clones derived from cultures of PBMC from atopic donors stimulated by allergen and IL-12 exhibited TH-1-like phenotype. In contrast, purified protein derivative (PPD)-specific T-cell lines and clones, which are typically of the TH-1 phenotype, were shifted by culture with neutralizing α-IL-12 antiserum to a TH-0 or TH-2 phenotype (Manetti *et al.*, 1993). A direct effect of IL-12 on TH-1 differentiation was also demonstrated in a murine model. TH-1 differentiation *in vitro* of native T cells from transgenic mice with an ovalbumin-specific T-cell receptor was shown to be dependent on IL-12 (Hsieh *et al.*, 1993). In addition to a developmental role in differentiation toward the TH-1 phenotype, IL-12 was shown to promote the growth of T cells of TH-1, but not of TH-2, phenotype (Germann *et al.*, 1993). Together, these studies suggest that IL-12 is central in the differentiation of the TH-1 and TH-2 subsets.

In studies examining the response of mice immunized with a hapten–protein conjugate (TNP-KLH) under conditions that normally promote a Th-2 response, McKnight *et al.* (1994) observed that IL-12 administration resulted in an inhibition of IL-4, and an enhancement of IFN-γ production from splenocytes stimulated *ex vivo* with antigen. Depletion of NK cells by pretreatment of mice with an anti-asialo GM1 antibody inhibited IFN-γ production but did not abrogate the effect of IL-12. The effects of IL-12 were not inhibited by anti-IFN-γ antibody. Conversely, anti-IL-12 treatment reduced serum IgG2 levels in TNP-KLH-vaccinated mice, and IFN-γ production by antigen-stimulated spleen cells was also reduced. In total, these results suggest that IL-12 can also promote TH-1 development *in vivo*. Compelling evidence for a key role of IL-12 in promoting TH-1 development *in vivo* is provided by the murine model of leishmaniasis. Treatment of susceptible mice with recombinant murine IL-12 during the first week of infection prevents the development of progressive, fatal disease and decreases parasite burden (Sypek *et al.*, 1993; Heinzel *et al.*, 1993). Cure of the parasitic infection is associated with a depression in IL-4 levels and a preservation of IFN-γ production *ex vivo* in the T lymphocytes isolated from draining lymph nodes of infected lesions. These findings are indicative of a protective TH-1 response. Anti-IFN-γ treatment abrogated the protective effect of IL-12 therapy, indicating that this cytokine is necessary for the antiparasitic effects of IL-12 therapy (Sypek *et al.*, 1993; Heinzel *et al.*, 1993). Thus, a component of the antiparasitic efficacy induced by IL-12 may be the induction of IFN-γ.

Significant antitumor and antimetastic activity has also been demonstrated in studies of murine IL-12 directed against a number of tumors in mice (Brunda *et al.*, 1993). IL-12 treatment markedly reduced experimental metastases or subcutaneous growth of a metastatic melanoma (B16F10), a reticulum cell sarcoma (M5076), and a renal cell adenocarcinoma (Renca) and resulted in a significant increase in survival (Brunda, 1994). Suppression of tumor growth in all models and regression in the Renca model could be achieved even when treatment was initiated as late as 14 days following injection of tumor cells. The mechanism of action of IL-12 in these models remains to be established. However, experiments have suggested the importance of a T-cell response and IFN-γ in the suppressive activity. IL-12 was effective in NK-deficient beige mice and anti-asialo GM1-depleted mice, indicating that NK cells are not the primary effector cells mediating the antitumor activity (Brunda *et al.*, 1993). However, the therapeutic efficacy of IL-12 was reduced in nude mice and in mice depleted of $CD8^+$ cells. Depletion of $CD4^+$ cells did not diminish suppression of tumor growth by IL-12 (Brunda *et al.*, 1993). In addition, neutralizing monoclonal antibodies to IFN-γ, but not those to TNF-α, abrogated the antitumor effects of IL-12 (Brunda *et al.*, 1993).

Although IL-12 was cloned on the basis of its ability to induce IFN-γ production and CTL maturation, our understanding of its biological functions has contributed to the understanding of immune development. Nevertheless, many questions remain, such as the regulation of IL-12 expression and the association of IL-12 expression with disease states. As a necessary cytokine in promoting TH-1 differentiation and in inducing IFN-γ to support the development of these cells, appropriately administered IL-12 is likely to be an effective vaccine adjuvant and/or therapeutic agent for developing a cellular immune response to pathogens. IL-12 also has the potential to ameliorate or prevent the development of allergic responses. The sustained and antigen-specific IFN-γ production may be key to the antitumor and antimicrobial activity of IL-12. IFN-γ induced by IL-12 has been found to be critical for the suppression of tumor growth and shown to be critical in IL-12-induced protection against leishmaniasis. The understanding and potential control of the immune response offered by the discovery and development of IL-12 suggest that it may have a role in manipulating the immune response for clinical benefit in diseases of humans (Wolf *et al.*, 1994; Brunda, 1994).

11. COMBINATION CHEMOTHERAPY AND IMMUNOTHERAPY

Because the cytokines and growth factors have unique mechanisms of action, they are ideal candidates for combination with chemotherapeutic agents. However, knowledge and consideration of the potential interactions between these two classes of drugs are necessary to design optimal treatment regimens for clinical use. How does one decide which combination of agents and what dose and schedule should be tested in the clinical trials? Clinical development relies heavily on preclinical animal model data. However, because of the sense of urgency to the development of cytokines, the necessary preclinical data are often not obtained prior to clinical entry of many of these therapeutic combinations. Similarly, in many instances the preclinical models used to profile the combination strategies have been predicated on the identification of a model to demonstrate activity rather than using a rigorous model to determine if there is therapeutic activity. In this review we have chosen to discuss the use of HDT and stem cell rescue as the ultimate in cytoreductive therapy and posttransplant immunotherapy. As shown later in this review, the latter provides one of the few statistically supported demonstrations of therapeutic efficacy related to T-cell augmentation [comparison of allogeneic (AoBMT) to autologous transplantation (AuBMT)]. Thus, strategies to upregulate T-cell function after autologous stem cell transplantation provide one of the major focuses for cytokine and interleukin therapy posttransplantation. The development of a functional and preferentially an augmented immune response after transplant is critical for the survival of the patient, because infections with bacteria, viruses, and/or fungi may occur as a result of the immune deficit created by the chemo/radiotherapy (Bhalla *et al.*, 1992; Oldham, 1982; Golomb *et al.*, 1988; Te Velde *et al.*, 1988). In addition, an augmented immune response and one that can overcome the immunosuppression and/or immune anergy may have therapeutic potential for patients with a reduced tumor burden. In patients receiving an AoBMT, a significant and prolonged period of immune deficiency has been demonstrated (Talmadge and Herberman, 1986; Mihich, 1986; Golomb *et al.*, 1988; Garman and Fan, 1983; Kawakami *et al.*, 1988; Herrmann *et al.*, 1988), although the exact mechanism for this deficit remains unclear. The return of immunologic function in AuBMT and AuBMT patients follows a pattern of reconstitution with general functions preceding more specific immunity in these patients (Te Velde *et al.*, 1988). The persistent elevation of relative and absolute numbers of HLA-Dr$^+$ and CD8$^+$ T cells has been well documented (Garman and Fan, 1983; Kawakami *et al.*, 1988). This is accompanied by depressed numbers of CD4$^+$ T cells, a low CD4:CD8 ratio, and depressed cellular responses as assessed using *in vitro* assays. This includes depressed mixed lymphocyte responses (MLR) and poor proliferative responses to standard mitogens or specific antigens (Widmer *et al.*, 1987; Essner *et al.*, 1989). Patients receiving BMT appear to have normal levels of functional NK cells (Te Velde *et al.*, 1990; Kotik and Mier, 1992), and IL-2-activated LAK, which have been shown to inhibit the growth of autologous leukemic cells (Mackinnon *et al.*, 1990; Bengtsson *et al.*, 1989). The first immunocompetent cells to repopulate the immune system after

AuBMT have γ/δ^+ T-cell receptors (TCR) and cytolytic functions similar to those seen both early in the ontogeny of the thymus and in primitive vertebrate immune systems i.e., increased NK, mitogen-induced cytotoxicity, and ADCC (antibody-dependent cell-mediated cytotoxicity) activity (Bengtsson *et al.*, 1989; Saito *et al.*, 1988). It appears that the immunologic deficits observed in these patients return to normal levels between 3 months and 1 year posttransplant, but may persist longer in patients developing GVHD following AoBMT (Te Velde *et al.*, 1988).

The origin of the immunosuppression following chemotherapy with or without stem cell support has not been addressed. One hypothesis regarding the origin of the immunosuppression posttransplantation is a change in the proportion of TH-1 and TH-2 cells. Several immunosuppressive cytokines, as discussed above, are produced from the TH-2 subset of helper T cells including IL-4 and IL-10. These cytokines, alone or together, might be involved in the downregulation of effector T cells following stem cell transplantation. Similarly, TGF-β may also be involved in suppressing T-cell function. TGF-β has been shown to inhibit antigen-specific T-cell responses to tumor cells, but only at the initiation and not at the effector cell level (Inge *et al.*, 1992). The mechanism of activity may include an indirect suppression of cytokine production as well as a direct antiproliferative effect on the induction of CTLs. Evidence from the literature indicates that macrophages can also function as suppressor cells through the release of reactive nitrogen intermediates which downregulate the proliferative responses of T cells (Schleifer and Mansfield, 1993). In addition, activated macrophages may also release prostaglandins (PG) which act synergistically to suppress peripheral responses by T cells. In contrast to the production by TH-2 cells of IL-4 and IL-10, TH-1 cells secrete IL-2 and IFN-γ and preferentially induce macrophage activation and DTH (a measure of T-cell activity) (Fiorentino *et al.*, 1991). Alternatively, the immune dysfunction that occurs following stem cell transplantation may be associated with the lack of an immune augmenting cytokine (see discussion above). For example, IL-7 (Welch *et al.*, 1989) supports the maturation of thymic T cells and can also augment a T-cell response. Similar to IL-2, IL-12 has been shown to exert effects on development of antigen-specific T cells (Manetti *et al.*, 1993). In addition, it upregulates the production of IFN-γ mRNA in T-cell blasts as well as augmenting NK cell activity (Carella *et al.*, 1992).

11.1. Graft-versus-Tumor Reactions in AoBMT

The role of T cells in controlling (or ablating) neoplastic disease has been demonstrated in allotransplanted patients and described as a graft-versus-tumor (GVT) reaction. A significantly higher risk of relapse is associated with the use of *in vitro* T-cell-depleted BM cells or the clinical use of cyclosporine A to prevent GVHD as observed in acute and chronic leukemia and lymphoma (Barrett *et al.*, 1989; Apperley *et al.*, 1986; Goldman *et al.*, 1988). It has been postulated that T-lymphocyte depletion increases leukemia relapse by removing the cells responsible for the GVT effect (Holden, 1993). Similar relapse rates are observed in recipients of non-T-cell-depleted transplants receiving cyclosporine A (CSA), suggesting that it inhibits the same GVT cells that are removed by T-cell depletion. Clearly, GVHD can also have unfavorable effects on transplant-related mortality (Schleifer and Mansfield, 1993; Carella *et al.*, 1992; Barrett *et al.*, 1989; Apperley *et al.*, 1986; Maraninchi *et al.*, 1987; Bortin *et al.*, 1979; Sullivan *et al.*, 1989; Clift *et al.*, 1990; Weiden *et al.*, 1979, 1981). In first remission, the decreased relapse rate with acute and/or chronic GVHD is more than offset by the increased risk of death from other causes (Carella *et al.*, 1992). Consequently, patients with GVHD have a lower risk of treatment failure, but an increased risk of morbidity from GVHD (Schleifer and Mansfield, 1993; Carella *et al.*, 1992; Apperley *et al.*, 1986; Weiden *et al.*, 1981). In other studies, a GVT effect in patients has been inferred from the retrospective observation that the probability of recurrent leukemia after AoBMT is about 2.5-fold lower in patients having acute GVHD than in those without GVHD (Bortin *et al.*, 1979; Sullivan *et al.*, 1988, 1989; Clift *et al.*, 1990; Weiden *et al.*, 1979, 1981; Mitsuyasu *et al.*, 1986). Chronic GVHD has also been suggested to contribute to improving long-term survival (Sullivan *et al.*, 1989; Weiden *et al.*, 1981). At present, it appears that the *ex vivo* marrow depletion of alloreactive donor T cells reduces the incidence of GVHD but increases the risk of graft failure and relapse of leukemia (Schleifer and Mansfield, 1993; Sullivan *et al.*, 1988; Mitsuyasu *et al.*, 1986). In a placebo-controlled study, a chronic GVHD could not be distinguished from a GVT effect (Clift *et al.*, 1990). Patients with chronic GVHD who remain subclinical throughout therapy have a 55% probability of relapse, as compared with 27% among patients with clinical manifestations of chronic GVHD (Clift *et al.*, 1990). Thus, the development of clinical chronic GVHD may be required for a GVT effect (Clift *et al.*, 1990).

The hypothesis that therapeutic activity following transplantation is associated with a T-cell response (GVT) was supported by the International Bone Marrow Transplantation Registry study of patients with early stage leukemia. The greatest antileukemic effect occurred with patients in whom chronic GVHD developed (Ringden and Horowitz, 1989). In this multicenter study to determine whether GVT reactions were important in preventing leukemia recurrence after BMT, 2254 transplants were studied (Horowitz *et al.*, 1990). Four groups were studied in detail: recipients of non-T-cell-depleted allografts with and without GVHD, recipients of T-cell-depleted allografts, and recipients of genetically identical twin transplants. A decrease in the relapse rate was observed in recipients of non-T-cell-depleted allografts with acute, chronic, or both acute and chronic GVHD as compared with recipients of non-T-cell-depleted allografts without GVHD. Acute myelogenous leukemic (AML) patients who received identical twin transplants had an increased probability of relapse compared with allograft recipients without GVHD, suggesting an antileukemic effect of allograft GVHD. Chronic myelogenous leukemia (CML) patients who received T-cell-depleted transplants with or without GVHD, also had a higher probability of relapse than recipients of non-T-cell-depleted allografts without GVHD suggesting an antileukemic effect of GVHD that is altered by T-cell depletion (Sullivan *et al.*, 1988).

11.2. GVT in AuBMT

While a GVT reaction might be expected following AoBMT, the ability to stimulate a T-cell antitumor response following AuBMT is less obvious. However, a syndrome similar to GVHD has been reported to occur spontaneously in about 8% of patients receiving autologous or syngeneic BMT (Hood *et al.*, 1987). GVHD after autologous or syngeneic BMT clinically and histologically resembles GVHD after AoBMT, but it is a mild self-limiting disease, generally involving only the skin. Whether GVHD could develop after AuBMT was controversial until Hess and colleagues demonstrated the same clinical and histological effect in animal models of the disease (Glazier *et al.*, 1983; Skorski *et al.*, 1990; Geller *et al.*, 1989). GVHD can be induced in rats or mice undergoing syngeneic BMT by treatment with CSA. In this model, GVHD appears to be mediated by autoreactive CTL directed against abnormal class II major histocompatibility complex (MHC) antigens (Hess *et al.*, 1985). The clinical induction of GVHD following AuBMT was demonstrated in non-Hodgkin's lymphoma (NHL) and Hodgkin's disease lymphoma patients who received CSA daily for 28 days following BMT. Histologically proven, class I–II GVHD developed in the skin of all patients at a median of 11 days following BMT (Jones *et al.*, 1989). This clinical observation was recently confirmed by Carella *et al.* (1991) with AuBMT and PSCT patients; 12 patients received CSA for 28 days following transplantation, starting on the day of transplantation. Histologically proven, acute GVHD of the skin occurred in 7 of the patients beginning 9 to 14 days following BMT and lasted 7 to 11 days. The CSA-induced GVHD after AuBMT resembled a mild GVHD following AoBMT. Yeager *et al.* (1992) recently extended their original observation of dermal GVHD in AML patients receiving AuBMT and CSA for 28 days. They found that 15 of 19 patients developed cutaneous histopathological grade 2 GVHD at a median of 33 days. However, a recent comment by Beyer *et al.* (1992) noted that the incidence of cutaneous GVHD was not assessed in control patients, although historically only 7% of patients at this institute have grade 2 cutaneous GVHD.

Another preclinical strategy to induce GVT was reported by Mazumder and colleagues (Charak *et al.*, 1990), who administered IL-2 following infusion of BM cells which had been coincubated with IL-2 to reduce contaminating tumor cells (Charak *et al.*, 1990). In these studies, a GVT activity was induced by the injection of r-IL-2 immediately following AuBMT with the induction of significant therapeutic activity (Charak *et al.*, 1990, 1991). This murine model of AML demonstrated that the administration of IL-2 following AuBMT significantly prolonged survival compared to AuBMT alone. The studies also showed that initiating r-IL-2 therapy immediately following BMT had significantly better therapeutic activity than initiating r-IL-therapy 1, 2, or 3 weeks following AuBMT (Charak *et al.*, 1991). These preclinical therapeutic results were confirmed by Ackerstein *et al.* (1991) and others (Kwak *et al.*, 1992) using r-IL-2 with a B-cell leukemia model and AuBMT. Recently, Mazumder and colleagues (Charak *et al.*, 1992) extended their preclinical observations in a combination therapy protocol with IL-2 and CSA for B-16 melanoma and C-1498

(AML), demonstrating significant therapeutic activity. Mazumder and colleagues (Charak *et al.*, 1993a) have also undertaken a clinical study based on their preclinical results discussed above. In this clinical trial they used IL-2-activated BM cells to transplant lymphoma patients with high-risk/resistant disease. BM cells were activated by incubating the cells with 1000 U/Ml IL-2 for 24 hr in gas-permeable bags (Charak *et al.*, 1993a). This resulted in a significant increase in NK and LAK cell activity as well as an upregulation of CD-25. The patients were infused with an average of 10^7 cell/kg and 10^4 CFU-GM/kg and achieved >500 ANC on average 23 days following transplantation. In addition, patients received a continuous infusion of r-IL-2 after transplantation. Interestingly, the majority of these patients developed an erythematous skin rash which histologically revealed changes suggestive of a grade II GVHD. A significant proportion of the patients also presented with symptoms associated with gastrointestinal GVHD. The preliminary data suggest that extensive GVHD can be induced with the use of *ex vivo* expanded BM NK cells from frozen marrow and subsequent T/NK cell support with continuous infusion of r-IL-2 after transplantation.

In other clinical studies using r-IL-2 alone following BMT, postinfusion lymphocytosis, an increase in NK cell phenotype and function, and the expected toxicity profile (Higuchi *et al.*, 1991; Blaise *et al.*, 1990; Negrier *et al.*, 1991; Soiffer *et al.*, 1992; Bosly *et al.*, 1992) have been observed. In one such study (Negrier *et al.*, 1991) with 18 evaluable patients, three responses were observed: one a CR of short duration in NHL, one a CR of 24+ months' duration, and one a PR of 6 months' duration in patients with metastatic gastric adenocarcinoma. In another study at the Dana Farber Cancer Institution and Harvard Medical School, r-IL-2 was infused following both AuBMT and AoBMT for a median of 85 days at a dose of 2×10^5 units/M^2 per day (Soiffer *et al.*, 1992). Toxicity was minimal and the treatment could be undertaken in an outpatient setting via a Hickman catheter. In this study no patient developed any signs of GVHD, hypotension, or pulmonary capillary leak syndrome. The treatment did not affect the absolute neutrophil count or hemoglobin level, although eosinophilia was observed. Despite the administration of this very low dose of r-IL-2, significant immunological changes were noted in all 13 of the patients with 5- to 40-fold increase in NK cell number. Phenotypically, the majority of these cells were CD56 bright, CD16$^+$, and CD3$^-$. In addition, there was a significant augmentation of *ex vivo* cytotoxicity against K-562 and colon tumor targets. In a similar study, it was shown that following continuous infusion of r-IL-2 in patients receiving AuBMT, the CD3$^+$ and CD16$^+$ cells secrete increased levels of IFN-γ and TNF, following *in vitro* culture, and that there was a significant increase in serum levels of IFN-γ but not TNF following the administration of r-IL-2 (Heslop *et al.*, 1989).

Similar clinical strategies with r-IFN-α also have been undertaken post-transplantation, with the observation of a reduced risk of relapse and an increase in myelosuppression (Klingemann *et al.*, 1991; Meyers *et al.*, 1987; Higano *et al.*, 1992). The Seattle Group (Higano *et al.*, 1992) reported an early study of the prophylactic use of r-IFN-α following AoBMT, and that adjuvant treatment with IFN-α had no effect on the probability or severity of cytomegalovirus (CMV) infections or GVHD in ALL patients who were in remission at the time of transplantation. However, in this large study, there was a significant reduction in the probability of relapse in the r-IFN-α recipients (p=0.004) as compared to transplant patients who did not receive r-IFN-α, although survival rates did not differ between the r-IFN-α recipients and control patients. It was suggested that the administration of r-IFN-α following transplantation reduced the risks of relapse but did not affect CMV infection, perhaps because r-IFN-α was not initiated until a median of 18 days following transplantation and was not administered chronically. For a review of immunoaugmenting strategies following BMT, see Klingemann and Phillips (1991). Recently, Ratanatharathom *et al.* (1994) extended the approach of the induction of a GVT reaction to a combination study which utilized both CSA-induced GVHD and IFN-α augmentation of this effect in autologous transplant patients. This trial used r-Hu-IFN-α2a at either 1 or 3 × 10^6 units given daily by s.c. administration beginning on day 0 of BMT and continuing for 28 days. CSA was also administered over the same time period at 1 mg/kg per day. Of 22 patients enrolled, 17 were considered evaluable. Thirteen of the patients who received r-Hu-IFN-α2a developed GVHD regardless of whether they received CSA, whereas only 2 of the 4 patients who received CSA alone developed detectable GVHD. Patient receiving 1×10^6 units/day of r-Hu-IFN-α2a concurrent with CSA showed a trend toward increased severity of clinical GVHD as compared to patients receiving CSA alone (p=0.06). It was concluded from this study that a r-Hu-IFN-α2a dose of 1×10^6 units/day following AuBMT and in combination with CSA is the highest dose of r-Hu-IFN-α2a that can be tolerated. It appears therefore that IFN-α administration can be safely started on day 0 of AuBMT and can both induce AuGVHD as a single agent and enhance the AuGVHD induced by CSA.

The studies by Jones *et al.* (1989) reporting the induction of GVHD following autologous transplantation for lymphoma and CSA also demonstrated the presence of posttransplant lymphocytes which were cytotoxic for pretransplant lymphocyte targets. They demonstrated that the cytotoxicity could be blocked by preincubation of target cells with an antibody against the public domain of the MHC class II antigen. Therefore, the hypothesis has been proposed that the upregulation of HLA-Dr antigen may render tumor cells more sensitive to autologous GVH activity. This was supported by Noga *et al.* (1992) who hypothesized that treatment with IFN-γ could potentiate the GVT effect associated with CSA-induced AuGVHD in a rat plasmacytoma model. This resulted in prolonged survival in animals exposed to AuGVHD and IFN-γ. Recently, Kennedy *et al.* (1994) investigated whether r-Hu-IFN-γ could augment CSA-induced GVHD following AuBMT in women with metastatic breast cancer. This was proposed because breast cancers are known to frequently express class II MHC antigen (HLA-Dr) (Bernard *et al.*, 1984) and may therefore be targets for such a cytotoxic effect. Furthermore, these investigators had recently completed a study of CSA following HDT and autologous BM infusion for women with metastatic breast cancer and shown that CSA will induce GVHD in this setting in a dose-dependent fashion with acceptable toxicity (Kennedy *et al.*, 1993). In their study

(Kennedy *et al.*, 1994) of IFN-γ and CSA, GVHD was induced in 56% of patients. The severity of GVHD was greater than their historical control population which had been treated with CSA alone. Stage III rash was seen in 36% of patients, compared with 3% in the historical control population. However, no severe visceral GVHD was observed. They suggest that although the incidence of GVHD seen in this study was similar to their prior Phase I trial of CSA alone at 2.5 mg/M^2, the extent of the GVHD rash was much greater, clinical stage III rash being seen in 36 versus 3% of historical controls (p=0.0007). Thus, IFN-γ appears to extenuate the severity of the cutaneous GVHD as compared to extending the frequency of patients developing GVHD. Furthermore, BM engraftment and peripheral blood reconstitution occurred rapidly with no readily apparent effect by either the CSA or the IFN-γ.

12. CONCLUSION

In the last 20 years, nonspecific immunostimulation has progressed from the initial trials with crude microbial mixtures and extracts to more sophisticated uses with a large collection of immunopharmacologically active compounds (only some of which are discussed here) having diverse actions on the immune system. A body of immunopharmacologic knowledge has evolved which shows substantial divergence from conventional pharmacology, particularly in terms of the relationship of dosing schedules to immunopharmacodynamics. This knowledge is important in evaluating agents and predicting appropriate use. While much remains to be learned and new compounds to be extracted and/or cloned, the future of immunotherapy seems bright, particularly in the context of immunorestoration in secondary or iatrogenic cellular immune deficiency.

The major opportunities for the exploitation of immunoregulatory proteins with therapeutic activities are likely to be predicated on combination treatments. Such strategies include the combination of proteins that are clinically efficacious with cytotoxic agents or antibiotics, e.g., IFN-α or β, zidovudine, and GM-CSF (Krown *et al.*, 1992) or a combination of proteins such as IFN-α or IL-2 and TNF. It should be noted that although the growth factors prevent or reduce the depth or duration of neutropenia and reduce the morbidity and mortality associated with secondary infection, there does not appear to be any increased therapeutic efficacy of such combination protocols. Nonetheless, there remains the potential for increased therapeutic efficacy due to an increased number of chemotherapy cycles or dose intensity associated with the support of myeloid augmentation by growth factors.

In summary, a number of the cytokines have been licensed having shown significant therapeutic activity in humans. However, they have as a class general deficiencies including pharmacokinetic liabilities which has stimulated an interest in the development of orally active peptide mimetics. In theory, synthetic BRMs would have significant pharmacologic advantages in that they have a potential to be orally active. While synthetic peptides may not have the same high level of biological activity compared to the cytokines and growth factors that they induce, their lower level of activity is compensated for by the ease of administration as well as the potential to induce *in situ* the "correct" cocktail of cytokines for optimal immunoregulatory or hematostimulatory activity. Clearly, the latter "hypothesis" has not been adequately tested; regardless, it is becoming clear, as discussed previously, that combinations of growth factors, cytokines, and BRMs will have optimal activity when used as adjuvants with more traditional therapeutic modalities.

REFERENCES

Ackerstein, A., Kedar, E., and Slavin, S., 1991, Use of recombinant human interleukin-2 in conjunction with syngenic bone marrow transplantation in mice as a model for control of minimal residual disease in malignant hematologic disorders, *Blood* **78:**1212–1215.

Aderka, D., Le, J., and Vilcek, J., 1989, IL-6 inhibits lipopolysaccharide-induced tumor necrosis factor production in cultured human monocytes, U937 cells, and in mice, *J. Immunol.* **143:**3517–3523.

Akahane, K., and Pluznik, D. H., 1992, Interleukin-4 inhibits interleukin-1α-induced granulocyte–macrophage colony-stimulating factor gene expression in a murine B-lymphocyte cell line via downregulation of RNA precursor, *Blood* **79:**3188–3195.

Alper, J., 1988, Cetus' proleukin in cancer—the excitement grows, *SCRIP* **1363:**24.

Ambrus, J. L., Jr., Chesky, L., Chused, T., Young, K. R., Jr., McFarland, P., August, A., and Brown, E. J., 1991. Intracellular signaling events associated with the induction of proliferation of normal human B lymphocytes by two different antigenically related human B cell growth factors [high molecular weight B cell growth factor (HMW-BCGF) and complement factor Bb], *J. Biol. Chem.* **266:**3702–3708.

Ambrus, J. L., Jr., Pippin, J., Joseph, A., Xu, C., Blumenthal, D., Tamayo, A., Claypool, K., McCourt, D., Srikiatchatochorn, A., and Ford, R. J., 1993, Identification of a cDNA for a human high-molecular-weight B-cell growth factor, *Proc. Natl. Acad. Sci. USA* **90:**6330–6334.

Aoki, T., Tashiro, K., Miyatake, S. I., Kinashi, T., Nakano, T., Oda, Y., Kikuchi, H., and Honjo, T., 1992, Expression of murine interleukin 7 in a murine glioma cell line results in reduced tumorigenicity in vivo, *Proc. Natl. Acad. Sci. USA* **89:**3850–3854.

Apperley, J. F., Jones, L., Hale, G., Waldmann, H., Hows, J., Rombos, Y., Tsatalas, C., Marcus, R. E., Goolden, A. W., Gordon-Smith, E. C., Catovsky, D., Galton, D. A. G., and Goldman, J. M., 1986, Bone marrow transplantation for patients with chronic myeloid leukaemia: T-cell depletion with CampaTH-1 reduces the incidence of graft-versus-host disease but may increase the risk of leukaemic relapse, *Bone Marrow Transplant.* **1:**53–66.

Arend, W. P., 1991, Interleukin-1 receptor antagonist. A new member of the interleukin-1 family, *J. Clin. Invest.* **88:**1445–1451.

Arend, W. P., 1993, Interleukin-1 receptor antagonist, *Adv. Immunol.* **54:**167–227.

Asher, A., Mule, J. J., Reichert, C. M., Shiloni, E., and Rosenberg, S. A., 1987, Studies on the antitumor efficacy of systemically administered recombinant tumor necrosis factor against several murine tumors in vivo, *J. Immunol.* **138:**963–974.

Ashkenazi, A., Marsters, S. A., Capon, D. J., Chamow, S. M., Figari, I. S., Pennica, D., Goeddel, D. W., Palladino, M. A., and Smith, D. H., 1991, Protection against endotoxic shock by a tumor necrosis factor receptor adhesion, *Proc. Natl. Acad. Sci. USA* **88:**10535–10539.

Atkins, M. B., Vachino, G., Tilg, H. J., Karp, D. D., Robert, N. J., Kappler, K., and Mier, J. W., 1992, Phase I evaluation of twice-daily intravenous bolus interleukin-4 in patients with refractory malignancy, *J. Clin. Oncol.* **10:**1802–1809.

Balkwill, F. R., Lee, A., Aldam, G., Moodie, E., Thomas, J. A., Tavernier, J., and Fiers, W., 1986, Human tumor xenografts treated with recombinant human tumor necrosis factor alone or in combination with interferons, *Cancer Res.* **46:**3990–3993.

Bamford, R. N., Grant, A. J., Burton, J. D., Peters, C., Kurys, G., Goldman, C. K., Brennan, J., Roessler, E., and Waldmann, T. A., 1994, The interleukin (IL) 2 receptor b chain is shared by IL-2 and a cytokine, provisionally designated IL-T that stimulates T-cell proliferation and the induction of lymphokine-activated killer cells, *Proc. Natl. Acad. Sci. USA* **91:**4940–4944.

Bargetzi, M. J., Lantz, M., Smith, C. G., Torti, F. M., Olsson, I., Eisenberg, S. P., and Starnes, H. F., Jr., 1993, Interleukin-1b induces interleukin-1 receptor antagonist and tumor necrosis factor binding protein in humans, *Cancer Res.* **53:**4010–4013.

Barrett, A. J., Horowitz, M. M., Gale, R. P., Biggs, J. C., Camitta, B. M., Dicke, K. A., Bluckman, E., Good, R. A., Herzig, R. H., Lee, M. B., Marmont, A. M., Masaoka, T., Ramsay, N. K. C., Rimm, A. A., Speck, B., Zwaan, F. E., and Bortin, M. M., 1989, Marrow transplantation for acute lymphoblastic leukemia: Factors affecting relapse and survival, *Blood* **74:**862–871.

Barton, B. E., and Jackson, J. V., 1993, Protective role of interleukin 6 in the lipopolysaccharide-galactosamine septic shock model, *Infect. Immun.* **61:**1496–1499.

Bengtsson, M., Totterman, T. H., Smedmyr, B., Festin, R., Oberg, B., and Simonsson, B., 1989, Regeneration of functional and activated NK and T sub-subset cells in the marrow and blood after autologous bone marrow transplantation: A prospective phenotypic study with 2/3-color FACS analysis, *Leukemia* **3:**68–75.

Ben-Sasson, S. Z., LeGros, G., Conrad, D. H., Finkelman, F. D., and Paul, W. E., 1990, IL-4 production by T cells from naive donors: IL-2 is required for IL-4 production, *J. Immunol.* **140:**1127.

Bernard, D., Maurizis, J. C., Ruse, F., Chassagne, J., Chollet, P., Sauvezie, B., deLatour, M., and Plagne, R., 1984, Presence of HLA-D/DR antigens on the membrane of breast tumor cells, *Clin. Exp. Immunol.* **56:**215–221.

Beyer, J., Schwerdtfeger, R., and Siegert, W., 1992, Graft-versus-host disease or graft-versus-host-like syndrome, *Blood* **80:**2948–2950.

Bhalla, K., Birkhofer, M., Grant, S., and Graham, G., 1989, The effect of recombinant human granulocyte–macrophage colony-stimulating factor (rGM-CSF) on 3′-deoxythymidine (AZT)-mediated biochemical and cytotoxic effects on normal human myeloid progenitor cells, *Exp. Hematol.* **17:** 17–20.

Bhalla, K., Tang, C., Lbrado, A. M., Grant, S., Tourkina, E., Holladay, C., Hughes, M., Mahoney, M. E., and Huang, Y., 1992, Granulocyte–macrophage colony-stimulating factor/interleukin-3 fusion protein (pIXY 321) enhances high-dose ara-C-induced programmed cell death or apoptosis in human myeloid leukemia cells, *Blood* **80:**2883–2890.

Black, P. L., Phillips, H., Tribble, H. R., Pennington, R. W., Schneider, M., and Talmadge, J. E., 1993, Antitumor response to recombinant murine interferon γ correlates with enhanced immune function of organ-associated, but not recirculating cytolytic T lymphocytes and macrophages, *Cancer Immunol. Immunother.* **37:**299–306.

Blaise, D., Olive, D., Stoppa, A. M., Viens, P., Pourreau, C., Lopez, M., Attal, M., Jasmin, C., Monges, G., Mawas, C., Mannoni, P., Palmer, P., Franks, C., and Phillip, T., 1990, Hematologic and immunologic effects of the systemic administration of recombinant interleukin-2 after autologous bone marrow transplantation, *Blood* **76:**1092–1097.

Bortin, M. M., Truitt, R. L., Rimm, A. A., and Bach, F. M., 1979, Graft-versus-leukaemia reactivity induced by alloimmunisation without augmentation of graft-versus-host reactivity, *Nature* **281:**490–491.

Bosly, A., Guillaume, T., Brice, P., Humblet, Y., Staquet, P., Doyen, C., Chatelain, B., Franks, C. R., Gisselbrecht, C., and Symann, M., 1992, Effects of escalating doses of recombinant human interleukin-2 in correcting functional T-cell defects following autologous bone marrow transplantation for lymphomas and solid tumors, *Exp. Hematol.* **20:**962–968.

Braunschweiger, P. G., Jones, S. A., Johnson, C. S., and Furmanski, P., 1991, Potentiation of mytomycin C and porfiromycin anti tumour activity in solid tumor models by recombinant human interleukin-1 a, *Cancer Res.* **51:**5454–5460.

Brunda, M. J., 1994, Interleukin-12, *J. Leukocyte Biol.* **55:**280–288.

Brunda, M. J., Luistro, L., Warrier, R. R., Wright, R. B., Hubbard, B. R., Murphy, M., Wolf, S. F., and Gately, M. K., 1993, Antitumor and antimetastatic activity of interleukin-12 against murine tumors, *J. Exp. Med.* **178:**1223–1230.

Bruno, E., Briddell, R. A., Cooper, R. J., Brandt, J. E., and Hoffman, R., 1992, Recombinant GM-CSF/IL-3 fusion protein: Its effect on in vitro human megakaryocytopoiesis, *Exp. Hematol.* **20:**494–499.

Bunn, P. A., Foon, K. A., Ihde, D. C., Longo, D. L., Eddy, J., Winkler, C. F., Veach, S. R., Zeffren, J., Sherwin, S., and Oldham, R., 1984, Recombinant leukocyte A interferon: An active agent in advanced cutaneous T-cell lymphomas, *Ann. Intern. Med.* **101:**484–487.

Burke, F., Naylor, M. S., Davies, B., and Balkwill, F., 1993, The cytokine wall chart, *Immunol. Today* **14:**165–169.

Burton, J. D., Bamford, R. N., Peters, C., Grant, A. J., Kurys, G., Goldman, C. K., Brennan, J., Roessler, E., and Waldmann, T. A., 1994, A lymphokine, provisionally designated interleukin T and produced by a human adult T-cell leukemia line, stimulates T-cell proliferation and the induction of lymphokine-activated killer cells, *Proc. Natl. Acad. Sci. USA* **91:**4935–4939.

Bush, H. W., 1984, The importance of dose intensity in chemotherapy of metastatic breast cancer, *J. Clin. Oncol.* **2:**1281–1288.

Busse, R., and Mulsch, A., 1990, Induction of nitric oxide syntheses by cytokines in vascular smooth muscle cells, *FEBS Lett.* **275:**87–90.

Caligiuri, M. A., Murray, C., Robertson, M. J., Wang, E., Cochran, K., Cameron, C., Schow, P., Ross, M. E., Klumpp, T. R., Soiffer, R. J., Smith, K. A., and Ritz, J., 1993, Selective modulation of human natural killer cells in vivo after prolonged infusion of low dose recombinant interleukin 2, *J. Clin. Invest.* **91:**123–132.

Cantell, K., and Hirvonen, S., 1977, Preparation of human leukocyte interferon for clinical use, *Tex. Rep. Biol. Med.* **35:**138–144.

Carella, A. M., Gaozza, E., Conjiu, A., Carlier, P., Nati, S., Truini, M., Castellaneta, A., and Viale, M., 1991, Cyclosporine-induced graft-versus-host disease after autologous bone marrow transplantation in hematological malignancies, *Ann. Hematol.* **6:**156–159.

Carella, A. M., Frassoni, F., van Lint, M. T., Gualandi, F., Occhini, D., Carlier, P., Pollicardo, N., Pungolino, E., Fagioli, F., Santini, G., Conjiu, A., Nati, S., Raffo, M. R., Podesta, M., Corvo, R., Vitale, V., Gallamini, A., Pogliani, E. M., Lanzi, E., Bacigalupo, A., and Marmont, A., 1992, autologous and allogeneic bone marrow transplantation in acute myeloid leukemia in first complete remission: An update of the Genoa experience with 159 patients, *Ann. Hematol.* **64:**128–131.

Castelli, M. P., Black, P. L., Schneider, M., Pennington, R., Abe, F., and Talmadge, J. E., 1988, Protective, restorative and therapeutic properties of recombinant human interleukin-1 in rodent models, *J. Immunol.* **140:**3830–3837.

Charak, B. S., Brynes, R. K., Groshen, S., Chen, S. C., and Mazumder, A., 1990, Bone marrow transplantation with interleukin-2-activated bone marrow followed by interleukin-2 therapy for acute myeloid leukemia in mice, *Blood* **76:**2187–2190.

Charak, B. S., Brynes, R. K., Katsuda, S., Groshen, S., Chen, S. C., and Mazumder, A., 1991, Induction of graft versus leukemia effect in bone marrow transplantation: Dosage and time schedule dependency of interleukin 2 therapy, *Cancer Res.* **51:**2015–2020.

Charak, B. S., Agah, R., and Mazumder, A., 1992, Synergism of interleukin-2 and cyclosporine A in induction of a graft-versus-tumor effect without graft-versus-host disease after syngeneic bone marrow transplantation, *Blood* **80:**179–184.

Charak, B. S., Areman, E. M., Dickerson, S. A., Choudhary, G. D., Sacher, R., Kotula, P. L., Brown, E. G., and Mazumder, A., 1993a, A novel approach to immunomodulation of frozen human bone marrow with interleukin-2 for clinical application, *Bone Marrow Transplant.* **11:**147–154.

Charak, B., Verma, U., Cahill, R., and Mazumder, A., 1993b, Autologous bone marrow transplantation with interleukin-2-activated bone marrow, *Blood* **10:**628a.

Chen, L., Mory, Y., Zilberstein, A., and Revel, M., 1988, Growth inhibition of human breast cancer carcinoma and leukemia/lymphoma cell lines by recombinant interferon-B2, *Proc. Natl. Acad. Sci. USA* **85:**8037–8041.

Chiu, C. P., and Lee, F., 1989, IL-6 is a differentiation factor for M1 and WEH1-3B myeloid cells, *J. Immunol.* **142:**1909–1912.

Clark, J. W., Smith, J. W., II, Steis, R. G., Urba, W. J., Crum, E., Miller, R., McKnight, J., Beman, J., Stevenson, H. C., Creekmore, S., Stewart, M., Conlon, K., Sznol, M., Kremers, P., and Longo, D. L., 1990, Interleukin-2 and lymphokine-activated killer cell therapy: Analysis of a bolus interleukin-2 and a continuous infusion interleukin-2 regimen, *Cancer Res.* **50:**7343–7350.

Clift, R. A., Buckner, C. D., Appelbaum, R. F., Bearman, S. E., Petersen, F. B., Fisher, L. D., Anasetti, C., Beatty, P., Bensinger, W. I., Doney, K., Hill, R. S., McDonald, G. B., Martin, P., Sanders, J., Singer, J., Stewart, P., Sullivan, K. M., Witherspoon, R., Storb, R., Hansen, J. A., and Thomas, E. D., 1990, Allogeneic marrow transplantation in patients with acute myeloid leukemia in first remission: A randomized trial of two irradiation regimens, *Blood* **76:**1867–1871.

Creekmore, S. P., Harris, J. E., Ellis, T. M., Braun, D. P., Cohen, I. I., Bhoopalam, N., Jassak, P. F., Cahill, M. A., Canzoneri, C. L., and Fisher, R. I., 1989, A phase I clinical trial of recombinant interleukin-2 by periodic 24-hour intravenous infusions, *J. Clin. Oncol.* **7:**276–284.

Crown, J., Jakubowski, A., and Gabrilove, J., 1993, Interleukin-1: Biological effects in human hematopoiesis, *Leuk-Lymphoma* **9:**433–440.

Crum, E. D., and Kaplan, D. R., 1991, In vivo activity of solid phase interleukin 2, *Cancer Res.* **51:**875.

Damia, G., Komschlies, K. L., Futami, H., Back, T., Gruys, M. E., Longo, D. L., Keller, J. R., Ruscetti, F. W., and Wiltrout, R. H., 1992a, Prevention of acute chemotherapy-induced death in mice by recombinant human interleukin 1:Protection from hematological and nonhematological toxicities, *Cancer Res.* **52:**4082–4089.

Damia, G. K. L., Komschlies, K. L., Faltynek, C. R., Ruscetti, F. W., and Wiltrout, R. H., 1992b, Administration of recombinant human interleukin-7 alters the frequency and number of myeloid progenitor cells in the bone marrow and spleen of mice, *Blood* **79:**1121–1129.

Davis, I., Maher, D., Cebon, J., Dyer, W., McKendrick, J., Bogley, G., Woodruff, R., Green, M., Fox, R., Rallings, M., Bonnem, E., Boyd, A., and Morslyn, G., 1991, Pharmacokinetic and clinical studies of interleukin-4 (IL-4) in patients with malignancy, *Proc. Am. Assoc. Clin. Oncol.* **10:**287.

Davis, S., Aldrich, T. H., Stahl, N., Pan, L., Taga, T., Kishimoto, T., Ip, N. Y., and Yancopoulos, G. D., 1993, LIFR beta and gp130 as heterodimerizing signal transducers of the tripartite CNTF receptor, *Science* **260:**1805–1808.

Dean, J. H., Cornacoff, J. B., Barbolt, T. A., Gossett, K. A., and LaBrie, T., 1992, Pre-clinical toxicity of IL-4: A model for studying protein therapeutics, *Int. J. Immunopharmacol.* **14:**391–397.

Del Prete, G. F., DeCarli, M., Mastromauro, C., Biagiotti, R., Macchia, D., Falagiani, P., Ricci, M., and Romagnani, S., 1991, Purified protein derivative of Mycobacterium tuberculosis and excretory-secretory antigen(s) of Toxocara canis expand in vitro human T cells with stable and positive (type 1 T helper or type 2 T helper-profile of cytokine production, *J. Clin. Invest.* **88:**346–350.

Dennis, D., Chachoua, A., Caron, D., Garrison, L., Liebes, L., Furnanski, P., Wiprovnick, J., Peace, D., Oratz, R., Spayer, J., and Blum, R. H., 1992, Biologic activity of interleukin 1 (IL-1) alpha in patients with refractory malignancies, *Proc. Am. Assoc. Clin. Oncol.* **11:**255.

Dinarello, C. A., 1991, Interleukin-1 and interleukin 1 antagonism, *Blood* **77:**1627–1652.

Dinarello, C. A., and Thompson, R. C., 1991, Blocking IL-1: Interleukin-1 receptor antagonists in vivo and in vitro, *Immunol. Today* **12:**404–410.

Ditonno, P., Tso, C. L., Sakata, T., Dekernion, J. B., and Belldegruin, A., 1992, Regulatory effects of interleukin-7 on renal tumor infiltrating lymphocytes, *Urol. Res.* **20:**205–210.

Editorial, 1994, Synergen drops Antril for sepsis, *SCRIP* **1942:**19.

Ellenberg, S. S., 1993, Surrogate endpoints, *Br. J. Cancer* **68:**457–459.

Engelmann, H., Aderka, D., Rubinstein, M., Rotman, D., and Wallach, D., 1989, A tumor necrosis factor-binding protein purified to homogeneity from human urine protects cells from tumor necrosis factor toxicity, *J. Biol. Chem.* **264:**11974–11980.

Essner, R., Rhoades, K., McBride, W. H., Morton, D. L., and Economou, J. S., 1989, IL-4 down-regulates IL-1 and TNF gene expression in human monocytes, *J. Immunol.* **142:**3857–3861.

Finkelman, F. D., Holmes, J., Katona, I. M., Urgan, J. F., Jr., Beckmann, M. P., Park, L. S., Schooley, K. A.,

Coffman, R. L., Mosmann, T. R., and Paul, W. E., 1990, Lymphokine control of in vivo immunoglobulin isotope selection, *Annu. Rev. Immunol.* **8:**303.

Fiorentino, D. F., Zlotnik, A., Vieira, P., Mosmann, T. R., Howard, M., Moore, K. W., and O'Garra, A., 1991, IL-10 acts on the antigen-presenting cell to inhibit cytokine production by Thl cells, *J. Immunol.* **46:**3444–3451.

Florentin, D. F., Bond, M. W., and Mosmann, T. R., 1989, Th2 clones secrete a factor that inhibits cytokine production by Thl clones, *J. Exp. Med.* **170:**2081.

Foon, K. A., Bottino, G., and Abrams, P. G., 1985, Phase II trial of recombinant leukocyte A interferon in patients with advanced chronic lymphocytic leukemia, *Am. J. Med.* **78:**216–220.

Freimann, J., Estrov, Z., Itoh, K., Talpaz, M., Estey, E., Kantarjian, H., O'Brien, S., Hunter, C., Sutterman, J., and Markowitz, A., 1991, Phase 1 studies of recombinant human interleukin-4 (IL-4), *Proc. Am. Assoc. Clin. Oncol.* **10:**216.

Garman, R. D., and Fan, D. P., 1983, Characterization of helper factors distinct from IL-2 necessary for the generation of allospecific cytotoxic T lymphocytes, *J. Immunol.* **130:**756–762.

Gearing, D. P., Comeau, M. R., Friend, D. J., Gimpel, S. D., Thut, C. J., McGourty, J., Brasher, K. K., King, J. A., Gillis, S., Mosley, B., Ziegler, S. F., and Cosman, D., 1992, The IL-6 signal transducer, gp130: An oncostatin M receptor and affinity converter for the LIF receptor, *Science* **255:**1434–1437.

Geller, R. B., Esa, A. H., Beschorner, W. E., Frondoza, C. G., Santos, G. W., and Hess, A. D., 1989, Successful in vitro graft-versus-tumor effect against an Ia-bearing tumor using cyclosporine-induced syngeneic graft-versus-host disease in the rat, *Blood* **74:**1165–1171.

Germann, T., Gately, M. K., Schoenhaut, D. S., Lohoff, M., Mattner, F., Fischer, S., Jin, S., Schmitt, E., and Rude, E., 1993, Interleukin-12/T cell stimulating factor, a cytokine with multiple effects on T helper type 1 (THl) but not on TH2 cells, *Eur. J. Immunol.* **23:**1762–1770.

Ghosh, A. K., Dazzi, H., Thatcher, N., and Moore, M., 1989, Lack of correlation between peripheral blood lymphokine-activated killer (LAK) cell function and clinical response in patients with advanced malignant melanoma receiving recombinant interleukin 2, *Int. J. Cancer* **43:**410–414.

Gilleece, M. H., Scarffe, J. H., Ghosh, A., Heyworth, C. M., Bonnem, E., Testa, N., Stem, P., Dexter, T. M., 1992, Recombinant human interleukin 4 (IL-4) given as daily subcutaneous injections—A phase 1 dose toxicity trial, *Br. J. Cancer* **66:**204–210.

Givon, T., Slavin, S., Haran-Ghera, N., Michalevicz, R., and Revel, M., 1992, Antitumor effects of human recombinant interleukin-6 on acute myeloid leukemia in mice and cell cultures, *Blood* **79:**2392–2398.

Glazier, A., Tutschka, P. J., Farmer, E. R., and Santos, G. W., 1983, Graft-versus-host disease in cyclosporin A-treated rats after syngeneic and autologous bone marrow reconstitution, *J. Exp. Med.* **158:**1–8.

Goldman, J. M., Gale, R. P., Horowitz, M. M., Biggs, J. C., Champlin, R. E., Gluckman, E., Hoffmann, R. G., Jacobsen, S. J., Marmont, A. M., McGlave, P. B., Messner, H. A., Rimm, A. A., Rozman, C., Speck, B., Tura, S., Weiner, R. W., and Borton, M. M., 1988, Bone marrow transplantation for chronic myelogenous leukemia in chronic phase. Increased risk for relapse associated with T-cell depletion, *Ann. Intern. Med.* **108:**806–814.

Golomb, H. M., Fefer, A., Golde, D. W., Ozer, H., Portlock, C., Silber, R., Rappeport, J., Ratain, M. J., Thompson, J., Bonnem, E., Spiegel, R., Tensen, L., Burke, J. S., and Vardiman, J. W., 1988, Report of a multi-institutional study of 193 patients with hairy cell leukemia treated with interferon-a 2b, *Semin. Oncol.* **15:**7–9.

Golumbek, P. T., Lazenby, A. J., Levitsky, H. I., Jaffee, L. M., Karasuyama, H., Baker, M., and Pardoll, D. M., 1991, Treatment of established renal cancer by tumor cells engineered to secrete interleukin-4, *Science* **254:**713–716.

Gore, M. E., Galligioni, E., Keen, C. W., Sorio, R., Loriaus, E. M., Grobben, H. C., and Franks, C. R., 1994, The treatment of metastatic renal cell carcinoma by continuous intravenous infusion of recombinant interleukin-2, *Eur. J. Cancer* **30A:**329–333.

Grabstein, K. H., Eisenman, J., Shanebeck, K., Rauch, C., Srinivasan, S., Fung, V., Beers, C., Richardson, J., Schoenborn, M. A., Ahdieh, M., Johnson, L., Alderson, M. R., Watson, J. D., Anderson, D. M., and Firi, J. G., 1994, Cloning of a T cell growth factor with the b chain of the interleukin-2 receptor, *Science* **264:**965–968.

Groopman, J. E., Gottlieb, M. S., Goodman, J., Mitsuyasu, R. T., Conant, M. A., Prince, H., Fahey, J. L., Derezin, M., Weinstein, W. M., Casavante, C., Rothman, J., Rudnick, S., and Volberding, P. A., 1984, Recombinant a-2 interferon therapy for Kaposi's sarcoma associated with the acquired immunodeficiency syndrome, *Ann. Intern. Med.* **100:**671–676.

Grzegorzewski, K., Komschlies, K. L., Mori, M., Kaneda, K., Usui, N., Faltynek, C. R., Keller, J. R., Ruscetti, F. W., and Wiltrout, R. H., 1994, Administration of rhIL-7 to mice induces the exportation of myeloid progenitor cells from the bone marrow to peripheral sites, *Blood* **83:**377–385.

Gubler, U., Chua, A. O., Schoenhaut, D. S., Dwyer, C. M., McComas, W., Motyka, R., Nabavi, N., Walitzky, A. G., Quinn, P. M., Familletti, P. C., and Gately, M. K., 1991, Co-expression of two distinct genes is required to generate secreted bioactive cytotoxic lymphocyte maturation factor, *Proc. Natl. Acad. Sci. USA* **88:**4143–4147.

Hanauske, A. R., Degen, D., Marshall, M. H., Hilsenback, S. G., Banks, P., Stuckey, J., Leahy, M., and Von-Hoff, D. D., 1992, Effect of recombinant human interleukin-a on clonogenic growth of primary human tumors *in vitro, J. Immunother.* **11:**155–158.

Heinzel, F. P., Schoenhaut, D. S., Rerko, R. M., Rosser, L. E., and Gately, M. K., 1993, Recombinant interleukin 12 cures mice infected with Leishmania major, *J. Exp. Med.* **177:**1505–1509.

Herberman, R. B., 1989a, Interleukin-2 therapy of human cancer: Potential benefits versus toxicity, *J. Clin. Oncol.* **7:**1–4.

Herberman, R. B., 1989b, Clinical cancer therapy with IL-2, *Cancer Invest.* **7:**515–516.

Herrmann, F., Schulz, G., Lindemann, A., Meyenburg, W., Krumwieh, D., and Mertelsmann, R., 1988, Yeast-expressed granulocyte–macrophage colony-stimulating factor in cancer patients: A phase 1b clinical study, *Behring Inst. Mitt.* **83:**107–118.

Heslop, H. E., Gottlieb, D. J., Bianchi, A. C. M., Meager, A., Prentice, H. G., Mehta, A. B., Hoffbrand, A. V., and Brenner, M. K., 1989, In vivo induction of gamma interferon and tumor necrosis factor by interleukin-2 infusion following intensive chemotherapy or autologous marrow transplantation, *Blood* **74:**1374–1380.

Hess, A. D., Horwitz, L., Beshorner, W. E., and Santos, G. W., 1985, Development of graft-vs-host disease-like syndrome in cyclosporine-treated rats after syngeneic bone marrow transplantation. Development of cytotoxic T lymphocytes with apparent polyclonal anti-Ia specificity, including autoreactivity, *J. Exp. Med.* **161:**718–730.

Higano, C. S., Raskind, W. H., and Singer, J. W., 1992, Use of alpha interferon for the treatment of relapse of chronic myelogenous leukemia in chronic phase after allogeneic bone marrow transplantation, *Blood* **80:**1437–1442.

Higuchi, C. M., Thompson, J. A., Petersen, F. B., Buckner, C. D., and Fefer, A., 1991, Toxicity and immunomodulatory effects of interleukin-2 after autologous bone marrow transplantation for hematologic malignancies, *Blood* **77:**2561–2568.

Hirayama, F., Katayama, N., Neben, S., Donaldson, D., Nickbarg, E. B., Clark, S. C., and Ogawa, M., 1994, Synergistic interaction between interleukin-12 and Steel factor in support of proliferation of murine lymphohemopoietic progenitors in culture, *Blood* **83:**92–98.

Hirose, K., Longo, D. L., Oppenheim, J. J., and Matsushima, K., 1993, Overexpression of mitochondrial manganese superoxide dismutase promotes the survival of tumor cells exposed to interleukin-1, tumor necrosis factor, selected anticancer drugs, and ionizing radiation, *FASEB J.* **7:**361–368.

Hock, H., Dorsch, M., Diamantstein, T., and Blankenstein, T., 1991, Interleukin 7 induces $CD4^+$ T cell-dependent tumor rejection, *J. Exp. Med.* **174:**1291–1298.

Holden, C., 1993, FDA okays surrogate markers, *Science* **259:**32.

Hood, A. F., Vogelsang, G. B., Black, L. P., Farmer, E. R., and Santos, G. W., 1987, Acute graft-vs.-host disease. Development following autologous and syngeneic bone marrow transplantation, *Arch. Dermatol.* **123:**745–750.

Horohov, D. W., Crim, J. A., Smith, P. L., and Siegel, J. P., 1988, IL-4 (B cell stimulatory factor 1) regulates multiple aspects of influenza virus-specific cell-mediated immunity, *J. Immunol.* **141:**4217–4223.

Horowitz, M. M., Gale, R. P., Sondel, P. M., Goldman, J. M., Kersey, J., Kolb, H. J., Rimm, A. A., Ringden, O., Rozman, C., Speck, B., Truitt, R. L., Swaan, F. E., and Bortin, M. M., 1990, Graft-versus-leukemia reactions after bone marrow transplantation, *Blood* **75:**555–562.

Hryniuk, W., and Levine, M. N., 1986, Analysis of dose intensity for adjuvant chemotherapy trials in stage II breast cancer, *J. Clin. Oncol.* **4:**1162–1167.

Hsieh, C., Macatomia, S. E., Tripp, C. S., Wolf, S. F., O'Garra, A., and Murphy, K. M., 1993, Development of T_H1 $CD4^-$ T cells through IL-12 produced by listeria-induced macrophages, *Science* **260:**547–549.

Inge, T. H., Hoover, S. K., Susskind, B. M., Barrett, S. K., and Bear, H. D., 1992, Inhibition of tumor-specific cytotoxic T-lymphocyte responses by transforming growth factor beta-1, *Cancer Res.* **52:**1386–1392.

Jacobsen, S. E. W., Veiby, O. P., and Smeland, E. B., 1993, Cytotoxic lymphocyte maturation factor (interleukin 12) is a synergistic growth factor for hematopoietic stem cells, *J. Exp. Med.* **178:**413–418.

Jaffe, H. S., and Herberman, R. B., 1988, Rationale for recombinant human IFN-a adjuvant immunotherapy for cancer, *J. Natl. Cancer Inst.* **80:**616–619.

Jicha, D. L., Mule, J. J., and Rosenberg, S. A., 1991, Interleukin 7 generates anti-tumor cytotoxic lymphocytes against murine sarcomas with efficacy in cellular adoptive immunotherapy, *J. Exp. Med.* **174:**1511–1515.

Johnson, C. S., Chang, M. J., Braunscheriger, P. G., and Furmanski, P., 1992, Acute hemorrhagic necrosis of tumours induced by interleukin-1 a: Effects independent of tumour necrosis factor, *J. Natl. Cancer Inst.* **83:**843–848.

Jones, G. J., and Itri, L. M., 1986, Safety and tolerance of recombinant interferon alpha-2a (Roferon-A) in cancer patients, *Cancer* **57:**1709–1715.

Jones, R. J., Vogelsang, G. B., Hess, A. D., Farmer, E. R., Mann, R. B., Geller, R. B., Piantadosi, S., and Santos, G. W., 1989, Induction of graft-versus-host disease after autologous bone marrow transplantation, *Lancet* **1:**754–757.

Jujjwara, T., Sakagami, K., Matsuoka, J., Shiozaki, S., Uchida, S., Fujioka, K., Takada, Y., Onoda, T., and Orita, K., 1990, Application of an interleukin-2 slow delivery system to the immunotherapy of established murine colon 26 adenocarcinoma liver metastases, *Cancer Res.* **50:**7003.

Kawakami, Y., Rosenberg, S. A., and Lotze, M. T., 1988, Interleukin-4 promotes the growth of tumor-infiltrating lymphocytes cytotoxic for human autologous melanoma, *J. Exp. Med.* **168:**2183–2191.

Kawakami, Y., Custer, M. C., Rosenberg, S. A., and Lotze, M. T., 1989, IL-4 regulates IL-2 induction of lymphokine-activated killer activity from human lymphocytes, *J. Immunol.* **142:**3452–3461.

Kennedy, M. J., Vogelsang, G. B., Beveridge, R. A., Farmer, E. R., Altomonte, V., Huelskamp, A. M., and Davidson, N. E., 1993, Phase I trial of intravenous cyclosporine to induce graft-vs-host disease in women undergoing autologous bone marrow transplantation for breast cancer, *J. Clin. Oncol.* **11:** 478–484.

Kennedy, M. J., Vogelsang, G. B., Jones, R. J., Farmer, E. R., Hess, A. D., Altomonte, V., Huelskamp, A. M., and Davidson, N. E., 1994, Phase I trial of interferon gamma to potentiate cyclosporine-induced graft-versus-host disease in women undergoing autologous bone marrow transplantation for breast cancer, *J. Clin. Oncol.* **12:**249–257.

Kilbourn, R. G., Gross, S. S., Lodato, R. F., Adams, J., Levi, R., Miller, L. L., Lachman, L. B., and Griffith, O. W., 1992, Inhibition of interleukin-1-alpha-induced nitric oxide synthase in vascular smooth muscle and full reversal of interleukin-1-alpha-induced hypotension by N-amino-L-argentine, *J. Natl. Cancer Inst.* **84:**1008–1016.

Kilian, P. L., Kaffka, K. L., Biondi, D. A., Lipman, J. M., Benjamin, W. R., Feldman, D., and Campen, C. A., 1991, Antiproliferative effect of interleukin-1 on human ovarian carcinoma cell line (NIH:OVAR3), *Cancer Res.* **51:**1923–1928.

Kishimoto, T., Akira, S., and Taga, T., 1992, Interleukin-6 and its receptors: A paradigm for cytokines, *Science* **258:**593–597.

Kishimoto, T., Taga, T., and Akira, S., 1994, Cytokine signal transduction, *Cell* **76:**253–262.

Klingemann, H. G., and Phillips, G. L., 1991, Immunotherapy after bone marrow transplantation, *Bone Marrow Transplant.* **8:**73–81.

Klingemann, H. G., Grigg, A. P., Wilkie-Boyd, K., Barnett, M. J., Eaves, A. C., Reece, D. E., Shepherd, J. D., and Phillips, G. L., 1991, Treatment with recombinant interferon (alpha-2b) early after bone marrow transplantation in patients at high risk for relapse, *Blood* **78:**3306–3311.

Kobayashi, M., Kitz, L., Ryan, M., Hewick, R. M., Clark, S. C., Loudon, R., Sherman, F., Perussia, B., and

Trinchieri, G., 1989, Identification and purification of natural killer cell stimulatory factor (NKSF), a cytokine with multiple biologic effects on human lymphocytes, *J. Exp. Med.* **170:**827–845.

Kohno, T., Brewer, M. T., Baker, S. L., Schwartz, P. E., King, M. W., Hale, K. K., Squires, C. H., Thompson, R. C., and Vannice, J. L., 1990, A second tumor necrosis factor receptor gene product can shed a naturally occurring tumor necrosis factor inhibitor, *Proc. Natl. Acad. Sci. USA* **87:**8331–8335.

Kondo, M., Takeshita, T., Ishii, N., Nakamura, M., Watanabe, S., Arai, K. I., and Sugamura, K., 1993, Sharing of the interleukin 2 (IL-2) receptor gamma chain between receptors for IL-2 and IL-4, *Science* **262:**1874–1877.

Konrad, M. W., Hamstreet, G., Hersh, E. M., Mansell, P. W. A., Mertelsmann, R., Kolitz, J. E., and Bradley, E. C., 1990, Pharmacokinetics of recombinant interleukin-2 in humans, *Cancer Res.* **50:**2009–2017.

Koschlies, K. L., Gregoria, T. A., Gruys, M. E., Back, T. C., Faltynek, C. R., and Wiltrout, R. H., 1994, Administration of recombinant human IL-7 to mice alters the composition of B-lineage cells and T cell subsets, enhances T cell function, and induces regression of established metastases, *J. Immunol.* **152:**5776–5785.

Kotik, A., and Mier, J. W., 1992, Selective cytokine in mRNA destabilization: A contributing factor in IL-4 mediated suppression of IL-2-induced IL-1b synthesis, *Int. J. Immunopathol. Immunopharmacol.* **4:**123–134.

Krown, S. E., Paredes, J., Buindow, D., Polsky, B., Gold, J. W. M., and Flomernberg, N., 1992, Interferon-B, zidovudine, and granulocyte–macrophage colony-stimulating factor: A phase 1 AIDS clinical trials group study in patients with Kaposi's sarcoma associated with AIDS, *J. Clin. Oncol.* **10:**1344–1351.

Kuga, T., Komatsu, Y., Yamasaki, M., Sekine, S., Miyaki, H., Nishi, T., Sato, M., Yokoo, Y., Asano, M., Okabe, M., and Itoh, S., 1989, Mutagenesis of human granulocyte colony stimulating factor, *Biochem. Biophys. Res. Commun.* **159:**103–111.

Kwak, L. W., Campbell, M. J., and Levy, R., 1992, Tumor resistance induced by syngenic bone marrow transplantation and enhanced by interleukin-2: A model for the graft versus leukemia reaction, *Cancer Res.* **52:**4117–4120.

Lane, L. C., Feinberg, J., Davey, V., Deyton, L., Baseler, M., Manischewitz, J., Masur, H., Kovacs, J. A., Herpin, B., Walker, R., Metcalf, J. A., Salzman, N., Quinnan, G., and Fauci, A. S., 1988, Anti-retroviral effects of interferon-α in AIDS-associated Kaposi's sarcoma, *Lancet* **2:**1218–1222.

Lee, A. M., Vadhan-Raj, S., Hamilton, R. F., Jr., Scheule, R. K., and Holian, A., 1993, The in vivo effects of rhIL-la therapy on human monocyte activity, *J. Leukocyte Biol.* **54:**314–321.

Lienard, D., Ewalenko, P., Delmotte, J. J., Renard, N., and Lejeune, F. J., 1992, High-dose recombinant tumor necrosis factor alpha in combination with interferon gamma and melphalan in isolation perfusion of the limbs for melanoma and sarcoma, *J. Clin. Oncol.* **10:**52–60.

Lim, S. H., Newland, A. C., Kelsey, S., Bell, A., Offerman, E., Rist, C., Gozzard, D., Bareford, D., Smith, M. P., and Goldstone, A. H., 1992, Continuous intravenous infusion of high-dose recombinant interleukin-2 for acute myeloid leukemia—A phase II study, *Cancer Immunol. Immunother.* **34:**337–342.

Londei, M., Verhoef, A., Hawrylwicz, C., Groves, J., De, B. P., and Feldmann, M., 1990, Interleukin 7 is a growth factor for mature human T cells, *Eur. J. Immunol.* **20:**425–428.

Lotscher, H., Pan, Y. E., Lahm, H. W., Gentz, R., Brockhaus, M., Tabuchi, H., and Leslauer, W., 1990, Molecular cloning and expression of the human 55kD tumor necrosis factor receptor, *Cell* **61:**351–360.

Lotze, M. T., Chang, A. E., Seipp, C. A., Simpson, C., Vetto, S. J., and Rosenberg, S. A., 1986, High-dose recombinant interleukin 2 in the treatment of patients with disseminated cancer. Responses, treatment-related morbidity and histologic findings, *J. Am. Med. Assoc.* **256:**3117–3124.

Lu, H. S., Boone, T. C., Souza, L. M., and Lai, P. H., 1989, Disulfide and secondary structures of recombinant human granulocyte colony stimulating factor, *Arch. Biochem. Biophys.* **268:**81–92.

Lu, L., Zhou, Z., Wu, B., Xiao, M., Shen, R. N., Williams, D. E., Kim, Y. J., Kwon, B. S., Ruscetti, S., and Broxmeyer, H. E., 1992, Influence of recombinant human interleukin (IL)-7 on disease progression in mice infected with Friend virus complex, *Int. J. Cancer* **52:**261–265.

Lynch, D. H., and Miller, R. E., 1994, Interleukin 7 promotes long-term in vitro growth of antitumor cytotoxic T lymphocytes with immunotherapeutic efficacy in vivo, *J. Exp. Med.* **179:**31–42.

Lynch, D. H., Namen, A. E., and Miller, R. E., 1991, In vivo evaluation of the effects of interleukin 2, 4, and 7 on enhancing the immunotherapeutic efficacy of anti-tumor cytotoxic T lymphocytes, *Eur. J. Immunol.* **21:**2977–2985.

Mackinnon, S., Hows, J. M., and Goldman, J. M., 1990, Induction of a syngeneic graft-versus-leukemia effect following bone marrow transplantation for chronic myeloid leukemia, *Leukemia* **4:**287–291.

McKnight, A. J., Zimmer, G. J., Fogelman, I., Wolf, S. F., and Abbas, A. K., 1994, Effects of interleukin-12 on helper T cell-dependent immune response in vivo, *J. Immunol.* **152:**2172–2179.

Maluish, A. E., Ortaldo, J. R., Conlon, J. C., Sherwin, S. A., Leavitt, R., Strong, D. M., Weirnik, P., Oldham, R. K., and Herberman, R. B., 1983, Depression of natural killer cytotoxicity after in vivo administration of recombinant leukocyte interferon, *J. Immunol.* **37:**236–244.

Maluish, A. E., Urba, W. J., Longo, D. L. O., Overton, W. R., Coggin, D., Crisp, E. R., Williams, R., Sherwin, S. A., Gordon, K., and Steis, R. G., 1988, The determination of an immunologically active dose of interferon-gamma in patients with melanoma, *J. Clin. Oncol.* **6:**434–445.

Manetti, R., Parronchi, P., Giudizi, M. G., Piccinni, M. P., Maggi, E., Trinchieri, G., and Romagnani, S., 1993, Natural killer cell stimulatory factor [interleukin 12 (IL-12)] induces T helper type 1 (Th1)-specific immune responses and inhibits the development of IL-4-producing Th cells, *J. Exp. Med.* **177:**1199–1204.

Maraninchi, D., Gluckman, E., Blaise, D., Guyotat, D., Rio, B., Pico, J., Leblond, V., Michallet, M., Dreyfus, F., and Ifrah, N., 1987, Impact of T-cell depletion on outcome of allogeneic bone marrow transplantation for standard-risk leukaemias, *Lancet* **2:**175–178.

Marcus, S. G., Perry-Lalley, D., Mule, J. J., Rosenberg, S. A., and Yang, J. C., 1994, The use of interleukin-6 to generate tumor-infiltrating lymphocytes with enhanced in vivo antitumor activity, *J. Immunother.* **15:**105–112.

Marumo, K., Tachibana, M., Deguchi, N., and Tazaki, H., 1992, Enhancement of lymphokine-activated killer activity induction *in vitro* by interleukin-1 administered in patients with urological malignancies, *J. Immunother.* **11:**191–197.

Mayer, P., Schulze, E., and Lam, C. H., 1992, Protective activity of IL-6 in infections and reduction of human tumor xenograft growth in nude mice, in: *IL-6: Physiopathology and Clinical Potentials* (M. Revel, ed.), Raven Press, New York, pp. 281–292.

Meyers, J. D., Flournoy, N., Sanders, J. E., McGuffin, R. W., Newton, B. A., Fisher, L. D., Lum, L. G., Appelbaum, F. R., Doney, K., Sullivan, K. M., Storb, R., Buckner, C. D., and Thomas, E. D., 1987, Prophylactic use of human leukocyte interferon after allogeneic marrow transplantation, *Ann. Intern. Med.* **107:**809–816.

Mihich, E., 1986, Future perspectives for biological response modifiers: A viewpoint, *Semin. Oncol.* **13:**234–254.

Misset, J. L., Mathe, G., Gastiaburu, J., Goutner, A., Dorval, T., Gouveia, J., Schwarzenberg, L., Machover, D., Ribaud, P., and de Vassal, F., 1982, Treatment of leukemias and lymphomas by interferons: II. Phase II of the trial treatment of chronic lymphoid leukemia by human interferon α^+, *Biomed. Pharmacother.* **39:**112–116.

Mitchell, L. C., Davis, L. S., and Lipsky, P., 1989, Promotion of human T lymphocyte proliferation by IL-4, *J. Immunol.* **142:**1548–1557.

Mitsuyasu, R. T., Champlin, R. E., Gale, R. P., Ho, W. G., Lenarsky, C., Winston, D., Selch, M., Elashoff, R., Giorgi, J. V., Wells, J., Terasaki, P., Billing, R., and Feig, S., 1986, Treatment of donor bone marrow with monoclonal anti-T-cell antibody and complement for the prevention of graft-versus-host disease. A prospective, randomized, double-blind trial, *Ann. Intern. Med.* **105:**20–26.

Miyajima, A., Kitamura, T., Harada, N., Yokota, T., and Arai, K. I., 1992, Cytokine receptors and signal transduction, *Annu. Rev. Immunol.* **10:**295–331.

Miyajima, A., Mui, A. L., Ogorochi, T., and Sakamaki, K., 1993, Receptors for granulocyte–macrophage colony-stimulating factor, interleukin-3, and interleukin-5, *Blood* **82:**1960–1974.

Miyaura, C., Onozaki, K., Akiyamma, Y., Taniyama, T., Hirano, T., Kishimoto, T., and Suda, T., 1988, Recombinant human interleukin-6 (B-cell stimulatory factor 2) is a potent inducer of differentiation of mouse myeloid leukemia cells (M1), *FEBS Lett.* **234:**17–21.

Moertel, C. G., 1986, On lymphokines, cytokines and breakthroughs, *J. Am. Med. Assoc.* **256:**3141.

Mohler, K. M., Torrance, D. T., Young, D. M., Callis, G., Roux, E. R., and Jacobs, C. A., 1991, Immunotherapeutic potential of soluble cytokine receptors in inflammatory disease, *FASEB Proc.* **5:**1086a.

Moormeier, J., Ratain, M., Westbrook, C., Vardiman, J., Daly, K., and Golomb, H. M., 1988, Low dose interferon in the treatment of hairy cell leukemia, *Proc. Am. Assoc. Cancer Res.* **29:**215.

Morrissey, P. J., Conlon, P., Braddy, S., Williams, D., Namen, A. E., and Mochizuki, D. Y., 1991a, Administration of IL-7 to mice with cyclophosphamide-induced lymphopenia accelerates lymphocyte repopulation, *J. Immunol.* **146:**1547–1552.

Morrissey, P. J., Conlon, P., Charrier, K., Braddy, S., Alpert, A., Williams, D., Namen, A. E., and Mochizuki, D., 1991b, Administration of IL-7 to normal mice stimulates B lymphopoiesis and peripheral lymphoadenopathy, *J. Immunol.* **147:**561–568.

Mosmann, T. R., and Moore, K. W., 1991, The role of IL-10 in crossregulation of Th1 and Th2 responses, *Immunol. Today* **12:**A49.

Mosmann, T. R., Cherwinski, H., Bond, M. W., Giedlin, M. A., and Coffman, R. L., 1986, Two types of murine helper T cell clone. I. Definition according to profiles of lymphokine activities and secreted proteins, *J. Immunol.* **136:**2348–2357.

Mule, J. J., McIntosh, J. K., Jablons, D. M., and Rosenberg, S. A., 1990, Antitumor activity of recombinant interleukin-6 in mice, *J. Exp. Med.* **171:**629–636.

Mule, J. J., Custer, M. C., Travis, W. D., and Rosenberg, S. A., 1992, Cellular mechanisms of the antitumour activity of recombinant IL-6 in mice, *J. Immunol.* **148:**2622–2629.

Mullen, C. A., Coale, M. M., Levy, A. T., Stetler-Stevenson, W. G., Liotta, L. A., Brandt, S., and Blaese, R. M., 1992, Fibrosarcoma cells transduced with the IL-6 gene exhibit reduced tumorigenic, increased immunogenicity, and decreased metastatic potential, *Cancer Res.* **52:**6020–6024.

Muss, H. B., 1987, Interferon therapy for renal cell carcinoma, *Semin. Oncol.* **14:**36–42.

Naume, B., and Espevik, T., 1991, Effects of IL-7 and IL-2 on highly enriched CD56-natural killer cells. A comparative study, *J. Immunol.* **147:**2208–2214.

Negrier, S., Ranchere, J. Y., Phillip, I., Merrouche, Y., Biron, P., Blaise, D., Attal, M., Rebattu, P., Clavel, M., Pourreau, C., Palmer, P., Favrot, M., Jasmin, C., Maraninchi, D., and Phillip, T., 1991, Intravenous interleukin-2 just after high dose BCNU and autologous bone marrow transplantation. Report of a multicentric French pilot study, *Bone Marrow Transplant.* **8:**259–264.

Nemunaitis, J., Appelbaum, F. R., Lilleby, K., Buhles, W. C., Rosenfeld, C., Zeigler, Z. R., Shadduck, R. K., Singer, J. W., Meyer, W., and Buckner, C. D., 1994, Phase I study of recombinant interleukin-1b in patients undergoing autologous bone marrow transplantation for acute myelogenous leukemia, *Blood* **83:**3474–3479.

Neta, R., Perlstein, R., Vogel, S. N., Ledney, G. D., and Abrams, J., 1992, Role of interleukin-6 (IL-6) in protection from irradiation and in endocrine responses to IL-1 and tumour necrosis factor, *J. Exp. Med.* **175:**689–694.

Neville, M. E., Pezella, K. M., Schmidt, K., Galbraith, W., and Ackerman, N., 1990, *In vivo* inhibition of tumor growth of B16 melanoma by recombinant interleukin 1 beta II. Mechanism of inhibition: The role of polymorphonuclear leukocytes, *Cytokine* **2:**456–463.

Nishioka, Y., Sone, S., Orino, E., Nii, A., and Ogura, T., 1991, Down-regulation by interleukin-4 of activation of human alveolar macrophages to the tumoricidal state, *Cancer Res.* **51:**5526–5531.

Noga, S. J., Horwitz, L., Kim, H., Laulis, M. K., and Hess, A. D., 1992, Interferon-γ potentiates the antitumor effect of cyclosporine-induced autoimmunity, *J. Hematother.* **1:**75–84.

Noguchi, M., Nakamura, Y., Russell, S. M., Ziegler, S. F., Tsang, M., Cao, X., and Leonard, W. L., 1993, Interleukin-2 receptor gamma chain: A functional component of the interleukin-7 receptor, *Science* **262:**1877–1880.

Nophar, Y., Kempter, O., Brakebusch, C., Engelmann, H., Zwang, R., Aderka, D., Holtmann, H., and Wallach, D., 1990, Soluble forms of tumor necrosis factor receptors (TNF-Rs). The cDNA for the type I TNF-R, cloned using amino acid sequence data of its soluble form, encodes both the cell surface and a soluble form of the receptor, *EMBO J.* **9:**3269–3278.

North, R. J., Neubauer, R. H., Huang, J. H., Newton, R. C., and Loveless, S. E., 1988, Interleukin-1-induced, T cell mediated regression of immunogenic murine tumors, *J. Exp. Med.* **168:**2031–2043.

O'Connell, M. J., Colgan, J. P., Oken, M. M., Ritts, R. E., Jr., Kay, N. E., and Itri, L. M., 1986, Clinical trial of recombinant leukocyte A interferon as initial therapy for favorable histology non-Hodgkin's lymphomas and chronic lymphocytic leukemia. An Eastern Cooperative Oncology Group pilot study, *J. Clin. Oncol.* **4:**128–136.

Oldham, O., Maleckar, J., West, W., and Yannelli, J., 1989, Il-2 and cellular therapy: Lymphokine-activated killer cells and tumor-derived activated cell. Cytokines in hematopoiesis malignant melanoma receiving recombinant interleukin-2, *Int. J. Cancer* **43:**410–414.

Oldham, R. K., 1982, Biological response modifiers program, *J. Biol. Resp. Mod.* **1:**81–100.

Orr, D., Oldham, R., Lewis, M., Ogden, J., Liao, S. K., Leung, K., Duperi, S., Birch, R., and Avner, B., 1989, Phase I study of the sequenced administration of etoposide (VP-16) and recombinant tumor necrosis factor (rTNF: Cetus) in patients with advanced malignancy, *Proc. Am. Soc. Clin. Oncol.* **8:**A741.

Paul, W. E., 1988, Interleukin 4/B cell stimulatory factor 1: One lymphokine, many functions, *FASEB J.* **1:**456.

Porgador, A., Tzehoval, E., Katz, A., Vadai, E., Revel, M., Feldman, M., and Eisenbach, L., 1992, Interleukin-6 gene transfection into Lewis lung carcinoma cells suppresses the malignant phenotype and confers immunotherapeutic competence against parental metastatic cells, *Cancer Res.* **52:**3679–3686.

Poutsiaka, D. D., Clark, B. D., Vannier, E., and Dinarello, C. A., 1991, Production of interleukin-1 receptor antagonist and interleukin-1b by peripheral blood mononuclear cells is differentially regulated, *Blood* **78:**1275–1281.

Quesada, J. R., Reuben, J., Manning, J. T., Hersh, E. M., and Gutterman, J. U., 1984, Alpha interferon for induction of remission in hairy-cell leukemia, *N. Engl. J. Med.* **310:**15–18.

Quesada, J. R., Rios, A., Swanson, D., Trown, P., and Gutterman, J. U., 1985, Antitumor activity of recombinant-derived interferon alpha in metastatic renal cell carcinoma, *J. Clin. Oncol.* **3:**1522–1528.

Ratanatharathorn, V., Uberti, J., Karanes, C., Lum, L. G., Abella, E., Dan, M. E., Hussein, M., and Sensenbrenner, L. L., 1994, Phase I study of alpha-interferon augmentation of cyclosporine-induced graft versus host disease in recipients of autologous bone marrow transplantation, *Bone Marrow Transplant.* **13:**625–630.

Rich, B. E., Campos-Torres, J., Tepper, R. I., Moreadith, R. W., and Leder, P., 1993, Cutaneous lymphoproliferation and lymphomas in interleukin 7 transgenic mice, *J. Exp. Med.* **177:**305–316.

Ringden, O., and Horowitz, M. M., 1989, Graft-versus-leukemia reactions in humans, *Transplant. Proc.* **21:**2989–2992.

Rios, A., Mansell, P., Newell, G. R., Reuben, J. M., Hersh, E. M., and Gutterman, J. U., 1985, Treatment of acquired immunodeficiency syndrome-related Kaposi's sarcoma with lymphoblastoid interferon, *J. Clin. Oncol.* **3:**506–512.

Rosenberg, S. A., Grimm, E., McGrogan, M., Doyle, M., Kawasaki, E., Koths, K., and Mark, D. F., 1984, Biological activity of recombinant human interleukin-2 produced in Eschericia coli, *Science* **223:**1412–1415.

Rosenberg, S. A., Lotze, M. T., Yang, J. C., Topalian, S. L., Chang, A. E., Schwartzentruben, D. J., Aebersold, P., Leitman, S., Linehan, W. M., and Seipp, C. A., 1993, Prospective randomized trial of high-dose interleukin-2 alone or in conjunction with lymphokine-activated killer cells for the treatment of patients with advanced cancer, *J. Natl. Cancer Inst.* **85:**622–632.

Rudolph, A., Krigel, R., and Zamkoff, K., 1989, Pharmacokinetics of human recombinant tumor necrosis factor (hr-TNF) in rats, monkeys, and humans, *Proc. Am. Soc. Clin. Oncol.* **8:**A757.

Russell, S. M., Keegan, A. D., Harada, N., Nakamura, Y., Noguchi, M., Leland, P., Friedmann, M. C., Miyajima, A., Puri, R. K., Paul, W. I., and Leonard, W. J., 1993, Interleukin-2 receptor gamma chain: A functional component of the interleukin-4 receptor, *Science* **262:**1880–1883.

Saito, H., Hatake, K., Dvorak, A. M., Leiferman, K. M., Dannenberg, A. D., Arai, N., Ishizaka, K., and Ishizaka, T., 1988, Selective differentiation and proliferation of hematopoietic cells induced by recombinant human interleukins, *Proc. Natl. Acad. Sci. USA* **85:**2288–2292.

Salmon, S. E., Young, L., Scuderi, P., and Clark, B., 1987, Antineoplastic effects of tumor necrosis factor alone and in combination with gamma-interferon on tumor biopsies in clonogenic assay, *J. Clin. Oncol.* **5:**1816–1821.

Samaridis, J., Casorati, G., Traunecker, A., Iglesias, A., Gutierrez, J. C., Muller, U., and Palacios, R., 1991, Development of lymphocytes in interleukin 7-transgenic mice, *Eur. J. Immunol.* **21:**453–460.

Sano, T., Saijo, N., Sasaki, Y., Shinkai, T., Eguchi, K., Tamura, T., Sakurai, M., Takahashi, H., Nakano, H., Nakagawa, K., and Hong, W. S., 1988, Three schedules of recombinant human interleukin-2 in the treatment of malignancy: Side effects and immunologic effects in relation to serum level, *Jpn. J. Cancer Res.* **79:**131–143.

Sato, N., Sakamaki, K., Terada, N., Arai, K., and Miyajima, A., 1993, Signal transduction by the high-affinity GM-CSF receptor: Two distinct cytoplasmic regions of the common beta subunit responsible for different signaling, *EMBO. J.* **12:**4181–4189.

Schall, T. J., Lewis, M., Koller, K. J., Lee, A., Rice, G. C., Wong, G. H. W., Catanaga, T., Granger, G. A., Lentz, R., Raab, H., Kohr, W. J., and Goeddel, D., 1990, Molecular cloning and expression of a receptor for human tumor necrosis factor, *Cell* **61:**361–370.

Scheid, C., Young, R., McDermott, R., Fitzsimmons, L., Scarffe, J. H., and Stern, P. L., 1994, Immune function of patients receiving recombinant human interleukin-6 (IL-6) in a phase I clinical study: Induction of C-reactive protein and IgE and inhibition of natural killer and lymphokine-activated killer cell activity, *Cancer Immunol. Immunother.* **38:**119–126.

Schiller, J. H., Storer, B. E., Witt, P. L., Alberti, D., Tombes, M. B., Arzoomanian, R., Proctor, R. A., McCarty, D., Brown, R. R., and Voss, S. D., 1991, Biological and clinical effects of intravenous tumor necrosis factor-α administered three times weekly, *Cancer Res.* **51:**1652–1658.

Schleifer, K. W., and Mansfield, J. M., 1993, Suppressor macrophages in African trypanosomiasis inhibit T cell proliferative responses by nitric oxide and prostaglandins, *J. Immunol.* **151:**5492–5503.

Schnidler, R., Mancilla, J., Endres, S., Chorbani, R., Clark, S. C., and Dinarello, C. A., 1990, Correlations and interactions in the production of interleukin-6 (IL-6), IL-1, and tumor necrosis factor (TNF) in human blood mononuclear cells: IL-6 suppresses IL-1 and TNF, *Blood* **75:**40–47.

Seckinger, P., Isaaz, S., and Dayer, J. M., 1988, A human inhibitor of tumor necrosis factor α, *J. Exp. Med.* **167:**1511–1516.

Sherman, M. L., Spriggs, D. R., Arthur, K. A., and Kufe, D. W., 1992, Enhanced myelosuppression in a phase I trial of recombinant human tumor necrosis factor in combination with etoposide, *Proc. Am. Assoc. Cancer Res.* **33:**245.

Skorski, T., Kawalec, M., Ratajczak, M., Szczyylik, C., and Kawiak, J., 1990, Return of immunohematopoietic impairment a long time after murine syngeneic bone marrow transplantation, *Bone Marrow Transplant.* **6:**315–319.

Smalley, R. V., Anderson, S. A., Tuttle, R. L., Connors, J., Thurmond, L. M., Huang, A., Castle, K., Magers, C., and Whisnant, J. K., 1991, A randomized comparison of two doses of human lymphoblastoid Interferon-α in hairy cell leukemia, *Blood* **78:**3133–3141.

Smith, J. W., Urba, W. J., Curti, B. D., Elwood, L. J., Steis, R. G., Janik, J. E., Sharfman, W. H., Miller, L. L., Fenton, R. G., and Conlon, K. C., 1992, The toxic and hematologic effects of interleukin-1 alpha administered in a phase 1 trial to patients with advanced malignancies, *J. Clin. Oncol.* **10:**1141–1152.

Smith, J. W., Longo, D. L., Alvord, W. G., Janik, J. E., Sharfman, W. H., Guase, B. L., Curti, B. D., Creekmore, S. P., Holmlund, J. T., and Fenton, R. G., 1993, The effects of treatment with interleukin-1 alpha on platelet recovery after high-dose carboplatin, *N. Engl. J. Med.* **328:**756–761.

Soiffer, R. J., Murray, C., Cochran, K., Cameron, C., Wang, E., Schow, P. W., Daley, J. F., and Ritz, J., 1992, Clinical and immunologic effects of prolonged infusion of low-dose recombinant interleukin-2 after autologous and T-cell-depleted allogeneic bone marrow transplantation, *Blood* **79:**517–526.

Sondel, P. M., Kohler, P. C., Hank, J. A., Moore, K. H., Rosenthal, N. S., Sosman, J. A., Bechhofer, R., and Storer, B., 1988, Clinical and immunological effects of recombinant interleukin-2 given by repetitive weekly cycles to patients with cancer, *Cancer Res.* **48:**2561–2567.

Sosman, J. A., Kohler, P. C., Hank, J. A., Moore, K. H., Bechhofer, R., Storer, B., and Sondel, P. M., 1988, Repetitive weekly cycles of interleukin-2. II. Clinical and immunologic effects of dose, schedule, and addition of indomethacin, *J. Natl. Cancer Inst.* **80:**1451–1461.

Sozzani, S., Zhou, D., Locati, M., Rieppi, M., Proost, P., Magazin, M., Vita, N., Van Damme, J., and Mantovani, A., 1994, Receptors and transduction pathways for monocyte chemotactic protein-2 and monocyte chemotactic protein-3, *J. Immunol.* **152:**3615–3622.

Spits, H., Yssel, H., Paliard, X., Kastelein, R., Figdor, C., and deVries, J. E., 1988, IL-4 inhibits IL-2-mediated induction of human lymphokine-activated killer cells, but not the generation of antigen-specific cytotoxic T lymphocytes in mixed leukocyte cultures, *J. Immunol.* **141:**29–36.

Stein, R. C., and Dalgleish, A. G., 1994, Immunomodulatory agents: The cytokines, *Eur. J. Cancer* **30A:**400–404.

Stern, A. S., Podlaski, F. J., Hulmes, J. D., Pan, Y. E., Quinn, P. M., Wolitzky, A. G., Familletti, P. C., Stremlo, C. L., Truitt, T., Chizzonite, R., and Gately, M. K., 1990, Purification to homogeneity and partial characterization of cytotoxic lymphocyte maturation factor from human B-lymphoblastoid cells, *Proc. Natl. Acad. Sci. USA* **87:**6808–6812.

Stevenson, H. C., Creekmore, S., Stewart, M., Conlon, K., Sznol, M., Kremers, P., Cohen, S., and Longo, D. L., 1990, Interleukin-2 and lymphokine-activated killer cell therapy: Analysis of bolus interleukin 2 and a continuous infusion interleukin 2 regimen, *Cancer Res.* **50:**7343–7350.

Subhash, C., Gautam, C. N. F., and Hamilton, T. A., 1992, Anti-inflammatory action of IL-4, *Am. Assoc. Immunol.* **148:**1411–1415.

Sugarman, B. J., Aggarwal, B. B., Hass, P. E., Figari, I. S., Palladino, M. A., Jr., and Shepard, H. M., 1985. Recombinant human tumor necrosis factor-α: Effects on proliferation of normal and transformed cells in vitro, *Science* **230:**943–945.

Sullivan, K. M., Witherspoon, R. P., Storb, R., Weiden, P., Flournoy, N., Dahlberg, S., Deeg, A. J., Sanders, J. E., Doney, K. C., Applebaum, F. R., McGuffin, R., McDonald, G. B., Meyers, J., Schubert, M. M., Gauvreau, J., Shulman, D. M., Sale, G. E., Anasetti, C., Laughman, T. P., Strom, S., Nemes, J., and Thomas, E. D., 1988, Prednisone and azathioprine compared with prednisone and placebo for treatment of chronic graft-v-host disease: Prognostic influence of prolonged thrombocytopenia after allogeneic marrow transplantation, *Blood* **72:**546–554.

Sullivan, K. M., Weiden, P. L., Storb, R., Witherspoon, R. P., Fefer, A., Fisher, L., Buckner, C. D., Anasetti, C., Applebaum, F. R., Badger, C., Bealty, P., Bensinger, W., Berenson, R., Bigelow, C., Cheever, M. A., Clift, R., Deeg, A. J., Doney, K., Greenberg, P., Hansen, J. A., Hill, R., Laughman, T., Martin, P., Neiman, P., Peterson, F. B., Sanders, J., Singer, J., Stewart, P., and Thomas, E. D., 1989, Influence of acute and chronic graft-versus-host disease on relapse and survival after bone marrow transplantation from HLA-identical siblings as treatment of acute and chronic leukemia, *Blood* **73:**1720–1728.

Sypek, J. P., Chung, C. L., Mayor, S. E. H., Subramanyam, J. M., Goldman, S. J., Sieburth, D. S., Wolf, S. F., and Schaub, R. G., 1993, Resolution of cutaneous leishmaniasis: Interleukin 12 initiates a protective T helper type 1 immune response, *J. Exp. Med.* **177:**1797–1802.

Takai, S., Yamada, K., Hirayama, N., Miyajima, A., and Taniyama, T., 1994, Mapping of the human gene encoding the mutual signal-transducing subunit (beta-chain) of granulocyte–macrophage colony-stimulating factor (GM-CSF), interleukin-3 (IL-3), and interleukin-5 (IL-5) receptor complexes to chromosome 22q13.1, *Hum. Genet.* **93:**198–200.

Talmadge, J. E., and Herberman, R. B., 1986, The preclinical screening laboratory. Evaluation of immunomodulatory and therapeutic properties of biological response modifiers, *Cancer Treat. Res.* **70:**171–182.

Talmadge, J. E., Tribble, H. R., Pennington, R. W., Phillips, H., and Wiltrout, R. H., 1987a, Immunomodulatory and immunotherapeutic properties of recombinant γ-interferon and recombinant tumor necrosis factor in mice, *Cancer Res.* **47:**2563–2570.

Talmadge, J. E., Phillips, H., Schindler, J., Tribble, H., and Pennington, R., 1987b. Systematic preclinical study on the therapeutic properties of recombinant human interleukin-2 for the treatment of metastatic disease, *Cancer Res.* **47:**5725–5732.

Talpaz, M., Kantarjian, H. M., McCredie, K., Trujillo, J. M., Keating, M. J., and Gutterman, J. V., 1986, Hematologic remission and cytogenic improvement induced by recombinant human interferon alpha A in chronic myelogenous leukemia, *N. Engl. J. Med.* **314:**1065–1069.

Tannock, I. F., Boyd, N. F., DeBoer, G., Erlichman, C., Fine, S., Larocque, G., Mayers, C., Perrault, D., and Sutherland, H., 1988, A randomized trial of two dose levels of cyclophosphamide, methotrexate, and fluorouracil chemotherapy for patients with metastatic breast cancer, *J. Clin. Oncol.* **6:**1377–1387.

Teichmann, J. V., Sieber, G., Ludwig, W. D., and Ruehl, H., 1988, Modulation of immune functions by long-term treatment with recombinant interferon-α2 in a patient with hairy-cell leukemia, *J. Interferon Res.* **8:**15–24.

Tepper, R. I., Pattengale, P. K., and Leder, P., 1989, Murine interleukin-4 displays potent anti-tumor activity in vivo, *Cell* **57:**503–512.

Te Velde, A. A., Yard, B. A., Klomp, J. P. G., de Vries, J. E., and Figdor, C. G., 1988, Modulation of phenotypic and functional properties on human peripheral blood monocytes by interleukin-4 (IL-4), *J. Immunol.* **140:**1548–1554.

Te Velde, A. A., Huijbens, R. J. F., Heije, K., de Vries, J. E., and Figdor, C. G., 1990, Interleukin-4 (IL-4) inhibits secretion of IL-1B, TNF alpha, and IL-6 by human monocytes, *Blood* **76:**1392–1397.

Thompson, J. A., Lee, D. J., Lindgren, C. G., Benz, L. A., Collins, C., Levitt, D., and Fefer, A., 1988, Influence of dose and duration of infusion of interleukin-2 on toxicity and immunomodulation. *J. Clin. Oncol.* **6:**669–678.

Thompson, J. A., Shulman, K. L., Benyunes, M. C., Lindgren, G., Collins, C., Lange, P. H., Bush, W. H., Jr., Benz, L. A., and Fefer, A., 1992, Prolonged continuous intravenous infusion interleukin-2 and lymphokine-activated killer-cell therapy for metastatic renal cell carcinoma, *J. Clin. Oncol.* **10:** 960–968.

Tilg, H., Mier, J. W., Vogel, W., Aulitzky, W. E., Wiedermann, C. J., Vannier, E., Huber, C., and Dinarello, C. A., 1993, Induction of circulating IL-1 receptor antagonist by IFN treatment, *J. Immunol.* **150:**4687–4692.

Tilg, H., Shapiro, L., Vannier, E., Poutsiaka, D. D., Trehu, E., Atkins, M. B., Dinarello, C. A., and Mier, J. W., 1994a, Induction of circulating IL-1 and TNF antagonists by IL-2 administration and their effects on IL-2-induced cytokine production in vitro, *J. Immunol.* **152:**3189–3198.

Tilg, H., Trehu, E., Atkins, M. B., Dinarello, C. A., and Mier, J. W., 1994b, Interleukin-6 (IL-6) as an anti-inflammatory cytokine: Induction of circulating IL-1 receptor antagonist and soluble tumor necrosis factor receptor p55, *Blood* **83:**113–118.

Tomlinson, E., 1989, Site-specific drugs and delivery systems: Toxicological and regulatory implications, in: *Topics in Pharmaceutical Sciences* (D. D. Breimer, D. J. A. Crommelin, and K. K. Midha, eds.), Federation International Pharmaceutic, The Hague, pp. 661–671.

Tomlinson, E., 1991, Site-specific proteins, in: *Polypeptide and Protein Drugs: Production, Characterization and Formulation* (R.C. Hider and D. Barlow, eds.), Ellis Horwood, Chichester, pp. 251–364.

Torti, F. M., Shortliffe, L. D., Williams, R. D., Pitts, W. C., Kempson, R. L., Ross, J. C., Palmer, J., Meyers, F., Ferrari, M., Hannigan, J., Spiegel, R., McWhirter, K., and Freiha, F., 1988, Alpha-interferon in superficial bladder cancer: A Northern California Oncology Group Study, *J. Clin. Oncol.* **6:**476–483.

Turner, M., Chantry, D., Katsikis, P., Berger, A., Brennan, F. M., and Feldmann, M., 1991, Induction of the interleukin-1 receptor antagonist protein by transforming growth factor-β, *Eur. J. Immunol.* **21:**1635–1639.

Ulich, T. R., Yin, S., Guo, K., Yi, E. S., Remick, D., and del Castillo, J., 1991, Intratracheal injection of endotoxin and cytokines. II. Interleukin-6 and transforming growth factor beta inhibit acute inflammation, *Am. J. Pathol.* **138:**1097–1101.

Vadhan-Raj, S., Kudelka, A. P., Garrison, L., Gano, J., Edwards, C. L., Freedman, R. S., and Kavanagh, J. J., 1994, Effects of interleukin-1a on carboplatin-induced thrombocytopenia in patients with recurrent ovarian cancer, *J. Clin. Oncol.* **12:**707–714.

Vannier, E., Miller, L. C., and Dinarello, C. A., 1992, Coordinated anti-inflammatory effects of interleukin-4: Interleukin-4 suppresses interleukin-1 production but up-regulates gene expression and synthesis of interleukin-1 receptor antagonist, *Proc. Natl. Acad. Sci. USA* **89:**4076–4080.

Vlasveld, L. T., Rankin, E. M., Hekman, A., Rodenhuis, S., Beijnen, J. H., Hilton, A. M., Dubbelman, A. C., Vyth-Dreese, F. A., and Melief, C. J. M., 1992, A phase I study of prolonged continuous infusion of low dose recombinant interleukin-2 in melanoma and renal cell cancer. Part I: Clinical aspects, *Br. J. Cancer* **65:**744–750.

Vlasveld, L. T., Hekman, A., Vyth-Dreese, F. A., Rankin, E. M., Scharenberg, J. G. M., Voordouw, A. C., Sein, J. J., Dellemijn, T. A. M., Rodenhuis, S., and Melief, C. J. M., 1993, A phase I study of prolonged continuous infusion of low dose recombinant interleukin-2 melanoma and renal cell cancer. Part II: Immunological aspects, *Br. J. Cancer* **68:**559–567.

Vose, J. M., Anderson, J. R., Kessinger, A., Biermann, P. J., Coccia, P., Reed, E. D., Gordon, B., and Armitage, J. O., 1993, High-dose chemotherapy and autologous hematopoietic stem cell transplantation for aggressive non-Hodgkin's lymphoma, *J. Clin. Oncol.* **11:**1846–1851.

Voss, S. D., Hong, R., and Sondel, P. M., 1994, Severe combined immunodeficiency, interleukin-2 (IL-2), and the IL-2 receptor: Experiments of nature continue to point the way, *Science* **83:**626–635.

Walsh, C. E., Liu, J. M., Anderson, S. M., Rossio, J. L., Niehuis, A. W., Young, N. S., 1992, A trial of recombinant human interleukin-1 in patients with severe refractory aplastic anaemia, *Br. J. Haematol.* **80:**106–110.

Weber, J., Yang, J. C., Topalian, S. L., Parkinson, D. R., Schwartzentruber, D. S., Ettinghausen, S. E., Gunn, H., Mixon, A., Kim, H., and Cole, D., 1993, Phase 1 trial of subcutaneous interleukin-6 in patients with advanced malignancies, *J. Clin. Oncol.* **11:**499–506.

Weiden, P. L., Flournoy, N., Thomas, E. D., Prentice, R., Fefer, A., Buckner, C. D., and Storb, R., 1979, Antileukemic effect of graft-versus-host disease in human recipients of allogeneic-marrow grafts, *N. Engl. J. Med.* **300:**1068–1073.

Weiden, P. L., Sulbran, K. M., Fluornoy, N., Storb, R., and Thomas, E. D., 1981, Antileukemic effect of chronic graft-versus-host disease: Contribution to improved survival after allogeneic marrow transplantation, *N. Engl. J. Med.* **304:**1529–1533.

Welch, N. S., Tullai, J., Guido, E., McMahon, M., Jolliffe, L. K., Lopez, A. F., Vadas, M. A., Lowry, P. A., Quesenberry, P. J., and Rosen, J., 1993, Interleukin-3/erythropoietin fusion proteins: In vitro effects on hematopoietic cells, *Exp. Hematol.* **21:**647–655.

Welch, P. A., Namen, A. E., Goodwin, R. G., Armitage, R., and Cooper, M. D., 1989, Human IL-7: A novel T cell growth factor, *J. Immunol.* **143:**3562–3567.

West, W. H., Tauer, K. W., Yannelli, J. R., Marshall, G. D., Orr, D. W., Thurman, G. B., and Oldham, R. K., 1987, Constant-infusion recombinant interleukin-2 plus lymphokine-activated killer cells in metastatic renal cancer, *N. Engl. J. Med.* **316:**898–905.

Widmer, M. D., Acres, R. B., Sassenfeld, H. M., and Grabstein, K. H., 1987, Regulation of stimulatory factor 1 (interleukin 4), *J. Exp. Med.* **166:**1447–1451.

Williams, D. E., Broxmeyer, H. E., Curtis, B. M., Dunn, J., Price, V., Craig, V., March, C. J., Cosman, D., and Park, L. S., 1990, Enhanced biological activity of a human GM-CSF/Il-3 fusion protein (abstract), *Exp. Hematol.* **18:**615.

Wolf, S. F., Temple, P. A., Kobayashi, M., Young, D., Dicig, M., Lowe, L., Dzialo, R., Fitz, L., Ferenz, C., Hewick, R. M., Kelleher, K., Herrmann, S. H., Clark, S. C., Azzoni, L., Chan, S. H., Trinchieri, G., and Perussia, B., 1991, Cloning of cDNA for natural killer cell stimulatory factor, a heterodimeric cytokine with multiple biologic effects on T and natural killer cells, *J. Immunol.* **146:**3074–3081.

Wolf, S. F., Sicburth, D., and Sypek, J., 1994, Interleukin 12: A key modulator of immune function, *Stem Cells* **12:**154–168.

Woodman, R. C., Richard, W., Rae, J., Jaffe, H. S., and Curnutte, J. T., 1992, Prolonged recombinant interferon-γ therapy in chronic granulomatous disease: Evidence against enhanced neutrophil oxidase activity, *Blood* **79:**1558–1562.

Yeager, A. M., Vogelsang, G. B., Jones, R. J., Farmer, E. R., Altomonte, V., Hess, A. D., and Santos, G. W., 1992, Induction of cutaneous graft-versus-host disease by administration of cyclosporine to patients undergoing autologous bone marrow transplantation for acute myeloid leukemia, *Blood* **79:**3031–3035.

CHAPTER 4

IMMUNOPHARMACOLOGY OF ANTICANCER AGENTS

M. JANE EHRKE and ENRICO MIHICH

1. INTRODUCTION

The initial attempts to alter the progression of neoplastic diseases in patients with certain types of cancer through the application of maximally tolerated doses of cytotoxic agents took place 40 to 50 years ago. Since that time impressive successes have been achieved in a number of malignancies. Nevertheless, there remain frequently occurring neoplasms for which there is no curative treatment. The failures are related mainly to the fact that the agents available to date are not sufficiently selective in their antitumor action; therefore, even a relatively small degree of natural or acquired resistance cannot be overcome by dose escalation without incurring unacceptable toxicity. Although the search for new cytotoxic agents with improved antitumor selectivity is continuing, alternative therapeutic approaches are also being aggressively sought in several different directions. As an example, the increasing knowledge of the molecular mechanisms regulating the cancer cell provides new sites for which it should be possible to rationally design new agents with unique anticancer specificities. Likewise, based on information about the interactions between tumor and host, approaches that exploit both the immunological and the nonimmunological phenomena involved in these interactions are being tested. This chapter is concerned with the possibility of exploiting antitumor host defenses of the immunological type

M. JANE EHRKE and ENRICO MIHICH • Grace Cancer Drug Center, Roswell Park Cancer Institute, Buffalo, New York 14263.

Immunopharmacology Reviews, Volume 2, edited by John W. Hadden and Andor Szentivanyi. Plenum Press, New York, 1996.

through the action of anticancer agents capable of inducing therapeutically favorable immunomodulation.

The successful development of immunochemotherapy requires that certain tenets of chemotherapy be reexamined. Thus, if a functioning host antitumor response is to be an integrated component of an overall therapeutic design, the inclusion during immunochemotherapy of maximally tolerated doses of chemotherapeutic agents, whose dose limiting toxicities often include bone marrow suppression, must be carefully weighed. Similarly, patients with advanced disease who have disease-related severe immunosuppression most likely would require therapeutic designs different from those effective in less (or non) immunodepressed patients. The therapeutic exploitation of host defenses introduces several new layers of complexity/opportunity for the development of effective regimens. For example, the complex interactive circuitry of cells and soluble factors comprising the mechanism of immune response offers multiple sites for possible immunopharmacological intervention. Conversely, an attempt to manipulate toward therapeutic advantage one component of this complex interactive circuitry may initiate other changes in the system leading to undesired effects. Careful attention must also be paid to the, as yet incompletely studied, pharmacological determinants of drug selectivity within the myeloid and/or lymphoid cell populations and to specific drug interactions within these populations. Using only a few examples to illustrate and discuss each point, an attempt is made in this chapter to focus attention on concepts illustrating the exciting potential of immunochemotherapeutic approaches in the treatment of neoplastic disease. The experimental examples cited are drawn in large part, but not exclusively, from our laboratory experience.

2. SITES OF IMMUNOPHARMACOLOGICAL INTERVENTION BASED ON THE MECHANISMS OF THE IMMUNE RESPONSE

The explosion over the past decade of knowledge on the mechanisms of immune responses has expanded enormously the understanding of this complex system and has provided multiple opportunities for therapeutic intervention. Although exciting work is under way investigating many new approaches in immunotherapy, such as the utilization of specific cytokines as immune mediators or effectors, the customizing of monoclonal antibodies to improve their utilization (Waldmann, 1992; Burton and Barbas, 1994), and immunization with specific 8- to 12-mer peptides derived from a known antigenic structure and selected to maximize insertion and retention in the peptide groove of the MHC molecule (Engelhard, 1994; Boon *et al.* 1994), these and other approaches are not discussed herein. Two examples of T-cell maturation and differentiation have been chosen for brief consideration within this chapter to highlight the potential for therapeutic intervention provided by such advances in mechanistic understanding. The two examples are (1) the maturation of MHC-restricted T cells and (2) the specific development of T-helper cell subsets.

2.1. Maturation of MHC-Restricted T Cells

The multistep process of intrathymic/extrathymic maturation of T cells into exquisitely specific, MHC restricted, self-tolerant effector cells has received a great deal of attention in the last two decades (Robey and Fowlkes, 1994). Steps critical to T-cell maturation can be summarized as follows: (1) production of a functional multicomponent T-cell receptor; (2) acquisition of class specificity (i.e., CD4 or CD8); (3) elimination of self-reactive cells; (4) acquisition of antigen specificity. Each step may involve multiple phenomena. Certainly that is true for the first step, since this involves rearrangement of the alpha and beta chains' V genes, production of and insertion of the gene products into the plasma membrane, and completion of links with intracellular signaling mechanisms (Robey and Fowlkes, 1994). Although several questions remain about the order and locations of many of the steps involved in deriving the repertoire of mature circulating T cells (see Matzinger, 1993, 1994; Robey and Fowlkes, 1994), ~90% of the cells generated within the thymus are eliminated during the maturational process prior to the exiting of the selected cells into the peripheral circulation (McPhee *et al.*, 1979). Thus, it would seem that there must be a number of rigorous checkpoints to ensure that each cell has appropriately accomplished each step. Tolerization (i.e., deletion and/or anergy) of self-peptide/MHC-reactive cells appears to occur not only in the thymus, but also (albeit to a lesser extent) in the periphery (Hammerling *et al.*, 1993; see also Matzinger, 1994). In large part, the cells designated for elimination receive signals that cause them to undergo apoptosis, a morphologically defined form of programmed cell death. The cells surviving all selection checkpoints enter the peripheral circulation and have the capacity to respond not only to self MHC/peptide complexes but also to allogeneic MHC alleles [i.e., alloreactive and antigen-reactive (self MHC-restricted) cells are now thought to be the same (Matzinger, 1993)]. Regardless of which antigens they respond to, they maintain their specificity for the class of MHC they had been programmed to recognize during maturation.

Even based only on the brief outline given above, it is clear that T cells undergoing maturational steps would make up a rather large array of biochemically/phenotypically distinguishable subsets. In support of this, changes in the expression of certain plasma membrane markers identify specific stages in the maturational sequence [i.e., from most immature to most mature (for more details see Matzinger, 1993; Robey and Fowlkes, 1994)], namely: $CD3^-,4^-,8^-,44^+$ (bone marrow T-cell precursors and early thymic immigrants) $\Rightarrow$ $CD3^-,4^-,8^-,44^-$ (medullar immature T cells) $\Rightarrow$ $CD3^-,4^+,8^+,44^-$ (cortical T cells) $\Rightarrow$ $CD3^{lo},4^+,8^+,44^-$ (cortical T cells) $\Rightarrow$ $CD3^{hi},4^+,8^-,44^-$ or $CD3^{hi},4^-,8^+,44^-$ (both thymic medullar and splenic T cells) $\Rightarrow$ $CD3^{hi},4^+,8^-,44^+$ or $CD3^{hi},4^-,8^+,44^+$ (both thymic medullar and splenic T cells). It is reasonable to predict that each subset might be uniquely sensitive/resistant to a specific agent.

Experimentation carried out recently demonstrated that, in fact, Adriamycin (ADM; doxorubicin) and cyclosporin A selectively delete distinct subsets of thymocytes (Zaleskis *et al.*, 1994b, 1995). In preliminary experiments it was shown that up to 40% of thymocytes exposed to 500 nM ADM for 24 hr in culture underwent apoptosis versus 12% of those in control cultures or 70% of those in cultures exposed to 100 nM dexamethasone (used as a positive control). At concentrations one log higher or one log lower, ADM did not have this effect. The cells shown to be decreased in the populations exposed to either ADM (500 nM) or dexamethasone had the $CD4^+,8^+$ phenotype. No differences were detected in the amount of ADM associated with/taken up by different thymocytes. Flow cytometric analysis showed that following administration of ADM (5 or 10 mg/kg, i.v., Day −5) to mice, as well as following *in vitro* exposure to ADM (500 nM, 24 hr), the $CD4^+,8^+$ subset in the thymus population was reduced; *in vivo* this subset was reduced from representing ~80% of the thymic population from the control mice (2×10^8 thymocytes) to ~0.5% of the population from the treated mice. Nevertheless, cells undergoing apoptosis were not detected in fresh cell preparations from the ADM-treated mice; this may be related to rapid elimination of apoptotic cells *in vivo* by phagocytes (Boyd and Hugo, 1991). In support of this possibility, thymocytes obtained 48 hr after ADM injection and then cultured for an additional 48 hr showed significantly higher levels of apoptosis than cultured thymocytes from untreated mice. Cyclosporin A treatment (20 mg/kg in olive oil, i.p., every other day for 3 weeks, i.e., a cumulative dose of 220 mg/kg in a total of 11 injections) resulted in decreased numbers of single positive $CD4^+,8^-$ (from 1.5×10^7 in controls to 0.13×10^7 in treated mice) or $CD4^-,8^+$ (from 0.9×10^7 in controls to 0.4×10^7) cells per mouse, with little or no effect on the numbers of double positive $CD4^+,8^+$ or double negative $CD4^-,8^-$ cells. The relative frequencies of thymocyte subpopulations from mice receiving the vehicle, olive oil, alone were essentially the same as those from naive control mice. Thus, there was no injection stress-induced depletion of even the most glucocorticoid-sensitive $CD4^+,8^+$ population.

From the results mentioned above, it is clear that cyclosporin A and ADM have contrasting effects on the cells of the mouse thymus. These effects led to an overall decrease of the $CD4^+/CD8^+$ ratio with cells taken from the thymus of cyclosporin A-treated mice and an increase of that ratio with cells from ADM-treated mice. In fact, the $CD3^-,4^+,8^+$ and $CD3^{lo},4^+,8^+$ populations were most susceptible to ADM and the $CD3^+,4^+,8^-$ cells were most susceptible to cyclosporin. One major exception to the inverse relationship of thymocyte sensitivity to the two agents was that neither cyclosporin A nor ADM affected $CD3^+,4^-,8^-$(TCR$\gamma\delta$) cells. There are fundamental differences between the development of TCR$\gamma\delta$ and TCR$\alpha\beta$ T subsets in the thymus. In contrast to TCR$\alpha\beta$ cells, the TCR$\gamma\delta$ subset apparently undergoes MHC selection extrathymically (Itohara *et al.*, 1993; Allison, 1993). Therefore, at the stage that this cell subset is phenotypically identifiable, it is destined to leave the thymus without further selection, which apparently occurs in the periphery. It is possible that at the point of leaving the thymus, these cells are relatively insensitive to signals inducing programmed cell death; a mechanism apparently operating in the ADM-induced selective deletion. Similarly, cyclosporin A is known to impair TCR/MHC interactions (Jenkins *et al.*, 1988); subsets bearing the TCR$\alpha\beta$ which fail to interact with self MHC intrathymically are eliminated/tolerized. However, TCR$\gamma\delta$ subsets are not subjected to this selection within the thymus and would not be affected by cyclosporin A-induced inhibition.

As will be discussed extensively later in this chapter, ADM has the capacity to modulate many host defense systems. In fact, it has been reported recently that ADM in combination with prolonged administration of IL-2 is a safe and effective immunomodulation-dependent therapeutic regimen for the treatment of ADM-resistant EL4 lymphoma in syngeneic C57BL/6 mice, yielding up to 80% long-term survivors (Ho *et al.*, 1993a,b). In fact, the efficacy of this treatment was shown to be completely dependent on the presence of functioning specific anti-EL4 CD8$^+$ T-cell effectors. It is tempting to speculate that ADM-induced depletion of double positive thymic cells results in the influx of new precursors, yielding an enlarged pool of cells potentially capable of reacting to the tumor-associated antigens during their maturational steps. This influx of potentially antigen-responsive precursors together with the prolonged administration of IL-2 may then result in the aggressive, prolonged anti-EL4 response shown to be responsible for the eradication of established tumor.

2.2. Development of Specific T-Helper Cell Subsets

The second example of a site of potential immunopharmacological intervention is the differentiation of T-helper subsets. The development of an effective, specific immune reactivity capable of controlling or eliminating the source of a foreign antigen always involves the production of either a cell-mediated or a humoral immune response. It has long been recognized that, in general, when a strong humoral response is elicited, little or no cellular response is seen and vice versa. Only very recently was it realized that this is determined, at least in part, by the nature of the CD4$^+$ T cells that develop after antigen recognition. It is now known that, subsequent to interaction with antigen, T-helper cells having distinct cytokine production/release profiles develop and that their function is determined by the repertoire of their cytokines (Mosmann and Coffman, 1989). The two subsets of cells that have been most extensively characterized are those called T_H1 and T_H2. It is currently thought that they arise from a common naive CD4$^+$ cell which produces only IL-2 on stimulation. T_H1 and T_H2 both apparently produce GM-CSF, IL-3, and TNF-α but are characterized by the panel of cytokines each uniquely produces. Thus, the T_H1 cells, which play a critical role in cellular responses, produce IFN-γ, IL-2, and TNF-β and the T_H2 cells, which mediate humoral responses, produce IL-4, 5, 6, and 10. There are activated CD4$^+$ cells which do not fall into either of these designations; in fact, CD4$^+$ clones that secrete other sets of cytokines appear rather frequently (Fitch *et al.*, 1993).

The accumulated evidence suggests that the secreted cytokines, the antigen-presenting cell type, and the antigen dose all contribute to the regulation of the differentiation and functional maturation of the T-helper cells (Mosmann and Coffman, 1989; O'Garra and Murphy, 1994). Thus, the presence of either IL-4 or 10 supports the generation of T_H2 cells and suppresses the development of T_H1. IFN-γ inhibits the development of T_H2 cells and the presence of IFN-γ + IL-2 is required, but is not sufficient (i.e., other factors are needed), to support the generation of T_H1 cells. In at least some systems IL-12 appears to be the other required factor promoting the development of T_H1 cells (O'Garra and Murphy, 1994). There are pathological conditions that respond best to humoral immune responses and others that are most responsive to cell-mediated responses. A recent report (Afonso *et al.*, 1994) has demonstrated the dramatic effect on disease outcome (*Leishmania major* infection of BALB/c mice) that can result from inducing T_H1 rather than T_H2 differentiation by adding IL-12 into an otherwise ineffective vaccine consisting of soluble leishmanial antigen.

That immunotherapeutic strategies involving the manipulation of T_H1 versus T_H2 differentiation may have antineoplastic potential is suggested by the following examples from relatively recent reports. Katz *et al.* (1989) demonstrated that, in the reticulum cell sarcoma–SJL/J mouse model, $CD4^+$ $V\beta17a^+$ T cells are essential to disease progession in vivo and monoclonal antibody-mediated elimination of $V\beta17a^+$ T cells completely inhibited tumor growth. These authors interpret their findings to indicate that the requisite $CD4^+$ T cells are providing a factor or factors necessary to sustain tumor growth; however, it seems equally plausible that the $CD4^+$ subset induced by the tumor actually suppresses the development of an antitumor immune response. North and Awwad (1990) actually demonstrated that this was the case in the L5178Y lymphoma–B6D2F1 mouse model. Thus, they found that the selective elimination of tumor-induced $CD4^+$ cells by a single injection of vinblastine (VLB) resulted in complete regression of advanced tumors. The tumor regression was dependent on the antitumor function of $CD8^+$ T cells and could be prevented by infusing VLB-sensitive $CD4^+$ T cells from a nontreated tumor-bearing donor. Mokyr and co-workers have demonstrated the importance of $TCR^-V\beta8^+$ $CD8^+$ T cells for tumor eradication following a low dose of melphalan in the MOPC-315–BALB/c mouse model (Mokyr *et al.*, 1993). Based on these findings they recently examined whether staphylococcal enterotoxin B, known to activate $TCR^-V\beta8^+$ T cells, could be exploited to improve the cure rate in the above model (Rubin *et al.*, 1994). It was found that staphylococcal enterotoxin B enhanced anti-MOPC-315 activity and, although this could occur through promoting the differentiation and/or the expansion of an effector cell population, the authors suggest that an alternative/additional mechanism might be through the inactivation/deletion of a subset of T cells that impairs the immune response to the tumor. Thus, it is known that $CD4^+$ T cells having downregulatory activity for anti-MOPC-315 CTL do occur (Mokyr *et al.*, 1993) and that staphylococcal enterotoxin B treatment can induce anergy of $V\beta8^+$ $CD4^+$ T cells (Rubin *et al.*, 1994). Yamamura *et al.* (1993) carried out PCR on mRNA derived from biopsy specimens of basal cell carcinoma and of seborrheic keratosis to characterize distinct patterns of local cytokine production in the two diseases. The mRNAs coding for IL-4, 5, and 10 and GM-CSF were strongly expressed in basal cell carcinoma and weakly in seborrheic keratosis lesions. Conversely, IL-2, IFN-γ, and lymphotoxin mRNAs were strongly expressed in seborrheic keratosis and weakly in basal cell carcinoma lesions. Thus, the local cytokine response associated with the malignant growth was T_H2-like and that associated with the benign growth was T_H1-like. The possibility that altered local cytokine production may contribute to the pathogenesis of cancer is suggested when, as these authors point out, their findings are considered together with the fact that, although Langerhans cells of the epidermis can present antigen to both T_H1 and T_H2 cells, following UV irradiation they preferentially activate only $CD4^+$ cells of the T_H2 type (Simon *et al.*, 1990).

These few examples indicate how the increase in our understanding of T cell maturation and differentiation provides exciting new sites for possible immunopharmacological intervention. Similar opportunities can be identified in multiple other areas of the host antitumor system in which our understanding of the mechanisms involved, also, are undergoing rapid expansion. The challenge now is to find ways to exploit these opportunities to therapeutic advantage; as indicated by the examples cited below, anticancer chemotherapeutic agents may prove to be useful in this respect.

3. CHEMOTHERAPEUTIC AGENT-INDUCED IMMUNOMODULATION

As alluded to above, in the immune system each cell type and function is likely to exhibit unique biochemical characteristics. Considering the knowledge acquired on the biochemical pharmacological basis of the selectivity of antitumor action of anticancer drugs, it is reasonable to postulate that some of these agents can exert immunomodulating effects based on specific interactions with biochemical determinants unique for a given target cell. Thus, selectivity of action on only certain cell types, or on cells at only certain stages of functional development, would be predicted. Such interactions can induce positive modulations which alter the balance between tumor and host to favor the host, with consequent tumor regression.

In order to design optimal treatments, questions must be asked for each tumor and for each stage of tumor progression. These questions include: which drug to use; how much to apply to interfere positively with the dynamics of the tumor–host relationship; and when to apply an agent during the evolution of the tumor–host interaction in order to have the desired effect. The large majority of the information available on the immunomodulating effects of anticancer drugs (Braun and Harris, 1981; Mihich and Ehrke, 1991) was acquired prior to and/or concurrent with the enormous acquisition of knowledge in virtually every aspect of immunology; therefore, certain findings need to be verified and/or extended in light of current information. Nevertheless, there is a large amount of data available on the interactions of anticancer agents with host anticancer responses.

Most of the anticancer chemotherapeutic agents known to date are generally considered to exert their effects through antiproliferative and cytotoxic actions. When used at maximally tolerated doses, many of these agents were shown to be immunosuppressive, probably as a consequence of actions involving the very mechanisms responsible for the antitumor effects. Therefore, it was assumed that their effects would be immunologically nonspecific in nature. This perception has persisted despite the fact that in the mid to late 1960s, it was documented that anticancer agents can augment immune responses and not just cause immunosuppression (Mihich, 1969, 1971). Those results as well as those obtained in the intervening years have been discussed in a number of reviews (e.g., Ehrke and Mihich, 1985; Ehrke *et al.*, 1989; Mihich and Ehrke, 1991).

Principles derived from previous studies established that the effects seen with any given chemotherapeutic agent are dependent on a number of variables which can be summarized as follows: (1) the timing of the drug administration with respect to antigenic stimulus, (2) the dose of drug used, (3) the dose of antigen, (4) the nature of the antigenic challenge (e.g., the route of administration, use of adjuvants, type of antigen), (5) the timing of response assessment relative to antigenic stimulus, and (6) the nature of the immune response assayed. Those studies established that certain anticancer drugs can cause therapeutically exploitable immunomodulations in experimental model systems, and provided initial suggestions that analogous phenomena may occur in humans. The reader is referred to the earlier reviews (Ehrke and Mihich, 1985; Ehrke *et al.*, 1989; Mihich and Ehrke, 1991) for detailed accounts of studies reported before 1989. The large majority of those studies were carried out with single agents and, despite the demonstration of significant positive modulation of host antitumor responses, in most cases where immunomodulating doses of a single agent were tested in syngeneic mouse/tumor models, significant long-term antitumor effects (i.e., "cures") were not obtained. This, however, should not be too surprising based on the experience gained in the development of effective chemotherapy. With very few exceptions, effective chemotherapy involves combinations of agents that alone have limited effects. Recently, increased attention has been given to combination chemoimmunotherapy studies. The findings derived from some of these recent studies will be reviewed here.

The two chemotherapeutic agents that have been most extensively studied as single agents in terms of their capacity to induce immunomodulation are cyclophosphamide (CY) and ADM; these studies have been reviewed recently (Ehrke *et al.*, 1989; Mihich and Ehrke, 1991). In summary, the immunomodulating effects reported to be induced by ADM include: stimulation of CTL responses; stimulation of LAK cell generation with cells from tumor bearers; inhibition of T regulatory cells; stimulation of monocyte/macrophage differentiation; inhibition of splenic NK cells; stimulation of NK cells within the PEC population; stimulation of IL-1 and 2 production; and stimulation of TNF and PGE_2 production. Those reported for CY seem to be almost exclusively linked to the ability of this agent to selectively inhibit T-suppressor cell development perhaps by elimination of precursor cells and/or of the helper/inducer cells needed for their maturation. This interference with immune regulation has been shown to lead to potentiation of humoral and cellular immunity to new antigens and/or a breach of natural and acquired tolerance. At least in part based on the fact that their immunomodulating properties had been most extensively characterized, these two agents have been used in the majority of the studies combining chemotherapeutic agents and other immunomodulators. Results obtained with these two agents are discussed first and then studies are summarized involving a number of other agents including: melphalan, vinca alkaloids, taxol, platinum compounds, fluoropyrimidines, mitomycin C, and nitrosoureas.

3.1. Adriamycin

The immunomodulation induced by ADM was studied extensively in nontumor systems and only recently has a comprehensive report on its effects on host defenses in a syngeneic tumor/mouse model been published (Maccubbin *et al.*, 1992; Ho *et al.*, 1993a,b). The model system used in this study was the EL4 T-cell lymphoma in syngeneic C57BL/6 mice. This model is a rigorous one because the EL4 line used is extremely aggressive and not overtly immunogenic. Immune-mediated effects on tumor growth, therefore, are difficult to demonstrate. In fact, the inoculation of as few as ten cells results in 100% mortality. Further evidence of the weak immunogenicity of this EL4 line is shown by the fact that a syngeneic CTL response can be generated only with spleen cells from EL4 tumor-bearing animals (i.e., cells primed *in vivo*) following restimulation in culture with x-irradiated EL4 and only when these cultures are supplemented with a low concentration of IL2 (Maccubbin *et al.*, 1989). In addition to its lack of immunogenicity, it was shown that all of the cell-mediated antitumor defense functions examined were inhibited as tumor growth progressed and that the inhibition of these various functions was the consequence of effects of tumor (Maccubbin *et al.*, 1989). The immunomodulating effects induced by ADM in C57BL/6 mice bearing EL4 tumor were compared to those induced in C57BL/6 mice bearing an ADM-resistant variant of EL4, EL4/ADM (Maccubbin *et al.*, 1992). EL4/ADM was developed *in vivo* and is approximately 10-fold more resistant to ADM than the parental EL4 (Ujházy *et al.*, 1990). The doses of ADM tested were 2, 4, and 6 mg/kg, administered i.v. on Days 1 and 8 after tumor inoculation. These doses and schedule were selected for the following reasons. First, they are within the reported therapeutic range for ADM in mice but are not curative in the EL4–C57BL/6 model. Second, higher doses of ADM resulted in apparently "cured" 60-day survivors; however, (1) by 120 days up to 70% of these mice had died of delayed drug toxicity, (2) the survivors at 60 days did not have detectable specific anti-EL4 immunity, and (3) under these conditions ADM has little effect on the progression of disease in EL4/ADM-bearing mice. Third, earlier studies had suggested that, if multiple injections of ADM were to be given, a 7-day interval might be advantageous and ADM administration once every 7 days is a clinically used schedule.

Spleen cells from the ADM-treated EL4- or EL4/ADM-tumor-bearing mice were compared with those from untreated control tumor-bearing mice in terms of their ability to respond to appropriate stimuli and develop a panel of different tumoricidal effector cells. Evaluations were carried out at different times between Days 10 and 23.

The tumoricidal effector functions assessed included specific anti-EL4 CTLs, LAKs, splenic macrophages, and peritoneal macrophages. The results from this study (Maccubbin *et al.*, 1992) established that the administration of ADM, at the doses indicated, on Days 1 and 8 did not suppress the development of tumoricidal functions, and that at the time cells from untreated tumor-bearing mice had become unresponsive because of progressive disease the responsiveness of cells from the ADM-treated mice was retained or actually augmented. Even though there were significant increases in the life spans of ADM-treated mice bearing either tumor, there were no long-term survivors. Since earlier studies had indicated that cells from ADM-treated mice produce increased amounts of IL-2 (Ehrke *et al.*, 1986), it was decided to examine the effect of IL-2 plus ADM treatment in the EL4– and EL4/ADM–C57BL/6 models.

Considerable toxicity was seen with either high-dose IL-2 or high-dose ADM alone; however, an effective treatment without apparent toxicity was developed by combining a moderate dose of ADM (4 mg/kg, i.v., Days 1 and 8 or only Day 8) with prolonged administration of a moderate dose of IL-2 (2 μg, b.i.d., i.p., Days 9 to 40). This treatment resulted in up to 80% long-term survivors among mice inoculated on Day 0 with EL4 lymphoma (5×10^4 cells). Neither agent, when administered singly under these conditions, induced long-term survivors. The survivors induced by the combination treatment had developed protective immunity as demonstrated by their ability to resist reimplantation with EL4 tumor. This resistance to tumor reimplantation could be transferred into naive mice with spleen cells from tumor-bearing mice receiving the combination treatment. The exposure of mice to sublethal, immunosuppressive, whole-body irradiation prior to tumor implantation completely abrogated the efficacy of the combination treatment. The treatment according to a protocol involving ADM injection on Day 8 only, but not on Days 1 and 8, was equally effective in inducing long-term survivors among EL4/ADM-bearing mice (Ho *et al.*, 1993b).

Subsequent studies established that the effectiveness of the combination treatment was dependent on the presence of $CD8^+$ cells (Ho *et al.*, 1993a). Thus, the induction of long-term survivors was completely ablated by pretreatment of mice with anti-CD8 monoclonal antibody (MAb), whereas pretreatment with anti-CD4 MAb only partially inhibited the therapeutic effects and anti-NK1.1 MAb had no effect or increased the number of survivors. A close association between survival, an increase in phenotypically identified $CD8^+$ cells, and an increase in specific anti-EL4 cytolytic activity was demonstrated with cells from the tumor site. No association was observed between survival and modulations in NK, LAK, or tumoricidal macrophage activity. The results of these studies established that, in this model, the most relevant correlate of a therapeutically effective, combination treatment-induced, host antitumor response is the level of specific EL4 tumor killing by cytolytic T lymphocytes present at the tumor site.

LoRusso *et al.* (1990) have carried out somewhat similar studies with other syngeneic murine tumor models. They found that the combination of various doses of ADM with high-dose IL-2 over a short period (ending Day 14) was ineffective in a mammary adenocarcinoma model. In contrast, the combination of dacarbazine with IL-2 was effective against the colon adenocarcinoma No. 11 tumor, but in this case they did not terminate IL-2 administration until Day 35. This suggests, as was seen in the studies by Ho *et al.* (1993a,b), that the prolongation of IL-2 administration may be critical for a therapeutic effect to be achieved. Two groups have examined the effect of the combination of ADM plus IL-2 in the murine Renca renal cell carcinoma model. Salup *et al.* (1987) were able to "cure" mice with the combination of high-dose ADM, plus IL-2 and LAK cell transfer; however, they did not find any evidence that these mice had developed specific tumor immunity. On the other hand, Gautam *et al.* (1991) used a lower dose of ADM plus IL-2 in the same model and found that the surviving animals displayed specific anti-Renca immunity. These results suggest that equally effective eradication of a tumor may be attained with a combination protocol involving either a high or a moderate dose of a chemotherapeutic agent, but with the lower dose, a more optimal biological response modifying dose, there is decreased probability of untoward toxicities and increased likelihood of developing long-lasting protective antitumor immunity.

Thus, it has become clear from all of these studies that ADM, at moderate doses but, nevertheless, doses within the defined therapeutic range, can initiate changes in host tumor interactions that, in combination with a second biological response modifier, can be exploited to therapeutic advantage. There remain, however, intriguing questions as to the actual mechanism of action by which the immunomodulations are induced. A few recent studies may provide some insight into these questions.

The kinetics of detectable intracellular ADM in lymphoma cells from the intraperitoneal cavity of C57BL/6 mice and in lymphocytes infiltrating the tumor ascites were evaluated (Zaleskis *et al.*, 1994c). It was found that both ADM-sensitive parental EL4 lymphoma cells and their ADM-resistant variant, EL4/ADM, had taken up equivalent amounts of ADM at 4 hr. The amount of ADM taken up by the lymphoma cells at 4 hr was greater than that taken up by the lymphocytes isolated from the intraperitoneal cavity in conjunction with the tumor cells; however, when an approximation of cell size/volume was used to derive an estimation of "concentration," it was seen that all of the cell types had similar intracellular ADM "concentrations." Despite the fact that the intracellular "concentration" of ADM at 4 hr was equal in the three cell types, at 24 hr and later marked differences were noted: thus, at 24 hr the total number of EL4 cells recovered was reduced by nearly twofold, the number of $CD3^+$ lymphocytes was unchanged, and the number of EL4/ADM was approximately doubled. At the same time the intracellular concentration of ADM was nearly double that seen at 4 hr in both EL4 cells and lymphocytes but reduced to nearly undetectable levels in the EL4/ADM cells. Since both EL4 and EL4/ADM were equally responsive to the combination chemoimmunotherapy, i.e., ADM plus IL-2 (Ho *et al.*, 1993a,b), these findings further confirm that a major role of ADM in this therapy must not be linked to direct toxicity to the lymphoma. Furthermore, the fact that no change in the number of $CD3^+$ cells was seen at a time when clear changes, both up and down, in the number of lymphoma cells were observed, suggests that immunomodulation also may not be the consequence of a relatively nonspecific elimination/stimulation of the lymphocyte pool.

A survey of ADM uptake by lymphoid organs indicated that peak levels were not attained in thymus until Day 3 while they were attained in all other organs on Day 1. Early studies had established that ADM immunomodulation was greatest 5 days after injection (Ehrke *et al.*, 1983). These findings suggested the possibility that ADM might be selectively affecting cells of the thymus. Studies *in vitro* established that concentrations of ADM that had been shown to be immunomodulating (Tomazic *et al.*, 1980) caused thymocyte apoptosis whereas immunosuppressive concentrations one log higher caused necrosis (Zaleskis *et al.*, 1994a). Cells induced to undergo apoptosis *in vitro* were shown to be those bearing both the CD4 and CD8 markers (i.e., the double positive thymocytes). Although *in vivo* apoptotic cells are rapidly removed by the reticuloendothelial system and, therefore, nearly impossible to detect in cell populations from fresh tissue samples, it was possible to show that 4 days after ADM injection double positive cells were reduced in the thymus from treated mice. Even though treatment with IL-2 alone had no effect on the numbers of double positive thymocytes recovered 4 days after starting treatment, the mice receiving the combination treatment had even fewer double positive thymocytes than those treated with ADM alone. It was suggested that combination-induced depletion of double positive cells within the thymus results in the maturation of increased numbers of new clones of positively selected progenitors which are then sustained by IL-2 in the periphery. Additionally, Huber and Moraska (1992) have shown that following ADM treatment there are detectable alterations in the antigenicity of myocytes which lead to the production of specific immune responses. It is possible, therefore, that ADM may also play a role by potentiating the antigenicity of the lymphoma cells which have taken it up in rather high amounts in the first 4 hr. Observations, in the EL4 model system, made by Sykes *et al.* (1993) indicate that in IL-2-treated mice, selective inhibition by IL-2 of CD4 cell activity can occur which results in ablation of graft-versus-host disease but retention of graft-versus-lymphoma activity. Such selective effects on subsets of $CD4^+$ cells may be crucial to the effective syngeneic anti-EL4 response.

3.2. Cyclophosphamide

The immunomodulation induced by CY has been studied extensively in a large number of systems (Ehrke and Mihich, 1985; Ehrke *et al.*, 1989; Mihich and Ehrke, 1991). CY, a product of rational drug development in the late 1950s, was designed as a prodrug that requires enzymatic cleavage *in vivo* to become active and is itself nontoxic. Following administration, CY is rapidly converted to the highly cytotoxic 4-hydroxy CY by liver mixed-function oxygenases. Because of this requirement for enzymatic activation, the large majority of studies of CY-induced immunomodulation have been carried out *in vivo*. It was first studied for its immunosuppressive activities, but by the late 1960s it was already established that, at low doses, it could function as an immunopotentiating agent. These early studies have been repeatedly reviewed (see Ehrke *et al.*, 1989; Mihich and Ehrke, 1991).

CY can potentiate both cellular and humoral immune responses in animal models. The initial studies of immunomodulation in animal models not involving tumors were quickly followed by those in a variety of syngeneic tumor models. The critical factors determining whether CY depresses or potentiates an immune response in these models were determined to be the timing of the CY with respect to antigen and the dose of CY. CY was most effective when it was administered 1 to 3 days before antigen and at doses lower than those at which it is generally used therapeutically as a directly cytotoxic agent against tumors. Nevertheless, positive effects were noted over a wide range of doses (15 to 300 mg/kg) in different models (see Ehrke and Mihich, 1985). Although never specifically examined in this context, it is tempting to speculate that the large diversity in effective doses seen in different murine models may reflect, at least to some degree, the reported differences in the levels of inducible liver mixed-function oxygenase activity found between strains of mice (Gurtoo *et al.*, 1978). Another suggestion is that the differences in effective doses reflect a requirement for at least minimal direct tumor cell kill and that this by some, as yet undefined, mechanism increases the host's recognition of the tumor and its ability to mount an antitumor response. In this regard, Bonmassar (D'Atri *et al.*, 1989) has long been a proponent of the concept of immunological xenogenization of tumor cells by chemical agents. Thus, based on such arguments, it is reasonable that what is a minimally effective (i.e., low) dose in one model might be a relatively high dose in another model.

Regardless of the model in which low-dose CY-induced immunological augmentation was studied, in the large majority of cases the findings led to the conclusion that selective deletion/inhibition of downregulating cells having the capacity to suppress immunity must have a role in the positive effect of the drug. In fact, Gershon and co-workers (Askenase *et al.*, 1975; Schwartz *et al.*, 1978) included low-dose CY-induced effects as crucial components in a series of experiments establishing the validity of the concept of T-suppressor cells. Subsequently, the availability of chemically synthesized 4-hydroperoxycyclophosphamide (4-OOHCY) (Colvin *et al.*, 1973), which decomposes in aqueous solution into 4-hydroxy CY (the initial, active metabolite of CY formed by liver microsomal activation), permitted the examination of the cellular basis of these effects in experiments in which cells were treated *in vitro*. Initial studies demonstrated that augmented cellular response to sheep erythrocytes in a mouse delayed-type hypersensitivity model was related to the selective inhibition of suppressor T-cell development by low concentrations of 4-OOHCY (Diamanstein *et al.*, 1981). In studies of culture-induced $CD8^+$ T-cell-mediated suppression of a murine allogeneic CTL response, Cowens *et al.* (1983) obtained results indicating that a low concentration of 4-OOHCY induced elimination of a $CD4^+$ inducer of suppression. This treatment did not result in the elimination of the $CD4^+$ helper/inducer required for the CTL generation, the $CD8^+$ precursor of the alloantigen-activated

CTL, or the mature CD8$^+$ suppressor cell. This same group, utilizing human peripheral blood lymphocytes, also established that low concentrations of 4-OOHCY selectively ablated formation of Con A-activated T cells capable of suppressing either pokeweed mitogen-stimulated polyclonal immunoglobulin secretion or induction of proliferation and allospecific CTL activation in mixed lymphocyte cultures (Ozer *et al.*, 1982; Smith *et al.*, 1987). In each case the evidence suggested that the 4-OOHCY-sensitive cell was a CD4$^+$ inducer cell. Conditions used to eliminate/inhibit this cell subset did not affect the ability of other cells in the population to be induced to produce immunoglobulin or to become activated CTL, and the CD4$^+$ helper cells required for both of those responses remained functional. Thus, these experiments established the exquisite selectivity of CY action on lymphoid cells, in that it was possible to eliminate a subset from a phenotypically defined population leaving other subset(s) within that population functionally unaffected in both the murine and human systems. Furthermore, these findings provided evidence of the existence of two subsets of CD4$^+$ helper/inducer cells. It is possible that the CY-sensitive helper/inducer cell is the T_H2 cell; if so, CY should be useful in further characterization of T-helper subsets. Furthermore, it can be suggested that low-dose CY might be considered in certain disease states in which T_H2 are implicated, such as early HIV infection (Romagnani and Maggi, 1994).

Although the majority of the *in vivo* studies of CY-induced immunomodulation involved the administration of CY 2 to 3 three days before antigen injection, evidence for the validity of the use of low-dose CY to facilitate immunologically mediated regression of established tumors has been obtained in murine systems. In the MOPC-315 tumor–BALB/c mouse model, a very low dose (15 mg/kg) of CY given when the tumors were large ($\geqslant$20 mm), but not when they were small (nonpalpable), resulted in 95% long-term survivors (Mokyr *et al.*, 1982). The level of induction of long-term survivors by a higher, but still moderate, dose (100 mg/kg) was similar to that obtained with the low dose but was not dependent on tumor size at time of injection (i.e., it was equally effective against nonpalpable and large tumors). The antitumor effects of the low-dose CY, in this model, were shown to be dependent on blocking of suppressor cells and potentiation of T-cell immunity, and those with the higher dose were much less dependent on a functioning host response. Other tumors, perhaps less sensitive to CY alone and/or less immunogenic, responded to moderate doses of CY in combination with another therapeutic modality. Thus, in the RPC-5–BALB/c (Laude *et al.*, 1993), FBL-3–C57BL/6 (Greenberg, 1991), and Meth A–BALB/c (Awwad and North, 1989) tumor–mouse models, treatment with either CY (100 to 150 mg/kg) or immune cells alone was ineffective, but when the treatments were combined (plus IL-2 in the FBL-3 model) marked therapeutic effects were seen. Somewhat similar results were obtained when the effect of CY + TNF was examined in the EL4–C57BL/6 model (Ehrke *et al.*, 1995; Krawczyk *et al.*, 1995). A low dose of CY, such as that which was effective alone in the MOPC-315 system, was ineffective with or without TNF in the EL4 system; however, a moderate dose (e.g., 150 mg/kg) of CY on Day 12 after tumor injection, which alone caused 20 to 40% long-term survivors, in combination with multiple injections of TNF (1000 units/mouse, Days

13, 16, 18, 21, and 23), which alone were ineffective, induced 60 to 80% long-term survivors. In each of these four models, evidence was obtained that tumor regressions were immunologically mediated. Survivors induced by the combination of CY plus TNF in the EL4 model have been followed for up to 2 years, at which time the mice were still able to reject a reimplantation of 5×10^4 EL4 cells (injection of naive mice with as few as 10 cells kills 100% of them). In parallel with the rechallenge studies, splenocytes and thymocytes from age-matched long-term survivors were found to develop significant specific anti-EL4 CTL activity when assessed *ex vivo*, this despite the fact that aliquots of the same splenocytes were only able to develop a marginal allo-CTL response. The significance of an effective therapy that induces in the survivor long-term specific immunological memory becomes apparent when one considers studies such as that of Hawkins *et al.* (1990). They investigated 749 deaths occurring among 4082 patients surviving at least 5 years after the diagnosis of childhood cancer. Of those assessable, 550 (74%) died of recurrent tumor and, among those classified as unrelated to tumor, infection was identified as a leading cause of death. These findings and others (see Ehrke, 1991) indicate that immunological alterations induced by "curative" treatments may last for many years and the potential of long-term untoward effects (e.g., increased susceptibility to infection or of delayed recurrent disease) must be considered. This suggests that treatments that include the host's own defense mechanism as an active component should be considered once a sound preclinical experimental basis has been established.

3.3. Adriamycin or Cyclophosphamide in Clinical Immunopotentiation Protocols

There is a paucity of reported clinical studies designed to evaluate the efficacy of treatments incorporating the potentiation of the patient's antitumor defense mechanisms. There have been a limited number of studies determining the functional and compositional changes in human peripheral blood lymphocytes induced by *in vivo* exposure to a potentially immunomodulating dose of a chemotherapeutic agent. The large majority of reported studies combining an anticancer cytotoxic agent with a cytokine and/or vaccine have taken one or more of the agents to maximally tolerated doses (i.e., toxicity). A few of these studies are briefly mentioned below.

Arinaga *et al.* (1985) reported that the capacity of peripheral blood lymphocytes from cancer patients to be converted to alloantigen-specific cytotoxic cells was significantly augmented 5, 7, and 10 days (peak on day 7) after a single dose of ADM (25 mg/m^2, i.v.), when compared to that of cells obtained before ADM treatment. Furthermore, similar to what was seen in the murine system, in response to ADM treatment there was evidence of an increase in: (1) immature, nonadherent monocyte/macrophages, (2) CD8$^+$ T cells, and (3) levels of IL-2 production (Arinaga *et al.*, 1986). These results indicated that a moderate dose of ADM can induce potentially useful immune modulations in cancer patients. Subsequently, a number of studies have examined treatments combining ADM with IL-2 with and without various other immunomodulators (e.g., Paciucci *et al.*, 1991; Clamon *et al.*, 1993; Oka *et al.*, 1994).

In each of these initial clinical investigations, toxicities attributable to one or more of the components were encountered, indicating that near-maximally tolerated doses were used. Nevertheless, responses were reported to have occurred in most studies, but they were generally short-lived. Based on the experience gained in the murine models, the following comments can be made: (1) effective immunotherapy generally is achieved with combinations of agents at doses that do not cause detectable toxicities; (2) when IL-2 treatment is terminated prematurely, tumor regrowth and death occur shortly thereafter (e.g., long-term survivors did not occur until IL-2 administration was prolonged to $\geqslant$ Day 35); (3) high-dose IL-2 sustains NK/LAK cells but low-dose IL-2 sustains CTL; (4) there is considerable evidence in the murine system and perhaps also in the human system that, if elicited and sustained for an adequate period of time, a specific antitumor CTL response is extremely effective in tumor eradication. Thus, the experience gained in the mouse still needs to be properly verified in humans.

The effects of *in vivo* exposure to CY on the composition and function of human peripheral blood lymphocytes have been studied by several groups. The most comprehensive and systematic investigation was carried out by Berd and colleagues (see Ehrke *et al.*, 1989; Berd *et al.*, 1990, 1994a). High-dose CY (1000 mg/m^2) caused marked depletion of circulating lymphocytes, whereas low-dose CY (300 mg/m^2) did not. Both high- and low-dose CY impaired the generation of nonspecific (Con A-induced) suppressor T cells without impairing the proliferative response to PHA. Neither dose caused significant reproducible changes in CD8$^+$ or CD4$^+$ T cells or their ratios. Treatment of melanoma patients with the low dose of CY plus vaccine every 28 days resulted in a progressive decrease in CD4$^+$ T cells expressing the 2H4 antigen, which identifies inducers of suppression. Significant depletion of this subset was not seen until Day 49, following two courses of CY plus vaccine. In contrast, potentiation of DTH was achieved when antigen was administered as early as 3 days after CY, at which time PBL exhibited reduction of Con A-inducible T suppressor activity. The authors postulated that the discordant results may be reconciled by assuming that the major effect of CY on suppressor-inducer cells is inhibitory, rather than lytic. Thus, this subset of cells may be functionally impaired within 3 days, but may not be depleted until considerably later. Alternatively, since the authors mention that patients receiving the vaccine but no CY exhibit increased, not decreased, percentages of CD4$^+$ cells expressing 2H4, one might postulate that CY deletes a phenotypically undefined precursor of the CD4$^+$2H4$^+$ T subset. If, in response to antigen, the development of suppression were dependent on an increase in 2H4$^+$ cells, elimination of the precursor cells would prevent it.

Following the acquisition of the information mentioned above, Berd and coworkers tried to develop immunotherapy treatments with CY followed by vaccination (Berd *et al.*, 1986). They used irradiated autologous tumor cells as vaccine in their initial clinical studies of the effects of vaccine plus low-dose CY. Surgically incurable, metastatic melanoma patients received the vaccine every 28 days and CY was given 3 days prior to each vaccine injection. Using this treatment they confirmed that CY pretreatment markedly augmented the development of DTH to melanoma-associated antigens, and that the resultant immunity could cause regression of metastatic tumors; however, the response rates were low. Subsequently, they have utilized hapten (DNP)-modified irradiated autologous tumor cells as a vaccine (Berd *et al.*, 1991). Although DNP-vaccine plus CY regularly induced tumor inflammatory responses involving infiltration of $CD8^+$ T lymphocytes, clinically defined tumor regressions were uncommon. However, when this strategy was applied to patients with stage 3 melanoma, all of whom had been rendered disease-free by resection of lymph node metastases, 2-year total survival and disease-free survival were high, namely, 60 and 78%, respectively (Berd *et al.*, 1994b). Furthermore, most of the relapses occurred in the first 6 months when melanoma immunity may not have been fully developed. Thus, using the approach of DNP-modified tumor cells as a vaccine in combination with low-dose CY, it is possible to induce clinically meaningful immune responses against unmodified tumor cells.

3.4. Immunomodulation by Other Chemotherapeutic Agents

Other agents have been studied and in nearly every case when carefully examined, they have been found to cause immunomodulation (see Mihich and Ehrke, 1991).

3.4.1. Melphalan

Mokyr and co-workers have examined the alkylating agent melphalan (L-phenylalanine mustard) extensively in their MOPC-315–BALB/c model (Mokyr *et al.*, 1993, 1994; Gorelik *et al.*, 1994; Weiskirch *et al.*, 1994). Low-dose melphalan-induced effects were found to mimic those of CY in the induction of long-term survivors and the mechanism by which this occurs was shown to require the participation of $CD8^+$ (but not $CD4^+$) T-cell-dependent antitumor immunity. In recent studies of this effective treatment they have demonstrated: (1) the importance of $V\beta8^+/CD8^+$ cells for the curative effect; (2) that these cells are specifically cytolytic for MOPC-315 cells, excrete large amounts of IFN-γ, and that both responses are MHC class 1 restricted; (3) that concurrent with the increase in IFN-γ production there is a decrease in IL-10 production by the tumor. Thus, low-dose melphalan treatment of mice bearing a large MOPC-315 tumor leads to a shift in the cytokine milieu in the vicinity of the tumor from T_H2-like to T_H1-like and this shift may be critical for the acquisition of antitumor immunity in otherwise nonresponsive mice. Finally, they have found that production of TGF-β by the tumor is ablated following low-dose melphalan.

3.4.2. Vinca Alkaloids

The immunomodulating potentials of the vinca alkaloids and other microtubulin network disruptive agents have been examined at least to a limited extent. The large majority of these studies have already been reviewed (see Ehrke and Mihich, 1985). Briefly, when examined in culture, VLB was found to inhibit the development of a cell culture-induced T-cell activity that suppresses allo-CTL development, but VLB was found to also inhibit other T-cell responses. Vincristine (VCR), structurally very similar to VLB but differing broadly in tumor target profile, was far less effective in inhibiting the culture-induced suppressor T-cell activity and did not reduce other T-cell responses. When antitumor humoral responses were assessed following administration of these vinca alkaloids at equitoxic doses (½ LD_{10}—3 mg VLB/kg and 1.5 mg VCR/kg) to tumor-challenged mice, VLB-induced augmentation (200 to 250%) was observed 6 days later, whereas VCR reduced the response or had no effect. In contrast, VCR caused augmentation of development of specific antitumor CTL (~25-fold more lytic units/culture) 14 days later, whereas following VLB administration CTL development was inhibited on Day 10 and essentially at control levels on Day 14. It was suggested based on these findings that by inhibiting B-cell responses VCR was augmenting T-cell responses and the converse for VLB (Ryoyama *et al.*, 1982; Ehrke and Mihich, 1985). In light of the current knowledge of immune response regulation, it can now be suggested that VCR may be facilitating a T_H1-like response and VBL a T_H2-like response. North and Awwad (1990) reported findings in a study of relatively high-dose (7.5 mg/kg) VLB in an advanced murine lymphoma model indicating that tumor regression depended on drug-mediated elimination of $CD4^+$ suppressor T cells that are replicating and sparing of nonreplicating $CD8^+$ effector cells. It is not clear whether experimental differences (e.g., dose of drug used) can explain the inconsistent conclusions; however, both sets of findings implicate selective effects on the same or similar subset of cells. Although further experimentation is required to clarify these points there are a few recent papers that provide some relevant information. Ferrua, Manie, and co-workers (Ferrua *et al.*, 1990; Manie *et al.*, 1993) have reported that the microtubule-disrupting agents, VCR, colchicine, and to a lesser extent VLB, can induce IL-1 production and release by the myelomonocytic THP-1 cell line. Using colchicine in further studies, they found that PKA, but not PKC, had a role in induction of IL-1 production, and taxol, a stabilizer of microtubule bundles, antagonized the induction of IL-1 production by colchicine, but not by LPS. They also determined that colchicine did not induce production of IL-6 or TNF. Ding *et al.* (1990) had shown earlier that taxol can cause release of TNF from murine macrophages. Chuang *et al.* (1994) found that taxol inhibited activation of lymphocytes with IL-2 and implicated microtubules in this function. Taken together these findings suggest that microtubule assembly/disassembly plays a critical role(s) in stimulation of hematopoietic cells to carry out a number of functions including the production of regulatory cytokines.

3.4.3. Cisplatin, 5-Fluorouracil, and Mitomycin C

Relatively early in the development of cisplatin as an anticancer agent, it was suggested that the host defense had a role in the overall efficacy of this agent (Conran and Rosenberg, 1972). Since then there have been several reports of enhanced immune responses induced by cisplatin (see Ehrke and Mihich, 1985; Mihich and Ehrke, 1991) as well as reports of cytokine-induced potentiation of the direct anti-tumor activities of certain platinum analogues (Chang *et al.*, 1994). Recently, Allavena *et al.* (1990) have investigated the effect of cisplatin on the generation of LAK cells. They found that exposure of human PBL to cisplatin concentrations $\geq 6\ \mu M$ for periods greater than 1 hr resulted in inhibition of the generation of LAK cells but not of the lytic activity of fully activated LAK cells. When compared to those collected before treatment, PBL collected from ovarian adenocarcinoma patients 1 hr after the i.v. administration of 50 mg cisplatin/m^2 were not inhibited; in fact, the cells from two of the five patients examined developed augmented levels of activity.

There have been a few reports of immune response augmentation induced by 5-fluorouracil, but many others in which only inhibition was observed (see Mihich and Ehrke, 1991). Scheper and co-workers (Claessen *et al.*, 1989) have recently shown that, when continuously released from an osmotic pump at the "antigen sensitization site," 5-fluorouracil or etoposide induced strong potentiation of cell mediated immunity. Although similar results were obtained with locoregional daily injection of etoposide, 5-fluorouracil was ineffective when administered in this manner. It is possible, therefore, that the inconsistent findings reported to date with 5-fluorouracil may be related, at least in part, to failure in some cases to sustain effective levels of the drug for an adequate period of time. Immunochemotherapy studies with 5-fluorouracil in combination with other cytotoxic/cytostatic agents (carboplatin and/or mitomycin C) and an immunomodulating agent (interferon α plus β or OK-432) have been carried out in colorectal cancer patients (Klein *et al.*, 1991) and in a model of human colon cancer in nude mice (Furukawa *et al.*, 1993). The results obtained in these studies indicate that the combination of moderate to low doses of cytotoxics/cytostatics with an immunomodulating agent was much more effective than either alone against primary tumor and in the nude mouse model the combination was quite effective against hepatic metastases which were resistant to either treatment alone. In the latter model it is unlikely that T cells are involved in the response but more likely that the macrophages and NK cells known to be abundant in the nude mouse play an active role.

3.4.4. Nitrosureas

It has been reported that 1,3-bis(2-chloroethyl)-1-nitrosourea (BCNU) induces tumoricidal macrophages, increased CTL activity, and a higher percentage of T_H1 cells in tumor-bearing mice (Nagarkatti *et al.*, 1988, 1990; Selvan *et al.*, 1990). The results obtained in two recent chemoimmunotherapy studies utilizing BCNU plus IL-2 indicate that the combination is more effective than BCNU alone and that IL-2 alone was completely ineffective in either model (Farone and Cox, 1992; Acerbis *et al.*, 1992). Farone and Cox (1992) showed that heat inactivated IL-2 could not substitute for IL-2 in the combination therapy and that the combination therapy-induced survivors were specifically resistant to rechallenge by the primary tumor. In the model studied by Acerbis *et al.* (1992), chemoimmunotherapy was used as an adjuvant after surgical removal of the primary M5076 tumor. In order to mimic the clinical situation, they chose to use BCNU, which they found to be most effective against the tumor. BCNU alone resulted in 10 to 20% survival and combination treatment resulted in 50 to 70% survival at 120 days. Without treatment or with IL-2 alone all mice died of liver metatases by Day 47. Thus, these results again indicate that the combination of a chemotherapeutic agent with a cytokine can be highly effective even against advanced disease.

4. CONCLUDING REMARKS

As discussed above, the increasing knowledge of the mechanisms of regulation of the immune response and of the action of immune effectors offers new opportunities for selective intervention toward the development of therapies of cancer based on the participation of antitumor defense mechanisms. Thus, it is now possible to design treatments with immunomodulating agents that hold promise of therapeutic success, particularly in combination with other modalities of treatment. The opportunities in this regard will increase further when the mechanisms involved in the suppression of immune responses by cancer are better understood, as this will allow for the design of treatments also including a reduction of the untoward effects of tumor.

The results summarized in this chapter clearly indicate that certain anticancer drugs, given according to certain regimens, can exert marked and rather well-defined immunomodulating effects. These effects are in some cases based on the selective inhibition or elimination of negative control mechanisms and in some cases on an actual direct augmentation of the immune response. These immunomodulating effects can be usefully exploited when the drugs are used in combination with such biological agents as specific cytokines or therapeutically used vaccines. Indeed, recently good progress has been made in developing "vaccines" with tumor cells transfected with certain cytokine genes, which are much more effective than killed unmodified cells. Combinations of anticancer drugs with certain cytokines have already been shown to be therapeutically effective in experimental tumor models, and the successful use of immunomodulating doses of CY in conjunction with tumor vaccines for the treatment of malignant melanoma in humans has been demonstrated (see above).

Based on the information discussed in this chapter, it is reasonable to expect that certain anticancer drugs can be used for their immunomodulating activity in immunochemotherapeutic regimens. A fundamental requirement in the design of such regimens would be that the agents employed be used at the optimal biological response modifier dose (OBRMD) and not at the maximum tolerated dose (MTD). The need for the use of biological response modifiers (BRMs) at OBRMD, and the difficulties in defining these doses in humans were extensively discussed several years ago (Mihich and Fefer, 1983). Indeed, the OBRMD should be defined based on the modification of those immune phenomena that are responsible for the antitumor effect; BRMs, including anticancer drugs when considered for their immunomodulating action, typically exert pleiotropic effects on the immune response and it is always difficult, both in experimental tumor models and in cancer patients, to identify the effects that are responsible for a given antitumor action. The difficulties in the clinic are compounded by the fact that at least certain human tumors exert relatively specific negative effects on the immune system. These effects can be expected to vary in a quantitative, and perhaps also qualitative, way with tumor progression, namely, at different stages of the neoplastic disease. It is not too surprising, therefore, that the determination of OBRMDs in the clinic has met with major obstacles which in many cases have not been overcome.

Realistically, one has to state that another set of obstacles is related to the well-developed cancer chemotherapy practice to administer anticancer drugs at the MTD. In fact, the opportunity to do so in combination chemotherapy has been one of the main reasons for the therapeutic successes achieved to date in the treatment of cancer. Nevertheless, the use of these drugs at the MTD unavoidably causes immunosuppression; whereas in some cases it is reasonable to assume that the immunosuppression is relatively transient and that sequential treatments with cytoreductive chemotherapy and immunochemotherapy could be successfully established in other cases a recovery from hematopoietic toxicity does not necessarily reflect a recovery of those elements of the immune response that are the targets of positive immunomodulation.

Although the clinical use of certain anticancer drugs at relatively low doses has been attempted in the past for the development of treatments inducing tumor cell differentiation, it has not been overtly successful especially in comparison with the effects of more specific differentiation inducers such as the retinoids. Regardless of this experience, based on the results of studies in preclinical tumor models such as those discussed herein, it seems reasonable to expect that the use of immunomodulating regimens of anticancer drugs may be more promising than the use of differentiation inducing regimens with similar drugs. It therefore seems ethically justified and clinically possible to investigate the effects of rationally and cautiously designed regimens with relatively low doses of anticancer drugs, particularly in combination with certain cytokines and/or therapeutically used vaccines, that would be aimed at treating the tumor through an augmentation of immune responses directed against the tumor itself.

Acknowledgments. The authors thank Drs. Ujházy, Berleth, Verstovšek and Ms. Doty-Henn for having read the manuscript and provided extremely useful comments. The skillful assistance of Ms. Jane M. Meer in the preparation of the manuscript is gratefully acknowledged. The investigations, described herein, carried out by the authors laboratory group have been supported in part by grants CA15142, CA13038, CA24538, and CA16056, NCI, USDHHS.

REFERENCES

Acerbis, G., Cleris, L., Rodolfo, M., Parmiani, G., and Formelli, F., 1992, Post surgical adjuvant chemo-immunotherapy with recombinant interleukin-2 and 1,3-bis-(2-chloroethyl)-1-nitrosurea on spontaneous metastases of a non-immunogenic murine tumour, *Cancer Immunol. Immunother.* **34**:383–388.

Afonso, L. C. C., Scharton, T. M., Vieira, L. Q., Wysocka, M., Trinchieri, G., and Scott, P., 1994, The adjuvant effect of interleukin-2 in a vaccine against *Leishmania major*, *Science* **263**:235–237.

Allavena, P., Pirovano, P., Bonazzi, C., Colombo, N., Mantovani, A., and D'Inacalci, M., 1990, In vitro and in vivo effects of cisplatin on the generation of lymphokine-activated killer cells, *J. Natl. Cancer Inst.* **82**:139–142.

Allison, J. P. 1993, $\gamma\delta$ T-cell development, *Curr. Opin. Immunol.* **5**:241–246.

Arinaga, S., Akiyoshi, T., and Tsuji, H., 1985, Augmentation of the cell-mediated cytotoxic response induced in mixed cell culture by adriamycin, *Jpn. J. Cancer Res.* **76**:414–419.

Arinaga, S., Akiyoshi, T., and Tsuji, H., 1986, Augmentation of the generation of cell mediated cytotoxicity after a single dose of adriamycin in cancer patients, *Cancer Res.* **46**:4213–4216.

Askenase, P. W., Hayden, B. J., and Gershon, R. K., 1975, Augmentation of delayed-type hypersensitivity by doses of cyclophosphamide which do not affect antibody responses, *J. Exp. Med.* **141**:697–703.

Awwad, M., and North, R. J., 1989, Cyclophosphamide-induced immunologically mediated regression of a cyclophosphamide resistant murine tumor: A consequence of eliminating precursor L3T4^{+} suppressor T-cells, *Cancer Res.* **49**:1649–1654.

Berd, D., Maguire, H. C., Jr., and Mastrangelo, M. J., 1986, Induction of cell-mediated immunity to autologous melanoma cells and regression of metastases after treatment with a melanoma cell vaccine preceded by cyclophosphamide, *Cancer Res.* **46**:2572–2576.

Berd, D., Maguire, H. C., Jr., McCue, P., and Mastrangelo, M. J., 1990, Treatment of metastatic melanoma with an autologous tumor cell vaccine: Clinical and immunological results in 64 patients, *J. Clin. Oncol.* **8**:1858–1867.

Berd, D., Murphy, G., Maguire, H. C., Jr., and Mastrangelo, M. J., 1991, Immunization with haptenized autologous tumor cells induces inflammation of human melanoma metastases, *Cancer Res.* **51**:2731–2736.

Berd, D., Maguire, H. C., Jr., Mastrangelo, M. J., and Murphy, G., 1994a, Activation markers on T cells infiltrating melanoma metastases after therapy with dinitrophenyl-conjugated vaccine, *Cancer Immunol. Immunother.* **39**:141–147.

Berd, D., Sato, T., Lattime, E. C., Maguire, H. C., Jr., and Mastrangelo, M. J., 1994b, Immunization with hapten-modified tumor cells: A strategy for the treatment of human melanoma, *Proc. AACR.* **35**:667–668.

Boon, T., Cerottini, J.-C., Van den Eynde, B., van der Bruggen, P., and Van Pel, A., 1994, Tumor antigens recognized by T lymphocytes, *Annu. Rev. Immunol.* **12**:337–365.

Boyd, R. L., and Hugo, P., 1991, Towards an integrated view of thymopoiesis, *Immunol. Today* **12**:71–79.

Braun, D., and Harris, J. E., 1981, Modulation of the immune response by chemotherapy, *Pharmacol. Ther.* **14**:89–122.

Burton, D. R., and Barbas, C. F., III, 1994, Human antibodies from combinatorial libraries, *Adv. Immunol.* **57**:191–280.

Chang, M.-J., Yu, W.-D., Reyno, L. M., Modzelewski, R. A., Egorin, M. J., Erkmen, K., Vlock, D. R., Furmnaski, P., and Johnson, C. S., 1994, Potentiation by interleukin 1α of cisplatin and carboplatin antitumor activity: Schedule-dependent and pharmokinetic effects in the RIF-1 tumor model, *Cancer Res.* **54**:5380–5386.

Chuang, L. T., Lotzova, E., Heath, J., Cook, K. R., Munkarah, A., Morris, M., and Wharton, J. T., 1994, Alteration of lymphocyte microtubule assembly, cytotoxicity, and activation by the anticancer drug taxol, *Cancer Res.* **54**:1286–1291.

Claessen, A. M. E., Valster, H., Bril, H., Meyer, S., and Scheper, R. J., 1989, Cell-mediated immunity is enhanced by cytostatic drugs continuously released at the site of antigenic stimulation, *Cancer Immunol. Immunother.* **28**:131–135.

Clamon, G., Herndon, J., Perry, M. C., Ozer, H., Kreisman, H., Maher, T., Ellerton, J., and Green, M. R.,

1993, Interleukin-2 activity in patients with extensive small-cell lung cancer: A phase II trial of Cancer and Leukemia Group B, *J. Natl. Cancer Inst.* **85**:316–320.

Colvin, M., Padgett, A. C., and Fenselou, C., 1973, A biologically active metabolite of cyclophosphamide, *Cancer Res.* **33**:915–922.

Conran, P. B., and Rosenberg, B., 1972, The role of host defense in the regression of sarcoma-180 in mice treated with cis-dichlorodiammineplatinum(II), in: *Antimicrobial and Antineoplastic Chemotherapy* (M. Semonsky, M. Hejzlar, and S. Masal, eds.), University Park Press, New York, pp. 235–236.

Cowens, J. W., Ozer, H., Ehrke, M. J., Colvin, M., and Mihich, E., 1983, Inhibition of the development of suppressor cells in culture by 4-hydroperoxycyclophosphamide, *J. Immunol.* **132**:95–100.

D'Atri, S., Tricarico, M., Margison, G.P., Allegrucci, M., Fuschiotti, P., Grohman, U., Giglietti, S., and Bonmassar, E., 1989, Antigenic changes of cancer cells following interaction with antitumour agents, in: *Drug Resistance: Mechanisms and Reversal.* (E. Mihich, ed.), John Libbey and Co., Rome, pp.271–294.

Diamanstein, T., Klos, M., Hahn, H., and Kaufmann, S. H. E., 1981, Direct in vitro evidence for different susceptibilities to 4-hydroperoxycyclophosphamide of antigen-primed T cells regulating humoral and cell-mediated immune responses to sheep erythrocytes, *J. Immunol.* **126**:1717–1722.

Ding, A. H., Porteu, F., Sanchez, E., and Nathan, C. F., 1990, Shared actions of endotoxin and taxol on TNF receptors and TNF release, *Science* **248**:370–372.

Ehrke, M. J., 1991, Effect of cancer therapy on host response and immunobiology, *Current Opin. Oncol.* **3**:1070–1077.

Ehrke, M. J., and Mihich, E., 1985, Immunoregulation by cancer chemotherapeutic agents, in: *The Reticuloendothelial System: A Comprehensive Treatise*, Volume VIII (J. W. Hadden and A. Szentivanyi, eds.), Plenum Press, New York, pp.309–347.

Ehrke, M. J., Tomazic, V., Ryoyama, K., Cohen, S. A., and Mihich, E., 1983, Adriamycin induced immunomodulation: Dependence upon time of administration, *Int. J. Immunopharmacol.* **5**:43–48.

Ehrke, M. J., Maccubbin, D., Ryoyama, K., Cohen, S. A., and Mihich, E., 1986, Correlation between adriamycin-induced augmentation of interleukin 2 production and of cell mediated cytotoxicity, *Cancer Res.* **46**:54–60.

Ehrke, M. J., Mihich, E., Berd, D., and Mastrangelo, M. J., 1989, Effects of anticancer agents on the immune system in man, *Semin. Oncol.* **16**:230–253.

Ehrke, M. J., Krawczyk, C., Maccubbin, D., and Mihich, E., 1991, Therapeutic efficacy of cyclophosphamide (CY) and TNF therapy in a murine tumor model: Possible role of specific thymic CTL activity, *Third Int. Workshop on Cytokines* **3**:488.

Ehrke, M. J., Verstovšek, S., Krawczyk, C. M., Ujházy, P., Zaleskis, G., Maccubbin, D., and Mihich, E., 1995, Cyclophosphamide plus tumor necrosis factor-α chemoimmunotherapy cured mice: Life-long immunity and rejection of re-implanted primary lymphoma, *Int. J. Cancer* **63**:463–471.

Engelhard, V. H., 1994, Structure of peptides associated with class I and class II MHC molecules, *Annu. Rev. Immunol.* **12**:181–207.

Farone, A. L., and Cox, D. C., 1992, 1,3-bis(2-chloroethyl)-1-nitrosurea (BCNU)/interleukin-2 chemoimmunotherapy of murine L1210 leukemia, *Cancer Immunol. Immunother.* **34**:279–281.

Ferrua, B., Manie, S., Doglio, A., Shaw, A., Sonthonnax, S., Limouse, M., and Schaffar, L., 1990, Stimulation of human interleukin 1 production and specific mRNA expression by microtubule-disrupting drugs, *Cell. Immunol.* **131**:391–397.

Fitch, F. W., McKisic, M. D., Lancki, D. W., and Gajewski, T. F., 1993, Differential regulation of murine lymphocyte subsets, *Annu. Rev. Immunol.* **11**:29–48.

Furukawa, T., Kubota, T., Watanabe, M., Kuo, T.-H., Kase, S., Saikawa, Y., Tanino, H., Teramoto, T., Ishibiki, K., Kitajima, M., and Hoffman, R. M., 1993, Immunochemotherapy prevents human colon cancer metastases after orthotopic onplantation of histologically-intact tumor tissue in nude mice, *Anticancer Res.* **13**:287–292.

Gautam, S. C., Chikkala, N. F., Ganapathi, R., and Hamilton, T. A., 1991, Combination therapy with adriamycin and interleukin 2 augments immunity against murine renal cell carcinoma, *Cancer Res.* **51**:6133–6137.

Gorelik, L., Prokhorova, A., and Mokyr, M. B., 1994, Low-dose melphalan-induced shift in the production of a Th2-type cytokine to a Thl-type cytokine in mice bearing a large MOPC-315 tumor, *Cancer Immunol. Immunother.* **39:**117–126.

Greenberg, P. D., 1991, Adoptive T cell therapy of tumors: Mechanisms operative in the recognition and elimination of tumor cells, *Adv. Immunol.* **49:**281–355.

Gurtoo, H. L., Dahms, R. P., Kanter, P., and Vaught, J. B., 1978, Association and dissociation of the Ah locus with the metabolism of aflatoxin B_1 by mouse liver, *J. Biol. Chem.* **253:**3952–3961.

Hammerling, G. J., Schonrich, G., Ferber, I., and Arnold, B., 1993, Peripheral tolerance as a multi-step mechanism, *Immunol. Rev.* **133:**93–104.

Hawkins, M. M., Kingston, J. E., and Kinnier Wilson, L. M., 1990, Late deaths after treatment for childhood cancer, *Arch. Dis. Child.* **65:**1356–1363.

Ho, R. L. X., Maccubbin, D., Ujhazy, P., Zaleskis, G., Eppolito, C., Mihich, E., and Ehrke, M. J., 1993a, Immunological responses critical to the therapeutic effects of adriamycin plus interleukin 2 in C57BL/6 mice bearing syngeneic EL4 lymphoma, *Oncol. Res.* **5:**363–372.

Ho, R. L. X., Maccubbin, D., Zaleskis, G., Krawczyk, C., Wing, K., Mihich, E., and Ehrke, M. J., 1993b, Development of a non-toxic adriamycin plus interleukin 2 therapy effective against both adriamycin sensitive and resistant lymphomas, *Oncol. Res.* **5:**373–381.

Huber, S. A. and Moraska, A., 1992, Cytolytic T lymphocytes and antibodies to myocytes in adriamycin-treated BALB/c mice, *Am. J. Path.* **140:**233–242.

Itohara, S., Mombaerts, P., Lafaille, J., Iacomini, J., Nelson, A., Clarke, A. R., Hooper, M. L., Farr, A., and Tonegawa, S., 1993, T cell receptor δ gene mutant mice: Independent generation of αβ T cells and programmed rearrangements of γδ TCR genes, *Cell* **72:**337–348.

Jenkins, M. K., Schwartz, R. H., and Pardoll, D. M., 1988, Effects of cyclosporin A on T cell development and clonal deletion, *Science* **241:**1655–1658.

Katz, J. D., Lebow, L. T., and Bonavida, B., 1989, The in vivo depletion of $V\beta17a^+$ T cells results in the inhibition of reticulum cell sarcoma growth in SJL/J mice, *J. Immunol.* **143:**1387–1394.

Klein, H. O., Golbach, G., Voigt, P., Coerper, C., and Bernhardt, C., 1991, Combination of interferons and cytostatic drugs for treatment of advanced colorectal cancer, *J. Cancer. Res. Clin. Oncol.* **117**(Suppl. IV):S214–S220.

Krawczyk, C. M., Verstovšek, S., Ujházy, P., Maccubbin, D., and Ehrke, M. J., 1995, Protective immunity induced by cyclophosphamide plus TNF-α combination treatment of EL4 lymphoma-bearing C57BL/6 mice, *Cancer Immunol. Immunother.* **40:**347–357.

Laude, M., Russo, K. L., Mokyr, M. B., and Dray, S., 1993, Cure of mice bearing a late-stage, highly metastatic, drug-resistant tumor by adoptive chemoimmunotherapy, *Cancer Immunol. Immunother.* **36:**229–236.

LoRusso, P.M., Aukerman, S. L., Polin, L., Redman, B. G., Valdivieso, M., Biernat, L., and Corbett, L. H., 1990, Antitumor efficacy of interleukin-2 alone and in combination with adriamycin and dacarbazine in murine solid tumor systems, *Cancer Res.* **50:**5876–5882.

Maccubbin, D., Mace, K., Ehrke, M. J., and Mihich, E., 1989, Modification of host antitumor defense mechanisms in mice by progressively growing tumor, *Cancer Res.* **49:**4216–4224.

Maccubbin, D., Wing, K., Mace, K., Ho, R. L. X., Ehrke, M. J., and Mihich, E., 1992, Adriamycin-modulation of host defenses in tumor bearing mice, *Cancer Res.* **52:**3572–3576.

McPhee, D., Pye, J., and Shortman, K., 1979, The differentiation of T lymphocytes: V. Evidence for intrathymic death of most thymocytes, *Thymus* **1:**151–159.

Manie, S., Schmid-Alliana, A., Kubar, J., Ferrua, B., and Rossi, B., 1993, Disruption of microtubule network in human monocytes induces expression of interleukin-1 but not that of interleukin-6 nor tumor necrosis factor-α, *J. Biol. Chem.* **268:**13675–13681.

Matzinger, P., 1993, Why positive selection? *Immunol. Rev.* **135:**81–131.

Matzinger, P., 1994, Tolerance, danger, and the extended family, *Annu. Rev. Immunol.* **12:**991–1045.

Mihich, E., 1969, Modification of tumor regression by immunologic means, *Cancer Res.* **29:**2345–2350.

Mihich, E., 1971, Preclinical evaluation of the interrelationships between cancer chemotherapy and immunity, in: *Prediction of Response in Cancer Therapy* (T. C. Hall, ed.), Natl. Cancer Inst. Monogr. No. 34, pp.90–102.

Mihich, E., and Ehrke, M. J., 1991, Immunomodulation by anticancer drugs, in: *Biologic Therapy of Cancer: Principles and Practice* (V. T. DeVita, Jr., S. Hellman, and S. A. Rosenberg, eds.), Lippincott, Philadelphia, pp.776–786.

Mihich, E., and Fefer, A., 1983, *Biological Response Modifiers: Subcommittee Report*, Natl. Cancer Inst. Monogr. No. 63, U.S. Government Printing Office, Washington, DC.

Mokyr, M. B., Hengst, J. C. D., and Dray, S., 1982, The role of antitumor immunity in cyclophosphamide-induced rejection of subcutaneous non-palpable MOPC-315 tumors, *Cancer Res.* **42:**974–979.

Mokyr, M. B., Rubin, M., Newell, K. A., Prokhorova, A., and Bluestone, J. A., 1993, Involvement of TCR-V beta 8.3$^+$ cells in the cure of mice bearing a large MOPC-315 tumor by low dose melphalan, *J. Immunol.* **151:**4838–4846.

Mokyr, M. B., Prokhorova, A., Rubin, M., and Bluestone, J. A., 1994, Insight into the mechanism of TCR-V beta 8$^+$/CD8$^+$ T cell-mediated MOPC-315 tumor eradication, *J. Immunol.* **153:**3123–3134.

Mosmann, T. R., and Coffman, R. L., 1989, Thl and Th2 cells: Different patterns of lymphokine secretion lead to different functional properties, *Annu. Rev. Immunol.* **7:**145–173.

Nagarkatti, M., Nagarkatti, P. S., and Kaplan, A. M., 1988, Differential effect of BCNU on T cell, macrophage, natural killer and lymphokine-activated killer cell activities in mice bearing a syngeneic tumor, *Cancer Immunol. Immunother.* **27:**38–46.

Nagarkatti, M., Clary, S. R., and Nagarkatti, P. S., 1990, Characterization of tumor infiltrating CD4$^+$ T cells as Thl cells based on lymphokine secretion and functional properties, *J. Immunol.* **144:**4898–4904.

North, R. J., and Awwad, M., 1990, Elimination of cycling CD4$^+$ suppressor T cells with an anti-mitotic drug releases non-cycling CD8$^+$ T cells to cause regression of an advanced lymphoma, *Immunol.* **71:**90–95.

O'Garra, A., and Murphy, K., 1994, Role of cytokines in determining T-lymphocyte function, *Curr. Opin. Immunol.* **6:**458–466.

Oka, M., Hazama, S., Yoshino, S., Shimoda, K., Suzuki, M., Shimizu, R., Yano, K., Nishida, M., and Suzuki, T., 1994, Intraarterial combined immunochemotherapy for unresectable hepatocellular carcinoma: Preliminary results, *Cancer Immunol. Immunother.* **38:**194–200.

Ozer, H., Cowens, J. W., Colvin, M., Nussbaum-Blumenson, A., and Sheedy, D., 1982, In vitro effect of 4-hydroperoxycyclophosphamide on human immunoregulatory T subset function, *J. Exp. Med.* **155:** 276–281.

Paciucci, P. A., Bekesi, J. G., Ryder, J. S., Odchimar, R., Chahinian, P. A., and Holland, J. F., 1991, Immunotherapy with IL2 by constant infusion and weekly doxorubicin, *Am. J. Clin. Oncol.* **14:**341–348.

Robey, E., and Fowlkes, B. J., 1994, Selective events in T cell development, *Annu. Rev. Immunol.* **12:**675–705.

Romagnani, S., and Maggi, E., 1994, Thl versus Th2 responses in AIDS, *Curr. Opin. Immunol.* **4:**616–622.

Rubin, M., Bluestone, J. A., Newell, K. A., Prokhorova, A., and Mokyr, M. B., 1994, Cooperation between staphylococcal enterotoxin B and low dose melphalan in the cure of mice bearing a large MOPC-315 tumor and extensive metastases, *J. Immunol.* **152:**3522–3529.

Ryoyama, K., Mace, K., Ehrke, M. J., and Mihich, E., 1982, The differential sensitivity of T-cell immune functions to vincristine and vinblastine, *Int. J. Immunopharmacol.* **4:**187–194.

Salup, R. R., Back, T. C., and Wiltrout, R. H., 1987, Successful treatment of advanced murine renal cell cancer by bicompartmental adoptive chemoimmunotherapy, *J. Immunol.* **138:**641–647.

Schwartz, A., Askenase, P. W., and Gershon, R. K., 1978, Regulation of delayed-type hypersensitivity reactions by cyclophosphamide-sensitive cells, *J. Immunol.* **121:**1573–1579.

Selvan, R. S., Nagarkatti, P. S., and Nagarkatti, M., 1990, Role of IL-2, IL-4 and IL-6 in the growth and differentiation of tumor-specific CD4$^+$ T helper and CD8$^+$ T cytotoxic cells, *Int. J. Cancer* **45:**1096–1102.

Simon, J. C., Cruz, P. D., Bergstresser, P. R., and Tigelaar, R. E., 1990, Low dose ultraviolet B-irradiated Langerhans cells preferentially activate CD4$^+$ cells of the T helper 2 subset, *J. Immunol.* **145:**2087–2091.

Smith, J. J., Mihich, E., and Ozer, H., 1987, In vitro effects of 4-hydroperoxycyclophosphamide on human immunoregulatory T subset function, *Meth. Find. Exp. Clin. Pharm.* **9:**555–568.

Sykes, M., Abraham, V. S., Harty, M. W., and Pearson, D. A., 1993, IL-2 reduces graft-versus-host disease and preserves a graft-versus-leukemia effect by selectively inhibiting CD4$^+$ T cell activity, *J. Immunol.* **150:**197–205.

Tomazic, V., Ehrke, M. J., and Mihich, E., 1980, Modulation of the cytotoxic response against allogeneic tumor cells in culture by adriamycin, *Cancer Res.* **40:**2748–2755.

Ujházy, P., Chen, Y., Fredericks, W., Ho, R., Baker, R., Mihich, E., and Ehrke, M. J., 1990, The relationship between multidrug resistance and tumor necrosis factor resistance in an EL4 cell line model, *Cancer Commun.* **2:**181–188.

Waldmann, T. A., 1992, Immune receptors: Targets for therapy of leukemia/lymphoma, autoimmune diseases and for the prevention of allograft rejection, *Annu. Rev. Immunol.* **10:**675–704.

Weiskirch, L. M., Bar-Dagan, Y., and Mokyr, M. B., 1994, Transforming growth factor-beta-mediated down-regulation of antitumor cytotoxicity of spleen cells from MOPC-315 tumor-bearing mice engaged in tumor eradication following low-dose melphalan therapy, *Cancer Immunol. Immunother.* **38:**215–224.

Yamamura, M., Modlin, R. L., Ohmen, J. D., and Moy, R. L., 1993, Local expression of antiinflammatory cytokines in cancer, *J. Clin. Invest.* **91:**1005–1010.

Zaleskis, G., Berleth, E., Ehrke, M. J., and Mihich, E., 1994a, Doxorubicin induced DNA degradation in murine thymocytes, *Mol. Pharmacol.* **46:**901–908.

Zaleskis, G., Ehrke, M. J., Verstovsek, S., Tzai, T. S., and Mihich, E., 1994b, Doxorubicin and cyclosporin A exhibit opposite immunophenotype toxicity in hematopoietic cells, *Proc. AACR* **35:**389.

Zaleskis, G., Ho, R. L. X., Diegelman, P., Maccubbin, D., Ujhazy, P., Mihich, E., and Ehrke, M. J., 1994c, Intracellular doxorubicin kinetics in lymphoma cells and lymphocytes infiltrating the tumor area in vivo: A flow cytometric study, *Oncol. Res.* **6:**183–194.

Zaleskis, G., Verstovsek, S., Tzai, T.-S., Mihich, E., and Ehrke, M. J., 1995, Doxorubicin and cyclosporin A affect murine lymphoid cell expressing different antigenic determinants, *Oncol. Res.* **7:**307–316.

PART III

MICROBIAL IMMUNOPHARMACOLOGY

CHAPTER 5

VIRUS-INDUCED IMMUNOSUPPRESSION

TAMMIE L. KEADLE, SANDRA DANIEL, BARRY T. ROUSE, and DAVID W. HOROHOV

1. INTRODUCTION

The recent emergence of the AIDS epidemic has rekindled interest in human infectious disease and has been a stimulus for studies designed to ascertain the mechanisms by which viruses cause disease and in particular immunosuppression. Traditional studies on viral pathogens had largely focused on agents that appeared to cause disease by directly injuring cells in which they replicated. Rarely is the immune system a primary target for direct injury by viruses, but when it is, the outcome is usually immunosuppression. Currently, we are aware that injury to the immune system more commonly results from secondary consequences of the many fundamental interactions that occur between viruses and cells. Thus, malfunction of the immune system can be the consequence of a virus replicating in cells other than those involved in immunity and viruses that do replicate in cells of the immune system may do so without overt signs such as direct cell killing. Functional changes may occur giving rise to sequelae such as immunopathology, autoimmunity, neoplasia, and immunosuppression. In this brief review we survey some of the better understood mechanisms of immune suppression that result from viral infections, focusing on retroviruses and emphasizing those rare examples where a molecular understanding of suppression

---

TAMMIE L. KEADLE • Department of Ophthalmology, Washington University School of Medicine, St. Louis, Missouri 63130. SANDRA DANIEL and BARRY T. ROUSE • Department of Microbiology, College of Veterinary Medicine, University of Tennessee, Knoxville, Tennessee 37916. DAVID W. HOROHOV • Department of Microbiology, College of Veterinary Medicine, Louisiana State University, Baton Rouge, Louisiana 70803.

Immunopharmacology Reviews, Volume 2, edited by John W. Hadden and Andor Szentivanyi. Plenum Press, New York, 1996.

appears to be at hand. Clearly, the aim is to unravel the mechanistic nature of immunosuppression so that rational approaches to therapy can be devised.

2. IMMUNOSUPPRESSION THROUGH DIRECT DESTRUCTION OR DAMAGE TO IMMUNE CELLS

With viruses that replicate in cells of the immune system, immunosuppression may result from direct destruction of cells. The actual mechanism of damage can be variable and may include cell membrane disruption, toxicity of viral nucleic acids, alteration of host cell biosynthetic pathways, inappropriate intracellular signaling following virus–receptor interactions, as well as cytotoxicity resulting from excessive production of viral protein or nucleic acids (reviewed in Mims, 1986; Potgieter, 1986). Direct destruction of lymphocytes is the consequence when parvoviruses replicate as occurs for example with feline panleukopenia (reviewed in Rouse and Horohov, 1986). Several paramyxoviruses such as measles virus may cause lympholysis which results in immunosuppression (McChesney and Oldstone, 1989; Pasternak, 1987). Similarly, infectious bursal disease virus produces necrotic lesions in the bursa of Fabricius of birds and may destroy mature B cells leading to impaired humoral immune responses (Sharma *et al.*, 1994). Currently, most interest, however, is focused on human immunodeficiency virus (HIV), the causative agent of AIDS. It is well established that the primary target cells for HIV infection are $CD4^+$ T cells, particularly within lymphoid tissues where virus may be concentrated. From *in vitro* studies it is evident that following a complete replication cycle (productive infection) cells usually die (reviewed in Schnittman and Fauci, 1994). Thus, direct lymphocyte destruction could be one of the causes of the profound immunosuppression observed in AIDS. Immunosuppression may be potentiated severalfold, however, if $CD4^+$ T-cell precursors or trophic cells are also destroyed by HIV infection (Stanley *et al.*, 1992; Schnittman *et al.*, 1990).

The molecular mechanism of cell killing by HIV is not clear but a number of mechanisms have been hypothesized. These include formation of holes in the cell membrane resulting from virus budding, inhibition of host cell synthetic capacity, ion fluxes and decreased cell viability caused by insertion of viral envelope proteins into the cell membrane, accumulation of unintegrated viral DNA in the cytoplasm, and accumulation of gp160–CD4 complexes around the nuclear pores of HIV-infected $CD4^+$ cells (reviewed in Haseltine, 1991; Schnittman and Fauci, 1994). Apparently, more than one mechanism may be occurring and some of these mechanisms may only operate when factors other than HIV infection are brought into play. It is also likely that HIV-infected cells which express surface gp120 can fuse with large numbers of $CD4^+$ lymphocytes to generate syncytia which become nonviable in a short period of time (reviewed in Schnittman and Fauci, 1994; Takai *et al.*, 1988). Apoptosis or programmed cell death of HIV/gp120-primed $CD4^+$ cells may contribute further to $CD4^+$ T-cell depletion in AIDS (Schnittman and Fauci, 1994). Of interest, feline immunodeficiency virus (FIV), a lentivirus that closely resembles HIV with regard to viral pathogenesis, is known to cause lysis of infected T cells and to mediate apoptosis (Bendinelli *et al.*, 1995).

In addition to virus-induced direct lytic effects, killing of HIV-infected cells may also proceed via immune-mediated mechanisms. Moreover, experiments by the Reinherz group and others (Lanzavecchia *et al.*, 1988; Siliciano *et al.*, 1988) indicate that uninfected $CD4^+$ cells may take up and process the HIV envelope protein, gp120, into peptides which can associate with MHC class II proteins and render cells susceptible to cytotoxicity by antigen-specific $CD4^+$ cytotoxic T lymphocytes (CTL). Probably a similar form of cytotoxicity mediated by $CD4^+$ or even $CD8^+$ CTL occurs *in vivo* and serves to destroy infected cells. In the initial phases of HIV pathogenesis, the $CD8^+$ CTL response is likely protective and functions to remove the minor population of infected $CD4^+$ cells that express antigen (Hoffenbach *et al.*, 1989; Plata *et al.*, 1987), but later the CTL response may contribute to immunosuppression through destruction of uninfected "bystander" cells including antigen-presenting cells (Emilie *et al.*, 1994). Indeed, some researchers have hypothesized that HIV-associated immunosuppression results primarily from virus-specific CTL activity and not HIV-mediated cytolysis (Zinkernagel and Hengartner, 1994).

In addition to depletion of $CD4^+$ cells, it appears that HIV-stimulated destruction of the microenvironment of lymphoid organs plays a significant contributory role in the progression of AIDS. This damage may be caused directly by infection with HIV or indirectly by immunopathologic mechanisms (Emilie *et al.*, 1994; Fauci, 1993). Thus, destruction of lymph node architecture and follicular dendritic cells, thymic epithelial cells, and bone marrow stromal cells may be key to induction of intractable immunosuppression with terminal consequences (reviewed in Fauci, 1993).

Although the idea that immune-mediated lymphoid destruction and eventual immunosuppression is hypothesized to occur in AIDS, better evidence for the operation of such an immune-mediated mechanism of immunosuppression is available from other systems. One of the better studied systems is murine infection with lymphocytic choriomeningitis virus (LCMV). This virus replicates in mononuclear phagocytes and lymphocytes but is not cytotoxic for them. Instead, immunosuppression appears to result from an anti-LCMV $CD8^+$ T-cell response which destroys LCMV-infected T-helper and antigen-presenting cells (Roost *et al.*, 1988; Odermatt *et al.*, 1991). These results emphasize the pivotal role that virus-specific cytolytic immune responses can play in exacerbation of immunosuppression, particularly in the case of lymphotropic viruses (Reibnegger *et al.*, 1987).

3. FUNCTIONAL IMPAIRMENT RESULTING FROM VIRAL INFECTION

Lymphotropic viruses may cause immunosuppression by inhibitory mechanisms other than being cyto-destructive. This is certainly true in infections with measles virus (MV), a paramyxovirus, and cytomegalovirus (CMV), a herpesvirus, where lymphocytes or macrophages taken from infected individuals can be shown to display impaired functional activity as measured by diminished effector cell activity or suppressed responses on stimulation by antigens or mitogens (reviewed in Horohov and Rouse, 1986; McChesney and Oldstone, 1989). In MV and its canine counterpart, canine distemper virus (CDV), immunosuppression may be profound and long lasting following acute infection. Direct lympholysis occurs, but this is not the whole story, since immunosuppression persists long after demonstrable virus has disappeared and circulating cell numbers appear normal. Hence, lymphocyte or monocyte responsiveness may be impaired and curious patterns of inactivity are observed in which some but not all antigens are recognized (Esolen *et al.*, 1993; Horohov and Rouse, 1986; McChesney and Oldstone, 1989). Lymphocytes taken from MV-infected individuals may also be markedly impaired in their ability to undergo proliferation and produce cytokines in response to stimulation by nonspecific mitogens (Ward and Griffin, 1993; Horohov and Rouse, 1986; McChesney and Oldstone, 1989). Some favor the idea that prolonged suppression in MV and CDV represents overactive suppressor cells, although how this effect is mediated is unclear.

A host of factors may potentially contribute to impaired immune function following viral infection and defy review here. One possibility, however, is functional depression resulting from cytokine dysregulation. Functional depression resulting from viral infection has been noted with several retroviruses and the notion that immunosuppression may be the outcome of a series of events that involve changes in cytokine gene expression has been gathering adherents (Joag and Narayan, 1993; Jolicoeur, 1991; Ward and Griffin, 1993; Gazzinelli *et al.*, 1992). Since cytokines play an integral role in regulating the type and duration of an immune response, specific disturbances in their production, secretion, or function could result in frank immunosuppression. Alterations in cytokine expression following cell stimulation have been noted with many retrovirus models (Jolicoeur, 1991; Lewis *et al.*, 1990; Faxvaag *et al.*, 1993; Gazzinelli *et al.*, 1992). Much of the earlier work was done with oncornaviruses such as murine leukemia virus (MLV) and feline leukemia virus (FeLV), but recently the focus has been on lentiviruses, particularly HIV.

Cytokine dysregulation in HIV infection is complex. Accordingly, observed cytokine profiles may depend on the stage of disease (Clerici and Shearer, 1994), the presence of coinfections (Gosselin *et al.*, 1992), the anatomic location under study (Emilie *et al.*, 1994), and *in vitro* culture conditions (Lotz and Seth, 1993; Ameglio *et al.*, 1994). Recently, a model has been proposed that correlates transition from T-helper (Th) 1-related cytokine expression (IFN, IL-2 and IL-12) and cell-mediated immune responses to Th2-related cytokine expression (IL-4, IL-5, IL-6, and IL-10) and humoral immune responses with increased disease severity (Clerici and Shearer, 1994). It has been postulated that preferential apoptosis of Thl cells or cofactors generated in the course of coincidental infectious episodes may induce the switch from Thl to Th2, thus ending the latent phase of HIV infection and resulting in the progression of AIDS (Clerici and Shearer, 1994). Evidence for this theory is provided by examining cytokine profiles of serum and cells from AIDS patients at various stages of the disease (Pantaleo and Fauci, 1995; Navikas *et al.*, 1994; Dalgleish, 1995; Clerici and Shearer, 1994). Of interest, some HIV-exposed seronegative people retain their ability to make IL-2 in response to HIV antigens and HIV-infected long-term nonprogressors are noted for persistence of cell-mediated immune responses (Oppenheim and Neta, 1994; Pantaleo and Fauci, 1995).

In addition to global changes in cytokine patterns that may occur during the course of AIDS, typical cytokine profiles for individual cell types may be disrupted. For example, LPS-stimulated and unstimulated monocytes from HIV-infected individuals were shown to differentially express the monokines TNF-α, IL-1β, and IL-6 dependent on the disease stage (Lathey *et al.*, 1994a,b). Similarly, CD4 cross-linking by HIV gp160 resulted in induction of IFN-α in the absence of IL-2 secretion in PBMC from normal individuals (Hu *et al.*, 1994).

Whatever the mechanisms, a number of cytokines have been shown to be elevated in blood or lymphoid tissue of HIV-infected individuals. These include TNF-α, IL-1, IL-6, IFN, IL-10, and TGF-β (Lotz and Seth, 1993; Fan *et al.*, 1993; Ameglio *et al.*, 1994; Emilie *et al.*, 1994). Conversely, serum levels of IL-2 and production of IL-12 by HIV-infected PBMC may be depressed (Emilie *et al.*, 1994; Fan *et al.*, 1993; Chehimi *et al.*, 1994). Effects of a single cytokine on immune function may vary with timing, location, level of expression, and the presence of other cytokines. Thus, circulating cytokine levels are difficult to interpret. Minimally, however, individual cytokines may be assessed with regard to their effects on virus replication and immunologic responses leading to immunosuppression.

3.1. Interferon and Immunosuppression

Initially known for their antiviral effects, it became apparent, especially from work by the Gresser group, that the IFNs express a wide array of immunomodulatory activities some of which can be considered as immunosuppressive (Gresser, 1977). Most of our understanding of the immunomodulatory effects of IFNs came from *in vitro* studies and rarely are molecular explanations available for the effects observed. Some observations do imply that IFNs may mediate immunosuppression *in vivo*. Accordingly, some viruses may induce levels of IFN which appear responsible for suppressing protective immune responses to coinfecting viruses (Brenan and Zinkernagel, 1983; Freidman, 1988). The mediator of suppression is assumed to be IFN because the effect could be mimicked by administering purified IFN or IFN inducers and could be reversed by giving specific anti-IFN serum (Brenan and Zinkernagel, 1983). How IFN causes immunosuppression is not well understood particularly at a molecular level. However, candidate mechanisms include antiproliferative effects, changes in membrane expression of various molecules involved in immune recognition, functional changes in antigen-presenting cells (APC), and opposition of the activities of other cytokines (reviewed in Horohov and Rouse, 1986).

Despite the fact that increased expression of IFN-α and -γ have been noted in the circulation and cells of HIV-infected individuals, the role of interferons in HIV-associated immunosuppression is unclear (Ameglio *et al.*, 1994; Emilie *et al.*, 1994). Thus, *in vitro* IL-2 production of peripheral blood leukocytes (PBL) from ARC/AIDS patients may be partially restored by anti-IFN-α antibodies (Zagury *et al.*, 1985), IFN-γ may increase HIV expression from chronically infected monocytic cells in contrast to other interferons (Biswas *et al.*, 1992), and IFN-γ upregulates apoptotic FAS antigen expression (Itoh *et al.*, 1991). In addition, anti-IFN effects of other cytokines may moderate IFN actions *in vivo* (Lotz and Seth, 1993) and HIV infection or gp120 treatment reduces the ability of cells to produce IFN-γ on subsequent stimulation (Hu *et al.*, 1994; Murray *et al.*, 1984). In the latter two instances, IFN would appear to be a victim of immunosuppression rather than its cause. Some workers have made attempts to formulate a hypothesis explaining various effects of the IFNs during HIV infection (Kornbluth *et al.*, 1990), but more data are required before any hypothesis can be fully evaluated.

3.2. TGF-β Immunosuppression

Another endogenous cytokine likely important as a mediator of immunosuppression during HIV infection is TGF-β. Serum and plasma of AIDS patients have elevated levels of TGF-β (Allen *et al.*, 1991; Lotz and Seth, 1993) and PBL from HIV-infected donors show increased constitutive and induced TGF-β production *in vitro* when compared to uninfected control PBL (Kekow *et al.*, 1990). Additionally, *in vitro* treatment of freshly isolated PBL with gp160 results in increased expression of TGF (Hu *et al.*, 1994). Since TGF-β exerts potent inhibitory effects against many cellular and humoral immune functions *in vitro* (Kehrl *et al.*, 1991; Palladino *et al.*, 1990; Lotz and Seth, 1993; Ruscetti *et al.*, 1993), overexpression in HIV-positive patients could contribute to immunosuppression (Allen *et al.*, 1991).

In general, TGF-β activity reflects a pattern whereby it switches on resting cells and switches off activated cells (Oppenheim and Neta, 1994; Ruscetti *et al.*, 1993). Hence, TGF-β increases mRNA levels and the production of inflammatory cytokines including IL-1, TNF, and IL-6 in resting monocytes, while activated macrophages are subject to downregulation. The downregulatory effects of TGF-β may also account for its potent suppression of B-cell proliferation and immunoglobulin secretion (except IgA), T lymphocyte and large granular lymphocyte (LGL) proliferation, and CTL activity (Oppenheim and Neta, 1994).

Specific mechanisms to explain TGF-β mediated *in vivo* effects include inhibition of the constitutive expression of IL-1 receptors on selected cells, induction of IL-1 mRNA expression, inhibition of CTL induction, downmodulation of MHC class II antigen expression on antigen-presenting cells (APC), and decreased IL-2 receptor expression and proliferative responses to IL-2 (reviewed in Lotz and Seth, 1993; Oppenheim and Neta, 1994; Ruscetti *et al.*, 1993). TGF-β also acts as a chemotactic factor for monocytes and can reduce the production of H_2O_2 and nitric oxide by macrophages (Lotz and Seth, 1993). It is likely that inhibition of IL-1 receptor expression could result in cells exposed to TGF-β appearing to be functionally defective via their lack of responsiveness for IL-1-mediated events (Dubois *et al.*, 1990). This could contribute to immunosuppression since IL-1 functions as a potent immunoregulatory molecule in a variety of immune responses (Dinarello, 1989). Likewise, decreased IL-2 responsiveness, whether as a primary effect or secondary to a functional deficit of IL-1, would impede numerous immune responses (Howard *et al.*, 1993). In addition to the activities above, it has been reported that TGF-β may inhibit cellular proliferation through the induction of protein phosphatase 1 as well as a protein tyrosine phosphatase (Grupposo *et al.*, 1991). Thus, since protein phosphorylation plays a significant role in T-cell activation and function, the induction of a phosphatase activity could contribute to a state of cellular nonresponsiveness.

TGF-β's mediation of immunosuppression by inhibiting CTL induction has been demonstrated in the LCMV system (Fontana *et al.*, 1989), and it is possible that TGF-β overexpression in AIDS patients may play an important role in downregulating the development of CTL responses. TGF-β may also mediate immunosuppression in AIDS by compromising some of the functions of APCs such as MHC expression (Czarniecki *et al.*, 1988). The latter could result, in part, from TGF-β's antagonism of IFN-γ induced macrophage activation (reviewed in Lotz and Seth, 1993). Interestingly, TGF-β may suppress HIV replication and expression in premonocytic cells (Poli *et al.*, 1991). Thus, TGF-β potentially plays a dual role in HIV-infected monocytes, contributing to immunosuppression while simultaneously helping to eliminate the virus in these cells by restricting replication. This inhibition of HIV replication by TGF-β is not, however, consistently noted in other infected cell types (Lotz and Seth, 1993). Therefore, the cumulative effect of TGF-β overexpression *in vivo* is likely to be chronically increased virus replication resulting from its interference with antiviral host defense mechanisms.

3.3. IL-1, TNF-α, and IL-6 during HIV Infection

IL-1, TNF-α, and IL-6 are present at elevated levels in serum or tissue fluids at some stages during HIV infection (Berman *et al.*, 1994; Lahdvirta *et al.*, 1988; Chollet-Martin *et al.*, 1994; Lathey *et al.*, 1994a; Emilie *et al.*, 1994). In addition, the spontaneous release of IL-1 and IL-6 by HIV-infected macrophages has been demonstrated (Berman *et al.*, 1994), and HIV infection of some cell types has been found to directly induce TNF-α (Butera, 1993). These cytokines have been reported to upregulate HIV expression in monocytes (IL-6) or T lymphocytes and monocytes (IL-1 and TNF-α) (Fauci, 1993). TNF-α enhances HIV gene expression by stimulating the promoter region of HIV's long terminal repeat (LTR) via activation of transcription factors which bind to NFκB consensus sequences present in HIV's LTR (Schnittman and Fauci, 1994; Duh *et al.*, 1989; Osborn *et al.*, 1989). Thus, TNF-α functions in an autocrine/paracrine fashion in induction of HIV replication. IL-6, on the other hand, acts to enhance HIV replication by a posttranscriptional mechanism (Poli *et al.*, 1990a).

The overall importance of IL-1, TNF-α, and IL-6 on HIV replication and immune responses *in vivo* is unclear and is an active area of research. IL-1 acts as an accessory molecule for T-lymphocyte activation, mediates inflammation, and acts in synergy with other cytokines as an inducer of B-cell maturation, proliferation, and immunoglobulin production (Dinarello, 1989; Durum and Oppenheim, 1993). Its immunosuppressive effects could stem from its ability to induce secretion of other cytokines such as TNF-α, IL-4, and IL-6 or its role in inducing cell activation, a necessity for HIV replication. The cytokine TNF-α is extremely pleiotropic and many of its activities can be considered to be proinflammatory rather than immunosuppressive (Chouaib *et al.*, 1991; Durum and Oppenheim, 1993). The role of TNF-α in disease progression is controversial since in some systems it has marked antimicrobial activity when a Thl-like cytokine profile is dominant and may be immunopathologic when a Th2-like profile is dominant (Dalgleish, 1995). The association of TNF-α with AIDS suggests that TNF-α may also be detrimental during a Th2 response to HIV. IL-6, while also a mediator of inflammation, additionally induces differentiation of B cells in to antibody-secreting plasma cells, which in HIV may contribute to hypergammaglobulinemia and autoantibody formation, thus contributing to immunosuppression (Durum and Oppenheim, 1993).

3.4. IL-10 and HIV Infection

Increased IL-10 levels have been associated with the later stages of HIV infection (Dalgleish, 1995; Oppenheim and Neta, 1994). Additionally, gp120 treatment of resting PBMC results in increased IL-10 expression (Ameglio *et al.*, 1994). This cytokine has been shown to increase or decrease HIV replication in monocytes/macrophages depending on the system studied (Fauci, 1993).

IL-10 is a cross regulatory cytokine produced by several cell types including Th2 cells (Moore *et al.*, 1993). Its potential for immunosuppression lies in its ability to block accessory cell functions of macrophages and induction of other cytokines such as IFN-α and IL-2 (Moore *et al.*, 1993). Hence, increased IL-10 expression may enhance Th2 responses to the detriment of protective Thl immune responses during the course of HIV infection. As with other cytokines, the *in vivo* role of IL-10 requires further study.

3.5. Interactions between Cytokines and HIV during HIV Infection

Agonistic and antagonistic relationships may exist between cytokines with respect to immune responses and HIV expression. More than likely, if we fully understand how cytokines and HIV cross-influence each other, we may be better able to control these interactions and perhaps curtail or reverse immunosuppression. HIV suppression of IL-2 production serves to diminish overall immunological defenses including the ability to eliminate HIV (Lane *et al.*, 1985; Murray *et al.*, 1984). HIV apparently inhibits IL-2 gene expression by interfering with signal transduction and/

or secondary messenger formation following activation of the CD3–TCR, thus interfering with IL-2 gene activation (Oyaizu *et al.*, 1990). Several investigators have demonstrated that HIV-infected CD4$^+$ T cells are defective in their ability to mobilize calcium following activation through the CD3–TCR complex (Hofmann *et al.*, 1990; Linette *et al.*, 1988; Pinching and Nye, 1990). In addition, since the 5′ regulatory region of the IFN-γ gene has homology with that of the IL-2 gene, HIV may downregulate IFN-γ gene expression by a mechanism similar to that for IL-2. However, further experimentation is necessary to unravel the exact mechanism by which HIV blocks signal transduction.

Cytokines do not mediate effects on HIV replication in isolation. This is perhaps best exemplified by the interactions between TNF-α, HIV, and other cytokines. TNF-α has been examined most closely with regard to its autocrine/paracrine enhancement of HIV replication (Poli *et al.*, 1990a,b). In addition to TNF-α's induction of HIV replication, reports suggest that HIV infection enhances TNF-α production *in vitro* and *in vivo* (Poli *et al.*, 1990; Osborn *et al.*, 1989; Butera, 1993). As previously discussed, TGF-β may be overexpressed during HIV infection resulting in upregulation of IL-1 expression (Lotz and Seth, 1993; Ruscetti *et al.*, 1993). If IL-1 receptors are functional on immune cells, overexpression of IL-1 would induce enhanced production of TNF-α [since these cytokines reciprocally induce each other's expression (Durum and Oppenheim, 1993)] which in turn could enhance HIV replication (Poli *et al.*, 1990a,b; Osborn *et al.*, 1989). Conversely, TGF-β is thought to antagonize most of the activities of TNF-α (Oppenheim and Neta, 1994) and to mediate HIV TAT-induced inhibition of IFN activity leading to increased viral replication (Lotz and Seth, 1993). In addition to TGF-β, IL-1, and IFN, IL-10 has been shown to affect TNF-α–HIV interactions. Accordingly, in a recent study IL-10 blocked HIV-induced TNF-α and IL-6 secretion (Weissman *et al.*, 1994). Thus, the net effect of any cytokine on HIV replication *in vivo* will depend on a complex interplay of responses elicited by many other factors.

While increased levels of these cytokines may be important for enhanced replication of HIV, the dysregulation of these cytokines could also be responsible for many of the clinical signs that are seen late in HIV infection. For instance, TNF-α, IL-1, and IL-6 are believed to contribute to the severe wasting of cachexia as well as CNS dysfunction which is seen in the terminal stages of AIDS, while IL-6 may be responsible for the nonspecific polyclonal B-cell activation and increased immunoglobulin levels observed in AIDS (reviewed in Merrill and Chen, 1991; Schnittman and Fauci, 1994; Durum and Oppenheim, 1993). Given the complex interactions that occur in the cytokine network, it should not be surprising that immune dysfunctions occur in HIV patients who are experiencing significant modulation of these important regulatory proteins. It is also likely that coinfection of HIV-seropositive individuals with other agents may contribute to the pathogenesis of immunosuppression, potentially by modulating cytokine levels. For instance, human herpesvirus 6 (HHV-6), which was first isolated from a patient infected with HIV (Salahuddin *et al.*, 1986), may also induce the production of IL-1-β and TNF-α (Flamand *et al.*, 1991; Gosselin *et al.*, 1992). HHV-6 has a tropism for many cells of the immune system, including CD4$^+$ T cells, B cells, monocytes/macrophages, and megakaryocytes (Ablashi *et al.*, 1987; Lusso *et al.*, 1988). Infection of these cells could lead to widespread immunosuppression via disturbances in regulation of cytokine gene expression. An example would be TNF-α production which in turn stimulates replication of HIV, an effect likely to be lethal to cells. It appears then that HHV-6 infection is one of many possible cofactors that influence the progression of an HIV infection from an asymptomatic nonimmunosuppressed state to full-blown AIDS.

3.6. Interference with Cytokine Signals

Since cytokines play essential roles in regulating immunity and mediating resistance, interfering with their function is expected to have immunosuppressive consequences. Two means of achieving this would be to inhibit their function with cytokine inhibitors (anti- or contracytokines) or generate an excess of soluble cytokine receptors which would compete with cell surface membrane receptors for cytokine binding, thus blocking cytokine binding and activation of its cell surface receptor. Both types of activities have been found to occur naturally and the prospect that cytokine function can be modulated therapeutically with soluble receptor molecules or anticytokines is an exciting one (Durum and Mealy, 1990; Arend and Dayer, 1990; Fauci, 1993; Howard *et al.*, 1993a,b). With regard to viral induction of contracytokines, most information is available for molecules generically termed contra-IL-1. A molecule with contra-activity is produced by EBV-transformed B cells (Scott *et al.*, 1989). Additional contra-IL-1 activities, differing in size characteristics, may be present in the sera of HIV-seropositive patients (Berman *et al.*, 1987) as well as produced by HIV-infected monocytes (Locksley *et al.*, 1988), and respiratory syncytial virus- or influenza virus-infected macrophages (Roberts *et al.*, 1986). A contra-IL-1 activity has also been reported in association with human CMV and Dengue virus infection (Moses and Garnett, 1990; Chang and Shaio, 1994). An anti-IL-1 inhibitor protein derived from monocytes that have been stimulated by nonviral factors has been cloned, sequenced, and expressed as recombinant proteins (Eisenberg *et al.*, 1990; Hannum *et al.*, 1990). This inhibitor appears to act as a pure receptor antagonist, binding to IL-1 receptors but not inducing any subsequent IL-1-mediated activities (Catania *et al.*, 1993; Hannum *et al.*, 1990).

Though reported anti-IL-1 proteins are receptor antagonists, it is also important to distinguish contra- or anticytokine effects from protease effects. With regard to the latter question, a recent study has shown that endopeptidase 24.11 (enkephalinase), a 95-kDa membrane-bound metalloproteinase, can inactivate IL-1 as measured by the thymocyte costimulation assay (Pierpart *et al.*, 1988). The role of endopeptidases as IL-1 inhibitors requires further exploration. Other IL-1 inhibitors that possess some of the attributes of IL-1 hint that IL-1 derivatives may sometimes serve as contra-IL-1s (Durum and Mealy, 1990; Durum *et al.*, 1991). As mentioned previously, an IL-1 inhibitor has been reported as present in the serum of patients with AIDS (Berman *et al.*, 1987). This inhibitor, of approximately 6 to 9 kDa, partially masked increased IL-1 production in these patients. Furthermore, this inhibitor was presumed to contribute to immunosuppression by blocking IL-1-dependent activation of T lymphocytes in AIDS patients.

The prospect that soluble cytokine receptor molecules could serve to inhibit cytokine function is a likely one, and several examples have now been reported. Indeed, members of the poxvirus family have been found to encode products homologous to receptors for IL-1, TNF-α, IFN-γ, or IL-8, with some viruses coding for more than one of these so-called "viroceptors" (Schreiber and McFadden, 1994; Upton *et al.*, 1991, 1992). Thus, vaccinia and cowpox encode IL-1R β homologues (Alcami and Smith, 1992; Spriggs *et al.*, 1992), Shope fibroma virus, myxoma virus, and cowpox virus encode TNF receptor homologues (Upton *et al.*, 1991; Hu *et al.*, 1994), myxoma virus T7 protein is homologous to the IFN-γ receptor (Upton *et al.*, 1992), and the swine pox genome may code for an IL-8 receptor homologue (Massung *et al.*, 1993)—the first example of a cell surface viroceptor. Secretion and biological activity of several of these viral cytokine receptors have been confirmed (Schreiber and McFadden, 1994; Mossman *et al.*, 1995; Alcami and Smith, 1992). As discussed previously, IL-1, TNF-α, and IFN-γ are potent immunoregulatory agents. Interfering with the function of these cytokines may help viruses evade host immunity and in addition serve to regulate the immune response to other antigens.

Artificial manipulation of cytokine responses, particularly during the course of HIV infection, may hold promise for controlling or reversing immunologic abnormalities associated with AIDS. Although, as described in the preceding sections, the interactions between HIV and cytokines are extremely complex and daunting, a number of therapeutic strategies are evolving. Most of these treatments are aimed at decreasing viral replication or restoring Th1/cell-mediated immune responses. Currently they include administration of anticytokine antibodies, contracytokines, soluble cytokine receptors, pharmacologic cytokine inhibitors, and Th1-like cytokines (reviewed in Fauci, 1993; Dalgleish, 1995). Undoubtedly, as more is learned about the role of cytokines in the pathogenesis of AIDS, these treatment strategies will be expanded, refined, and tailored more to the individual's disease stage.

4. IMMUNOSUPPRESSION MEDIATED BY VIRAL PRODUCTS

Of necessity, viruses are frugal. Because of their limited genomes, they must extract the maximum amount of use from each virus-encoded product. This implies that some viral proteins will subserve multiple functions and those that efficiently promote completion of the viral life cycle will be specifically retained. Thus, viral structural proteins may serve to promote viral replication or persistence in the face of an active immune response and viruses seem to have pirated various elements of the host's immune system in order to gain the advantage in their struggle for survival. The latter two phenomena are examined in the following sections.

4.1. Suppression by Viral Structural Proteins

From studies on many viruses, but especially retroviruses, it is apparent that viral proteins or polypeptides released from infected cells may affect the function of immune cells. This paracrine effect may result in immunosuppression and play a significant contributory role in disease pathogenesis. One of the earliest studied viral products that expressed immunosuppressive activities was p15E, the transmembrane portion of the envelope protein for the FeLV retrovirus (Rojko and Olsen, 1984; McChesney and Oldstone, 1987; Rojko *et al.*, 1988). A 26-amino-acid sequence of p15E of feline and murine leukemia viruses is conserved among the transmembrane envelope proteins of murine, feline, simian, and human T-cell leukemia retroviruses, and partially for HIV gp41 (Cianciolo *et al.*, 1984, 1985; Sonigo *et al.*, 1986). CKS-17, a 17-amino-acid peptide representing the conserved domain within this region, exerts a range of immunosuppressive effects including suppression of *in vitro* synthesis of IFN-γ and -α, TNF-α, and IL-2; depressed lymphocyte blastogenesis; diminished expression of membrane IL-2 receptors; decreased CTL, NK, and DTH responses; and modulation of B-cell immunoglobulin production (Cianciolo *et al.*, 1985; Rojko *et al.*, 1988; Rojko and Olsen, 1984; Haraguchi *et al.*, 1992, 1995; Chernukhin *et al.*, 1993; Good *et al.*, 1991). Effects of CKS-17 on monocytes also occur. These include dramatic changes in cell morphology and distribution, modulation of functions such as induced PGE_2 and TGF-β production, and depressive effects on monocyte progenitor cells in bone marrow (Good *et al.*, 1990; Chernukhin *et al.*, 1993). Recent work indicates that CKS-17's effects on monocytes and macrophages (key IL-10 and 12 producers) may precipitate an imbalance between Th1 and Th2-related cytokine production and thereby negatively influence cell-mediated immunity resulting in immunosuppression (Haraguchi *et al.*, 1995). Thus, CKS-17 downregulated stimulant-induced mRNA accumulation of IFN-γ, IL-2 and 12; upregulated induced mRNA accumulation of IL-10; and had no effect on IL-4, 5, 6, or 13. Furthermore, anti-IL-10 antibodies were able to restore IFN-γ but not IL-12 mRNA accumulation, suggesting that CKS-17 suppression of IFN-γ may be secondary to its enhancement of IL-10 expression and suppression of IL-12 (Haraguchi *et al.*, 1995). Thus, CKS-17 can potentially mediate immunosuppression in multiple ways. Studies on this peptide have revealed a possible molecular mechanism by which CKS-17 and p15E mediate their various immunosuppressive activities. Thus, p15E is believed to intercalate into cellular membranes and this may interfere with intracellular signal transduction such as triggering of Ca^{2+}/calmodulin-dependent activation of adenyl cyclase (Rojko and Olsen, 1984) in some cell types or Ca^{2+}-mediated protein kinase C activation in other cells (Dezzutti *et al.*, 1989; Gottlieb *et al.*, 1990). Studies have also demonstrated that exposure to CKS-17 results in interference with cellular signal transduction through protein kinase C-mediated pathways (Gottlieb *et al.*, 1990; Kadota *et al.*, 1991).

Another viral protein that may mediate paracrine immunosuppressive effects is the envelope glycoprotein of HIV, gp120. Effects on both mononuclear phagocytic cells and T cells have been documented (Diamond *et al.*, 1988; Oyaizu *et al.*, 1990; Theodore *et al.*, 1994; Liegler and Stites, 1994). For example, exposure of normal monocytes to purified HIV-1 or gp120 results in significantly impaired chemotactic responses, an effect that correlates with decreases in expression of surface receptors for the potent chemotactic ligands C5a and FMLP (Wahl *et al.*, 1989). As demonstrated in various experimental systems, the potentially immunosuppressive effects of gp120 on T-cell function include: decreased lymphoproliferation, reduced expression of IL-2 (Tyring *et al.*, 1991) and IL-2 receptors (Oyaizu *et al.*, 1990), decreased production of IFN-γ (Tyring *et al.*, 1991), and depressed chemotactic activity of $CD4^+$ T cells (Theodore *et al.*, 1994). Synthetic peptides corresponding to HIV envelope gp120 also enhance *in vitro* production of IL-1 and TNF, and depress production of IFN-α in freshly isolated PBMC (Tyring *et al.*, 1991).

The mechanism whereby gp120 peptide exerts its immunosuppressive effects is currently under investigation in a number of labs. Several possibilities exist, all of which may result in functional anergy. These include: (1) CD4 downregulation in infected (Weinhold *et al.*, 1989; Wahl *et al.*, 1989) and uninfected bystander cells (Theodore *et al.*, 1994), (2) inhibition of MHCII–CD4 interactions through direct physical blockade with gp120 (Clayton *et al.*, 1989; Mittler and Hoffman, 1989; Zagury *et al.*, 1994) or through proposed internal complexing between gp120 CD4 homologous sites (see Section 4.2) and MHCII molecules in infected macrophages (Zagury *et al.*, 1994), and (3) gp120-induced aberrations in receptor-mediated signal transduction (Chirmule *et al.*, 1990).

In addition to the gp120 region of the HIV precursor envelope protein, gp160, the transmembrane gp41 region may also possess immunosuppressive properties. Thus, in *in vitro* systems, peptide fragments of gp41 induce a variety of potentially suppressive events including depressed NK and CTL activity (Cauda *et al.*, 1988; Wang *et al.*, 1995), decreased proliferation of lymphocytes in response to several types of stimulation (Wang *et al.*, 1995), altered cytokine production patterns (Tyring *et al.*, 1991), and reduced protein kinase C activity and Ca^{2+} influx during signal transduction (Want *et al.*, 1995). The finding of gp120 (Oh *et al.*, 1992) and gp41 (Wang *et al.*, 1995) in the circulation of AIDS patients underscores the possible *in vivo* significance of the above experimental findings for gp120 and gp41, and the potential importance of HIV structural proteins in inducing dysfunction of uninfected immune cell populations.

In conclusion, there is substantial evidence that viral structural proteins can induce immunosuppression in the absence of whole infectious virions. The means by which these proteins may induce states of cellular dysfunction and immunosuppression are only now being elucidated. Many of them will undoubtedly share a common mechanism of action, that is, the ability to dysregulate cellular signal transduction. This dysregulation may result in anergy—the inability of a cell to respond to a given stimulus—and ultimately immunosuppression.

4.2. Molecular Mimicry and Immunosuppression

In recent years it has become increasingly clear that viruses employ molecular mimicry as a means of immune evasion. Viroceptors have already been described (Section 3.6). In addition, a number of other virus-encoded proteins have been shown to emulate selected aspects of host immune responses. Except for HIV, larger DNA viruses are often involved. Targets of this molecular counterfeiting include regulatory proteins and proteins involved in cell signaling pathways. In general, these viral products may have direct effects similar to their cellular counterparts or indirect effects resulting from interference with normal processes or induction of autoimmunity.

Current examples of virus-encoded regulatory protein homologues include cytokines, complement inhibitors, and serine protease inhibitors. Accordingly, IL-10 homologues have been identified in the genome of equine herpes virus type 2 (Rode *et al.*, 1993, 1994) and Epstein–Barr virus (Moore *et al.*, 1990). IL-10 is produced by stimulated Th2 cells and is a potent inhibitor of cytokine production by Th1 cells, particularly IFN-γ (reviewed in Moore *et al.*, 1993). As such, the IL-10 molecule is a potent regulator of immune responses inhibiting the immunoregulatory function of IFN-γ. The EBV IL-10 homologue, BCRF1, has been well studied and expresses many of the functions of IL-10. These include immunomodulating functions such as suppression of IFN-γ synthesis by murine Th1 clones and human PBMC, and suppressed induction of NK cells and CTL (Hsu *et al.*, 1990; Swaminathan *et al.*, 1993). IL-10 may also inhibit the antigen-presenting function of monocytes through downregulation of class II MHC on these cells (Moore *et al.*, 1993). These modulating effects may or may not help to ensure the survival of EBV in the immunologically hostile host, but the effects may be generally immunosuppressive and favor the survival or stimulate the activity of other infecting agents such as HIV.

Complement regulatory proteins have been identified in the genome of vaccinia virus (Kotwal and Moss, 1988), herpes simplex virus (Friedman *et al.*, 1984), and herpesvirus Saimiri (Albrecht *et al.*, 1992), and functional activity of secreted viral products have been demonstrated (Isaacs *et al.*, 1992; Harris *et al.*, 1990; Rother *et al.*, 1994). Presumably these complement regulatory proteins could subvert the normal antiviral functions of the complement cascade such as lysis of free virus or virally infected cells, virus opsonization or neutralization, and the elicitation of specific inflammatory immune responses (Liszewski and Atkinson, 1993). It seems likely that complement effects on unrelated pathogens might also be affected.

In addition to cytokines and complement regulatory proteins, virus-encoded serpins homologous to cellular products have been identified in the genome of several viruses (Macen *et al.*, 1993; Thompson *et al.*, 1993). Serpins belong to a superfamily of related proteins that regulate serine proteases (Carrell *et al.*, 1987). As such, viral serpins may act to inappropriately decrease inflammatory responses in favor of enhanced viral replication, spread, or persistence.

HIV infection provides a good example of molecular mimicry involving signal transduction pathways. Thus, homologies between HIV proteins and host proteins include (among others) CD4, MHC, and FAS (Dalgleish, 1995; Zagury *et al.*, 1993, 1994). The potential for immune suppression with such homologues may lie in the generation of aberrant cell signaling or autoimmunity. Thus, the CD4 identity sequence of gp120 strongly inhibited T-cell proliferation *in vitro* in the presence of antigen-primed macrophages (Zagury *et al.*, 1993). gp120 MHC identity segment also suppressed immune activation in this system but to a lesser extent. Presumably, direct physical blockade or delivery of negative signals could be responsible for the observed anergy. With regard to induction of autoimmunity by virus-encoded homologues, it is interesting to note that the blood of HIV-infected individuals contains both specific autoantibodies and CTLs directed against shared virus–cell CD4 sequences (Zagury *et al.*, 1993). Immune responses directed against gp120–MHC identity regions could potentially account for autoimmune reactivity to certain HLA types and alloantigen-like responses during the course of AIDS (Dalgleish, 1995). Immune responses to HIV-encoded CD4 and MHC homologues may result in elimination of uninfected immune cells thus further contributing to the immunosuppression seen in HIV infections (Schnittman and Fauci, 1994; Dalgleish, 1995).

With respect to the FAS identity of gp120 (Zagury *et al.*, 1994), it may be speculated that cells expressing FAS ligand preferentially undergo apoptosis on binding of the FAS homologue. Such a scenario has been proposed to explain selective depletion of FAS ligand-expressing Th1 cells during the course of HIV infection (Clerici and Shearer, 1994).

Viral mimicry of minor lymphocyte stimulating (MLS) antigens is another example of the advantageous use of cell signaling molecules by viruses. For over 20 years, researchers have investigated the role of MLS antigens, now termed "superantigens," in the mouse. These antigens were named for their ability to cause intense proliferation of $CD4^+$ cells *in vitro* in mixed lymphocyte cultures between murine strains that were identical at their major histocompatibility complex site. It is now clear that these murine alloantigens exert their proliferative effect by binding simultaneously to an MHC class II molecule and to all T-cell receptors that bear specific variable β chains (Herman *et al.*, 1991; Janeway, 1991). Several investigators have independently reported that MLS genes or "superantigens" appear to be encoded by the long terminal repeat of mouse mammary tumor retroviruses (Choi *et al.*, 1991; Dyson *et al.*, 1991; Frankel *et al.*, 1991; Fleischer, 1994). Such nonspecific activation events may serve to diminish specific immune responses thereby providing a state of partial immunosuppression. Additionally, expression of the superantigen may provide a selective advantage since many retroviruses replicate preferentially in activated cells. Thus, carrying its own superantigen may help these retroviruses gain a foothold during early infection. As speculated by Choi and colleagues (Choi *et al.*, 1991), the mouse mammary tumor virus may use this superantigen to stimulate T cells which then act as reservoirs for virus when the normal target reservoir, cells of the lactating mammary gland epithelium, are not dividing.

It remains to be investigated whether human retroviruses such as HIV encode some type of superantigen. At present, strong superantigenic activity has not been identified in association with HIV infection (Schnittman and Fauci, 1994; Dalgleish, 1995). However, it is noteworthy that regions of the HIV-1 envelope do stimulate normal cells and this may aid HIV infection by providing an actively proliferating target population (Dahlberg, 1988).

Discussions within this section have focused on the role of viral structural proteins and molecular mimicry in immunosuppression. Above all else, they demonstrate the extreme versatility and adaptability of viruses within their environment. Because the effector arms of the immune system are a powerful element of evolutionary pressure for eukaryotic viruses, it is likely that future studies will reveal many more instances of viral economy and molecular mimicry associated with enhancement of the viral life cycle and immunosuppression.

5. IMMUNOSUPPRESSION MEDIATED BY VIRUS-INDUCED SUPPRESSOR CELLS AND FACTORS

There is considerable literature concerning the probability that viruses in some instances mediate immunosuppression by inducing the overactivity of regulating suppressor cells or causing such cells to produce suppressor factors which in turn serve to down regulate immune cell activity (reviewed in Asherson, 1986; Horohov and Rouse, 1986). The field of suppression is complex and controversial and only a brief overview is offered here.

In general, different types of cells may work to suppress immune responses. The most common suppressor cells are T lymphocytes. Often, several T-suppressor cells sequentially interact with each other and antigen-presenting cells or factor-presenting cells to produce a final product. There are two types of suppressor factors associated with suppressor cells: antigen-specific suppressor factors and antigen-nonspecific suppressor factors (NS-SF). Antigen-specific suppressor factors may contain elements for antigen recognition and genetic restriction (Asherson, 1986; Horohov and Rouse, 1986). NS-SF, as the name implies, downregulate immune reactivity to any antigen in the effective concentration range of the factor. The latter compounds comprise a diverse and often ill-defined group which, in addition to more unique substances, may include cytokines such as prostaglandins, interferons, or interleukins (Asherson, 1986; Horohov and Rouse, 1986).

Suppressor cell activity in the influenza virus and HSV systems has received the most scrutiny (reviewed in Horohov and Rouse, 1986; Rouse and Horohov, 1986). Although a variety of immune responses may be subject to control by suppressor cells and factors (Asherson, 1986), most available information in viral systems relates to DTH and CTL responses. Hence, suppressor circuits controlling DTH and CTL responses have been extensively described for these two viruses. Depending on the system studied, suppressor cells act as necessary regulators of immune reactivity or contributors to immune pathology.

The topic most relevant to this work is how viruses and suppressor cells relate to immunosuppression and disease. Two answers may apply. First, suppressor cells induced by a given virus may cause suppression of immune responses directed to that same virus, thus initiating or enhancing related pathology. This may be the case in the well-studied HSV system wherein enhanced HSV-specific suppressor cell activity is associated with recurrent viral shedding and disease (Horohov and Rouse, 1986; Rinaldo and Torpey, 1993). While it is unclear whether enhanced suppressor activity is a cause or an effect of increased viral replication in this system, HSV-induced suppressor cells could inhibit protective cell-mediated immune responses and thus increase viral spread and lesion severity (Horohov and Rouse, 1986; Rouse and Horohov, 1986; Rinaldo and Torpey, 1993). Second, suppressor cells induced by a given virus may cause suppression of immune responses directed to unrelated pathogens. Thus, for example, cytomegalovirus (CMV)-dependent suppressor cells inhibit simian virus 40 (SV40)-specific CTL differentiation *in vitro* (Campbell *et al.*, 1989), and a NS-SF regulating HSV-specific CTL induction depresses lytic activity in influenza virus CTL induction cultures (Horohov *et al.*, 1985). Instances of generalized immunosuppression by viruses such as HSV, CMV, and EBV may have important implications with regard to patients with underlying immunosuppressive disorders, notably AIDS (Rinaldo and Torpey, 1993). In these cases, infection with herpesviruses could result in more severe clinical herpetic disease and exacerbation of existing immune deficits.

In summary, virus-induced suppressor cells and factors may mediate immunosuppression that results in detrimental effects on the host, but this is controversial in some systems. A secondary role in suppressing immune responses to other pathogens might prove more clinically relevant particularly in concurrent infections with HIV.

6. CONCLUSION

In the last 15 years our understanding of how viruses cause disease has advanced dramatically, and we are closer to achieving the ultimate objective of providing molecular explanations for the outcome of the interactions that occur between viruses and host cells. Although not recognized as human pathogens until recently, retroviruses have taken center stage since at least three of these viruses are pathogens of the immune system and give rise to complex, invariably lethal syndromes that include immunosuppression as a significant component. This review has focused on retroviruses, and we have attempted to document the various means by which immunosuppression is mediated, expecting that a mechanistic and molecular understanding will soon be followed by the development of novel and appropriate therapies.

It is evident that viruses may suppress immune function in many ways, but basically two patterns are recognizable. Viruses may directly damage or change the function of cells that they infect, or some of the viral products released from infected cells may inhibit the function of other immune cells. A recurring theme in studies on mechanisms of immunosuppression is that dyscrasia in the expression of one or more cytokines is involved. Assuming that the role of various cytokines during an immunosuppressive viral infection can be unraveled, the prospect of immunotherapy becomes a realistic one. Thus, many genetically engineered recombinant cytokines are available and could be used for reconstruction. This approach is already beginning, although apart from the requirement to accurately define which cytokines have impaired expression during a particular infection syndrome, there are some major obstacles to overcome. Thus, regular administration of the Th1-like cytokine, IL-2, increases the $CD4^+$ T-cell count in AIDS patients but is associated with toxicity and other adverse effects (Dalgleish, 1995). The therapeutic efficacy of IL-12 in HIV disease is currently being tested in clinical trials (Dalgleish, 1995). Initial results in murine tumor models and mice infected with *Leishmania major* (Heinzel *et al.*, 1993) and *Toxoplasma gondii* (Gazzinelli *et al.*, 1993) are promising.

Another potential means of modulating cytokines in situations where their activity needs to be blocked is to use molecules that bind to and inhibit cytokines, or to use molecules that bind to and block specific cytokine receptors on target cells. Hence, soluble TNF-α receptors have been shown to inhibit TNF-α-induced HIV transcription and expression *in vitro* and may hold promise for use in selected circumstances in HIV-infected individuals (Howard *et al.*, 1993). Another encouraging approach seems to be the use of soluble receptor binding antagonists. Therapeutic interest may be greatest in receptor binding antagonists since these block the biological activity of cytokines, and may lack the side effects of toxicity and immunogenicity (Arend and Dayer, 1990; Arend *et al.*, 1990; Durum and Mealy, 1990). One such molecule, a recombinant IL-1 protein that binds but does not activate IL-1 receptors, has been isolated and its gene cloned (Eisenberg *et al.*, 1990; Arend *et al.*, 1990). This IL-1 receptor antagonist has been shown to block the IL-1-dependent induction of HIV *in vitro* (Fauci, 1993), and reduce the severity of inflammation in several *in vivo* models of experimental disease (Catania *et al.*, 1993). In addition, clinical trials have utilized IL-1 receptor antagonist to block the tissue effects of IL-1 with some clinical benefit (Dinarello and Thompson, 1991).

Readjusting cytokine dyscrasia is not the only option available to deal with the immunosuppressive consequences of viral infection. Thus, if we fully understand the molecular consequences of exposure to some inhibitory viral component, then it may be possible to use drugs (immunomodulators) that reverse the process. One hopes that if viral immunologists succeed in providing biochemical explanations for immunosuppression, immunopharmacologists will be able to put the knowledge to good use and conjure up appropriate therapeutic modalities.

ACKNOWLEDGMENTS. We appreciate the expert help, patience, and constructive criticisms of many colleagues. The author's work is supported by EY07057-13, AI14981, and EY05093.

REFERENCES

Ablashi, D. V., Salahuddin, S. Z., Josephs, S. F., Lusso, P., Gallo, R. C., Hung, C., Lemp, J., and Markham, P. D., 1987, HBLV (or HHV-6) in human cell lines, *Nature* **329:**207–210.

Albrecht, J. C., Nicholas, J., Biller, D., Cameron, K. R., Biesinger, B., Newman, C., Wittmann, S., Craxton, M. A., Coleman, H., Fleckenstein, B., and Honess, R. W., 1992, Primary structure of the herpesvirus Saimiri genome, *J. virol.* **66:**5047–5058.

Alcami, A., and Smith, G. L., 1992, A soluble receptor for interleukin-1 beta encoded by vaccinia virus: A novel mechanism of virus modulation of the host response to infection, *Cell* **71**:153–167.

Allen, J. B., Wong, H. L., Gujre, P. M., Simon, G. L., and Wahl, S. M., 1991, Association of circulating receptor Fc gamma RIII positive monocytes in AIDS patients with elevated levels of transforming growth factor beta, *J. Clin. Invest.* **87**:1773–1779.

Ameglio, F., Capobianchi, M. R., Castilletti, C., Feis, P. C., Fais, S., and Trento, E., 1994, Recombinant gp120 induced IL-10 in resting peripheral blood mononuclear cells correlation with induction of other cytokines, *Clin. Exp. Immunol.* **95**:455–458.

Arend, W. P., and Dayer, J. M., 1990, Cytokines and cytokine inhibitors or antagonists in rheumatoid arthritis, *Arthritis Rheum.* **33**:305–315.

Arend, W. P., Welgus, H. G., Thompson, R. C., and Eisenberg, S. P., 1990, Biological properties of recombinant human monocyte-derived interleukin-1 receptor antagonist, *J. Clin. Invest.* **85**:1694–1698.

Asherson, G. L., 1986, An over view of T-suppressor cell circuits, *Annu. Rev. Immunol.* **4**:37–68.

Bendinelli, M., Pistello, M., Lombardi, S., Poli, A., Garzelli, C., Matteucci, D., Ceccherini-Nelli, L., Malvaldi, G., and Tozzini, F., 1995, Feline immunodeficiency virus: An interesting model for AIDS studies and an important cat pathogen, *Clin. Microbiol. Rev.* **8**:87–112.

Berman, M. A., Sandborg, C. I., Calabia, B. S., Andrews, B. S., and Friou, G. J., 1987, Interleukin 1 inhibitor masks high interleukin 1 production in acquired immunodeficiency syndrome (AIDS), *Clin. Immunol. Immunopathol.* **42**:133–140.

Berman, M. A., Zaldivar, F., Imfeld, K. L., and Kenney, J. S., 1994, HIV-1 infection of macrophages promotes long-term survival and sustained release of interleukins 1 alpha and 6, *AIDS Res. Hum. Retrovir.* **10**:529–539.

Biswas, P., Poli, G., and Kinter, A. L., 1992, Interferon-gamma induces the expression of human immunodeficiency virus in persistently infected promonocytic cells (U1) and redirects the production of virions to intracytoplasmic vacuoles in PMA-differentiated U1 cells, *J. Exp. Med.* **176**:739–750.

Brenan, M., and Zinkernagel, R. M., 1983, Influence of one virus infection on a second concurrent primary in vivo antiviral cytotoxic T cell response, *Infect. Immun.* **41**:470–478.

Butera, S. T., 1993, Cytokine involvement in viral permissiveness and the progression of HIV disease, *J. Cell. Biochem.* **53**:336–342.

Campbell, A. E., Slater, J. S., and Futch, W. S., 1989, Murine cytomegalovirus-induced suppression of antigen-specific cytotoxic T lymphocyte maturation, *Virology* **173**:268–275.

Carrell, R. W., Pemberton, P. A., and Boswell, D. R., 1987, The serpins: Evolution and adaptation in a family of protease inhibitors, *Cold Spring Harbor Symp. Quant. Biol.* **52**:527–535.

Catania, A., Manfredi, M. G., Airaghi, L., Ceriani, G., Gandino, A., and Lipton, J. M., 1993, Cytokine antagonists in infectious and inflammatory disorders, *Ann. N.Y. Acad. Sci.* **685**:149–158.

Cauda, R., Tumbarello, M., Ortona, L., Kanda, P., Kennedy, R. C., and Chanh, T. C., 1988, Inhibition of normal human natural killer cell activity by human immunodeficiency virus synthetic transmembrane peptides, *Cell. Immunol.* **115**:57–65.

Chang, D. M., and Shaio, M. F., 1994, Production of interleukin-1 (IL-1) and IL-1 inhibitor by human monocytes exposed to Dengue virus, *J. Infect. Dis.* **170**:811–817.

Chehimi, J., Starr, S. E., Frank, I., D'Andrea, A., Ma, X., MacGregor, R. R., Sennelier, J., and Trinchieri, G., 1994, Impaired interleukin 12 production in human immunodeficiency virus-infected patients, *J. Exp. Med.* **179**:1361–1366.

Chernukhin, I. V., Khaldoyanidi, S. K., Kozlov, V. A., and Gaidul, K. V., 1993, The influence of synthetic peptide from retroviral transmembrane protein p15E on murine spleen cell proliferation and bone marrow hemopoietic precursor colony formation, *Biomed. Pharmacother.* **47**:397–402.

Chirmule, N., Kalyanaraman, V. S., Oyaizu, N., Slade, H. B., and Pahwa, S., 1990, Inhibition of functional properties of tetanus antigen-specific T-cell clones by envelope glycoprotein gp120 of human immunodeficiency virus, *Blood* **75**:152–158.

Choi, Y., Kappler, J. W., and Marrack, P., 1991, A superantigen encoded in the open reading frame of the 3′ long terminal repeat of mouse mammary tumour virus, *Nature* **350**:203–207.

Chollet-Martin, S., Simon, F., Matheron, S., Joseph, C. A., Elbim, C., and Gougerot-Pocidalo, M. A., 1994,

Comparison of plasma cytokine levels in African patients with HIV-1 and HIV-2 infections, *AIDS* **8:**879–884.

Chouaib, S., Branellec, D., and Buurman, W. A., 1991, More insights into the complex physiology of TNF, *Immunol. Today* **12:**141–142.

Cianciolo, G. J., Kipnis, R. J., and Snyderman, R., 1984, Similarity between p15E of murine and feline leukaemia virus and p21 of HTLV, *Nature* **311:**515–520.

Cianciolo, G. J., Copeland, T. D., Oroszlan, S., and Snyderman, R., 1985, Inhibition of lymphocyte proliferation by a synthetic peptide homologous to retroviral envelope proteins, *Science* **230:**453–455.

Clayton, L. K., Sieh, M., Pious, D. A., and Reinherz, E. L., 1989, Identification of human CD4 residues affecting class II MHC versus HIV-1 gp120 binding, *Nature* **339:**548–552.

Clerici, M., and Shearer, G. M., 1994, The Th1–Th2 hypothesis of HIV infection: New insights, *Immunol. Today* **15:**575–581.

Czarniecki, C. W., Chiu, H. H., Wong, G. H. W., McCabe, S. M., and Palladino, M. A., 1988, Transforming growth factor beta modulates the expression of class II histocompatibility antigens on human cells, *J. Immunol.* **140:**4217–4223.

Dahlberg, J. E., 1988, An overview of retrovirus replication and classification, *Adv. Vet. Sci. Comp. Med.* **32:**1–36.

Dalgleish, A. G., 1995, The immune response to HIV: Potential for immunotherapy? *Immunol. Today* **16:**356–358.

Dezzutti, C. S., Wright, K. A., Lewis, M. G., Lafrado, L. J., and Olsen, R. G., 1989, FeLV-induced immunosuppression through alterations in signal transduction: Down regulation of protein kinase C, *Vet. Immunol. Immunopathol.* **21:**55–67.

Diamond, D. C., Sleckman, B. P., Gregory, T., Lasky, L. A., Greenstein, J. L., and Burakoff, S. J., 1988, Inhibition of CD4$^+$ T cell function by HIV envelope protein, gp120, *J. Immunol.* **141:**3715–3717.

Dinarello, C. A., 1989, Interleukin-1 and its biologically related cytokines, *Adv. Immunol.* **44:**153–210.

Dinarello, C. A., and Thompson, R. C., 1991, Blocking IL-1: Interleukin 1 receptor antagonists in vivo and in vitro, *Immunol. Today* **12:**404–410.

Dubois, C. M., Ruscetti, F. W., Palaszynski, E. W., Falk, L. A., Oppenheim, J. J., and Keller, J. R., 1990, Transforming growth factor beta is a potent inhibitor of interleukin 1 (IL-1) receptor expression: Proposed mechanism of inhibition of IL-1 action, *J. Exp. Med.* **172:**737–744.

Duh, E. J., Maury, W. J., Folks, T. M., Fauci, A. S., and Rabson, A. B., 1989, Tumor necrosis factor alpha activates human immunodeficiency virus type 1 through induction of nuclear factor binding to the NF-kB sites in the long terminal repeat, *Proc. Natl. Acad. Sci. USA* **86:**5974–5978.

Durum, S. K., and Mealy, K., 1990, Hilton Head revisited—Cytokine explosion of the 80's takes shape for the 90s, *Immunol. Today* **11:**103–106.

Durum, S. K., and Oppenheim, J. J., 1993, Proinflammatory cytokines and immunity, in: *Fundamental Immunology* (W. E. Paul, ed.), Raven Press, New York, pp. 801–836.

Durum, S. K., Quinn, D. G., and Meugge, K., 1991, New cytokines and receptors make their debut in San Antonio, *Immunol. Today* **12:**54–57.

Dyson, P. J., Knight, A. M., Fairchild, S., Simpson, E., and Tomonari, K., 1991, Genes encoding ligands for deletion of BV11 T cells cosegregate with mammary tumour virus genomes, *Nature* **349:**531–532.

Eisenberg, S. P., Evans, R. J., Arend, W. P., Verderber, E., Brewer, M. T., Hannum, C. H., and Thompson, R. C., 1990, Primary structure and functional expression from complementary DNA of human interleukin-1 receptor antagonist, *Nature* **343:**341–346.

Emilie, D., Fior, R., Jarrousse, B., Marfaing-Koka, A., Merrien, D., Devergne, O., Crevon, M. C., Maillot, M. C., and Galanaud, P., 1994, Cytokines in HIV infection, *Int. J. Immunopharmacol.* **16:**391–396.

Esolen, L. M., Ward, B. J., Moench, T. R., and Griffin, D. E., 1993, Infection of monocytes during measles, *J. Infect. Dis.* **168:**47–52.

Fan, J., Bass, H. Z., and Fahey, J. L., 1993, Elevated IFN gamma and decreased IL-2 gene expression are associated with HIV infection, *J. Immunol.* **150:**5031–5040.

Fauci, A. S., 1993, Multifactorial nature of human immunodeficiency virus disease: Implications for therapy, *Science* **262:**1011–1018.

Faxvaag, A., Espevik, T., and Dalen, A., 1993, Multiple derangements of cytokine homeostasis in mice infected with immunosuppressive retrovirus, *Cell. Immunol.* **150:**247–256.

Flamand, L., Gosselin, J., D'Addario, M., Hiscott, J., Ablashi, D. V., Gallo, R. C., and Menezes, J., 1991, Human herpesvirus 6 induces interleukin 1 beta and tumor necrosis factor alpha, but not interleukin 6, in peripheral blood mononuclear cell culture, *J. Virol.* **65:**5105–5110.

Fleischer, B., 1994, Superantigens, *Acta Pathol. Microbiol. Immunol. Scand.* **102:**3–12.

Fontana, A., Frie, K., Bodmer, S., Hofer, E., Schreier, M. H., Palladino, M. A., and Zinkernagel, R. M., 1989, Transforming growth factor beta inhibits the generation of cytotoxic T cells in virus-infected mice, *J. Virol.* **143:**3230–3234.

Frankel, W. N., Rudy, C., Coffin, J. M., and Huber, B. T., 1991, Linkage of Mls genes to endogenous mammary tumour viruses of inbred mice, *Nature* **349:**526–528.

Friedman, H. M., Cohen, G. H., Eisenbergh, R. J., Seidel, C. A., and Cines, D. B., 1984, Glycoprotein C of herpes simplex virus 1 acts as a receptor for C3b complement component on infected cells, *Nature* **309:**633–635.

Friedman, R. M., 1988, Interferons, in: *Textbook of Immunophysiology* (J. J. Oppenheim and E. M. Shevach, eds.), Oxford University Press, London, pp. 348–362.

Gazzinelli, R. T., Makino, M., Chattopadhyay, S. K., Snapper, C. M., Sher, S., and Hugin, A. W., 1992, CD4+ subset regulation in viral infection. Preferential activation of Th2 cells during progression of retrovirus-induced immunodeficiency in mice, *J. Immunol.* **148:**182–188.

Gazzinelli, R. T., Heiny, S., Wynn, T. A., Wolf, S., and Sher, A., 1993, Interleukin 12 is required for the T-lymphocyte-independent induction of interferon gamma by an intracellular parasite and induced resistance in T-cell deficient hosts, *Proc. Natl. Acad. Sci. USA* **90:**6115–6119.

Good, R. A., Ogasawara, M., Liu, W. T., Lorenz, E., and Day, N. K., 1990, Immunosuppressive actions of retroviruses, *Lymphology* **23:**56–59.

Good, R. A., Haraguchi, S., Lorenz, E., and Day, N. K., 1991, In vitro immunomodulation and in vivo immunotherapy of retrovirus-induced immunosuppression, *Int. J. Immunopharmacol.* **13**(Suppl. 1)**:**1–7.

Gosselin, J., Flamand, L., d'Addario, M., Hiscott, J., Stefanescu, I., Ablashi, D. V., Gallo, R. C., and Menezes, J., 1992, Modulatory effects of Epstein Barr, herpes simplex, and human herpes-6 viral infections and coinfections on cytokine synthesis, *J. Immunol.* **149:**181–187.

Gottlieb, R. A., Kleineman, E. S., O'Brian, C. A., Tsujimoto, S., Cianciolo, G. J., and Lennarz, W. J., 1990, Inhibition of protein kinase C by a peptide conjugate homologous to a domain of the retroviral protein p15E, *J. Immunol.* **145:**2566–2570.

Gresser, I., 1977, On the varied biologic effects of interferon, *Cell. Immunol.* **34:**406–415.

Gruppuso, P. A., Mikumo, R., Brautigan, D. L., and Braun, L., 1991, Growth arrest induced by transforming growth factor beta1 is accompanied by protein phosphatase activation in human keratinocytes, *J. Biol. Chem.* **266:**3444–3449.

Hannum, C. H., Wilcox, C. J., Arend, W. P., Joslin, F. G., Dripps, D. J., Heimdal, P. L., Armes, L. G., Sommer, A., Eisenberg, S., and Thompson, R. C., 1990, Interleukin-1 receptor antagonist activity of a human interleukin-1 inhibitor, *Nature* **343:**336–340.

Haraguchi, S., Good, R. A., Cianciolo, G. J., and Day, N. K., 1992, A synthetic peptide homologous to retroviral envelope protein down-regulates TNF-alpha and IFN-gamma mRNA expression, *J. Leukocyte Biol.* **52:**469–472.

Haraguchi, S., Good, R. A., James-Yarish, M., and Cianciolo, G. J., 1995, Differential modulation of Th1- and Th2-related cytokine mRNA expression by a synthetic peptide homologous to a conserved domain within retroviral envelope protein, *Proc. Natl. Acad. Sci. USA* **92:**3611–3615.

Harris, S. L., Frank, I., Yee, A., Cohen, G. H., Eisenberg, R. J., and Friedman, H. M., 1990, Glycoprotein C of herpes simplex virus type 1 prevents complement-mediated cell lysis and virus neutralization, *J. Infect. Dis.* **162:**331–337.

Haseltine, W. A., 1991, Molecular biology of the human immunodeficiency virus type 3, *FASEB J.***5:**2349–2360.

Heinzel, F. P., Schoenhaut, D. S., Rerko, R. M., Rosser, L. E., and Garely, M. K., 1993, Recombinant IL 12 cures mice infected with Leishmania major, *J. Exp. Med.* **177:**1505–1509.

Herman, A., Kappler, J. W., Marrack, P., and Pullen, A. M., 1991, Superantigens: Mechanism of T cell stimulation and role in immune responses, *Annu. Rev. Immunol.* **9:**745–772.

Hoffenbach, A., Langlade-Demoyen, P., Dadaglio, G., Vilmer, E., Michel, F., Mayaud, C., Autran, B., and Plata, F., 1989, Unusually high frequencies of HIV-specific cytotoxic T lymphocytes in humans, *J. Immunol.* **142:**452–462.

Hofmann, B., Nishanian, P., Baldwin, R. L., Insixiengmay, P., Nel, A., and Fahey, J. L., 1990, HIV inhibits the early steps of lymphocyte activation, including initiation of inositol phospholipid metabolism, *J. Immunol.* **145:**3699–3705.

Horohov, D. W., and Rouse, B. T., 1986, Virus-induced immunosuppression, *Vet. Med. Small Anim. Clin.* **16:**1097–1127.

Horohov, D. W., Moore, R. N., and Rouse, B. T., 1985, Production of soluble suppressor factors by herpes simplex virus-immune mice, *J. Virol.* **54:**798–803.

Howard, M. C., Miyajima, A., and Coffman, R., 1993, T cell derived cytokines and their receptors, in: *Fundamental Immunology* (W. E. Paul, ed.), Raven Press, New York, pp. 763–800.

Howard, O. M., Clouse, K. M., Smith, C., Goodwin, R. G., and Farrar, W. L., 1993, Soluble tumor necrosis factor receptor: Inhibition of human immunodeficiency virus activation, *Proc. Natl. Acad. Sci. USA* **90:**2335–2339.

Hsu, D., Malefyt, R. W., Fiorentino, D. F., Dang, M., Vieira, P., Devries, J., Spits, H., Mosmann, T. R., and Moore, K. W., 1990, Expression of interleukin-10 activity by Epstein–Barr virus protein BCRF1, *Science* **250:**830–832.

Hu, F. Q., Smith, C. A., and Pickup, D. J., 1994, Cowpox virus contains two copies of an early gene encoding a soluble secreted form of the type II TNF receptor, *Virology* **204:**343–356.

Hu, R., Oyaizu, N., Kalyanaraman, K., and Pahwa, S., 1994, HIV-1 gp 160 as a modifier of Th1 and Th2 cytokine response: gp 160 suppresses interferon gamma and interleukin-2 production concomitantly with enhanced interleukin-4 production *in vitro*, *Clin. Immunol. Immunopathol.* **73:**245–251.

Hugin, A. W., Vacchio, M. S., and Morse, H. C., III, 1991, A virus-encoded "superantigen" in a retrovirus-induced immunodeficiency syndrome of mice, *Science* **252:**424–427.

Isaacs, S. N., Kotwal, G. J., and Moss, B., 1992, Vaccinia virus complement-control protein prevents antibody-dependent complement-enhanced neutralization of infectivity and contributes to virulence, *Proc. Natl. Acad. Sci. USA* **89:**628–632.

Itoh, N., Yonehara, S., and Ishii, A., 1991, The polypeptide encoded by the DNA for human cell surface antigen Fas can mediate apoptosis, *Cell* **66:**233–243.

Janeway, C., 1991, Mls: Makes a little sense, *Nature* **349:**459–460.

Joag, S. V., and Narayan, O., 1993, Immunodeficiency-inducing retroviruses, *Curr. Opin. Immunol.* **5:**595–599.

Jolicoeur, P., 1991, Murine acquired immunodeficiency syndrome (MAIDS): An animal model to study the AIDS pathogenesis, *FASEB J.* **5:**2398–2405.

Kadota, J., Cianciolo, G. J., and Snyderman, R., 1991, A synthetic peptide homologous to retroviral transmembrane envelope proteins depresses protein kinase C mediated lymphocyte proliferation and directly inactivated protein kinase C: A potential mechanism for immunosuppression, *Microbiol. Immunol.* **35:**443–459.

Kehrl, J. H., Taylor, A., Kim, S., and Fauci, A. S., 1991, Transforming growth factor beta is a potent negative regulator of human lymphocytes, *Ann. N.Y. Acad. Sci.* **628:**345–353.

Kekow, J., Wachsman, W., McCutchan, J. A., Cronin, M., Carson, D. A., and Lotz, M., 1990, Transforming growth factor beta and noncytopathic mechanisms of immunodeficiency in human immunodeficiency virus infection, *Proc. Natl. Acad. Sci. USA* **87:**8321–8325.

Kornbluth, R. S., Oh, P. S., Munis, J. R., Cleveland, P. H., and Richman, D. D., 1990, The role of interferons in the control of HIV replication in macrophages, *Clin. Immunol. Immunopathol.* **54:**200–219.

Kotwal, G. J., and Moss, B., 1988, Vaccinia virus encodes a secretory polypeptide structurally related to complement control proteins, *Nature* **335:**176–181.

Lahdvirta, J., Maury, C. P. J., Teppo, A. M., and Repo, H., 1988, Elevated levels of circulating cachectin/tumor necrosis factor in patients with acquired immunodeficiency syndrome, *Am. J. Med.* **85:**289–291.

Lane, H. C., Depper, J. M., Greene, W. C., Whalen, G., Waldmann, T. A., and Fauci, A. S., 1985, Qualitative loss of immune function in patients with the acquired immunodeficiency syndrome. Evidence for a selective defect in soluble antigen recognition, *N. Engl. J. Med.* **313**:79–84.

Lanzavecchia, A., Roosnek, E., Gregory, T., Berman, P., and Abrignani, S., 1988, T cells can present antigens such as HIV gp120 targeted to their own surface molecules, *Nature* **334**:530–532.

Lathey, J. L., Kanangat, S., and Rouse, B. T., 1994a, Differential expression of tumor necrosis factor alpha and interleukin 1 beta compared with interleukin 6 in monocytes from human immunodeficiency virus-positive individuals measured by polymerase chain reaction, *J. AIDS* **7**:109–115.

Lathey, J. L., Kanangat, S., Rouse, B. T., Agosti, J. M., and Spector, S. A., 1994b, Dysregulation of cytokine expression in monocytes from HIV-positive individuals, *J. Leukocyte Biol.* **56**:347–352.

Lewis, M. G., Birx, D. L., Zack, P. M., Vahey, M. A., Redfield, R. R., Burke, D. S., and Jahrling, P. B., 1990, Elevated levels of circulating interleukin-6 are associated with infection with an acutely fatal simian immunodeficiency virus isolate (SIV sm/pbj), Abstr. 3rd Annu. Meet. NIH Natl. Coop. Drug Disc. Groups for Treatment of AIDS, Abstr. 43, p. 105.

Liegler, T. J., and Stites, D. P., 1994, HIV-1 gp120 and anti-gp120 induce reversible unresponsiveness in peripheral CD4 T lymphocytes, *J. AIDS* **7**:340–348.

Linette, G. P., Hartzman, R. J., Ledbetter, J. A., and June, C. H., 1988, HIV-1 infected T cells show a selective signaling defect after perturbation of CD3/antigen receptor, *Science* **241**:573–576.

Liszewski, M. K., and Atkinson, J. P., 1993, The complement system, in: *Fundamental Immunology* (W. E. Paul, ed.), Raven Press, New York, pp. 917–939.

Locksley, R. M., Crowe, S., Sadick, M. D., Heinzel, F. P., Gardner, K. D., McGrath, M. S., and Mills, J., 1988, Release of IL-1 inhibitory activity (contra-IL-1) by human monocyte-derived macrophages infected with human immunodeficiency virus in vitro and in vivo, *J. Clin. Invest.* **82**:2097–2105.

Lotz, M., and Seth, P., 1993, TGF beta and HIV infection, *Ann. N.Y. Acad. Sci.* **685**:501–511.

Lusso, P., Markham, P. D., Tschachler, D., Veronese, F. M., Salahuddin, Z., Ablashi, D. V., Pahwa, S., Krohn, K., and Gallo, R. C., 1988, In vitro cellular tropism of human B-lymphotropic virus (human herpesvirus-6), *J. Exp. Med.* **167**:1659–1670.

McChesney, M. B., and Oldstone, M. B. A., 1987, Viruses perturb lymphocyte functions: Selected principles characterizing virus-induced immunosuppression, *Annu. Rev. Immunol.* **5**:279–304.

McChesney, M. B., and Oldstone, M. B. A., 1989, Virus-induced immunosuppression: Infections with measles virus and human immunodeficiency virus, *Adv. Immunol.* **45**:335–380.

Macen, J. L., Upton, C., Nation, N., and McFadden, G., 1993, SERP1, a serine proteinase inhibitor encoded by myxoma virus is a secreted glycoprotein that interferes with inflammation, *Virology* **195**:348–363.

Massung, R. F., Jayaranna, V., and Moyer, R., 1993, DNA sequence analysis of conserved and unique regions of swinepox virus: Identification of genetic elements supporting phenotypic observations including a novel G protein-coupled receptor homologue, *Virology* **197**:511–528.

Merrill, J. E., and Chen, I. S. Y., 1991, HIV-1, macrophages, glial cells, and cytokines in AIDS nervous system disease, *FASEB J.* **5**:2391–2397.

Mims, C. A., 1986, Interactions of viruses with the immune system, *Clin. Exp. Immunol.* **66**:1–16.

Mittler, R. S., and Hoffman, M. K., 1989, Synergism between HIV and gp120 and gp120-specific antibody in blocking human T-cell activation, *Science* **245**:1380–1388.

Moore, K., Vieira, P., Fiorentino, D., Trounstine, M., Khan, T., and Mosmann, T., 1990, Homology of cytokine synthesis inhibitory factor (IL-10) to the Epstein–Barr virus gene BCRF1, *Science* **248**:1230–1234.

Moore, K. W., O'Garra, A., de Waal Malefyt, R., Vieira, P., and Mosmann, T. R., 1993, Interleukin-10, *Annu. Rev. Immunol.* **11**:165–190.

Moses, A. V., and Garnett, H. M., 1990, The effect of human cytomegalovirus on the production and biologic action of interleukin 1, *J. Infect. Dis.* **162**:381–388.

Mosmann, T. R., 1991, Role of a new cytokine, interleukin-10, in the cross regulation of T helper cells, *Ann. N.Y. Acad. Sci.* **628**:337–344.

Mossman, K., Upton, C., and McFadden, G., 1995, The myxoma virus-soluble interferon-gamma receptor homolog, M-T7, inhibits interferon-gamma in a species-specific manner, *J. Biol. Chem.* **270**:3031–3038.

Murray, H. W., Rubin, B. Y., Masur, H., and Roberts, R. B., 1984, Impaired production of lymphokines and immune (gamma) interferon in the acquired immunodeficiency syndrome, *N. Engl. J. Med.* **310:**883–889.

Navikas, V., Link, J., Wahren, B., Persson, C., and Link, H., 1994, Increased levels of interferon-gamma (IFN gamma), IL-4 and transforming growth factor-beta (TGF-beta) mRNA expressing blood mononuclear cells in human HIV infection, *Clin. Exp. Immunol.* **96:**59–63.

Odermatt, B., Eppler, M., Leist, T. P., Hengartner, H., and Zinkernagel, R. M., 1991, Virus-triggered acquired immunodeficiency by cytotoxic T-cell-dependent destruction of antigen-presenting cells and lymph follicle structure, *Proc. Natl. Acad. Sci. USA* **88:**8252–8256.

Oh, S. K., Cruikshank, W. W., and Raina, J., 1992, Identification of HIV-1 envelope glycoprotein in the serum of AIDS and ARC patients, *J. AIDS* **5:**251–256.

Oppenheim, J. J., and Neta, R., 1994, Pathophysiological roles of cytokines in development, immunity, and inflammation, *FASEB J.* **8:**158–162.

Osborn, L., Kunkel, S., and Nabel, G. J., 1989, Tumor necrosis factor alpha and interleukin 1 stimulate the human immunodeficiency virus enhancer by activation of the nuclear factor kappa B, *Proc. Natl. Acad. Sci. USA* **86:**2336–2340.

Oyaizu, N., Chirmule, N., Kalyanaraman, V. S., Hall, W. W., Good, R. A., and Pahwa, S., 1990, Human immunodeficiency virus type 1 envelope glycoprotein gp120 produces immune defects in CD4+ T lymphocytes by inhibiting interleukin 2 mRNA, Proc. Natl. Acad. Sci. USA **87:**2379–2383.

Palladino, M. A., Morris, R. E., Starnes, H. F., and Levinson, A. D., 1990, The transforming growth factor betas: A new family of immunoregulatory molecules, *Ann. N.Y. Acad. Sci.* **593:**181–187.

Pantaleo, G., and Fauci, A. S., 1995, New concepts in the immunopathogenesis of HIV infection, *Annu. Rev. Immunol.* **13:**487–512.

Pasternak, C. A., 1987, Viruses as toxins with selective reference to paramyxoviruses, *Arch. Virol.* **93:**169–184.

Pierpart, M. E., Najdovski, T., Applebloom, T. E., and Deschodt-Lanckman, M. M., 1988, Effect of human endopeptidase 24.11 ("enkephalinase") on interleukin 1 induced thymocyte proliferative activity, *J. Immunol.* **140:**3803–3811.

Pinching, A. J., and Nye, K. E., 1990, Defective signal transduction—A common pathway for cellular dysfunction in HIV infection? *Immunol. Today* **11:**256–259.

Plata, F., Autran, B., Perdroza-Martins, L., Wain-Hobson, S., Raphael, M., Mayaud, C., Denis, M., Guillon, J. M., and Debra, P., 1987, AIDS virus specific cytotoxic T lymphocytes in lung disorders, *Nature* **328:**348–351.

Poli, G., Bressler, P., Kinter, A., Duh, E., Timmer, W. C., Rabson, A., Justement, J. S., Stanley, S., and Fauci, A. S., 1990a, Interleukin 6 induces human immunodeficiency virus expression in infected monocytic cells alone and in synergy with tumor necrosis factor alpha by transcriptional and post-transcriptional mechanisms, *J. Exp. Med.* **172:**151–158.

Poli, G., Kinter, A., Justement, J. S., Kehrl, J. H., Bressler, P., Stanley, S., and Fauci, A. S., 1990b, Tumor necrosis factor alpha functions in an autocrine manner in the induction of human immunodeficiency virus expression, *Proc. Natl. Acad. Sci. USA* **87:**782–785.

Poli, G., Kinter, A. L., Justement, J. S., Bressler, P., Kehrl, J. H., and Fauci, A. S., 1991, Transforming growth factor beta suppresses human immunodeficiency virus expression and replication in infected cells of the monocyte/macrophage lineage, *J. Exp. Med.* **173:**589–597.

Potgieter, L. N., 1986, Pathogenesis of viral infections, *Vet. Clin. North Am. Small Anim. Pract.* **16:**1049–1074.

Reibnegger, G., Fuchs, D., Hausen, A., Werner, E. R., Dietrich, M. P., and Wachter, H., 1987, Theoretical implications of cellular immune reactions against helper lymphocytes infected by an immune system retrovirus, *Proc. Natl. Acad. Sci. USA* **84:**7270–7274.

Rinaldo, C. R., and Torpey, D. J., III, 1993, Cell-mediated immunity and immunosuppression in herpes simplex virus infection, *Immunodeficiency* **6:**33–90.

Roberts, N. J., Prill, A. H., and Mann, T. N., 1986, Interleukin 1 and interleukin 1 inhibitor production by human macrophages exposed to influenza virus or respiratory syncytial virus, *J. Exp. Med.* **163:**511–519.

Rode, H. J., Janssen, W., Rosen-Wolff, A., Bugert, J. J., Thein, P., Becker, Y., and Darai, G., 1993, The genome of equine herpesvirus type 2 harbors an interleukin 10 (IL10)-like gene, *Virus Genes* **7**:111–116.

Rode, H. J., Bugert, J. K., Handermann, M., Schnitzler, P., Kehm, R., Janssen, W., Delius, H., and Darai, G., 1994, Molecular characterization and determination of the coding capacity of the genome of equine herpesvirus type 2 between the genome coordinates 0.235 and 0.258 (the EcoRI DNA fragment N; 4.2 kbp), *Virus Genes* **9**:61–75.

Rojko, J., and Olsen, R. G., 1984, The immunobiology of the feline leukemia virus, *Vet. Immunol. Immunopathol.* **6**:107–165.

Rojko, J., Essex, M., and Trainin, Z., 1988, Feline leukemia/sarcoma viruses and immunodeficiency, *Adv. Vet. Sci. Comp. Med.* **32**:57–96.

Roost, H., Charan, S., Gobet, R., Ruedi, E., Hengartner, H., Althage, A., and Zinkernagel, R. M., 1988, An acquired immune suppression in mice caused by infection with lymphocytic choriomeningitis virus, *Eur. J. Immunol.* **18**:511–518.

Rother, R. P., Rollins, S. A., Fodor, W. L., Albrecht, J. C., Setter, E., Fleckenstein, B., and Squinto, S. P., 1994, Inhibition of complement-mediated cytolysis by the terminal complement inhibitor of herpesvirus Saimiri, *J. Virol.* **68**:730–737.

Rouse, B. T., and Horohov, D. W., 1986, Immunosuppression in viral infections, *Rev. Infect. Dis.* **8**:850–873.

Ruscetti, R., Varesio, L., Ochoa, A., and Ortaldo, J., 1993, Pleiotropic effects of transforming growth factor beta on cells of the immune system, *Ann. N.Y. Acad. Sci.* **685**:488–500.

Salahuddin, S. Z., Ablashi, D. V., Markham, P. D., Josephs, S. F., Sturzenegger, S., Kaplan, M., Halligan, G., Biberfield, D., Wong-Stall, F., Kramarsky, B., and Gallo, R. C., 1986, Isolation of a new virus, HTLV, in patients with lymphoproliferative disorders, *Science* **234**:596–601.

Schnittman, S. M., and Fauci, A. S., 1994, Human immunodeficiency virus and acquired immunodeficiency syndrome: An update, *Adv. Intern. Med.* **39**:305–355.

Schnittman, S. M., Denning, S. M., and Greenhouse, J. J., 1990, Evidence for susceptibility of intrathymic T-cell precursors and their progeny carrying T-cell antigen receptor phenotypes TCR alpha beta+ and TCR gamma delta+ to human immunodeficiency virus infection: A mechanism for $CD4^+$ (T4) lymphocyte depletion, *Proc. Natl. Acad. Sci. USA* **87**:7727–7731.

Schreiber, M., and McFadden, G., 1994, The myxoma virus TNF-receptor homologue (T2) inhibits tumor necrosis factor alpha in a species-specific fashion, *Virology* **204**:692–705.

Scott, D. M., Rodgers, B. C., Fecke, C., Buiter, J., and Sissons, J. G., 1989, Human cytomegalovirus and monocytes: Limited infection and negligible immunosuppression in normal mononuclear cells infected *in vitro* with mycoplasma-free virus strains, *J. Gen. Virol.* **70**:685.

Sharma, J. M., Karaca, K., and Pertile, T., 1994, Virus-induced immunosuppression in chickens, *Poult. Sci.* **73**:1082–1086.

Siliciano, R. F., Lawton, T., Knall, C., Karr, R. W., Berman, P., Gregory, T., and Reinherz, E. L., 1988, Analysis of host virus interactions in AIDS with anti-gp120 T cell clones: Effect of HIV sequence variation and a mechanism for CD4+ cell depletion, *Cell* **54**:561.

Sodroski, J. W., Goh, W. C., Rosen, C., Campbell, K., and Haseltine, W. A., 1986, Role of the HTLV-III/LAV envelope in syncytium formation and cytopathicity, *Nature* **322**:470–474.

Sonigo, P., Barker, C., Hunter, E., and Wain-Hobson, S., 1986, Nucleotide sequence of Mason-Pfizer monkey virus: An immunosuppressive D type retro virus, *Cell* **45**:375–385.

Spriggs, M., Hruby, D., Maliszewski, C., Pickup, D., Sims, J., Buller, R. B., and VanSlyke, J., 1992, Vaccinia and cowpox viruses encode a novel secreted interleukin 1 binding protein, *Cell* **71**:145–152.

Stanley, S. K., Kessler, S. W., and Justement, J. S., 1992, CD34+ bone marrow cells are infected with HIV in a subset of seropositive individuals, *J. Immunol.* **149**:689–697.

Swaminathan, S., Hesselton, R., Sullivan, J., and Kieff, E., 1993, Epstein–Barr virus recombinants with specifically mutated BCRF1 genes, *J. Virol.* **67**:7406–7413.

Takai, Y., Wong, G. G., Clark, S. C., Burakoff, S. J., and Herrmann, S. H., 1988, B cell stimulatory factor 2 is involved in the differentiation of cytotoxic T lymphocytes, *J. Immunol.* **140**:508–512.

Theodore, A. C., Kornfeld, H., Wallace, R. P., and Cruikshank, W. W., 1994, CD4 modulation of noninfected human T lymphocytes by HIV-1 envelope glycoprotein gp120: Contribution to the immunosuppression seen in HIV-1 infection by induction of CD4 and CD3 unresponsiveness, *J. AIDS* **7**:899–907.

Thompson, J. P., Turner, P. C., Ali, A. N., Crenshaw, B. C., and Moyer, R. W., 1993, The effects of serpin gene mutations on the distinctive pathobiology of cowpox and rabbitpox virus following intranasal inoculation of Balb/c mice, *Virology* **197**:328–338.

Tyring, S. K., Cauda, R., Tumbarello, M., Ortona, L., Kennedy, R. C., Chanh, T. C., and Kanda, P., 1991, Synthetic peptides corresponding to sequences in HIV envelope gp41 and gp120 enhance in vitro production of interleukin-1 and tumor necrosis factor but depress production of interferon alpha, interferon gamma and interleukin-2, *Viral Immunol.* **4**:33–42.

Upton, C., Macen, J. L., Schreiber, M., and McFadden, G., 1991, Myxoma virus expresses a secreted protein with homology to the tumor necrosis factor receptor gene family that contributes to viral virulence, *Virology* **184**:370–382.

Upton, C., Mossman, K., and McFadden, G., 1992, Encoding of a homolog of the IFN-gamma receptor by myxoma virus, *Science* **258**:1369–1372.

Wahl, S. M., Allen, J. B., Gartner, S., Orenstein, J. M., Popovic, M., Chenoweth, D. E., Arthur, L. O., Farrar, W. L., and Wahl, L. M., 1989, HIV-1 and its envelope glycoprotein down-regulate chemotactic ligand receptors and chemotactic function of peripheral blood monocytes, *J. Immunol.* **142**:3553–3559.

Wang, H., Nishanian, P., and Fahey, J. L., 1995, Characterization of immune suppression by a synthetic HIV gp41 peptide, *Cell. Immunol.* **161**:236–243.

Ward, B. J., and Griffin, D. E., 1993, Changes in cytokine production after measles virus vaccination: Predominant production of IL-4 suggests induction of a Th2 response, *Clin. Immunol. Immunopathol.* **67**:171–177.

Weinhold, K. J., Lyerly, H. K., Stanley, S. D., Austin, S. A., Mathews, T. J., and Bolognesi, D. P., 1989, HIV-1 gp120-mediated immune suppression and lymphocyte destruction in the absence of viral infection, *J. Immunol.* **142**:3091–3099.

Weissman, D., Poli, G., and Fauci, A. S., 1994, Interleukin 10 blocks HIV replication in macrophages by inhibiting the autocrine loop of tumor necrosis factor alpha and interleukin 6 induction of virus, *AIDS Res. Hum. Retrovir.* **10**:1199–1206.

Zagury, D., Gagne, I., and Reveil, B., 1985, Repairing the T-cell defect in AIDS, *Lancet* **1**:449–502.

Zagury, J. F., Bernard, J., Achour, A., Astgen, A., Lachgar, A., Fall, L., Carelli, C., Issing, W., Mbika, J. P., Picard, O., Carlotti, M., Callebaut, I., Mornon, J. P., Burny, A., Feldman, M., Bizini, B., and Zagury, D., 1993, Identification of CD4 and major histocompatibility complex functional peptide sites and their homology with oligopeptides from human immunodeficiency virus type 1 glycoprotein gp120: Role in AIDS pathogenesis, *Proc. Natl. Acad. Sci. USA* **90**:7573–7577.

Zagury, J. F., Lachgar, A., Achour, A., Chams-Harvey, V., Cho, Y. Y., Le Coq, H., Bizzini, B., Feldman, M., Burny, A., and Zagury, D., 1994, Pathogenic disorders involved in immunosuppression and T cell depletion characterizing AIDS, *Biomed. Pharmacother.* **48**:11–16.

Zinkernagel, R. M., and Hengartner, H., 1994, T-cell mediated immunopathology versus direct cytolysis by virus: Implications for HIV and AIDS, *Immunol. Today* **15**:262–268.

CHAPTER 6

IMMUNOTHERAPY OF MICROBIAL DISEASES

K. NOEL MASIHI

1. INTRODUCTION

Marvels of modern medicine have apparently tamed a multitude of microbial infections. Vaccination has had a major impact in the control of important diseases including smallpox, yellow fever, polio, measles, mumps, rubella, diphtheria, tetanus, and pertusis. It is, nonetheless, enlightening to note that immunotherapeutic intervention in the form of immunization predates the postulates of infection or immunology. Edward Jenner discovered the smallpox vaccination in 1780. Since then only around 25 vaccines against various infectious diseases have been licensed and general widespread use has been restricted to about 10 vaccines. It is disconcerting that there are a vast number of diseases afflicting humans and domestic mammals for which no vaccines or specific chemotherapy will be available in the near future. In addition, infections that caused ravages in the 19th century, such as tuberculosis, are resurging with vehemence. Recent episodes of plague, diphtheria, cholera, and Ebola virus, diseases long thought to be under control, have heightened public awareness of infectious diseases.

Resistance to antibiotics and infections in immunocompromised patients would persist as problems predictably even in the next millennium. The steady progression in the longevity of the population at large will be associated with a rising number of transplantations being performed and a concurrent increase in the incidence of opportunistic infections. Extended use of immunosuppressive and cytotoxic drugs as well as diseases such as AIDS manifest opportunistic infections as one of their most

K. NOEL MASIHI • Robert Koch Institute, Federal Institute for Infectious and Non-Communicable Diseases, D-13353 Berlin, Germany.

Immunopharmacology Reviews, *Volume 2*, edited by John W. Hadden and Andor Szentivanyi. Plenum Press, New York, 1996.

common complication. International, governmental, and private institutions concerned with public health will have to face up to the challenge posed by existing and emerging microbial infections.

The knowledge of the intricate interaction of microbes with the immune system has engendered the realization that simple straightforward strategies may not be adequate. Antigenic analysis of the molecular structures of microbial pathogens and application of monoclonal antibodies has led to the identification of immunodominant epitopes that are germane to protection. Weak immunogens such as viral subunits, synthetic peptides, and antigenic epitopes produced by recombinant gene technology will require optimal antigen presentation and effective immunomodulators capable of potentiating protective immune responses. New concepts acting as adjunct to established therapies are urgently needed.

A wide spectrum of strategies involving immunomodulators are currently being formulated for treating infectious diseases (Masihi, 1994). The bacterial cell surface has been like a Pandora's box in yielding many immunomodulators. Active moieties have been identified for peptidoglycans of most bacterial species, cord factors of mycobacteria, endotoxic liposaccharides of gram-negative bacteria, and lipoteichoic acids of certain gram-positive bacteria. Pyrogenicity and other undesirable side effects have been observed with many bacterial immunomodulators but clinically acceptable nonpyrogenic analogues have been synthesized. This review surveys and scrutinizes the gamut of approaches being taken in developing new or improved strategies using a variety of immunomodulators for immunotherapy against infectious diseases.

2. IMMUNOMODULATORS IN VIRAL INFECTIONS

2.1. Bacterium- and Virus-Derived Immunomodulators

Viable mycobacteria, in particular the attenuated vaccine strain of bacillus Calmette–Guérin (BCG), and heat-killed or formalin-inactivated *Propionibacterium* (*Corynebacterium*) *parvum*, have been employed as nonspecific first-generation microbial immunomodulators for enhancing resistance against several viral infections. These early empirical studies have been reviewed elsewhere (Masihi *et al.*, 1989b).

One of the more promising developments has rejuvenated BCG as a vehicle for a new generation of live recombinant vaccines. New molecular genetic technology has made it feasible to introduce foreign genes into BCG. A variety of HIV type 1 polypeptides have been expressed in BCG recombinants under the control of the mycobacterial hsp70 promoter. The HIV polypeptides produced in BCG are capable of inducing antibody and T-lymphocyte responses (Aldovini and Young, 1991).

Immunomodulator *muramyl dipeptide* (MDP), *N*-acetyl-muramyl-L-alanyl-D-isoglutamine, is a small glycopeptide that represents the minimal structure essential for mycobacterial adjuvanticity. Synthetic MDP and its analogues possess pleiotropic properties. An interesting biological activity of MDP is to enhance nonspecific resistance against microbial infections including viruses. As reviewed elsewhere (Masihi *et al.*, 1989b), MDP and certain analogues, alone or in combination with other agents, have been shown to be capable of conferring resistance against influenza, herpes simplex, Sendai, Semliki Forest, and vaccinia viruses. Mouse hepatitis virus type 3 (MHV-3) causes fatal hepatic necrosis in susceptible mice culminating in death within a matter of a few days. Hepatic necrosis liberates several enzymes that are present intracellularly within the liver into blood circulation. MDP and a non-pyrogenic analogue, Murametide, inhibited the steep elevation of serum trans-aminases induced by MHV-3, irrespective of whether the immunomodulators were administered before or after the infection. The histopathological examination of the liver revealed marked necrosis of the hepatic parenchymal cells and infiltration of the inflammatory cells in controls but not in MDP-treated animals (Masihi *et al.*, 1989a).

N-Acetylglucosaminyl-β (1–4)-*N*-acetylmuramyl tri- or tetrapeptides (GM) and lipophilic derivatives have been studied for nonspecific resistance against Sendai virus. The antiviral activity of GM derivatives was shown to increase with the chain length of the fatty acid combined with the diaminopimelyl group (Iida *et al.*, 1989). MDP-Lys(L18) (*N*-α-acetylmuramyl-L-alanyl-D-isoglutaminyl-*N*-ϵ-stearoyl-L-lysine) was shown to restore the resistance to HSV infection in cyclophosphamide-treated mice (Ishihara *et al.*, 1989). MDP-Lys(L18) and 6-*O*-L18-MDP(Me) could confer protection against Sendai virus infection in mice. MDP analogues 1-*O*-L18-(6-*O*-P)-MDP(Me) and 2-*N*-L18-MDP did not stimulate significant levels of cytokines or induce cytotoxic macrophages and did not protect against Sendai virus infection (Saiki *et al.*, 1988). MDP-Lys(L18) decreased murine cytomegalovirus titers in the target organs and conferred protection against systemic lethal infection (Eizuru *et al.*, 1992). MDP-Lys(L18) has been licensed in Japan under the trademark Romurtide, and has been shown to be effective for restoration of decreased neutrophils and platlets in cancer patients. The incidence of infectious diseases in the MDP-Lys(L18)-treated group has been observed to be lower than in the control groups during the clinical trials. MDP-Lys(L18) and another adjuvant, B30-MDP, were effective for the potentiation of antigenicity of Seoul-type hantaviruses strain B-1 inactivated vaccine (Azuma *et al.*, 1994) and recombinant hepatitis B virus surface antigen (Tamura *et al.*, 1995). A virosome vaccine consisting of B30-MDP, cholesterol, and influenza virus surface antigens has recently been confirmed as safe in Phase I clinical trial in humans (Azuma *et al.*, 1994). Mice administered MDP or murabutide 2 days and poly I:C 1 day prior to influenza A/Hong Kong/68 virus had reduced pulmonary virus titers and mortality (Wyde *et al.*, 1990). In earlier studies on immunomodulator-induced resistance against influenza, combination of MDP plus trehalose dimycolate (TDM) (Masihi *et al.*, 1985) and monophosphoryl lipid A (MPL) plus TDM (Masihi *et al.*, 1986b) led to a decrease in the lung virus titers on day 3 and to an earlier clearance of the virus to undetectable levels compared to controls.

An adjuvant formulation containing threonyl MDP has been shown to markedly reduce the incidence and severity of primary herpes simplex virus infection in guinea pigs (Byars *et al.*, 1994). Another MDP analogue, MTP-PE, has been used as an adjuvant immunomodulator in a number of studies. Immunization of herpes simplex virus-infected guinea pigs with a subunit glycoprotein vaccine containing MTP-PE reduced the incidence of recurrent disease up to 80% (Burke *et al.*, 1994). Recombinant HIV envelope protein administered with MTP-PE has been shown to generate cytotoxic T lymphocytes in mice (Bui *et al.*, 1994) and has induced specific binding antibodies and lymphoproliferative responses in human volunteers (Kahn *et al.*, 1994). Influenza virus vaccine containing lipophilic MTP-PE has been reported to cause chills, fever, nausea, and transient elevation of white blood cell counts and erythrocyte sedimentation (Keitel *et al.*, 1993).

Adamantylamide dipeptide (AdDP) is a novel hybrid entity combining pertinent components of both an antiviral and an immunomodulator in a single synthetic compound (Masek *et al.*, 1984). In an innovative approach, a group of compounds were synthesized where 1 amino-amantadine moiety was linked to the essential L-alanine-D-isoglutamine portion of immunomodulator MDP. Amantadine is a primary symmetric amine with an interesting tricyclic structure that has been extensively employed in humans since 1966 for the prophylaxis and chemotherapy of influenza and Parkinson's disease.

The effect of AdDP and amantadine on the infectivity of influenza virus was investigated using the sensitive Madin–Darby canine kidney (MDCK) cells. It could be shown that 50 μg/ml of either AdDP or amantadine completely inhibited the infection and replication of influenza virus inoculated at 10^{-5} to 10^{-7} dilutions. In contrast, the same dilutions produced detectable viral hemagglutination activity in the control cultures. The efficacy of AdDP was comparable to that of amantadine and even the highest dose (150 μg/ml) that was tested did not produce toxic effects (Masihi *et al.*, 1987).

The results of preclinical studies with immunomodulator AdDP demonstrate that the homotypic immunity induced by influenza subunit vaccines can be broadened to a heterologous immune response. Subunit vaccine containing A/Sichuan(H3N2) and $Al(OH)_3$ stimulated high antibody levels. Despite the presence of high circulating antibody, animals were not protected against heterologous H1N1 influenza A/PR/8/34 infection. Mice immunized with A/Sichuan vaccine containing AdDP induced lower levels of antibody than vaccine with $Al(OH)_3$ but were significantly protected against A/PR/8/34 challenge. Similar immunization with influenza B/Beijing vaccines containing $Al(OH)_3$ or AdDP induced barely detectable antibody on day 28 but animals receiving AdDP were partially protected against A/PR/8/34 challenge. Secondary immunization greatly boosted the antibody response to A/Sichuan in animals receiving the subunits with $Al(OH)_3$, but not in the AdDP group, when compared with subunit vaccine alone. However, protection against A/PR/8/34 reached 80% in the AdDP group whereas, despite high levels of HI antibody, it did not exceed 10% in the other two groups (Masihi *et al.*, 1990a, 1992).

The stimulation of host resistance mechanisms by immunomodulators apparently reduces the burden of peak amount of virus enabling the host to cope and survive. MDP analogues including murabutide, MTP-PE, and MDP-Lys(L18) are potent inducers of a variety of cytokines such as IL-1, IL-6, CSFs, TNF-α, and IFN-γ in mice and humans (Asano *et al.*, 1994; Azuma *et al.*, 1994; Bahr *et al.*, 1995).

HIV infection leads to a progressive decrease in cell-mediated immune functions which renders the patient susceptible to opportunistic infections. Common bacterial infections are increasingly being diagnosed in HIV-infected individuals. Cells of the monocyte–macrophage lineage kill invading bacterial pathogens and subsequently release immunoadjuvant components from the degraded cell walls. Since certain bacterial components possess immunomodulatory properties, an investigation of their effects on HIV-infected monocytes is of interest. MDP exhibited an inhibitory activity against HIV infection of CD4-positive H9 lymphocytes and U937 monocytoid cells. An inhibitor of viral reverse transcriptase, 2′,3′-dideoxyadenosine (ddA), produced potent inhibition in cultures that were similarly infected with HIV. MDP could partially reduce antigen production in persistently HIV-infected KE37/1 lymphocyte cultures. Although the inhibition induced by MDP on day 7 after infection did not reach the level obtained with specific retroviral reverse transcriptase inhibitor ddA, it is noteworthy that up to 67% reduction of p24 antigen could be attained. Moreover, a single application of 100 μg of MDP at the initiation of the culture containing persistently infected CD4-positive KE37/1 lymphocytes could induce an inhibition of up to 38% on day 14. The doses of MDP used in this investigation ranged from 10 to 1000 μg. The lower doses of MDP, i.e., 10 μg, were in general less effective in KE37/1 and U937 cell lines. The higher dosages were more effective and maintained their inhibitory activity even at later time points of culture (Masihi *et al.*, 1990b). Cultured monocyte-derived macrophages infected with HIV *in vitro* and treated with liposomal formulation of lipophilic MDP analogue MTP-PE were shown to have an inhibitory effect on virus production (Lazdins *et al.*, 1990). Interestingly, the MDP analogue MDP(Thr)-GDP has shown a complete lack of cellular transcription factor nuclear factor-κB (NF-κB) activation in various cell lines (Schreck *et al.*, 1992).

Cultures of lymphocytic KE37/1 cells infected with HIV and treated with AdDP or AZT inhibited production of various HIV antigens by 78 and 68%, respectively, on day 7 after infection as reflected by sensitive antigen capture ELISAs. Persistently HIV-infected KE37/1 cells cocultured with uninfected AdDP-treated or AZT-treated cells resulted respectively in 37 and 56% inhibition of p24 antigen production on day 3. Anti-HIV effects decreased to 11% inhibition by day 6 in cultures containing AZT-pretreated cells whereas in cultures containing AdDP-pretreated cells the inhibition remained stable at 38%. Inactive amounts of AdDP and AZT in the lymphocytic H9 cell line exhibited a significant synergistic effect of 60% reduction of HIV antigen production when both agents were used in combination. Treatment of monocytoid U937 cells with an inactive dose of AdDP and AZT dosage capable of inducing a 60% reduction could further increase the inhibition of HIV p24 antigen production to 92% (Masihi and Masek, 1993). A synthetic peptide derived from HIV-1 transmembrane region of glycoprotein gp41 when combined with AdDP in a liposome showed adjuvant activity comparable to that with Freund's complete adjuvant (Turnek *et al.*, 1994). These results make AdDP a worthy candidate warranting further investigations.

Mycobacterial TDM, and detoxified endotoxin, MPL, as well as activity of antiretroviral agents, such as AZT, 2′,3′-ddA and γ-interferon, were investigated in U937- HIV infection model. Antiretrovirals strongly inhibited p24 antigen production. Immunomodulators TDM and MPL could also reduce the replication of HIV in promonocytic cells at an early stage of infection (Rohde-Schulz *et al.*, 1990). Depressed chemiluminescence activity of animals injected intravenously with peptides representing epitopes of the main structural protein of HIV core, p24 and viral envelope glycoprotein gp120 could be overcome by MPL (Pohle *et al.*, 1990).

AZT, one of the primary drugs for the treatment of HIV, is associated with bone marrow toxicity. The termination of AZT treatment results in increased levels of viral antigen and decreased numbers of $CD4^+$ cells. Recombinant GM-CSFs have been used for bone marrow salvage in immunosuppressive chemotherapy but is also associated with dose-limiting side effects that occur in the therapeutic range. *In situ* induction of physiological levels of GM-CSF and other cytokines such as IL-1 which can act synergistically would appear to be a more rational approach toward reduction of AZT toxicity. MDP is an inducer of GM-CSF and IL-1. Evaluation of the effectiveness of pretreatment with MDP or liposomal MDP-GDP showed that while MDP is able to protect against AZT-induced bone marrow toxicity at doses up to 20 mg/kg AZT, liposomal MDP-GDP confers significant myeloid protection at up to 50 mg/kg AZT (Phillips *et al.*, 1990).

Polyclonal B-cell stimulation and macrophage activation can be induced by bacterial cell wall constituents. Synthetic derivatives of N-terminal lipopeptide of bacterial lipoprotein solely consisting of palmitic acid residues are potent immunoadjuvants. Unlike Freund's complete adjuvant, lipopeptides are nonpyrogenic and do not cause tissue lesions. *Lipopeptides* bind to defined B-lymphocyte membrane proteins including MHC. Changes in the intracellular calcium concentrations obtained using lipopeptides suggest action on intracellular calcium stores or plasma membrane calcium channels without signal-transducing mechanisms involving cAMP or cGMP or phosphatidylinositol. P3C analogues can stimulate protein and RNA biosynthesis and preferentially induce IgM, IgG2(a+b), and IgG plaque-forming cells. Coupling of lipopeptides to haptens or low-molecular-weight antigens induces a marked specific antibody response which can be further enhanced by introducing haplotype-specific T-helper cell epitopes into the conjugates and *in vivo* priming of cytotoxic T cells can be achieved by coupling to epitopes presented by MHC class I molecules (Bessler *et al.*, 1994). HIV peptides covalently coupled to lipopeptides induced antigen-specific IgM and IgG antibodies. Lipopeptide conjugates of foot-and-mouth virus disease induced protection against lethal virus infection in guinea pigs (Bessler *et al.*, 1990). Covalent association of lipopeptidic lauroyl-peptides to a peptide derived from the principal neutralizing domain of HIV-1 envelope glycoprotein has been reported recently. Trimexautide was able to efficiently induce a relevant virus-specific CTL response, while pimelautide was able to stimulate a strong antibody response to the linked peptide, or to a coinjected protein (Déprez *et al.*, 1995).

Lipid A has been identified as the active moiety exhibiting various immunopharmacological activities of bacterial lipopolysaccharide. Synthetic lipid A analogues GLA-59 and GLA-60 have been shown to confer protection against vaccinia virus infection (Ikeda *et al.*, 1990). GLA-60 could also confer complete protection to beige mice against murine CMV-associated mortality (Ikeda *et al.*, 1993). DT-5461, a synthetic lipid A-related compound, enhanced host resistance to Sendai virus infection (Yoshida *et al.*, 1994).

The novel amphiphile *BAG/LPS*, extracted from delipidated cells of *Mycobacterium bovis* BCG, has been identified in Japan. BAG/LPS is nonpyrogenic and consists mainly of sugars, such as mannose and moinositol, and fatty acids such as palmitic acid and tuberculostearic acid. Interestingly, chemical constituents such as hydroxymyristic acid, ketodeoxyoctanate, mycolic acids, muramic acids, and diaminopimelic acid which are frequently found in many bacterial immunomodulators have not been detected. BAG/LPS induced TNF and IFN-α and -β but not IFN-γ, in MDP-primed mice and showed a significant production of IL-1 in C3H/HeN mice. BAG/LPS generated tumoricidal macrophages and in combination with MDP caused hemorrhagic necrosis and complete cure in established Meth-A tumor-bearing mice (Kotani *et al.*, 1990). Effectiveness of BAG/LPS in infectious diseases such as vaccinia virus is under investigation.

Virus-derived immunomodulators have been mainly used in veterinary medicine. Inactivated poxvirus preparations such as *Baypamun* (PIND-ORF) have been shown to protect cattle against manifestation of clinical symptoms after an experimental infection with infectious bovine rhinotracheitis virus and reduce virus excretion by more than 99%; administration of Baypamun was associated with accelerated interferon synthesis (Strube *et al.*, 1989). Inactivated Newcastle disease virus mixed with endotoxin in Freund's incomplete adjuvant has been tested in field trials by treating 2782 calves and 4387 swine and comparing with a similar number of untreated animals. The clinical results showed significant reductions in the incidence and the duration of conditioned infections related to opportunistic organisms including those caused by IBR-, P13-, adeno-, and rotaviruses in the treated animals (Galassi *et al.*, 1986).

2.2. Fungus-Derived Immunomodulators

Lentinan is a chemically well-defined 1–3-β-D-glucan with 1–6-β-D-glucopyranoside branches and is isolated from an edible Japanese mushroom (Chihara, 1990; Maeda *et al.*, 1994). There are many reports on the antitumor activity of lentinan. The focus is now shifting to possible antiinfectious activities of lentinan and related yeast glucan, sulfated lentinan, and curdlan. The ability of polysaccharide immunomodulator lentinan to stimulate nonspecific resistance against respiratory viral infections was investigated. Significant protection was conferred by lentinan administered intranasally before lethal influenza virus infection and could be corroborated by a reduction of the lung virus titers. Since the lung is the target organ of influenza virus infection, lentinan was also administered by the intravenous route. Lentinan conferred complete protection against an LD_{75} challenge dose of virulent influenza virus and significantly prolonged the survival time after an LD_{100} challenge (Irinoda *et al.*, 1992). Enhanced chemiluminescence (CL) activity was present at an early stage in groups receiving lentinan. Significant nitric oxide activity could also be stimulated by culturing bronchoalveolar macrophages in the presence of lentinan. TNF actvity could not be detected in lung lavage but measurable IL-6 was produced already after 6 hr in animals administered lentinan alone and in lentinan-pretreated influenza virus-infected mice (Irinoda *et al.*, 1992).

Yeast *glucan* has been shown to enhance resistance against herpes simplex virus types I and II, and murine hepatitis virus (Chihara, 1990). Polysaccharide schizophyllan conferred protection to mice against lethal Sendai virus infection (Hotta *et al.*, 1993).

Natural polysaccharides possessing antitumor activity through host-mediated reaction were not effective against HIV. For instance, lentinan enhanced the inhibitory activity against HIV only in combination with AZT (Kaneko *et al.*, 1990). In contrast, sulfated polysaccharides exerted direct inhibitory activity on HIV replication but were not active as antitumor agents. Lentinan sulfate, arabinosyl curdlan sulfate, and galactosyl curdlan sulfate exhibited significant inhibitory activity against HIV (Yoshida *et al.*, 1989). Curdlan sulfate may exert inhibitory effect on HIV-1 infection by delaying the events that precede and/or include reverse transcription and by interfering with the membrane fusion process (Jagodzinski *et al.*, 1994).

AM3, a polysaccharide immunomodulator, given orally for 1 year to patients with chronic active hepatitis could clear serum HBV-DNA and HBeAg in 8 of 13 patients (Villarrubia *et al.*, 1992). AM3 was among the immunomodulators found to be capable of preventing death and other disease manifestations related to Punta Toro virus, a phlebovirus related to Rift Valley fever virus (Sidwell *et al.*, 1992) and against disease induced by Friend virus complex (Sidwell *et al.*, 1993). Recently, AM3 has been used as an adjuvant to hepatitis B revaccination in nonresponder healthy persons (Sánchez *et al.*, 1995)

2.3. Synthetic Compounds as Immunomodulators

Immunotherapy of AIDS-related complex (ARC) and asymptomatic HIV infection with a variety of immunomodulators has been competently reviewed elsewhere (Hadden, 1992).

A new synthetic purine immunomodulator, *5′-methyl inosine monophosphate* (MIMP), is a thymomimetic immunomodulator capable of inducing in human prothymocytes the expression of T-lymphocyte differentiation markers (CD3, CD4, CD8) and IL-2 receptor (CD25). MIMP has been shown to enhance mitogen-induced proliferation of lymphocytes, augment IgM plaque-forming cells, induce delayed-type hypersensitivity, and normalize an impaired response to IL-2. Depressed phytohemagglutinin responses of lymphocytes suppressed by an HIV-derived peptide, IFN-α, prostaglandin PGE_2, or lymphocytes from pre-AIDS (ARC) patients could be progressively restored by MIMP. The mean day death in mice infected with Friend leukemia virus, employed as a murine model of AIDS, could be significantly delayed by MIMP (Hadden *et al.*, 1991; Sosa *et al.*, 1994)).

Inosine pranobex (isoprinosine) has been shown to inhibit replication of echo-, rhino-, polio-, adeno-, herpes, and cytomegaloviruses and has been shown in two multicenter clinical trials to delay the progression of HIV infection to AIDS when $CD4^+$ counts are greater than 400 (reviewed in De Simone *et al.*, 1991).

Therapeutic approaches oriented toward improving the function of T lymphocytes include *diethyldithiocarbamate* (DTC). DTC was found to be effective in therapy of LP-BM5 murine retrovirus-induced lymphoproliferative immunodeficiency disease (Hersh *et al.*, 1991b). In multicenter double-blind placebo-controlled clinical trials in patients with ARC or AIDS, DTC was shown to decrease the occurrence of opportunistic infections (Hersh *et al.*, 1991a). However, in another trial no beneficial immunomodulatory effect of DTC could be demonstrated in HIV infection (Vanham *et al.*, 1993).

Synthetic immunomodulator *AS101* [ammonium trichloro(dioxyethylene-*O-O'*) tellurate] has been found to increase the secretion of cytokines such as IL-2 and CSF and to improve CD4:CD8 ratio in AIDS patients (Kalechman *et al.*, 1990). AS101 showed some activity against disease induced by Friend virus complex (Sidwell *et al.*, 1993). AS101 also restored significantly CSF and IL-6 production by BM cells in mice infected sublethally with murine cytomegalovirus (Sredni *et al.*, 1994).

Synthetic *poly A:poly U* is a complex consisting of polyribonucleotides polyadenylic acid and polyuridylic acid. It has been administered to over 1000 individuals and has shown beneficial effects in breast and gastric cancer patients. Poly A:poly U stimulates release of IFN-γ by activated T cells, induces increased levels of interferon-associated enzymes 2-5A synthetase and protein kinase, stimulates production of IL-1, TNF, IL-6, and colony stimulating activity, and activates macrophages as shown by phagocytosis, chemiluminescence, and H_2O_2 production. Poly A:poly U can enhance specific antibody responses to protein and polysaccharide antigens. Poly A:poly U is more potent than Freund's complete adjuvant in stimulating monoclonal antibodies to HIV-1 glycoprotein. Antibody to influenza A/New Jersey/76 monovalent vaccine was significantly enhanced by poly A:poly U. A preliminary clinical trial with human volunteers has confirmed the adjuvant effect of poly A:poly U in influenza vaccine (Tursz *et al.*, 1990). Spleen cells from poly A:poly U-treated mice inhibited the replication of murine cytomegalovirus in confluent monolayer cells of secondary mouse embryo fibroblasts at 37°C and even at hyperthermic 40°C conditions (Lee *et al.*, 1992). The antiviral activity of poly A:poly U appeared to be related mainly to the action of IFN-γ produced by T cells.

BCH-527, the lipophilic hydrochloride salt of octadecyl D-alanyl L-glutamine, significantly inhibited murine cytomegalovirus as shown by increased numbers of survivors and decreased titers of virus recoverable from tissues. Influenza A (H1N1) infection was weakly inhibited, with antiviral activity seen in lowered lung scores and lung weights and less decline in arterial oxygen saturation values. BCH-527 was stimulatory to cytotoxic T cells, natural killer (NK) cells, macrophages, and splenic B cells (Sidwell *et al.*, 1995).

A glucofuranose immunomodulator, *Substance WG 209*, *N*-[*N*-(1,2; 5,6-di-*O*-isopropylidene-D-glucofuranosyl-3-*O*-methylcarbonyl)-glycyl]-D-glutamic acid, administered intranasally as an aqueous preparation provided significant protection against aerosol influenza virus infection (Gruszecki *et al.*, 1988). Substance WG 209 has been shown to lack somnogenic and pyrogenic activities (Johannsen *et al.*, 1994).

Synthetic immunomodulator *DDA* (dimethyl dioctadecyl ammoniumbromide) could prolong survival of aged mice against influenza virus, and confer protective effects against murine hepatitis virus confirmed by liver histology and undetectable levels of serum transaminases (Masihi and Rohde-Schulz, 1990).

Immunomodulator *FCE 20696* is a dibenzopyran derivative that has been shown to confer protection against several viral infections. The severity of the lung lesions caused by influenza virus was decreased and survival against HSV-1 was increased by FCE 20696. This immunomodulator is effective parenterally and even by the oral route (Trizio *et al.*, 1990)

The thiazolopyrimidine nucleoside *7-thia-8-oxoguanosine* [5-amino-3-beta-D-ribofuranosylthiazolo (4,5-*d*) pyrimidine-2,7(3*H*,6*H*)-dione] prevented death in mice infected with Semliki Forest, San Angelo, and banzi viruses when administered prophylactically. Protection was conferred against HSV-1 and murine cytomegalovirus infections and against encephalitis induced by intracerebral inoculation of a human coronavirus in mice (Smee *et al.*, 1990). Immunomodulator 7-thia-8-oxoguanosine induces interferon and potentiates NK cell activity and also provided significant protection against encephalomyocarditis virus, rat coronavirus and showed moderate effectiveness against HSV-2 and vesicular stomatitis viruses. Another nucleoside analogue, 7-deazaguanosine, was found to be highly protective in mice inoculated with lethal doses of Semliki Forest or San Angelo viruses and lesser but still significant protective activity was evident against banzi and EMC viruses (Smee *et al.*, 1991).

Immunomodulator *CL246,738* [3,6-bis(2-piperidinoethoxy)acridine trichloride] is a synthetic heterocyclic of the acridine class and is a potent inducer of interferon and NK cells. CL246,738 protected mice from lethal Semliki Forest and banzi virus infections. Spleen cells of CL246,738-treated mice produced IFN-α whereas peritoneal exudate cells produced IFN-β. Treatment of CL246,738-treated mice with antiinterferon antibodies abrogated the protection against SFV encephalitis (Sazotti *et al.*, 1989).

An immunomodulatory agent designated *R837* was investigated in a guinea pig model of genital HSV-2 infection. Topical R837 application exhibited *in vivo* anti-HSV activity and reduced both acute and latent neural infections and recurrent genital disease (Bernstein and Harrison, 1989).

The steroidal glycoside *L-644,257* [6-(5-cholesten-3β-yloxy)hexyl 1-thio-β-D-mannopyranoside] conferred significant protection against HSV-1 when administered prior to challenge (Hagmann *et al.*, 1990).

Immunomodulator *LS 2616* (quinoline-3-carboxamide) is a potent inducer of NK cell activity. LS 2616 showed antiinflammatory effects in Coxsackie virus B3-induced myocarditis and increased the number of survivors and survival time (Ilbäck *et al.*, 1989).

Pretreatment with the synthetic peptide *FK565* [hepatanoyl-γ-D-glutamyl-(L)-*meso*-diaminopimelyl-(D)-alanine] significantly inhibited myocardial viral replication of encephalomyocarditis virus and increased survival (Sato *et al.*, 1992).

The new immunomodulator *pidotimod* [(*R*)-3-(*S*)-(5-oxo-2-pyrrolidinyl)-carbonyl-thiazolidine-4-carboxylic acid] significantly increased survival time after challenge with low doses of mengovirus, herpes simplex virus and influenza virus (Dianzani *et al.*, 1994).

An alkylpurine derivative, *9-alkylguanine*, was shown to confer protection against a lethal Semliki forest virus infection in mice (Michael *et al.*, 1994).

2.4. Endogenous Immunomodulators

2.4.1. Cytokines

Nonspecific first-generation microbial immunomodulators such as BCG and *Corynebacterium parvum* showed limited anecdotal efficacy in treatment of malignancies in early empirical studies which could not be reliably reproduced in randomized clinical trials. The general consensus among clinical investigators was that immunomodulatory treatments needed elucidation of underlying mechanisms and development of more specific immunotherapeutic agents. Recent advances in the monoclonal antibody and recombinant DNA technologies have led to availability of cytokines with defined immunomodulatory activities. The last decade has seen emergence of cytokines as promising therapeutic agents. Many adjuvant-active immunomodulators such as MDP and LPS may exert their activity, at least in part, by endogenous induction of cytokines (Asano *et al.*, 1994; Azuma *et al.*, 1994; Bahr *et al.*, 1995).

Evidence is accruing that cytokines are intimately involved in antimicrobial immune responses by modulation of the expression of major histocompatibility complex and various adhesion molecules regulating the activity of effector cells. Certain cytokines stimulate the production of other cytokines in synergistic or antagonistic networks. Synergistic and individual antiviral effects of cytokines produced by infiltrating cells appear to play an important role in control of viral infections.

Interleukin 1 (IL-1) molecules are important regulators of immunity and inflammation. They can be induced in a wide variety of cells including monocytes, macrophages, fibroblasts, endothelial and epithelial cells in response to antigens, toxins, and other cytokines. IL-1α pretreatment of WISH cells induced an antiviral state against

VSV infection (Ruggiero *et al.*, 1989). IL-1α could transiently suppress the late erythroid colony-forming units induced by a conventional strain of Friend leukemia virus (Johnson *et al.*, 1990). Substantial elevation of spontaneous *in vitro* production of IL-1β has been observed during IFN-α therapy resulting in the clearance of HBeAg in chronic carriers of hepatitis B (Daniels *et al.*, 1990). Calves administered bovine herpesvirus-1 vaccine in conjunction with recombinant bovine IL-1β showed increased serum neutralizing antibodies, cytotoxic responses and decreased virus excretion (Reddy *et al.*, 1990).

Interleukin 2 (IL-2) is synthesized and secreted by antigen- or mitogen-activated T lymphocytes. IL-2 acts as a potent growth factor for clonal expansion of T lymphocytes and stimulates lymphokine-activated killer cell and NK cell activities. Human and animal neonates are highly susceptible to herpes simplex virus (HSV) infection. Administration of human recombinant IL-2 protected neonatal mice from a lethal HSV infection. Protection was associated with macrophage-mediated antibody-dependent cellular cytotoxicity via helper T-cell-produced IFN-γ (Kohl *et al.*, 1989). Adoptive transfer of lymphocytes from animals infected with HSV-1 helped clear the virus more effectively when IL-2 was injected into the recipients (Rouse *et al.*, 1985). Protective effect of HSV crude extract or glycoprotein D subunit vaccines could be enhanced against HSV type 2 genital infection in guinea pigs by coadministration of recombinant IL-2 (Weinberg and Merigan, 1988). A truncated herpes simplex virus glycoprotein gene fused to the human IL-2 gene has been shown to induce superior antiherpes antibodies and to protect animals against herpes challenge (Hazama *et al.*, 1993). The potency of inactivated rabies virus vaccine could be increased by daily systemic administration of IL-2 as shown by enhanced protection following challenge with virulent rabies virus (Nunberg *et al.*, 1989). T lymphocytes from uremic patients not responding to hepatitis B vaccination produce inadequate amounts of IL-2. Administration of low-dose IL-2 with hepatitis B vaccine to uremic nonresponders resulted in a 70% seroconversion. IL-2 has also been applied *in vivo* for immunotherapy of established cytomegalovirus (Reddehase *et al.*, 1987). Human herpesvirus-6 (HHV-6) was isolated in 1986 from AIDS patients and is the etiologic agent of a childhood disease characterized by fever and skin rash, namely, exanthem subitum. Addition of recombinant IL-2 strongly inhibited the virus-induced cytopathic effect, reduced the number of infected cells, and produced an almost total absence of extracellular virions in treated cultures (Roffman and Frenkel, 1990). Several studies with IL-2 therapy in AIDS patients have generally yielded poor results despite elevation of some immunological parameters. In fact, IL-2 has been shown to increase the production within 24 hr of HIV *in vitro* by naturally infected mononuclear cells from seropositive donors (Todd *et al.*, 1991) and to enhance translocation of bacteria from intestines to other organs (Penn *et al.*, 1991).

Lymphokine-activated killer (LAK) cells are effector cells that are generated by culturing leukocytes in the presence of IL-2. LAK cells inoculated into suckling mice conferred protection against murine cytomegalovirus infection (Bukowski *et al.*, 1988). LAK cells have been shown to chemotactically migrate and accumulate at site of infection by mouse hepatitis virus or vaccinia virus (Natuk *et al.*, 1989). Administration of bovine recombinant IL-2 in calves induced LAK cells and increased their resistance against bovine herpesvirus-1 challenge (Reddy *et al.*, 1989). Adherent LAK cells, generated by cultivation of NK cells with IL-2, have been shown to kill monocytes infected with HIV for up to 7 days (Melder *et al.*, 1990).

The *colony-stimulating factors* (CSFs) are intimately involved in the production and differentiation of stem cells in the bone marrow to phagocytic cells. CSFs are classified into four major types, namely, IL-3, granulocyte–macrophage CSF (GM-CSF), macrophage CSF (M-CSF), and granulocyte CSF (G-CSF).

IL-3 is a multi-colony-stimulating factor that can stimulate the proliferation and differentiation of pluripotent progenitor cells common to different hematopoietic cell lineages. Primary mouse embryonic cells infected with HSV-1 showed a 1000-fold decrease in virus titer when cultured in the presence of IL-3. Protective effect could be reversed by antiinterferon antibodies suggesting production of interferon mediated by IL-3 (Chan *et al.*, 1990).

M-CSF secreted by mononuclear phagocytes, fibroblasts, and endothelial cells provides an autocrine differentiation signal for proliferation of committed hematopoietic progenitor cells to form macrophages. M-CSF can enhance the production of other cytokines such as interferons and TNF. Murine macrophages treated with M-CSF became resistant to VSV infection (Lee and Warren, 1987). Treatment of murine macrophages with M-CSF increased macrophage survival and reduced the amount of HSV-1 virus produced in cultures. Protective effect of M-CSF could be inhibited by antiinterferon antibodies indicating that the effect was related to the induction of endogenous interferon (Lee and Warren, 1987). In contrast to the HSV-1 virus model, monocytes cultured in recombinant human M-CSF were more than 400-fold more susceptible to HIV infection (Kalter *et al.*, 1991). The significantly enhanced susceptibility of human primary macrophages also reduced the anti-HIV activity of dextran sulfate and soluble CD4 (Bergamini *et al.*, 1994). This demonstrates that M-CSF can either confer protection or exacerbate disease development.

Pretreatment and presence of GM-CSF during culture of U937 human monocytic cells provided protection against HIV infection (Hammer *et al.*, 1986). A synergistic activity of GM-CSF with AZT could be obtained (Hammer and Gillis, 1987; Perno *et al.*, 1989) and toxic effect of AZT on human myeloid progenitor cells could be ameliorated (Bhalla *et al.*, 1989). Replication of HIV in monocytes may, however, be increased under certain experimental conditions by CSF (Perno *et al.*, 1989; Gendelman *et al.*, 1988). In another model, GM-CSF enhanced influenza virus infection of monocytes even though a more rapid release of IFN-α could be induced (Bender *et al.*, 1993).

IL-10, a regulator cytokine of both the lymphoid and myeloid cells, is produced by the Th2 subset of T-helper cells. Recombinant human IL-10 could inhibit HIV-1 replication in infected monocytes and peripheral blood mononuclear cells (Masood *et al.*, 1994) and in human macrophages (Akridge *et al.*, 1994).

IL-12 stimulated enhanced levels of IFN-γ but showed no protective effect in either prophylactic or therapeutic regimens against influenza virus or encephalomyocarditis virus (Gladue *et al.*, 1994).

TNF-α is a pleiotropic cytokine that is mainly produced by the macrophages. TNF exhibits potent immunomodulatory activities including proliferation of B and T lymphocytes, cytotoxic T cells, enhanced expression of MHC class I and II antigens, IL-2 receptors and augmentation of IL-2-stimulated immunoglobulin production and NK cell activity. TNF can also activate neutrophils, induce differentiation of hematopoietic cells, and synergize with other cytokines such as IFN-γ and IL-1. TNF has been shown to possess protective effects against a variety of microorganisms. Recombinant human TNF-α exhibited a distinct antiviral activity on HeLa cells infected with encephalomyocarditis virus (Arakawa *et al.*, 1987). TNF induced antiviral activity against VSV in HEP-2, WI-38, and HEL cell lines (Mestan *et al.*, 1986; Wong and Goeddel, 1986). Combination of TNF with low concentrations of IFN-β or IFN-γ exerted synergistic antiviral activity against VSV (Mestan *et al.*, 1988) and HSV-1 (Feduchi and Carrasco, 1991; Feduchi *et al.*, 1989). Pretreatment of WISH cells with TNF-α or -β or IL-1 induced an antiviral state against VSV infection (Ruggiero *et al.*, 1989). *In vivo* administration of TNF-α inhibited the yield of VSV in peripheral blood mononuclear cells from patients with malignancy by 99% (Nokta *et al.*, 1991). The neurotropic pseudorabies virus (PRV) replicates efficiently in all neural cell types. TNF-α induced a state of antiviral activity in astrocytes against a low dose of PRV (Schijns *et al.*, 1991). TNF has been used to treat chronic hepatitis B virus infection (Sheron *et al.*, 1990). Positive response to IFN-α therapy in chronic carriers of hepatitis B is accompanied by the clearance of HBeAg and substantial elevation in spontaneous *in vitro* production of TNF (Daniels *et al.*, 1990).

Response to TNF can be dichotomous and may be dependent on the pathogenesis caused by the disease state. TNF has been attributed with both beneficial and harmful effects. Bacterial LPS has been found to potentiate the production of TNF from influenza virus-infected (Nain *et al.*, 1990) or influenza neuraminidase-treated (Houde and Arora, 1990) macrophages. TNF production was found to be significantly reduced in patients with chronic hepatitis B (Mueller and Zielinski, 1990). Administration of recombinant human TNF to chronic hepatitis B virus patients not responsive to interferon treatment showed an initial reduction in serum HBV DNA at lower doses (10–15 $\mu g/m^2$) of TNF. Higher doses ($> 30\ \mu g/m^2$) of TNF in some patients enhanced the viral replication and raised HBV DNA and HBsAg. Administration of human recombinant TNF to mice with severe, but clinically inapparent lymphocytic choriomeningitis virus (LCMV) infection caused rapid death. In contrast, TNF given earlier in the course of disease prevented mortality and pretreatment protected against development of lethal disease (Doherty *et al.*, 1989). In another study, treatment of mice with recombinant TNF had no effect on LCM virus clearance (Klavinski *et al.*, 1989). Simian varicella virus (SVV)-infected monkeys given rHuTNF, at doses found to be nontoxic in uninfected monkeys, showed increased mortality (Soike *et al.*, 1989). Porcine monocytes treated with TNF showed an increase of African swine fever virus production (Esparza *et al.*, 1988). C57BL/6 mice pretreated with TNF showed prolonged survival after infection with HSV-1 (Rossol-Voth *et al.*, 1991), but persistently HSV-infected macrophages from the same strain of mice showed an increase of virus yield and cytopathic effects after treatment with TNF (Domke-Opitz and Kirchner, 1990). The exact molecular mechanisms responsible for protective or antagonistic activities of cytokines such as TNF remain to be elucidated.

TNF reduced the replication of HIV in HUT-78 cells (Wong *et al.*, 1988) but enhanced viral replication in MOLT-4 cells (Ito *et al.*, 1989). TNF treatment of the HUT-78 cell line chronically infected with simian immunodeficiency virus induced a two- to threefold increase in the viral reverse transcriptase activity (Lairmore *et al.*, 1991). Primary blood monocyte-derived macrophages treated with recombinant human TNF-α starting either before or after HIV-1 infection enhanced viral replication of both lymphocyte-tropic and macrophage-tropic strains (Mellors *et al.*, 1991). Recombinant TNF has been shown to activate HIV mRNA (Matsuyama *et al.*, 1989), increase replication (Folks *et al.*, 1989), and enhance syncytium formation (Vyakarnam *et al.*, 1990) in T cell lines. The activity of AZT against HIV can be inhibited by TNF (Ito *et al.*, 1990). Raised levels of both TNF and soluble TNF receptors are detected during HIV-1 infection in seropositive patients (Aukrust *et al.*, 1994). The role of TNF and other cytokines in HIV has been reviewed (Matsuyama *et al.*, 1991).

The evidence for a pathophysiological involvement of TNF has provided the rationale for development of potential therapeutic strategies based on interrupting the production of TNF. Antibodies against TNF and IL-6 abolished HIV-inductive capacity of B-cell cultures from HIV-infected patients with hypergammaglobulinemia (Rieckmann *et al.*, 1991). Cell surface Fas antigen is associated with TNF receptor. A cytotoxic monoclonal anti-Fas antibody selectively could kill HIV-infected cells mimicking the cytocidal action of TNF but without augmentation of HIV replication (Kobayashi *et al.*, 1990). A recent survey of several preclinical and clinical studies of pentoxifylline for the treatment of HIV infection showed that decreased TNF production correlated with changes in HIV load suggesting that pentoxifylline may inhibit HIV expression by suppressing TNF production (Dezube, 1994). Thalidomide, a selective inhibitor of TNF, also has been shown to suppress the replication of HIV in cell lines and in the peripheral blood mononuclear cells of patients with AIDS (Makonkawkeyoon *et al.*, 1993).

2.4.2. Prostaglandins

Prostaglandins are natural fatty acid products obtained as a result of enzymatic oxidation of arachidonic acid. Prostaglandin A (PGA) and related derivatives can exert inhibitory activity against viruses. The replication of HIV in a T-cell line was inhibited by PGA as shown by the number and size of virus-induced syncytia and the amount of viral antigen (Ankel *et al.*, 1991). PGA has shown interferon-independent antiviral activity against encephalomyocarditis virus (Ankel *et al.*, 1985) and inhibition of primary transcription of vesicular stomatitis virus (Bader and Ankel, 1990). Herpes simplex virus replication could be inhibited by PGA (Yamamoto *et al.*, 1987) and viral gene expression of vaccinia virus (Benavente *et al.*, 1984) and virus glycosylation in Sendai virus-infected cells (Santoro *et al.*, 1989) were selectively inhibited by PGA. A synthetic long-acting 16,16-dimethyl-PGA analogue exhibited activity against influenza virus in mice as shown by the increased survival of infected mice and by 40% decreased virus titers in the lungs (Santoro *et al.*, 1988). These studies indicate that PGA and analogues might be useful for therapy of viral disease, but further evaluation of the safety and antiviral efficacy *in vivo* are needed.

3. IMMUNOMODULATORS IN BACTERIAL INFECTIONS

3.1. Bacterium-Derived Immunomodulators

Heat-killed *Lactobacillus casei*, LC 9018, enhanced phagocytic functions and IL-1 production, and led to elimination of *Mycobacterium fortuitum* and *M. chelonae* at the site of infection when administered intramuscularly six times a week (Saito *et al.*, 1987). Combination of ofloxacin with *L. casei* in mice infected with *M. fortuitum* led to delay in incidence of spinning disease, decreased renal lesions, and an increase in the rate of elimination of organisms from the kidneys (Tomioka *et al.*, 1990). DEODAN, a lysozyme from *L. bulgaricus*, has been shown to increase the phagocytic activity, IL-1 and provide protection against *K. pneumoniae* and *L. monocytogenes* infections (Popova *et al.*, 1993).

TDM has been shown to enhance resistance against diverse bacterial infections including *E. coli*, *L. monocytogenes*, and *S. enteritidis* infections (reviewed in Masihi *et al.*, 1988) and against *K. pneumoniae* in neutropenic animals (Madonna *et al.*, 1989). TDM administered in combination with MDP could induce significant resistance against virulent *M. tuberculosis* (Masihi *et al.*, 1985).

Immunomodulator *GF 787* is a particulate fraction of *Propionibacterium acnes* consisting of cell wall peptidoglycan with attached glycoprotein. Treatment with GF 787 prolonged the survival of susceptible BALB/c mice expressing the *ity*^{s} gene on macrophages against *Salmonella typhimurium* infection. Kupffer cells from treated mice displayed resistance to *in vitro* lethal effects of *S. typhimurium* (Delfino *et al.*, 1990).

A natural immunomodulator, *L. monocytogenes factor Ei*, could induce non-specific resistance against *K. pneumoniae* infection (Franek and Malina, 1990).

Administration of synthetic *MDP* analogue muramyl tripeptide, MTP-PE, induced resistance against *K. pneumoniae* infection in mice; liposomal encapsulation of MTP-PE reduced by twofold the amount of immunomodulator required and decreased the toxic side effects by tenfold (Melissen *et al.*, 1992, 1994). Pretreatment of pigs with MTP-PE protected against development of septic leukocytopenia caused by experimental pneumococcemia, enhanced bacterial clearance, and significantly decreased mortality (Izbicki *et al.*, 1991). Nonspecific activation of the host defense system can be a helpful adjunct in supporting the failing antibiotic treatment in certain infectious diseases. Prophylactic treatment of mice with five doses of liposomal MTP-PE or IFN-γ increased survival from 0 to 65% in a model of *K. pneumoniae*-induced septicemia in mice. Administration of MTP-PE and IFN-γ coencapsulated in liposome resulted in 100% survival in this model (Ten Hagen *et al.*, 1995).

A recent study reported on a placebo-controlled double-blind clinical trial of GMDP for immunotherapy of septic complications arising after abdominal surgery (Khaitov *et al.*, 1994). Prophylactic administration of GMDP and postoperative treatment of patients who acquired infections showed decreased frequency of septic complications and reduced mortality. In a different investigation, the core body temperature of Sprague–Dawley rats was regulated at 32–40°C, and 24 hr after administration of MDP, a sublethal challenge with *E. coli* was given; high-dose MDP significantly accelerated peritoneal bacterial clearance but no interaction between MDP and core body temperature was observed (Stellato *et al.*, 1988). In another study, killed *E. coli* was given multiple times with MDP to cynomolgous monkeys in an attempt to enhance the effect of vaginal immunization against urinary tract infections; levels of urinary and serum immunoglobulins were reduced and no protective effect on induced cystitis was observed (Uehling *et al.*, 1990). An extracorporeal filter consisting of polystyrene fiber-bound polymyxin B has been used experimentally in treatment of gram-negative bacterial infection. Significant improvements in rats infected with *E. coli* occurred in groups pretreated with MDP and in animals treated with a combination of MDP, polystyrene fiber-bound polymyxin B, and gentamycin (Cheadle *et al.*, 1991). The growth of leprosy bacilli in the hybrid nude mouse strain Jcl:AF-nu could be completely inhibited by combination of the bacteriostatic DDS and either MDP or water-soluble lipoidal amine, CP-46665, mixed with the chow (Gidoh and Tsutsumi, 1989). Nonspecific resistance induced by MDP to bacterial infections has been reviewed elsewhere (Parant *et al.*, 1992).

Soluble protective antigen (SPA) extracted from *Salmonella enteritidis* can enhance the chemotactic activity and superoxide generation greater than that induced by MDP or LPS and has been evaluated as a bacterial-origin immunomodulator. SPA reduced the number of bacteria in liver and afforded increased resistance to *L. monocytogenes* infection (Uchiya and Sugihara, 1989).

Acetone-killed *Salmonella typhimurium* vaccine containing synthetic *lipopeptide* derivative of bacterial lipoprotein, Pam3Cys-Ser-Ser-Asn-Ala, provided protection against intraperitoneal challenge with *S. typhimurium* even when 90% of the bacterial component was replaced by the lipopeptide (Schlecht *et al.*, 1989). WS1279, another novel lipopeptide, has been shown to augment host resistance to *Staphylococcus aureus* in normal and immunosuppressed mice (Tanaka *et al.*, 1993).

3.2. Fungus-Derived Immunomodulators

Lentinan can confer protection against *Listeria* and prevent relapse of *Mycobacterium tuberculosis* (Chihara, 1990; Maeda *et al.*, 1994). *S. cerevisiae* glucan induced nonspecific resistance against *K. pneumoniae* infection and yeast glucan can protect patients from sepsis, bacteremia, and peritonitis resulting from *E. coli*, *Staphylococcus aureus*, and *Pseudomonas aeruginosa* infections (reviewed in Chihara, 1990).

The safety and efficacy of PGG-glucan in surgical patients at high risk for postoperative infection who underwent major thoracic or abdominal surgery were recently studied. Patients who received PGG-glucan had significantly fewer infectious complications (3.4 versus 1.4 infections per infected patient), decreased intravenous antibiotic requirement (10.3 versus 0.4 day) and shorter intensive care unit length of stay (3.3 versus 0.1 day). PGG-glucan appears to be effective in the further reduction of the morbidity and cost of major surgery (Babineau *et al.*, 1994).

Polysaccharide "*RBS*," an α-glucan, administered intraperitoneally to mice led to increased IL-1 production, an enhanced elimination of bacteria and protection against *L. monocytogenes* and *E. coli* infections (Takeda *et al.*, 1990).

A protein-bound polysaccharide, *PSK* (Krestin), induced significant activity against *E. coli* when mice were pretreated by intraperitoneal, subcutaneous, or intramuscular routes and also after repeated oral administration (Sakagami *et al.*, 1991).

3.3. Synthetic Compounds as Immunomodulators

A novel synthetic immunomodulator designated *FCE 24578* [2-cyano-3-(1,4-dihydro-1-phenyl-(1)-benzothiopyran(4,3-*c*)pyrazol-3-yl)-3-oxo-*N*-phenylpropanamide] was identified during a screening program. FCE 24578 can induce protection in normal mice against *Listeria monocytogenes* and *Shigella flexneri* and in cyclophosphamide-immunodepressed mice against opportunistic infection by *Pseudomonas aeruginosa* (Verini and Ungheri, 1989). Immunomodulator FCE 20696 showed some activity against *M. tuberculosis* when it was given orally twice weekly for 5 weeks during the course of the disease (Verini and Ungheri, 1989).

A glucofuranose immunomodulator, *Substance 209*, administered as a squalane-in-water preparation 4 weeks before aerosol challenge with virulent *M. tuberculosis* significantly restricted bacterial growth and reduced the number of viable counts by 3 $\log_{10}$ in pretreated mice (Gruszecki *et al.*, 1988).

Synthetic immunomodulators *AdDP* and *ML 310* also induced nonspecific resistance against *K. pneumoniae* infection (Franek and Malina, 1990).

Cross-bred calves vaccinated against *Pasteurella multocida* and administered *levamisole* by oral, subcutaneous, or transdermal route produced highly significant antibody titers during the primary humoral response (Sharma *et al.*, 1990).

The steroidal glycoside *L-644,257* [6-(5-cholesten-3β-yloxy)hexyl 1-thio-β-D-mannopyranoside] provided protection to cyclophosphamide-immunosuppressed mice against *P. aeruginosa*, *K. pneumoniae*, and *S. aureus* (Hagmann *et al.*, 1990).

3.4. Endogenous Immunomodulators: Cytokines

Treatment with recombinant murine *IL-1α* significantly enhanced resistance of mice to *Listeria monocytogenes*. Maximal antibacterial resistance was observed when intravenous IL-1 was given concurrently or intraperitoneal IL-1 was injected 48 hr before listerial challenge (Czuprynski and Brown, 1987). Recombinant human IL-1α administered 3 days and 1 day before infection with *Pseudomonas aeruginosa* most effectively protected animals from death (Ozaki *et al.*, 1987). Mice rendered granulocytopenic by cyclophosphamide, infected with *Pseudomonas aeruginosa* and given gentamicin 6 and 23 hr later showed increased survival when IL-1β was administered 24 hr before infection (Van der Meer *et al.*, 1988). Recombinant human IL-1α given intraperitoneally 24 hr before *P. aeruginosa* infection enhanced survival of neutropenic mice (Van der Meer *et al.*, 1989). Recombinant human IL-1α administered simultaneously and 1 day after infection with *Klebsiella pneumoniae* conferred maximal protection (Ozaki *et al.*, 1987); the protective activity of IL-1 was dose-dependent. Intravenous administration of recombinant human IL-1α to mice depressed the growth of *Brucella abortus* 19 in spleen and liver when given 4 hr before infection (Zhan *et al.*, 1991). IL-1 given to C3H/HeJ mice after but not prior to infection increased resistance to *Salmonella typhimurium* (Morrissey and Charrier, 1991). These studies show that IL-1 pretreatment prolongs survival in lethal infection in normal and in neutropenic mice. In a recent study, IL-1 could reduce circulating TNF-α and IL-6 as well as LPS-stimulated production of IL-1α and TNF-α (Vogels *et al.*, 1994). Upregulation of mRNA for the IL-1 receptor antagonist (IL-1Ra) was observed in several organs of IL-1-pretreated mice, suggesting that IL-1Ra could attenuate deleterious IL-1 effects. In addition, IL-1 pretreatment downregulated steady-state mRNA for the type I IL-1R and the type I TNFR in several organs at the time of infection, suggesting desensitization of target cells as an additional mechanism of IL-1-induced protection (Vogels *et al.*, 1994).

The lethal effects of endotoxin or septicemia are mediated mainly by TNF. Since large quantities of IL-1 are released soon after TNF in response to bacteremia or endotoxin, IL-1 has been suggested to be a comediator of endotoxin lethality (Alexander *et al.*, 1991). A receptor antagonist to IL-1 produced from IgG-adherent human monocytes has been sequenced and expressed in *E. coli* vector. Mice given a lethal *E. coli* endotoxin (LPS) challenge exhibited improved survival when treated with human recombinant receptor antagonist protein to IL-1 (Alexander *et al.*, 1991). The growth of virulent, but not avirulent, *E. coli* has been observed to be enhanced by IL-1β but can be blocked by IL-1 receptor antagonist (Porat *et al.*, 1991).

Recombinant human *IL-2* significantly reduced the total *Mycobacterium lepraemurium* counts in the footpad, lymph nodes, and liver of infected mice by 6 months (Jeevan and Asherson, 1988). A lack of local lymphokine production could account for the inability of infected macrophages to eliminate *M. leprae* in patients. Administration of recombinant human IL-2 in clinical studies induced an influx of T cells, enhanced cell-mediated immunity, and led to significant decrease in the total burden of *M. leprae* and degradation of leprosy bacilli (Kaplan, 1991). Administration of recombinant human IL-2 significantly reduced the viable counts of *Mycobacterium bovis* in the spleen by 60 days after BCG infection (Jeevan and Asherson, 1988). The number of viable *Mycobacterium avium* in splenic macrophages decreased when cultured in the presence of autologous sensitized T cells and recombinant IL-2

(Hubbard and Collins, 1991). Exposure of human monocyte-derived macrophages to IL-2-treated NK cells before infection with *M. avium* induced significant mycobactericidal activity (Bermudez and Young, 1991). Recombinant human IL-2 administered intravenously significantly enhanced resistance of mice against *L. monocytogenes*; IL-2 was protective when injected concurrently or up to 24 hr prior to listerial infection (Haak-Frendscho *et al.*, 1989). Administration of recombinant IL-2 daily for 7 days reduced *K. pneumoniae* counts in a dose-dependent manner and enhanced the clearance of bacteria from the lungs after aerosol exposure (Iizawa *et al.*, 1988).

Recombinant human IL-2 given prophylactically enhanced survival and conferred complete recovery from an otherwise lethal *E. coli* type O2 infection (Chong, 1987). Cell-mediated protection against fatal *E. coli* septicemia was enhanced by treatment with IL-2 (Goronzy *et al.*, 1989). However, patients who receive high doses of IL-2 acquire a profound defect in neutrophil chemotaxis and show a frequent complication of bacterial sepsis (Klempner *et al.*, 1990). A higher incidence of bacterial infections has been observed in AIDS patients receiving IL-2 (Murphy *et al.*, 1988). Recombinant human IL-2, even in concentrations as low as 1 U/ml, and recombinant human GM-CSF have been shown to enhance growth of a virulent, but not avirulent, strain of *E. coli* in tissue culture medium by two- to threefold suggesting that certain cytokines may act as growth factors for some virulent bacteria (Denis *et al.*, 1991).

IL-4 has been shown to increase the bacteriostatic activity of murine peritoneal macrophages against *M. avium* infection (Denis and Gregg, 1991).

Recombinant human *IL-6* given intraperitoneally 24 hr before *P. aeruginosa* infection showed some protective effect in neutropenic mice but only when a high dosage of 800 ng was used (Van der Meer *et al.*, 1989). IL-6 was 10–100 times less potent than IL-1 in protecting mice in this infection model. Since IL-6 can produce minute amounts of IL-1 *in vivo*, the protection induced by IL-6 may be mediated by IL-1.

Increased levels of IL-6 have been observed in various disease states including patients with bacterial infections (Bauer and Hermann, 1991). *Listeria monocytogenes* induces IL-6 production which shows direct correlation with the severity of the infection in mice (Havell and Sehgal, 1991). Treatment with bioengineered IL-6 receptors or anti-IL-6 antibodies may be a promising therapeutic approach. Anti-IL-6 monoclonal antibody pretreatment in a mouse model of septic shock by a lethal dose of intraperitoneal *E. coli* has been shown to protect animals from death (Starnes *et al.*, 1990).

IL-8 is a potent neutrophil-activating peptide-1. Microbial invasion induces migration of neutrophils to the site of infection and subsequent phagocytosis. Polymorphonuclear leukocytes showed induction of IL-8 mRNA on exposure to commonly encountered stimuli such as bacterial endotoxin at sites of infection and release of IL-8 after phagocytosis (Bazzoni *et al.*, 1991). Production of IL-8 by phagocytosing neutrophils strengthens the notion that neutrophils may enhance antimicrobial defense by facilitating recruitment of new cells.

IL-10 is a cytokine synthesis inhibitory factor produced by Th2 lymphocytes and is capable of suppressing IFN-γ production by Th1 cells. Release of reactive oxygen and nitrogen intermediates and cytokines such as TNF, which are important in antimicrobial defense, can also be suppressed by IL-10. This has led to the suggestion that macrophages treated with IL-10 may become permissive for growth of pathogens through inhibition or deactivation of IFN-γ (Bogdan *et al.*, 1991).

Effects of *IL-12* have been shown to be dependent on the invading organism. Animals pretreated with IL-12 had higher mortality following challenge with *E. coli* but enhanced survival and clearance after *L. monocytogenes* and *S. aureus* infections (Gladue *et al.*, 1994).

Administration of recombinant *TNF* has been shown to confer protection against *Klebsiella pneumoniae* and *Streptococcus pneumoniae* infections in mice (Parant, 1988). The clearance of *Legionella pneumophila* in mice could be speeded up by TNF-induced activation of polymorphonuclear leukocyte function (Blanchard *et al.*, 1988). TNF has been used for the treatment of experimental disseminated *Myobacterium avium* infection in mice (Bermudez *et al.*, 1989) and anti-TNF treatment during an early stage accelerated multiplication of *M. bovis* (Kindler *et al.*, 1989). Significant inhibition of growth of *M. avium* complex could also be observed in human macrophages treated with TNF (Suzuki *et al.*, 1994). TNF has been shown to be involved in early protection against *M. avium* (Appelberg *et al.*, 1994). Protective effect of recombinant TNF has been observed in murine salmonellosis (Nakano *et al.*, 1990). Injection of anti-TNF-α antiserum to resistant A/J mice exacerbated sublethal *Salmonella typhimurium* infection; anti-TNF-α treatment did not accelerate bacterial growth but the colony counts continued to increase past the plateau point indicating that TNF-α is important in mediating the plateau phase in a salmonella infection (Mastroeni *et al.*, 1991). Human recombinant TNF-α treatment enhanced resistance to *Listeria monocytogenes* infection in mice (Roll *et al.*, 1990) whereas anti-TNF antibody injection exacerbated sublethal infection with *L. monocytogenes* (Nakane *et al.*, 1988a).

Measurable levels of circulating TNF are observed in patients with septic shock syndrome (Casey *et al.*, 1993). Clinical trials in sepsis patients and in patients at risk have shown anti-TNF antibodies to be well tolerated (Saravolatz *et al.*, 1994). Further trials on efficacy and clinical utility of anti-TNF antibodies in sepsis are ongoing. Soluble TNF receptors capable of specifically inhibiting TNF, namely, soluble type I (p55) and type II (p75) TNF receptors (TNFR), are found circulating in blood. Elevated levels of soluble TNFR have been observed in patients with a clinical diagnosis of sepsis (van der Poll *et al.*, 1993) but the concentrations of TNFR are inadequate to prevent toxic reactions. Administration of TNFR to raise plasma concentration 1000-fold can prevent TNF-mediated damage (Moldawer, 1993).

Resident peritoneal macrophages treated with *M-CSF* exhibited enhanced phagocytosis and killing of *Listeria monocytogenes* (Cheers *et al.*, 1989). Recombinant murine *GM-CSF* administered to mice could confer protection against listerial infections (Magee and Wing, 1989; Shinomiya *et al.*, 1991). Administration of GM-CSF to mice enhanced clearance of *Salmonella typhimurium* (Morrissey *et al.*, 1989; Morrissey and Charrier, 1990). Significant inhibition of growth of *Mycobacterium avium* complex could be observed in human macrophages treated with GM-CSF (Suzuki *et al.*, 1994). *G-CSF* induced resistance in neutropenic animals to infections by *Pseudomonas aeruginosa* (Mooney *et al.*, 1988), *Staphylococcus aureus*, *Serratia marcescens*, or *C. albicans* (Cohen *et al.*, 1988; Matsumoto *et al.*, 1987).

Mice immunosuppressed with cyclosporin A can be protected against fatal infection by *L. monocytogenes* when treated with *IFN-γ* (Nakane *et al.*, 1988b) and endogenous production of IFN-γ is required for the resolution of listerial infection (Buchmeier and Schreiber, 1985). Bone marrow-derived macrophages treated with IFN-γ showed high bactericidal activity against *L. monocytogenes* (Denis, 1991a). Administration of IFN-γ can enhance resistance to *Francisella tularensis* (Leiby *et al.*, 1992). However, treatment with IFN-γ led to enhancement of growth in macrophages of *M. lepraemurium*, another intracellular pathogen (Denis, 1991b). Patients with chronic granulomatous disease are unable to generate oxidative respiratory burst. As a consequence, they develop recurring catalase-positive bacterial infections such as *Staphylococcus aureus*, *Pseudomonas cepacia*, and *Chromobacterium violaceum*. Multicenter clinical trials have shown that sustained administration of IFN-γ to chronic granulomatous disease patients markedly reduced the relative risk of serious infection (Gallin, 1991).

4. IMMUNOMODULATORS IN PARASITIC AND FUNGAL INFECTIONS

4.1. Bacterium-Derived Immunomodulators

Avirulent *Salmonella typhimurium*, strain SL3235, is blocked in the aromatic pathway. Three different C3H mouse strains, including defective C3H/HeJ, when treated with a single injection of *S. typhimurium* SL3235, but not viable BCG, induced the generation of activated macrophages capable of killing *L. major* (Schafer *et al.*, 1988).

Induction of immunity using soluble leishmanial antigen from *L. major* required concurrent injection of *Corynebacterium parvum* (Scott *et al.*, 1987).

Trehalose dimycolate (*TDM*) extracted from mycobacterial cell walls is a potent immunomodulator. Significant resistance against oral *Toxoplasma gondii* infection was induced by intraperitoneal pretreatment of mice with TDM (Masihi *et al.*, 1985) and corroborated by a significant reduction in the number of cysts in brains (Masihi *et al.*, 1986a). Partial protection comparable to that induced by specific immunization with nonpathogenic trophozoites against lethal intranasal infection by *Acanthamoeba culbertsoni* could be conferred by intravenous pretreatment with MDP (Masihi *et al.*, 1986a).

Multilamellar liposomes containing encapsulated MTP-PE and IFN-γ significantly reduced *Leishmania donovani* parasites in spleens of treated animals (Hockertz *et al.*, 1991). CDRI compound 86/448, a glycopeptide structurally related to MDP, was shown to be more potent in inhibiting *L. donovani* infection in hamsters and in improving the efficacy of sodium stibogluconate (Pal *et al.*, 1991).

A cloned protein containing sequences of the circumsporozoite antigen of *Plasmodium falciparum* induced strongest antibody responses in rabbits and monkeys when immunization was performed with alum-adsorbed liposomes containing *lipid A* and antigen (Richards *et al.*, 1988). Role of immunomodulators such as MDP analogues and lipid A have been reviewed (Siddiqui, 1990). Human antibody responses to *P. falciparum* circumsporozoite protein vaccine were shown to be superior when MPL and mycobacterial cell wall skeleton were used as adjuvants (Rickman *et al.*, 1991). In another study, a *P. falciparum* circumsporozoite protein recombinant fusion protein formulated with monophosphoryl lipid A, cell wall skeleton of mycobacteria, and squalane was administered to 12 volunteers. After the third dose of vaccine, significant amounts of antibodies were observed in sera of some volunteers who also did not develop parasitemia when challenged by the bite of mosquitoes carrying *P. falciparum* sporozoites (Hoffman *et al.*, 1994). Recently, complete protection from lethal *P. yoelii* malaria was produced by three immunizations with whole killed blood-stage parasite antigen in copolymer P1004 and detoxified RaLPS as adjuvants. The protection lasted for 9 months and was associated with an anamnestic rise in antibody titer of the IgG2a isotype during the challenge infection (Hunter *et al.*, 1995).

4.2. Fungus-Derived Immunomodulators

Lentinan can induce granuloma formation against *Schistosoma mansoni* and *S. japonicum*, and show a therapeutic effect against *Mesocestoides corti* (Chihara, 1990). Particulate glucan administered with glutaraldehyde-killed *T. cruzi* culture forms, but not glucan or killed trypanosomes alone, provided significant protection up to 275 days postchallenge (Williams *et al.*, 1989). Yeast *glucan* can prolong survival against parasitic infections by *Plasmodium berghei* and *Leishmania donovani* and exert antifungal activity against *Candida*, *Cryptococcus*, and *Sporotrichum* (Chihara, 1990). Glucan administered in combination with soluble *P. berghei* antigen (Maheshwari and Siddiqui, 1989) or fractions of *L. donovani* promastigotes (Obaid *et al.*, 1989) developed well-defined cell-mediated and humoral immune responses and conferred protection against challenge with live parasites.

4.3. Synthetic Compounds as Immunomodulators

Treatment with synthetic immunomodulator *LF-1695* increased oxygen metabolite production and cytotoxic activity of effector macrophages and platelets against *Schistosoma mansoni* and induced a higher degree of protection against parasite challenge (Thorel *et al.*, 1988).

The steroidal glycoside *L-644,257* [6-(5-cholesten-3β-yloxy)hexyl 1-thio-β-D-mannopyranoside] provided protection against *C. albicans* in cyclophosphamide-immunosuppressed mice (Hagmann *et al.*, 1990). An analogue of deoxyspergualin, N-563, was also shown to significantly prolong the survival time of cyclophosphamide-immunosuppressed mice against *C. albicans* (Aoyagi *et al.*, 1994).

Prophylactic administration of *isoprinosine* to mice could confer protection against *Trypanosoma cruzi* (Abath *et al.*, 1988).

Combination of pentostam with *levamisole* induced enhanced activity against *L. donovani* infection in hamsters and mice (Rifaat *et al.*, 1989). Guinea pigs infected with *L. enriettii* and treated with levamisole did not develop ulcerative lesions and showed no metastases, eosinophilia, or leukopenia (Rezai *et al.*, 1988). The severity of *L. major* infection in mice receiving levamisole was lower in comparison with controls (Rezai *et al.*, 1988). Levamisole has been reported to be active against *Strongyloides venezuelensis* infection in rats (Campos *et al.*, 1989). Levamisole administered prophylactically to mice could confer protection against *Trypanosoma cruzi* (Abath *et al.*, 1988). Mice infected for 45 days with *Schistosoma mansoni* and treated with levamisole exhibited increased resistance, which could be enhanced further by combination with praziquantel, to challenge with schistosoma cercariae (Botros *et al.*, 1989).

4.4. Endogenous Immunomodulators

4.4.1. Leukocyte-Derived Immunomodulator

Mucocutaneous candidal infection is frequently associated with a deficiency in cell-mediated immunity and oral candidiasis is an important clinical manifestation of HIV infection. Treatment with *IMREG-1*, a leukocyte-derived immunomodulator, improved control of oropharyngeal candida infection and decreased the occurrence of opportunistic infections. IMREG-1 can augment delayed-type hypersensitivity to recall antigens, enhance production of leukocyte migration inhibition factor, IFN-γ and expression of IL-2 receptors on $CD4^+$ helper lymphocytes (Gottlieb and Gottlieb, 1990).

4.4.2. Cytokines

Low doses of *IL-1* have been shown to inhibit parasitemia and protect mice against cerebral malaria caused by *Plasmodium berghei* (Curfs *et al.*, 1990). The growth of *C. albicans* in mice immunosuppressed with either cyclophosphamide or irradiation was significantly reduced when recombinant human IL-1α was administered 24 hr before, given simultaneously with or 6 hr after infection (Kullberg *et al.*, 1990). Prophylactic treatment with recombinant human IL-1β enhanced resistance of normal and cyclophosphamide-treated mice to systemic infection with *C. albicans* (Pecyk *et al.*, 1989).

Administration of *IL-2* has been shown to increase survival time of mice infected with *Trypanosoma cruzi* (Choromanski and Kuhn, 1985) and *Toxoplasma gondii* (Sharma *et al.*, 1985). Macrophages cultured with IL-2 and IFN-γ before infection with *L. major* develop resistance to infection which can be abrogated by anti-TNF antibodies. This suggests that IL-2 may act as a cofactor with IFN-γ for the induction of macrophage antimicrobicidal activity with TNF as the effector molecule (Belosevic *et al.*, 1990).

IL-4 has multiple biologic activities. Resistance against *Leishmania donovani* induced by IFN-γ in human monocytes is abrogated by IL-4 (Lehn *et al.*, 1989). Administration of anti-IL-4 monoclonal antibodies to neutralize IL-4 led to an attenuation of an otherwise fatal infection by *L. major* (Sadick *et al.*, 1990). IL-4, however, plays an important role in immunity to nematode parasites (Urban *et al.*, 1992).

In vivo injection of recombinant *TNF* has been shown to inhibit experimental infections with *Plasmodium* species (Taverne *et al.*, 1987; Clark *et al.*, 1987) and anti-TNF treatment is followed by an increase of *Plasmodium vinckei* parasitemia (Neifer *et al.*, 1989). Human recombinant TNF has an inhibitory effect on both virulent and nonvirulent strains of *Entamoeba histolytica* (Ghadirian, 1990). Administration of TNF-α can mediate protection against murine cutaneous leishmaniasis (Titus *et al.*, 1989; Liew *et al.*, 1990) although TNF does not exert direct leishmanicidal effect *in vitro* (Moll *et al.*, 1990). The Thl subset of CD4$^+$ T cells secreting IFN-γ are protective in murine cutaneous leishmaniasis, whereas the Th2 subset capable of producing IL-4 exacerbate the infection (Liew, 1991). Subcutaneous immunization induces Th2 cells while intraperitoneal or intravenous immunization generates Thl cells. Immunization with a *Leishmania major* peptide together with TNF-α prevented disease enhancement by the subcutaneous route and led to the desirable induction of Thl cells (Liew *et al.*, 1991).

Recombinant TNF induced protective effects against *Trypanosoma cruzi* and *Toxoplasma gondii* infections in mice (Black *et al.*, 1989). Murine recombinant TNF-α has been shown to enhance the expression of antimicrobicidal activity by IFN-γ primed macrophages cultured under low endotoxin conditions to kill or inhibit *Toxoplasma gondii* (Sibley *et al.*, 1991). Protection afforded by IFN-γ and TNF to mice infected with *Toxoplasma gondii* could be abrogated by anti-TNF antibodies (Chang *et al.*, 1990).

There is growing evidence from a number of studies that *IFN-γ* plays a central role in protection against *Toxoplasma gondii* (reviewed in Subauste and Remington, 1991). Administration of IFN-γ to athymic nude mice also prevented proliferation of the parasite in various organs and prolonged the survival of treated animals (Suzuki *et al.*, 1991). Mice rendered immunodeficient by selective depletion of CD4$^+$ cells and administered an aerosol of recombinant murine IFN-γ showed reduced intensity of *Pneumocystis carinii* infection (Beck *et al.*, 1991). IFN-γ is essential for the resolution of *Plasmodium berghei* infection in rodents (Schofield *et al.*, 1987) and human neutrophils treated with IFN-γ significantly augmented the killing of asexual blood forms of *Plasmodium falciparum* (Kumaratilake *et al.*, 1991). Mice infected with

Cryptosporidium showed greatly enhanced oocyst shedding when treated with anti-IFN-γ antibody (Ungar *et al.*, 1991). IFN-γ plays an important role in the control of pneumonia caused by *Chlamydia trachomatis* (Williams *et al.*, 1988) and represents a crucial host defense against *Rickettsia conorii* (Li *et al.*, 1987).

Treatment with *M-CSF* of human monocytes (Wang *et al.*, 1989) and elicited murine macrophages (Karbassi *et al.*, 1987) induces killing of *Candida albicans.* Human monocytes treated *in vitro* with recombinant human *IL-3* or *GM-CSF* were capable of inducing antifungal activity against *C. albicans* (Wang *et al.*, 1989). GM-CSF stimulates the oxidative respiratory burst and secretion of hydrogen peroxide in phagocytic cells (Sullivan *et al.*, 1989; Reed *et al.*, 1987), a host defense mechanism that could augment antimicrobicidal activity. Macrophages activated by GM-CSF exhibit enhanced capacity to kill *Leishmania donovani* (Weiser *et al.*, 1987), *L. tropica* (Handmann and Burgess, 1979) and *Trypanosoma cruzi* (Reed *et al.*, 1987). In other studies, human macrophages did not show killing activity against *Toxoplasma gondii* or bacterial infection by *Legionella pneumophila* (Nathan *et al.*, 1984; Jensen *et al.*, 1988).

Treatment of mice with GM-CSF increased the parasite burden and led to an exacerbation of leishmanial infection (Greil *et al.*, 1988). Antibodies to GM-CSF and IL-3 have been shown to dramatically decrease the incidence of neurological symptoms in cerebral malaria (Grau *et al.*, 1988).

IL-12, also known as NK cell-stimulating factor, is a heterodimeric cytokine produced by monocytes and B cells. It has multiple effects on T and NK cells and is a potent inducer of Th1 cytokine IFN-γ. Anti-IL-12 antibodies completely inhibited *T. gondii* or endotoxin-stimulated IFN-γ by NK cells. Treatment with IL-12 prolonged survival of SCID mice infected with *T. gondii* (Gazzinelli *et al.*, 1993). IFN-γ-dependent activation of macrophages by NK cells in SCID mice is essential for the development of natural immunity. Neutralization of IL-12 showed that heat-killed *L. monocytogenes* require IL-12 to stimulate IFN-γ production by SCID splenocytes (Tripp *et al.*, 1993). Treatment with murine IL-12 during the first week of infection with *L. major* cured the majority of the normally susceptible BALB/c mice and provided durable resistance against reinfection (Heinzel *et al.*, 1993). In contrast, administration of anti-IL-12 antibody at the time of infection to resistant C57BL/6 mice exacerbated disease (Sypek *et al.*, 1993). These observations suggest that IL-12 may prevent Th2 responses that are deleterious in certain infections and promote protective IFN-γ based Th1 responses.

Transforming growth factor beta (TGF-β) belongs to an ancestral evolutionary family of regulatory cytokines with potent growth inhibitory activities. It is produced at high levels by activated T lymphocytes, monocytes and macrophages among other cells, and during morphogenesis. Suppressive molecules such as TGF-β can down-regulate host response to intracellular pathogens. Production and release of TGF-β appears to be an important parasite escape mechanism. Impaired activity of macrophages has been observed in association with TGF-β in infections with *T. cruzi* (Silva *et al.*, 1991), *Leishmania* (Barral-Neto *et al.*, 1992), and *T. gondii* (Bermudez *et al.*,

1993). Anti-TGF-β antibody can partially inhibit TGF-β-induced downregulation and may represent an interesting intervention strategy. Host defense mechanisms within the brain, however, may vary. Microglial cells located within the brain are considered as ontogenic and functional equivalents of macrophages. Activation of microglia with IFN-γ plus TGF-β showed dose-dependent anti-*T. gondii* effect. Anti-TGF-β antibody inhibited antitoxoplasma activity of IFN-γ plus LPS-treated microglia suggesting a role for TGF-β in neural host defense function (Chao *et al.*, 1993).

5. CONCLUDING REMARKS AND FUTURE PROSPECTS

Immunomodulators are rapidly evolving to become a viable adjunct to established therapeutic modalities. This review highlights the recent application of a wide array of natural products of microbial origin, chemically synthesized molecules, and recombinant cytokines in prophylaxis and treatment of diverse diseases.

Therapeutic value of cytokines in infectious diseases is increasingly being recognized. IL-2, IL-12, TNF-α, and IFNs may be useful in potentiating host antimicrobial defense via stimulating the host effector cells. Other cytokines such as IL-1, IL-3, and hematopoietic growth factors alone and in combination are considered as being beneficial in treatment of infections associated with neutropenia, neonatal septicemia or in prevention of infections accompanying aplastic anemia, chemotherapy, immunodeficiency, or burn injury. Overall, the use of cytokines as therapeutic tools in the setting of infections has given rise to an optimistic view of the use of such reagents. Approaches based on neutralization of immunosuppressive cytokines in infectious diseases are also an area of considerable promise. Limitations of therapy with exogenous cytokines, however, have to be recognized. These are associated with the inherent toxicity of such material, their unclear pharmacological behavior, and their pleiotropic effects. Efficacy of exogenous cytokines capable of potentiating normal host defense mechanisms may be curtailed in immunocompromised patients lacking pertinent effector cells or containing disease-related factors preventing lymphocyte activation. Parasite, bacterial, and viral adaptations to the presence of cytokines pose new problems and approaches based on cytokine intervention will have to take these factors into account.

T-helper lymphocytes can be distinguished into two subtypes based on their response and ability to secrete a variety of mediators. Cytokines such as IFN-γ and TNF secreted by Th1-type cells are potent agents capable of limiting viral replication and controlling the multiplication of intracellular pathogens. Cytokines such as IL-4, IL-5, and IL-10 produced by Th2-type cells are capable of downregulating cell-mediated host defense effector mechanisms and can even exacerbate certain infections. On the other hand, IFN-γ has been shown to suppress protective mechanisms and IL-4 to play an important role in immunity to certain nematode parasites. Treatment regimens capable of manipulating the repertoire of cytokine cascade will be valuable in establishing effective immunotherapy. Selective stimulation by suitable immunomodulators of discrete lymphocyte subpopulations and cytokines important in protective effector mechanisms against a given infection is predicted to play an increasingly important role. Certain immunomodulators, MDP analogues for example, possess adjuvant activity whereas others more efficiently can induce CSFs and other cytokines. Identification of immunomodulators which can enhance the immunogenicity of antigens for both class I and class II MHC-restricted responses will also be important. Tailor-made immunomodulators produced by practical application of the advances in molecular biology and peptide synthesis will permit development of products based on scientific evidence rather than empiricism.

REFERENCES

Abath, F. G., Coutinho, E. M., Montenegro, S. M., Gomes, Y. M., and Carvalho, A. B., 1988, The use of non-specific immunopotentiators in experimental Trypanosoma cruzi infection, *Trans. R. Soc. Trop. Med. Hyg.* **82:**73–76.

Akridge, R. E., Oyafuso, L. K. M., and Reed, S. G., 1994, IL-10 is induced during HIV-1 infection and is capable of decreasing viral replication in human macrophages, *J. Immunol.* **153:**5782–5789.

Aldovini, A., and Young, R. A., 1991, Humoral and cell-mediated immune responses to live recombinant BCG-HIV vaccines, *Nature* **351:**479–482.

Alexander, H. R., Doherty, G. M., Buresh, C. M., Venzon, D. J., and Norton, J. A., 1991, A recombinant human receptor antagonist to interleukin 1 improves survival after lethal endotoxemia in mice, *J. Exp. Med.* **173:**1029–1032.

Ankel, H., Mittnacht, S., and Jacobsen, H., 1985, Antiviral activity of prostaglandin A on encephalomyocarditis virus-infected cells: A unique effect unrelated to interferon, *J. Gen. Virol.* **66:**2355–2364.

Ankel, H., Turriziani, O., and Antonelli, G., 1991, Prostaglandin A inhibits replication of human immunodeficiency virus during acute infection, *J. Gen. Virol.* **72:**2797–2800.

Aoyagi, K., Abe, F., Nemoto, K., Abe, S., Ishizuka, M., Takeuchi, T., and Yamaguchi, H., 1994, The novel immunostimulant N-563, an analogue of deoxyspergualin, promotes resistance to Candida albicans infection in mice, *J. Antibiot.* **47:**1077–1083.

Appelberg, R., Castro, A. G., Pedrose, J., Silva, R. A., Orme, I. M., and Minóprio, P., 1994, Role of gamma interferon and tumor necrosis factor alpha during T-cell-independent and -dependent phases of *Mycobacterium avium* infection, *Infect. Immun.* **62:**3962–3971.

Arakawa, T., Hsu, Y.-R., Toth, E, and Stebbing, N., 1987, The antiviral activity of recombinant human tumor necrosis factor, *J. Interferon Res.* **7:**103–105.

Asano, T., McWaters, A., An, T., Matsushima, K., and Kleinerman, E. S., 1994, Liposomal muramyl tripeptide up-regulates interleukin-1 alpha, interleukin-1 beta, tumor necrosis factor-alpha, interleukin-6 and interleukin-8 gene expression in human monocytes, *J. Pharmacol. Exp. Ther.* **268:**1032–1039.

Aukrust, P., Liabakk, N. M., Mueller, F., Lien, E., Espevik, T., and Froland, S.S., 1994, Serum levels of tumor necrosis factor-alpha TNF-alpha and soluble TNF receptors in human immunodeficiency virus type 1 infection—Correlations to clinical, immunologic, and virologic parameters, *J. Infect. Dis.* **169:**420–424.

Azuma, I., Yoo, Y. C., Tamura, M., Yoshida, R., Yoshimatsu, K., Arikawa, J., and Yamanishi, K., 1994, Protective activity of MDP-Lys(L18) on hantavitus infection in newborn mice and potentiation of antigenicity by B30-MDP and MDP-Lys(L18) of inactivated hantavirus strain B-1 vaccine and recombinant hepatitis B virus surface antigen, in: *Immunotherapy of Infections* (K. N. Masihi, ed.), Dekker, New York, pp. 191–203.

Babineau, T. J., Marcello, P., Swails, W., Kenler, A., Bistrian, B., and Forse, R. A., 1994, Randomized phase I/II trial of a macrophage-specific immunomodulator (PGG-glucan) in high-risk surgical patients, *Ann. Surg.* **220:**601–609.

Bader, T., and Ankel, H., 1990, Inhibition of primary transcription of vesicular stomatitis virus by prostaglandin A1, *J. Gen. Virol.* **71:**2823–2832.

Bahr, G., Darcissac, E., Bevec, D., Dukor, P., and Chedid, L., 1995, Immunopharmacological activities and clinical development of muramyl peptides with particular emphasis on murabutide, *Int. J. Immunopharmacol.* **17:**117–131.

Barral-Neto, M., Barral, A., Brownell, C. E., Skeiky, Y. A. W., Ellingwoth, L. R., Twardzik, D. R., and Reed, S. G., 1992, Transforming growth factor-beta in leishmanial infection: A parasite escape mechanism, *Science* **257:**545–548.

Bauer, J., and Hermann, F., 1991, Interleukin-6 in clinical medicine, *Ann. Hematol.* **62:**203–210.

Bazzoni, F., Cassatella, M. A., Rossi, F., Ceska, M., Dewald, B., and Baggiolini, M., 1991, Phagocytosing neutrophils produce and release high amounts of neutrophil-activating peptide 1/interleukin 8, *J. Exp. Med.* **173:**771–774.

Beck, J. M., Liggitt, H. D., Brunette, E. N., Fuchs, H. J., Shellito, J. E., and Debs, R. J., 1991, Reduction in intensity of Pneumocystis carinii pneumonia in mice by aerosol administration of gamma interferon, *Infect. Immun.* **59:**3859–3862.

Belosevic, M., Finbloom, D. S., Meltzer, M., and Nacy, C. A., 1990, IL-2. A cofactor for induction of activated macrophage resistance to infection, *J. Immunol.* **145:**831–839.

Benavente, J., Esteban, M., Jaffe, B. M., and Santoro, M. G., 1984, Selective inhibition of viral gene expression as the mechanism of the antiviral action of PGA1 in vaccinia virus-infected cells, *J. Gen. Virol.* **65:**599–608.

Bender, A., Amann, U., Jäger, R., Nain, M., and Gemsa, D., 1993, Effect of granulocyte/macrophage colony-stimulating factor on human monocytes infected with influenza A virus, *J. Immunol.* **151:**5416–5424.

Bergamini, A., Perno, C. F., Dini, L., Capozzi, M., Pesce, C. D., Ventura, L., Cappannoli, L., Falasca, L., Milanese, G., Caliò, R., and Rocchi, G., 1994, Macrophage colony-stimulating factor enhances the susceptibility of macrophages to infection by human immunodeficiency virus and reduces the activity of compounds that inhibit virus binding, *Blood* **84:**3405–3412.

Bermudez, L. E., and Young, L. S., 1991, Natural killer cell-dependent mycobacteriostatic and mycobactericidal activity in human macrophages, *J. Immunol.* **146:**265–270.

Bermudez, L. E. M., Stevens, P., Kolonoski, P., Wu, M., and Young, L. S., 1989, Treatment of experimental disseminated Mycobacterium avium complex infection in mice with recombinant IL-2 and tumor necrosis factor, *J. Immunol.* **143:**2996–3000.

Bermudez, L. E., Covaro, G., and Remington, J., 1993, Infection of murine macrophages with Toxoplasma gondii is associated with release of transforming growth factor beta and downregulation of expression of tumor necrosis factor receptors, *Infect. Immun.* **61:**4126–4130.

Bernstein, D. I., and Harrison, C. J., 1989, Effects of the immunomodulating agent R837 on acute and latent herpes simplex virus type 2 infections, *Antimicrob. Agents Chemother.* **33:**1511–1515.

Bessler, W. G., Kleine, B., Biesert, L., Schlecht, S., Schaude, R., Wiesmüller, K.-H., Metzger, J., and Jung, G., 1990, Bacterial surface components as immunomodulators, in: *Immunotherapeutic Prospects of Infectious Diseases* (K. N. Masihi and W. Lange, eds.), Springer-Verlag, Berlin, pp. 37–48.

Bessler, W., Beck, W., Wiesmüller, K. H., and Jung, G., 1994, Modulation of the immune system by bacterial products: Hapten-specific humoral immune responses induced by lipopeptides conjugated to T helper cell epitopes, in: *Immunotherapy of Infections* (K. N. Masihi, ed.), Dekker, New York, pp. 329–338.

Bhalla, K., Birkhofer, M., Grant, S., and Graham, G., 1989, The effect of recombinant human granulocyte–macrophage colony-stimulating factor on AZT-mediated biochemical and cytotoxic effects on normal human myeloid progenitor cells, *Exp. Hematol.* **17:**17–20.

Black, C. M., Israelski, D. M., Suzuki, Y., and Remington, J. S., 1989, Effect of recombinant tumor necrosis factor on acute infection in mice with Toxoplasma gondii or Trypanosoma cruzi, *Immunology* **68:**570–574.

Blanchard, D. K., Djeu, J. Y., Klein, T. W., Friedman, H., and Stewart, W. E., 1988, Protective effects of tumor necrosis factor in experimental Legionella pneumophila infections of mice via activation of PMN function, *J. Leukocyte Biol.* **43**:429–435.

Bogdan, C., Vodovotz, Y., and Nathan, C., 1991, Macrophage deactivation by interleukin 10, *J. Exp. Med.* **174**:1549–1555.

Botros, S. S., Hassan, S. I., El-Nahal, H. M., Azab, M. E., Shaker, Z. A., and El-Garem, A., 1989, Levamisole restored the compromised state of immunity after specific chemotherapy in experimental Schistosomiasis mansoni, *Immunopharmacol. Immunotoxicol.* **11**:611–629.

Buchmeier, N. A., and Schreiber, R. D., 1985, Requirement of endogenous interferon-gamma for resolution of Listeria monocytogenes infection, *Immunology* **82**:7404–7408.

Bui, T., Dykers, T., Hu, S. L., Faltynek, C. R., and Ho, R. K., 1994, Effect of MTP-PE liposomes and interleukin-7 on induction of antibody and cell-mediated immune responses to a recombinant HIV-envelope protein, *J. AIDS* **7**:799–806.

Bukowski, J. F., Yang, H., and Welsh, R. M., 1988, The antiviral effect of lymphokine-activated killer cells: characterization of the effector cells mediating prophylaxis, *J. Virol.* **62**:3642–3648.

Burke, R. L., Goldbeck, C., Ng, P., Stanberry, L., Ott, G., and Van Nest, G., 1994, The influence of adjuvant on the therapeutic efficacy of a recombinant genital herpes vaccine, *J. Infect. Dis.* **170**:1110–1119.

Byars, N. E., Fraser-Smith, E. B., Pecyk, R. A., Welch, M., Nakano, G., Burke, R. L., Hayward, A. R., and Allison, A. C., 1994, Vaccinating guinea pigs with recombinant glycoprotein D of herpes simplex virus in an efficacious adjuvant formulation elicits protection against vaginal infection *Vaccine* **12**:200–209.

Campos, R., Pinto, P. L., Amato, N. V., Matsubara, L., Miyamoto, A., de Carvalho, S. A., Takiguti, C. K., and Moreira, A. A., 1989, Treatment of experimental infection by Strongyloides venezuelensis in rats, with the use of injectable ivermectin and levamisole, *Rev. Inst. Med. Trop. Sao Paulo* **31**:48–52.

Casey, L. C., Balk, R. A. and Bone, R. C., 1993, Plasma cytokine and endotoxin levels correlate with survival in patients with the sepsis syndrome, *Ann. Intern. Med.* **119**:771–778.

Chan, W. L., Ziltener, H. J., and Liew, F. W., 1990, Interleukin-3 protects mice from acute herpes simplex virus infection, *Immunology* **71**:358–363.

Chang, H. R., Grau, G. E., and Pechere, J. C., 1990, Role of TNF and IL-1 in infections with Toxoplasma gondii, *Immunology* **69**:33–37.

Chao, C. C., Hu, S., Gekker, G., Novick, W. J., Remington, J. S., and Peterson, P. K., 1993, Effects of cytokines on multiplication of Toxoplasma gondii in microglial cells, *J. Immunol.* **150**:3403–3410.

Cheadle, W. G., Hanasawa, K., Gallinaro, R. N., Nimmanwudipong, T., Kodama, M., and Polk, H. C., 1991, Endotoxin filtration and immune stimulation improve survival from gram-negative sepsis, *Surgery* **110**:785–791.

Cheers, C., Hill, M., Haigh, A. M., and Stanley, E. R., 1989, Stimulation of macrophage phagocytic but not bactericidal activity by colony-stimulating factor 1, *Infect. Immun.* **57**:1512–1516.

Chihara, G., 1990, Lentinan and its related polysaccharides as host defence potentiators: Their application to infectious diseases and cancer, in: *Immunotherapeutic Prospects of Infectious Diseases* (K. N. Masihi and W. Lange, eds.), Springer-Verlag, Berlin, pp. 9–18.

Chong, K.-T., 1987, Prophylactic administration of interleukin-2 protects mice from lethal challenge with gram-negative bacteria, *Infect. Immun.* **55**:668–673.

Choromanski, L., and Kuhn, R., 1985, Interleukin-2 enhances specific and nonspecific immune responses in experimental Chagas disease, *Infect. Immun.* **50**:354–357.

Clark, I. A., Hunt, N. H., Butcher, G. A., and Cowden, W. B., 1987, Inhibition of murine malaria (Plasmodium chabaudi) in vivo by recombinant interferon-gamma or tumor necrosis factor, and its enhancement by butylated hydroxyanisole, *J. Immunol.* **139**:3493–3496.

Cohen, A. M., Hines, D. K., Korach, E. S., and Ratzkin, B. J., 1988, In vivo activation of neutrophil function in hamsters by recombinant human granulocyte colony-stimulating factor, *Infect. Immun.* **56**:2861–2865.

Curfs, J. H., Van der Meer, J. W., Sauerwein, R. W., and Eling, W. M., 1990, Low dosages of interleukin 1 protect mice against lethal cerebral malaria, *J. Exp. Med.* **172**:1287–1291.

Czuprynski, C. J., and Brown, J. F., 1987, Recombinant murine interleukin-1 alpha enhancement of nonspecific antibacterial resistance, *Infect. Immun.* **55:**2061–2065.

Daniels, H. M., Meager, A., Eddleston, A. L., Alexander, G. J., and Williams, R., 1990, Spontaneous production of tumor necrosis factor alpha and interleukin-1 beta during interferon alpha treatment of chronic HBV infection, *Lancet* **335:**875–877.

Delfino, D., Chiofalo, M. S., Altavilla, D., Arena, A., Iannello, D., and Mastroeni, P., 1990, Interaction of rat macrophages with Leishmania infantum: role of tumor necrosis factor, in: *Immunotherapeutic Prospects of Infectious Diseases* (K. N. Masihi and W. Lange, eds.), Springer-Verlag, Berlin, pp. 271–277.

Denis, M., 1991a, Growth of Listeria monocytogenes in murine macrophages and its modulation by cytokines, activation of bactericidal activity by interleukin-4 and interleukin-6, *Can. J. Microbiol.* **37:**253–257.

Denis, M., 1991b, Modulation of Mycobacterium lepraemurium growth in murine macrophages: Beneficial effect of tumor necrosis factor and granulocyte–macrophage colony-stimulating factor, *Infect. Immun.* **59:**705–707.

Denis, M., and Gregg, E. O., 1991, Modulation of Mycobacterium avium growth in murine macrophages: Reversal of unresponsiveness to interferon-gamma by indomethacin or interleukin-4, *J. Leukocyte Biol.* **49:**65–72.

Denis, M., Campbell, D., and Gregg, E. O., 1991, Interleukin-2 and granulocyte–macrophage colony-stimulating factor stimulate growth of a virulent strain of Escherichia coli, *Infect. Immun.* **59:**1853–1856.

Déprez, B., Gras-Masse, H., Martinon, F., Gomard, E., Lévy, J.-P., and Tartar, A., 1995, Pimelautide or trimexautide as built-in adjuvants associated with an HIV-1-derived peptide: Synthesis and *in vivo* induction of antibody and virus-specific cytotoxic T-lymphocyte-mediated response, *J. Med. Chem.* **38:**459–465.

De Simone, C., Famularo, G., Tzantzoglou, S., Moretti, S., and Jirillo, E., 1991, Inosine pranobex in the treatment of HIV infection: A review, *Int. J. Immunopharmacol.* **13**(Suppl. 1)**:**19–27.

Dezube, B. J., 1994, Pentoxifylline for the treatment of infection with human immunodeficiency virus, *Clin. Infect. Dis.* **18:**285–287.

Dianzani, C., Colangelo, D., Tonso, E., Guidotto, S., and Viano, I., 1994, In vivo antiviral effects of pidotimod, *Arzneim. Forsch.* **44:**1431–1433.

Doherty, P., Allan, J. E., and Clark, I. A., 1989, Tumor necrosis factor inhibits the development of viral meningitis or induces rapid death depending on the severity of inflammation at the time of administration, *J. Immunol.* **142:**3576 3580.

Domke-Opitz, I., and Kirchner, H., 1990, Stimulation of macrophage by endotoxin results in the reactivation of a persistent herpes simplex virus infection, *Scand. J. Immunol.* **32:**69–75.

Eizuru, Y., Nakagawa, N., Hamasuna, R., and Minamishima, Y., 1992, Protective effect of MDP-Lys(L18), a synthetic derivative of muramyldipeptide, on murine cytomegalovirus infection, *Nat. Immun.* **11:**225–236.

Esparza, I., Gonzalez, J. C., and Vinuela, E., 1988, Effect of interferon-alpha, interferon-gamma and tumour necrosis factor on African swine fever virus replication in porcine monocytes and macrophages, *J. Gen. Virol.* **69:**2973–2980.

Feduchi, E., and Carrasco, L., 1991, Mechanism of inhibition of HSV-1 replication by tumor necrosis factor and interferon gamma, *Virology* **180:**822–825.

Feduchi, E., Alonso, M. A., and Carrasco, L., 1989, Human gamma interferon and tumor necrosis factor exert a synergistic blockade on the replication of herpes simplex virus, *J. Virol.* **63:**1354–1359.

Folks, T. M., Clouse, K. A., Justement, J., Rabson, A., Duh, E., Kehrl, J. H., and Fauci, A. S., 1989, Tumor necrosis factor-alpha induces the expression of T-cell clone, *Proc. Natl. Acad. Sci. USA* **86:**2365–2368.

Franek, J., and Malina, J., 1990, Immunomodulatory capacity of drugs evaluated in a mouse model of Klebsiella pneumoniae infection, in: *Immunotherapeutic Prospects of Infectious Diseases* (K. N. Masihi and W. Lange, eds.), Springer-Verlag, Berlin, pp. 55–58.

Galassi, D., Galassi, P., Pelliccioni, A., and Semprini, P., 1986, Clinical results obtained in cattle and swine by means of biological immunostimulators, *Comp. Immun. Microbiol. Infect. Dis.* **9**:285–295.

Gallin, J. I., 1991, Interferon-gamma in the management of chronic granulomatous disease, *Rev. Infect. Dis.* **13**:973–978.

Gazzinelli, R. T., Hieny, S., Wynn, T. A., Wolf, S., and Sher, A,, 1993, Interleukin 12 is required for the T-lymphocyte-independent induction of interferon gamma by an intracellular parasite and induces resistance in T-cell-deficient hosts, *Proc. Natl. Acad. Sci. USA* **90**:6115–6119.

Gendelman, H. E., Orenstein, J. M., Martin, M. A., Ferrua, C., Mitra, R., Phipps, T., Wahl, L. A., Lane, H. C., and Fauci, A. S., 1988, Efficient isolation and propagation of human immunodeficiency virus on recombinant colony-stimulating factor 1-treated monocytes, *J. Exp. Med.* **167**:1428–1441.

Ghadirian, E., 1990, In vitro effect of human recombinant tumor necrosis factor on Entamoeba histolytica trophozoites, *Immunobiology* **180**:339–350.

Gidoh, M., and Tsutsumi, S., 1989, The inhibitory effects by combined doses of DDS and several immunostimulants on the growth of leprosy bacilli inoculated into footpads of hybrid nude mice, *Nippon Rai. Gakkai. Zasshi* **58**:241–249.

Gladue, R. P., Laquerre, A. M., Magna, H. A., Carrol, L. A., O'Donnell, M., Changelian, P. S., and Franke, A. E., 1994, In vivo augmentation of IFN-gamma with a rIL-12 human/mouse chimera: Pleiotropic effects against infectious agents in mice and rats, *Cytokine* **6**:318–328.

Goronzy, J., Weyand, C., Quan, J., Fathman, C. G., and O'Hanley, P., 1989, Enhanced cell-mediated protection against fatal Escherichia coli septicemia induced by treatment with recombinant IL-2, *J. Immunol.* **142**:1134–1138.

Gottlieb, A. A., and Gottlieb, M. S., 1990, Experience with IMREG-1, a leukocyte derived immunomodulator on candidiasis and progression of disease in patients with AIDS-related complex, in: *Immunotherapeutic Prospects of Infectious Diseases* (K. N. Masihi and W. Lange, eds.), Springer-Verlag, Berlin, pp. 121–128.

Grau, G. E., Kindler, J., Piguet, P. F., Lambert, P. H., and Vassali, P., 1988, Prevention of experimental cerebral malaria by anticytokine antibodies: IL-3 and granulocyte-macrophage colony-stimulating factor are intermediates in increased tumor necrosis factor production and macrophage accumulation, *J. Exp. Med.* **168**:1499–1504.

Greil, J., Bodendorfer, B., Rollinghoff, M., and Solbach, R., 1988, Application of recombinant granulocyte-macrophage colony-stimulating factor has a detrimental effect in experimental murine leishmaniasis, *Eur. J. Immunol.* **18**:1527–1533.

Gruszecki, W., Masihi, K. N., Labischinski, H., and Bradaczek, H., 1988, Synthesis and some biological activities of a novel glucofuranose immunomodulator, in: *Immunomodulators and Nonspecific Host Defence Mechanisms against Microbial Infections* (K. N. Masihi and W. Lange, eds.), Pergamon Press, New York, pp. 415–427.

Haak-Frendscho, M., Young, K. M., and Czuprynski, C. J., 1989, Treatment of mice with human recombinant interleukin-2 augments resistance to the facultative intracellular pathogen Listeria monocytogenes, *Infect. Immun.* **57**:3014–3021.

Hadden, J.W., 1992, Recent thoughts on the immunotherapy of infectious diseases including HIV infection, *Adv. Exp. Med. Biol.* **319**:13–22.

Hadden, J. W., Giner-Sorolla, A., and Hadden, E. M., 1991, Methyl inosine monophosphate (MIMP), a new purine immunomodulator for HIV infection, *Int. J. Immunopharmacol.* **13**(Suppl. 1):43–48.

Hagmann, W. K., Ponipipom, N. M., Jackson, J. J., Wood, D. D., Boltz, R. C., and Zweerink, H. J., 1990, Steroidal glycolipid, L-644,257, is a potent enhancer of nonspecific host resistance, *Int. J. Immunopharmacol.* **12**:241–246.

Hammer, S. M., and Gillis, J. M., 1987, Synergistic activity of granulocyte–macrophage colony-stimulating factor and 3′-azido-3′-deoxythymidine against human immunodeficiency virus in vitro, *Antimicrob. Agents Chemother.* **1987**:1046–1050.

Hammer, S. M., Gillis, J. M., Groopman, J. E., and Rose, R. M., 1986, In vitro modification of human immunodeficiency virus infection by granulocyte–macrophage colony-stimulating factor and gamma interferon, *Proc. Natl. Acad. Sci. USA* **83**:8734–8738.

Handmann, E., and Burgess, A. W., 1979, Stimulation by granulocyte–macrophage colony-stimulating factor of Leishmania tropica killing by macrophages, *J. Immunol.* **122:**1134–1137.

Havell, E. A., and Sehgal, P. B., 1991, Tumor necrosis factor-independent Il-6 production during murine listeriosis, *J. Immunol.* **146:**756–761.

Hazama, M., Mayumi-Aono, A., Asakawa, N., Kuroda, S., Hinuma, S., and Fujisawa, Y., 1993, Adjuvant-independent enhanced immune responses to recombinant herpes simplex virus type 1 glycoprotein D by fusion with biologically active interleukin-2, *Vaccine* **11:**629–636.

Heinzel, F. P., Schoenhaut, D. M., Rerko, R. M., Rosser, L. E., and Gately, M. K., 1993, Recombinant interleukin 12 cures mice infected with Leishmania major, *J. Exp. Med.* **177:**1505–1509.

Hersh, E. M., Brewton, G., Abrams, D., Bartlett, J., Galpin, J., Gill, P., Gorter, R., Gottlieb, M., Jonikas, J. J., and Landesman, S., 1991a, Ditiocarb sodium (diethyldithiocarbamate) therapy in patients with symptomatic HIV infection and AIDS, *J. Am. Med. Assoc.* **265:**1538–1544.

Hersh, E. M., Funk, C. Y., Ryschon, K. L., Petersen, E. A., and Mosier, D. E., 1991b, Effective therapy of LP-BM5 murine retrovirus-induced lymphoproliferative immunodeficiency disease with diethyldithiocarbamate, *AIDS Res. Hum. Retrovir.* **7:**553–561.

Hockertz, S., Franke, G., Paulini, I., and Lohmann-Matthes, M. L., 1991, Immunotherapy of murine visceral leishmaniasis with murine recombinant interferon-gamma and MTP-PE encapsulated in liposomes, *J. Interferon Res.* **11:**177–185.

Hoffman, S. L., Edelman, R., Bryan, J. P., Schneider, I., Davis, J., Sedegah, M., Gordon, D., Church, P., Gross, M., Silverman, C., Hollingdale, M., Clyde, D., Sztein, M., Losonsky, G., Paparello, S., and Jones, T. R., 1994, Safety, immunogenicity, and efficacy of a malaria sporozoite vaccine administered with monophosphoryl lipid A, cell wall skeleton of mycobacteria, and squalane as adjuvant, *Am. J. Trop. Med. Hyg.* **51:**603–612.

Hotta, H., Hagiwara, K., Tabata, K., Ito, W., and Homma, M., 1993, Augmentation of protective immune responses against Sendai virus infection by fungal polysaccharide schizophyllan, *Int. J. Immunopharmacol.* **15:**55–60.

Houde, M., and Arora, J. S., 1990, Stimulation of tumor necrosis factor secretion by purified influenza virus neuraminidase, *Cell. Immunol.* **129:**104–111.

Hubbard, R. D., and Collins, F. M., 1991, Immunomodulation of mouse macrophage killing of Mycobacterium avium in vitro, *Infect. Immun.* **59:**570–574.

Hunter, R. L., Kidd, M. R., Olsen, M. R., Patterson, P. S., and Lal, A. A., 1995, Induction of long-lasting immunity to *Plasmodium yoelii* malaria with whole blood-stage antigens and copolymer adjuvants, *J. Immunol.* **154:**1762–1769.

Iida, J., Saiki, I., Ishihara, C., and Azuma, I., 1989, Prophylactic activity against Sendai virus infection and macrophage activation with lipophilic derivatives of N-acetylglucosaminylmuramyl tri- or tetrapeptides, *Vaccine* **7:**225–228.

Iizawa, Y., Nishi, T., Kondo, M., Tsuchiya, K., and Imada, A., 1988, Effect of recombinant human interleukin-2 on the course of experimental chronic respiratory tract infection caused by Klebsiella pneumoniae in mice, *Infect. Immun.* **56:**45–50.

Ikeda, S., Matsuura, M., Nakatsuka, M., Homma, J. Y., Kiso, M., Hasegawa, A., and Nishimura, C., 1990, Non-specific protective activity of synthetic lipid A-subunit analogs against microbial infections is influenced by their 2-N- and 3-O-linked acyl substituents in the D-glucosamine backbone, *J. Clin. Lab. Immunol.* **32:**177–181.

Ikeda, S., Neyts, J., Matsuura, M., Kiso, M., Hasegawa, A., Nishimura, C., and De Clerck, E., 1993, Protective activity of the lipid A analogue GLA-60 against murine cytomegalovirus infection in immunodeficient mice, *J. Gen. Virol.* **74:**1399–1403.

Ilbäck, N.-G., Fohlman, J., Slorach, S., and Friman, G., 1989, Effects of the immunomodulator LS 2616 on lymphocyte subpopulations in murine coxsackievirus B3 myocarditis, *J. Immunol.* **142:**3225–3228.

Irinoda, K., Masihi, K. N., Chihara, G., Kaneko, Y., and Katori, T., 1992, Stimulation of microbicidal host defence mechanisms against aerosol influenza virus infection by lentinan, *Int. J. Immunopharmacol.* **14:**971–977

Ishihara, C., Iida, J., Mizukoshi, N., Yamamoto, N., Yamamoto, K., Kato, K., and Azuma, I., 1989, Effect of

N alpha-acetylmuramyl-L-alanyl-D-isoglutaminyl-N epsilon-stearoyl-L-lysine on resistance to herpes simplex virus type-1 infection in cyclophosphamide-treated mice, *Vaccine* **7**:309–313.

Ito, M., Baba, M., and Sato, A., 1989, Tumor necrosis factor enhances replication of human immunodeficiency virus in vitro, *Biochem. Biophys. Res. Commun.* **158**:306–312.

Ito, M., Baba, M., Mori, S., Hirabayashi, K., Sato, A., Shigeta, S., and De Clercq, E., 1990, Tumor necrosis factor antagonizes inhibitory effect of azidothymidine on human immunodeficiency virus (HIV) replication in vitro, *Biochem. Biophys. Res. Commun.* **166**:1095–1101.

Izbicki, J. R., Ziegler-Heitbrock, H. W., Luetticken R., Ruckdeschel, G., Wilker, D. K., and Schweiberer, L., 1991, Studies on post-splenectomy infection and immune activation by muramyl peptide. A new concept in the prevention of severe infections, *Chirurg* **6**:2–8.

Jagodzinski, P. P., Wiaderkiewicz, R., Kurazawski, G., Kloczewiak, M., Nakashima, H., Hyjek, E., Yamamoto, N., Uryu, T., Kaneko, Y., Posner, M. R., and Kozbor, D., 1994, Mechanism of the inhibitory effect of curdlan sulfate on HIV-1 infection in vitro, *Virology* **202**:735–745.

Jeevan, A., and Asherson, G. L., 1988, Recombinant interleukin-2 limits the replication of Mycobacterium lepraemurium and Mycobacterium bovis BCG in mice, *Infect. Immun.* **56**:660–664.

Jensen, W. A., Rose, R. M., Burke, R. H., Anton, K., and Remold, H. G., 1988, Cytokine activation of antibacterial activity in human pulmonary macrophages: Comparison of recombinant interferon gamma and granulocyte–macrophage colony-stimulating factor, *Cell. Immunol.* **117**:369–377.

Johannsen, L., Obal, F., Kapas, L., Kovalzon, V., and Krueger, J. M., 1994, Somnogenic activity of muramyl peptide-derived immune adjuvants, *Int. J. Immunopharmacol.* **16**:109–116.

Johnson, C. S., Chang, M. J., Thurlow, S. M., Pourbohloul, S. C., and Furmanski, P., 1990, Immunotherapeutic approaches to leukemia: The use of Friend virus-induced erythroleukemia model system, *Cancer Res.* **50**(Suppl):5682S–5686S.

Kahn, J. O., Sinangi, F., Baenziger, J., Murcar, N., Wynne, D., Coleman, R. L., Steimer, K. B., Dekker, C. L., and Chernoff, D., 1994, Clinical and immunologic responses to human immunodeficiency virus (HIV) type 1SF2 gp120 subunit vaccine combined with or without muramyl tripeptide dipalmitoyl phosphatidylethanolamine in non-HIV-infected human volunteers, *J. Infect. Dis.* **170**:1288–1291.

Kalechman, Y., Albeck, M., Oron, M., Sobelman, D., Gurwith, M., Sehgal, S. N., and Sredni, B., 1990, Radioprotective effects of immunomodulator AS101, *J. Immunol.* **145**:1512–1517.

Kalter, C. D., Nakamura, M., Turpin, J. A., Baca, L. M., Hoover, D. L., Dieffenbach, C., Ralph, P., Gendelman, H. E., and Meltzer, M. S., 1991, Enhanced HIV replication in macrophages colony-stimulating factor-treated monocytes, *J. Immunol.* **146**:298–306.

Kaneko, Y., Yamamoto, Y., and Uryu, T., 1990, Biological actions of polysaccharides and those derivatives against cancer and AIDS, in: *Immunotherapeutic Prospects of Infectious Diseases* (K. N. Masihi and W. Lange, eds.), Springer-Verlag, Berlin, pp. 109–119.

Kaplan, G., 1991, The role of rIL-2 in the modulation of cellular immunity in resistance to infection, *Immunol. Lett.* **30**:199–200.

Karbassi, A., Becker, J. M., Foster, J. S., and Moore, R. N., 1987, Enhanced killing of Candida albicans by murine macrophages treated with macrophage colony-stimulating factor: Evidence for augmented expression of mannose receptors, *Infect. Immun.* **139**:417–421.

Keitel, W., Couch, R., Bond, N., Adair, S., Van Nest, G., and Dekker, C., 1993, Pilot evaluation of influenza virus vaccine (IVV) combined with adjuvant, *Vaccine* **11**:909–913.

Khaitov, R. M., Pinegin, B. V., Butakov, A. A., and Andronova, T. M., 1994, Immunotherapy of infectious postoperative complications with glucosaminylmuramyl dipeptide, in: *Immunotherapy of Infections* (K. N. Masihi, ed.), Dekker, New York, pp. 205–211.

Kindler, V., Sappino, A. P., Grau, G. E., Piguet, P. F., and Vassalli, P., 1989, The inducing role of tumor necrosis factor in the development of bacterial granulomas during BCG infection, *Cell* **56**:731–740.

Klavinski, L. S., Geckeler, R., and Oldstone, M. B., 1989, Cytotoxic T lymphocyte control of acute lymphocytic choriomeningitis virus infection: Interferon gamma, but not tumour necrosis factor alpha, displays antiviral activity in vivo, *J. Gen. Virol.* **70**:3317–3325.

Klempner, M. S., Noring, R., Mier, J. W., and Atkins, M., 1990, An acquired chemotactic defect in neutrophils from patients receiving interleukin-2 immunotherapy, *N. Engl. J. Med.* **322**:959–965.

Kobayashi, N., Hamamoto, Y., Yamamoto, N., Ishii, A., Yonehara, M., and Yonehara, S., 1990, Anti-Fas monoclonal antibody is cytocidal to human immunodeficiency virus-infected cells without augmenting viral replication, *Proc. Natl. Acad. Sci. USA* **87:**9620–9624.

Kohl, S., Loo, L. S., Drath, D. B., and Cox, P., 1989, Interleukin-2 protects neonatal mice from lethal herpes simplex virus infection: A macrophage-mediated, gamma interferon-induced mechanism, *J. Infect. Dis.* **159:**239–247.

Kotani, S., Nagao, A., Tamura, T., Okamura, H., Nagata, K., Aoyama, K., Kusumoto, S., Kokeguchi, S., Kato, K., Fujii, N., Usami, H., Yoshida, T., Akagawa, K., Tanaka, S., Komuro, T., Ikeda-Fujita, T., Kato, Y., and Utsunomiya, J., 1990, Purification and endotoxin-like bioactivities of a novel amphiphile from Mycobacterium bovis BCG, in: *Immunotherapeutic Prospects of Infectious Diseases* (K. N. Masihi and W. Lange, eds.), Springer-Verlag, Berlin, pp. 19–36.

Kullberg, B.-J., Van't Wout, J. W., and Van Furth, R., 1990, Role of granulocytes in increased host resistance to Candida albicans induced by recombinant interleukin-1, *Infect. Immun.* **58:**3319–3324.

Kumaratilake, L. M., Ferrante, A., and Rzepczyk, C., 1991, The role of T lymphocytes in immunity to Plasmodium falciparum. Enhancement of neutrophil-mediated parasite killing by lymphotoxin and IFN-gamma: Comparisons with tumor necrosis factor effects, *J. Immunol.* **146:**762–767.

Lairmore, M. D., Post, A. A., Goldsmith, C. S., and Folks, T. M., 1991, Cytokine enhancement of simian immunodeficiency virus (SIV/mac) from a chronically infected cloned T-cell line (HuT-78), *Arch. Virol.* **121:**43–53.

Lazdins, J. K., Woods-Cook, K., Walker, M., and Alteri, E., 1990, The lipophilic muramyl peptide MTP-PE is a potent inhibitor of HIV replication in macrophages, *AIDS Res.* **10:**1157–1161.

Lee, B. K., Mohrman, M., Odean, M. J., Johnson, A. G., Morin, A., and Deschamps de Paillette, E., 1992, Polyadenylic: polyuridylic acid-induced determinants of host resistance to cytomegalovirus and their potentiation by hyperthermia, *J. Immunother.* **12:**105–114.

Lee, M., and Warren, M. K., 1987, CSF-1-induced resistance to viral infection in murine macrophages, *J. Immunol* **138:**3019–3022.

Lehn, M., Weiser, W. Y., Engelhorn, S., Gillis, S., and Remold, H. G., 1989, IL-4 inhibits H_2O_2 production and antileishmanial capacity of human cultured monocytes mediated by IFN-gamma, *J. Immunol.* **143:**3020–3024.

Leiby, D. A., Fortier, A. H., Crawford, R. M., Schreiber, R. D., and Nacy, C. A., 1992, In vivo modulation of the murine immune response to Francisella tularensis LVS by administration of anticytokine antibodies, *Infect. Immun.* **60:**84–89.

Li, H., Jerrells, T. R., Spitalny, G. L., and Walker, D. H., 1987, Gamma interferon as a crucial host defense against Rickettsia conorii in vivo, *Infect. Immun.* **55:**1252–1255.

Liew, F. Y., 1991, Role of cytokines in killing of intracellular pathogens, *Immunol. Lett.* **30:**193–198.

Liew, F. Y. C., Parkinson, S., Millot, A., Severn, A., and Carrier, M., 1990, Tumor necrosis factor (TNF-alpha) in leishmaniasis. I. TNF-alpha mediates host protection against cutaneous leishmaniasis, *Immunology* **69:**570–573.

Liew, F. Y., Li, Y., Yang, D. M., Severn, A., and Cox, F. E. G., 1991, TNF-alpha reverses the disease-exacerbating effect of subcutaneous immunization against murine cutaneous leishmaniasis, *Immunology* **74:**304–309.

Madonna, G. S., Ledney, G. D., Elliott, T. B., Brook, I., Ulrich, J. T., Myers, K. R., Patchen, M. L., and Walker, R. I., 1989, Trehalose dimycolate enhances resistance to infection in neutropenic animals, *Infect. Immun.* **57:**2495–2501.

Maeda, Y. Y., Yonekawa, H., and Chihara, G., 1994, Application of lentinan as cytokine inducer and host defense potentiator in immunotherapy of infectious diseases, in: *Immunotherapy of Infections* (K. N. Masihi, ed.), Dekker, New York, pp. 261–279.

Magee, D. M., and Wing, E. J., 1989, Secretion of colony-stimulating factors by T cell clones: Role in adoptive protection against Listeria monocytogenes, *J. Immunol.* **143:**2336–2341.

Maheshwari, R., and Siddiqui, M. U., 1989, Immunoprotection by beta-1,3 glucan antigen combination in Plasmodium berghei infection in mice, *Indian J. Med. Res.* **89:**396–403.

Makonkawkeyoon, S., Limson-Pobre, R. N., Moreira, A. L., Schauf, V, and Kaplan, G., 1993, Thalidomide inhibits the replication of human immunodeficiency virus type 1, *Proc. Natl. Acad. Sci. USA* **90:** 5974–5978.

Masek, K., Seifert, J., Flegel, M., Krojidlo, M., and Kolinsky, J., 1984, The immunomodulatory property of a novel synthetic compound adamantylamide dipeptide, *Meth. Find. Exp. Clin. Pharmacol.* **6:**667.

Masihi, K. N. (ed.), 1994, *Immunotherapy of Infections,* Dekker, New York.

Masihi, K. N., and Masek, K., 1993, Effect of the synthetic immunomodulator adamantylamide dipeptide on replication of human immunodeficiency virus alone and in combination with azidothymidine, *Int. J. Immunother.* **IX:**143–150.

Masihi, K. N., and Rohde-Schulz, B., 1990, Application of immunomodulators against infectious diseases, *Aerztl. Lab.* **36:**207–212.

Masihi, K. N., Brehmer, W., Lange, W., Werner, H., and Ribi, E., 1985, Trehalose dimycolate from various mycobacterial species induces differing anti-infectious activities in combination with muramyl dipeptide, *Infect. Immun.* **50:**938–940.

Masihi, K. N., Bhaduri, C. R., Werner, H., Janitschke, K., and Lange, W., 1986a, Effects of muramyl dipeptide and trehalose dimycolate on resistance of mice to Toxoplasma gondii and Acanthamoeba culbertsoni infections, *Int. Arch. Allergy Appl. Immunol.* **81:**112–117.

Masihi, K. N., Lange, W., Brehmer, W., and Ribi, E., 1986b, Immunobiological activities of nontoxic lipid A: Enhancement of nonspecific resistance in combination with trehalose dimycolate against viral infection and adjuvant effects, *Int. J. Immunopharmacol.* **8:**339–345

Masihi, K. N., Lange, W., Rohde-Schulz, B., and Masek, K., 1987, Antiviral activity of immunomodulator adamantylamide dipeptide, *Int. J. Immunother.* **III:**89.

Masihi, K. N., Lange, W., and Özel, M., 1988, Biomedical applications of chromatographic fraction containing trehalose dimycolate in squalane emulsion, *J. Chromatogr.* **440:**473–478.

Masihi, K. N., Kröger, H., Lange, W., and Chedid, L., 1989a, Muramyl peptides confer hepatoprotection against murine viral hepatitis, *Int. J. Immunopharmacol.* **11:**879–886.

Masihi, K. N., Lange, W., and Rohde-Schulz, B., 1989b, Stimulation of antiviral activity by immunomodulators, in: *Antiviral Drugs, Basic and Therapeutic Aspects* (R. Calio and G. Nistico, eds.), Pythagora Press, Rome, pp. 163–188.

Masihi, K. N., Lange, W., Schwenke, S., Gast, G., Huchshorn, P., Palache, A., and Masek, K., 1990a, Effect of immunomodulator adamantylamide dipeptide on antibody response to influenza subunit vaccines and protection against aerosol influenza infection, *Vaccine* **8:**159.

Masihi, K. N., Lange, W., Rohde-Schulz, B., and Chedid, L., 1990b, Muramyl dipeptide inhibits replication of human immunodeficiency virus in vitro, *AIDS Res. Hum. Retrovir.* **6:**393–399.

Masihi, K. N., Rohde-Schulz, B., Masek, K., and Palache, B., 1992, Antiviral and adjuvant activity of immunomodulator adamantylamide dipeptide, *Adv. Exp. Med. Biol.* **319:**275–286.

Masood, R., Lunardi-Iskander, Y., Moudgil, T., Zhang, Y., Law, R. E., Huang, C., Puri, R. K., Levine, A. M., and Gill, P. S., 1994, IL-10 inhibits HIV-1 replication and is induced by Tat, *Biochem. Biophys. Res. Commun.* **202:**374–383.

Mastroeni, P., Arena, A., Costa, G. B., Liberto, M. C., Bonina, L., and Hormaeche, C. E., 1991, Serum TNF-alpha in mouse typhoid and enhancement of a salmonella infection by anti-TNF-alpha antibodies, *Microb. Pathogen.* **11:**33–38.

Matsumoto, M., Matsubara, S., Matsuno, T., Tamura, M., Hattori, K., Nomura, H., Ono, M., and Yokota, T., 1987, Protective effect of human granulocyte colony-stimulating factor on microbial infection in neutropenic mice, *Infect. Immun.* **55:**2715–2720.

Matsuyama, T., Hamamoto, Y., Soma, G., Mizuno, D., Yamamoto, N., and Kobayashi, N., 1989, Cytocidal effect of tumor necrosis factor on cells chronically infected with human immunodeficiency virus (HIV): Enhancement of HIV replication, *J. Virol.* **63:**2504–2509.

Matsuyama, T., Kobayashi, N., and Yamamoto, N., 1991, Cytokines and HIV infection: Is AIDS a tumor necrosis factor disease? *AIDS* **5:**1405–1417.

Melder, R. J., Balachandran, R., Rinaldo, C. R., Gupta, P., Whiteside, T. L., and Herberman, R. B., 1990, Cytotoxic activity against HIV-infected monocytes by recombinant interleukin 2-activated natural killer cells, *AIDS Res. Hum. Retrovir.* **6:**1011–1015.

Melissen, P. M. B., van Vianen, W., Rijsbergen, Y., and Bakker-Woudenberg, I. A. J. M., 1992, Free versus liposome-encapsulated muramyl tripeptide phosphatidylethanolamide in treatment of experimental Klebsiella pneumoniae infection, *Infect. Immun.* **60:**95–101.

Melissen, P. M., van Vianen, W., and Bakker-Woudenberg, I. A., 1994, Treatment of Klebsiella pneumoniae septicemia in normal and leukopenic mice by liposome-encapsulated muramyl tripeptide phosphatidylethanolamide, *Antimicrob. Agents Chemother.* **38:**147–150.

Mellors, J. W., Griffith, B. P., Ortiz, M. A., Landry, M. L., and Ryan, J. L., 1991, Tumor necrosis factor-alpha/cachectin enhances human immunodeficiency virus type 1 replication in primary macrophages, *J. Infect. Dis.* **163:**78–82.

Mestan, J., Digl, W., Mittnacht, S., Hillen, H., Blohm, D., Möller, A., Jacobsen, H., and Kirchner, H., 1986, Antiviral effects of recombinant tumor necrosis factor, *Nature* **323:**816–819.

Mestan, J. M., Brockhaus, M., Kirchner, H., and Jacobsen, H., 1988, Antiviral activity of tumor necrosis factor. Synergism with interferons and induction of oligo-2′,5′-adenylate synthetase, *J. Gen. Virol.* **69:**3113–3120.

Michael, M. A., Cottam, H. B., Smee, D. F., Robins, R. K., and Kini, G. D., 1993, Alkylpurines as immunopotentiating agents. Synthesis and antiviral activity of certain alkylguanines, *J. Med. Chem.* **36:**3431–3436.

Moldawer L. L., 1993, Interleukin-1, TNF alpha and their naturally occuring antagonists in sepsis, *Blood Purification* **11:**128–133.

Moll, H., Binoeder, K., Bogdan, C., Solbach, W., and Röllinghoff, M., 1990, Production of tumor necrosis factor during murine cutaneous leishmaniasis, *Parasite Immunol.* **12:**483–494.

Mooney, D. P., Gameli, R. L., O'Reilly, M., and Herbert, J. C., 1988, Recombinant human granulocyte colony-stimulating factor and Pseudomonas burn wound sepsis, *Arch. Surg.* **123:**1353–1357.

Morrissey, P. J., and Charrier, K., 1990, GM-CSF administration augments the survival of ity-resistant A/J mice, but not ity-susceptible C57BL/6 mice, to a lethal challenge with Salmonella typhimurium, *J. Immunol.* **144:**557–561.

Morrissey, P. J., and Charrier, K., 1991, Interleukin-1 administration to C3H/HeJ mice after but not prior to infection increases resistance to Salmonella typhimurium, *Infect. Immun.* **59:**4729–4731.

Morrissey, P. J., Grabstein, K. H., Reed, S. G., and Conlon, P. J., 1989, Granulocyte/macrophage colony-stimulating factor: A potent activation signal for mature macrophages and monocytes, *Int. Arch. Allergy Appl. Immunol.* **88:**40–45.

Mueller, C., and Zielinski, C. C., 1990, Impaired lipopolysaccharide-inducible tumor necrosis factor production in vitro by peripheral blood monocytes of patients with viral hepatitis, *Hepatology* **12:**1118–1124.

Murphy, P. M., Lane, H. C., Gallin, J. I., and Fauci, A. S., 1988, Marked disparity in incidence of bacterial infections in patients with acquired immunodeficiency syndrome receiving interleukin-2 or interferon-gamma, *Ann. Intern. Med.* **108:**36–41.

Nain, M., Hinder, F., Gong, J. H., Schmidt, A., Bender, A., Sprenger, H., and Gemsa, D., 1990, Tumor necrosis factor production of influenza A virus-infected macrophages and potentiating effect of lipopolysaccharides, *J. Immunol.* **145:**1921–1928.

Nakane, A., Minagawa, T., and Kato, K., 1988a, Endogenous tumor necrosis factor (cachectin) is essential to host resistance against Listeria monocytogenes infection, *Infect. Immun.* **56:**2563–2569.

Nakane, A., Minagawa, T., Yasuda, I., Yu, C., and Kato, K., 1988b, Prevention by gamma interferon of fatal infection with Listeria monocytogenes infection, *Infect. Immun.* **56:**2011–2015.

Nakano, Y., Onozuka, K., Terada, Y., Shinomiya, H., and Nakano, M., 1990, Protective effect of recombinant tumor necrosis factor-alpha in murine salmonellosis, *J. Immunol.* **144:**1935–1941.

Nathan, C. F., Prendergast, T. J., Wiebe, M. E., Stanley, E. R., Platzer, E., and Remold, H. G., 1984, Activation of human macrophages: Comparison of other cytokines with interferon gamma, *J. Exp. Med.* **160:**600–605.

Natuk, R. J., Bukowski, J. F., Brubaker, J. O., and Welsh, R. M., 1989, Antiviral effect of lymphokine-activated killer cells: Chemotaxis and homing to sites of virus infection, *J. Virol.* **63:**4969–4971.

Neifer, S., Kremsner, P. G., and Bienzle, U., 1989, Application of anti-TNF to Plasmodium vinckei-infected mice is followed by an increase of parasitaemia, *Acta Trop.* **46:**273–275.

Nokta, M., Matzke, D., Jennings, M., Schlick, E., Nadler, P., and Pollard, R., 1991, In vivo administration of tumor necrosis factor alpha is associated with antiviral activity in human peripheral mononuclear cells, *Proc. Soc. Exp. Biol. Med.* **197**:144–148.

Nunberg, J. H., Doyle, M. V., York, S. M., and York, C. J., 1989, Interleukin 2 acts as an adjuvant to increase the potency of inactivated rabies virus vaccine, *Proc. Natl. Acad. Sci. USA* **86**:4240–4243.

Obaid, K. A., Ahmad, S., Khan, H. M., Mahdi, A. A., and Khanna, R., 1989, Protective effect of L. donovani antigens using glucan as an adjuvant, *Int. J. Immunopharmacol.* **11**:229–235.

Ozaki, Y., Ohashi, T., Minami, A., and Nakamura, S.-I., 1987, Enhanced resistance of mice to bacterial infection induced by recombinant human interleukin-1a, *Infect. Immun.* **55**:1436–1440.

Pal, R., Rizvi, S. Y., Kundu, B., Mathur, K. B., and Katiyar, J. C., 1991, Leishmania donovani in hamsters: Stimulation of nonspecific resistance by some novel glycopeptides and impact on therapeutic efficacy, *Experientia* **47**:486–490.

Parant, M., 1988, Effects of TNF in bacterial infections, *Ann. Inst. Pasteur Immunol.* **139**:301–304.

Parant, M. A., Parant, F. J., Le Contel, C., Lefrancier, P., and Chedid, L., 1992, MDP derivatives and resistance to bacterial infections in mice, *Adv. Exp. Med. Biol.* **319**:175–184.

Pecyk, R. A., Fraser-Smith, E. B., and Matthews, T. R., 1989, Efficacy of interleukin-1β against systemic Candida albicans infections in normal and immunosuppressed mice, *Infect. Immun.* **57**:3257–3258.

Penn, R. L., Nguyen, V. Q., Specian, R. D., Stevens, P., and Berg, R. D., 1991, Interleukin-2 enhances the translocation of Escherichia coli from the intestines to other organs, *J. Infect. Dis.* **164**:1168–1172.

Perno, C. F., Yarchoan, R., Cooney, D. A., Hartman, N. R., Webb, D. S., Hao, Z., Mitsuya, H., Johns, D. G., and Broder, S., 1989, Replication of HIV in monocytes: Granulocyte/macrophage colony-stimulating factor potentiates viral production yet enhances the antiviral effect mediated by AZT and other congeners of thymidine, *J. Exp. Med.* **169**:933–951.

Phillips, N. C., Tsoukas, C., and Chedid, L., 1990, Abrogation of azidothymidine-induced bone marrow toxicity by free and liposomal muramyl dipeptide, in: *Immunotherapeutic Prospects of Infectious Diseases* (K. N. Masihi and W. Lange, eds.), Springer-Verlag, Berlin, pp. 136–139.

Pohle, C., Rohde-Schulz, B., and Masihi, K. N., 1990, Effects of synthetic HIV peptides, cytokines and monophosphoryl lipid A on chemiluminescence response, in: *Immunotherapeutic Prospects of Infectious Diseases* (K. N. Masihi and W. Lange, eds.), Springer-Verlag, Berlin, pp. 144–149.

Popova, P., Guencheva, G., Davidkova, G., Bogdanov, A., Pacelli, E., Opalchenova, G., Kutzarova, T., and Koychev, C., 1993, Stimulating effect of DEODAN, an oral preparation from Lactobacillus bulgaricus ("LB51") on monocytes/macrophages and host resistance to experimental infections, *Int. J. Immunopharmacol.* **15**:25–37.

Porat, R., Clark, B. D., Wolff, S. M., and Dinarello, C. A., 1991, Enhancement of growth of virulent strains of Escherichia coli by interleukin-1, *Science* **254**:430–431.

Reddehase, M. J., Mutter, W., and Kozinowski, U. H., 1987, In vivo application of recombinant interleukin-2 in the immunotherapy of established cytomegalovirus, *J. Exp. Med.* **165**:650–656.

Reddy, P. G., Blecha, F., Minocha, H. C., Anderson, G. A., Morril, J. L., Fedorka-Cray, P. J., and Baker, P. E., 1989, Bovine recombinant interleukin-2 augments immunity and resistance to bovine herpesvirus infection, *Vet. Immunol. Immunopathol.* **23**:61–74.

Reddy, D. N., Reddy, P. G., Minocha, H. C., Fenwick, B. W., Baker, P. E., Davis, W. C., and Blecha, F., 1990, Adjuvanticity of recombinant bovine interleukin-1 beta: Influence on immunity, infection, and latency in a bovine herpesvirus-1 infection, *Lymphokine Res.* **9**:295–307.

Reed, S. G., Nathan, C. F., Pihl, D. L., Rodricks, P., Shanebeck, K., Conlon, P. J., and Grabstein, K. H., 1987, Recombinant granulocyte/macrophage colony-stimulating factor activates macrophages to inhibit Trypanosoma cruzi and release hydrogen peroxide: Comparison with interferon gamma, *J. Exp. Med.* **166**:1734–1746.

Rezai, H. R., Behbehani, A. B., Gettner, S., and Ardehali, S., 1988, Effect of levamisole on the course of experimental leishmaniasis in guinea-pigs and mice: Haematological and immunological findings, *Ann. Trop. Med. Parasitol.* **82**:243–249.

Richards, R. L., Hayre, M. D., Hockmeyer, W. T., and Alving, C. R., 1988, Liposomes, lipid A, and aluminium hydroxide enhance the immune response to a synthetic malaria sporozoite antigen, *Infect. Immun.* **56**:682–686.

Rickman, L. S., Gordon, D. M., Wistar, R., Krzych, U., Gross, M., Hollingdale, M. R., Egan, J. E., Chulay, J. D., and Hoffman, S. L., 1991, Use of adjuvant containing mycobacterial cell-wall skeleton, monophosphoryl lipid A, and squalane in malaria circumsporozoite protein vaccine, *Lancet* **337:**998–1001.

Rieckmann, P., Poli, G., Kehrl, J. H., and Fauci, A. S., 1991, Activated B lymphocytes from human immunodeficiency virus-infected individuals induce virus expression in infected T cells and a promonocytic cell line, U1, *J. Exp. Med.* **173:**1–5.

Rifaat, L. K., Mohammad, M. A., and Jawat, S. Z., 1989, Ivermectin, levamisole and thymic extract for chemotherapy and immunostimulation of visceral leishmaniasis in hamsters and mice, *Jpn. J. Med. Sci. Biol.* **42:**51–61.

Roffman, E., and Frenkel, N., 1990, Interleukin-2 inhibits the replication of human herpesvirus-6 in mature thymocytes, *Virology* **175:**591–594.

Rohde-Schulz, B., Masihi, K. N., and Lange, W., 1990, Reduced replication of human immunodeficiency virus in promonocytic cells by bacterial immunomodulators and anti-retroviral drugs at an early stage of HIV-infection, in: *Immunotherapeutic Prospects of Infectious Diseases* (K. N. Masihi and W. Lange, eds.), Springer-Verlag, Berlin, pp. 129–133.

Roll, J. T., Young, K. M., Kurtz, R. S., and Czuprynski, C. J., 1990, Human rTNF alpha augments anti-bacterial resistance in mice: Potentiation of its effects by recombinant human rIL-1 alpha, *Immunology* **69:**316–322.

Rossol-Voth, R., Rossol, S., Schett, K. H., Corridori, S., de Cian, W., and Falke, D., 1991, In vivo protective effect of tumor necrosis factor alpha against experimental infection with herpes simplex virus type 1, *J. Gen. Virol.* **72:**143–147.

Rouse, B. T., Miller, L. S., Turtinen, L., and Moore, R. N., 1985, Augmentation of immunity to herpes simplex virus by in vivo administration of interleukin-2, *J. Immunol.* **134:**926–930.

Ruggiero, V., Antonelli, G., Gentile, M., Conciatori, G., and Dianzani, F., 1989, Comparative study on the antiviral activity of tumor necrosis factor (TNF)-alpha, lymphotoxin/TNF-beta, and IL-1 in WISH cells, *Immunol. Lett.* **21:**165–170.

Sadick, M. D., Heinzel, F. P., Holaday, B. J., Pu, R. T., Dawkins, R. S., and Locksley, R. M., 1990, Cure of murine leishmaniasis with anti-interleukin 4 monoclonal antibody, *J. Exp. Med.* **171:**115–127.

Saiki, I., Saito, S., Fujita, C., Ishida, H., Iida, J., Murata, J., Hasegawa, A., and Azuma, I., 1988, Induction of tumoricidal macrophages and production of cytokines by synthetic muramyl dipeptide analogues, *Vaccine* **6:**238–244.

Saito, H., Tomioka, H., and Nagashima, K., 1987, Protective and therapeutic efficacy of Lactobacillus casei against experimental murine infections due to Mycobacterium fortuitum complex, *J. Gen. Microbiol.* **133:**2843–2851.

Sakagami, H., Aoki, T., Simpson, A., and Tanuma, S., 1991, Induction of immunopotentiation activity by a protein-bound polysaccharide, PSK [review], *Anticancer Res.* **11:**993–1000.

Sánchez, L., Peña, E., Civantos, A., Sada, G., Alvarez, M. M., Chirigos, M. A., and Villarrubia, V. G., 1995, AM3, an adjuvant to hepatitis B revaccination in non-responder healthy persons, *J. Hepatol.* **22:**119

Santoro, M. G., Favalli, C., Mastino, A., Jaffe, B. M., Esteban, M., and Garaci, E., 1988, Antiviral activity of a synthetic analog of prostaglandin A in mice infected with influenza A virus, *Arch. Virol.* **99:** 89–100.

Santoro, M. G., Amici, C., Elia, G., Benedetto, A., and Garaci, E., 1989, Inhibition of virus glycosylation as the mechanism of the antiviral action of prostaglandin A in Sendai virus-infected cells, *J. Gen. Virol.* **70:**789–800.

Saravolatz, L. D., Wherry, J. C., Spooner, C., Markowitz, N., Allred, R., and Remick, D., 1994, Clinical safety, tolerability, and pharmacokinetics of murine monoclonal antibody to human tumor necrosis factor-alpha, *J. Infect. Dis.* **169:**214–217.

Sato, Y., Maruyama, S., Kawai, C., and Matsumori, A., 1992, Effect of immunostimulant therapy on acute viral myocarditis in an animal model, *Am. Heart J.* **124:**428–434.

Sazotti, M., Coppenhaver, D. H., Singh, I. P., Poast, J., and Baron, S., 1989, The in vivo antiviral effect of CL246,738 is mediated by the independent induction of interferon-alpha and interferon beta, *J. Interferon Res.* **9:**265–274.

Schafer, R., Nacy, C. A., and Eisenstein, T. K., 1988, Induction of activated macrophages in C3H/HeJ mice by avirulent Salmonella, *J. Immunol.* **140:**1638–1644.

Schijns, V. E., Van der Neut, R., Haagmans, B. L., Bar, D. R., Schnellekens, H., and Horzinek, M. C., 1991, Tumour necrosis factor alpha, interferon-gamma and interferon-beta exert antiviral activity in nervous tissue cells, *J. Gen. Virol.* **72:**809–815.

Schlecht, S., Wiesmueller, K. H., Jung, G., and Bessler, W. G., 1989, Enhancement of protection against Salmonella infection in mice mediated by a synthetic lipopeptide analogue of bacterial lipoprotein in S. typhimurium vaccines, *Int. J. Med. Microbiol.* **1:**271.

Schofield, L., Villaquiran, J., Ferreira, A., Schellekens, H., Nussenzweig, R., and Nussenzweig, V., 1987, Gamma interferon, CD8+ T cells and antibodies required for immunity to malaria sporozoites, *Nature* **330:**664–666.

Schreck, R., Bevec, D., Dukor, P., Baeurle, L., Chedid, L., and Bahr, G.M., 1992, Selection of a muramyl peptide based on its lack of activation of nuclear factor-kB as a potential adjuvant for AIDS vaccines, *Clin. Exp. Immunol.* **90:**188–193.

Scott, P., Pearce, E., Natovitz, P., and Sher, A., 1987, Vaccination against cutaneous leishmaniasis in a murine model. I. Induction of protective immunity with a soluble extract of promastigotes, *J. Immunol.* **139:**221–227.

Sharma, L. K., Jagadish, S., and Mulbagal, A. N., 1990, Effects of haemorrhagic septicaemia vaccination and levamisole administration on the humoral response in cross-bred calves, *J. Vet. Pharmacol. Ther.* **13:**23–28.

Sharma, S. D., Hoffin, J. M., and Remington, J. S., 1985, In vivo recombinant interleukin-2 administration enhances survival against a lethal challenge with Toxoplasma gondii, *J. Immunol.* **135:**4160–4163.

Sheron, N., Lau, J. Y., Daniels, H. M., Webster, J., Eddleston, A. L., Alexander, G. J., and Williams, R., 1990, Tumour necrosis factor to treat chronic hepatitis B virus infection, *Lancet* **336:**321–322.

Shinomiya, N., Tsuru, S., Katsura, Y., Kayashima, S., and Nomoto, K., 1991, Enhanced resistance against Listeria monocytogenes achieved by pretreatment with granulocyte colony-stimulating factor, *Infect. Immun.* **59:**4740–4743.

Sibley, L. D., Adams, L. B., Fukutomi, Y., and Krahenbuhl, J. L., 1991, Tumor necrosis factor-alpha triggers antitoxoplasmal activity of IFN-gamma primed macrophages, *J. Immunol.* **147:**2340–2345.

Siddiqui, W. A., 1990, Role of adjuvants in malaria vaccines, in: *Immunotherapeutic Prospects of Infectious Diseases* (K. N. Masihi and W. Lange, eds.), Springer-Verlag, Berlin, pp. 325–335.

Sidwell, R. W., Huffman, J. H., Smee, D. F., Gilbert, J., Gessaman, A., Pease, A., Warren, R. P., Huggins, J., and Kende, M., 1992, Potential role of immunomodulators for treatment of phlebovirus infections of animals, *Ann. N.Y. Acad. Sci.* **653:**344–355.

Sidwell, R. W., Morrey, J. D., Okleberry, K. M., Burger, R. A., and Warren, R. P., 1993, Immunomodulator effects on the Friend virus infection in genetically defined mice, *Ann. N.Y. Acad. Sci.* **685:**432–446.

Sidwell, R. W., Smee, D. F., Huffman, J. H., Bailey, K. W., Warren, R. P., Burger, R. A., and Penney, C. L., 1995, Antiviral activity of an immunomodulatory lipophilic desmuramyl dipeptide analog, *Antiviral Res.* **26:**145–159.

Silva, J. S., Twrdzik, D. R., and Reed, S. G., 1991, Regulation of Trypanosoma cruzi infections in vitro and in vivo by transforming growth factor beta (TGF-beta), *J. Exp. Med.* **174:**539–545.

Smee, D. F., Alaghamandan, H. A., Cottam, H. B., Jolley, W. B., and Robins, R. K., 1990, Antiviral activity of the novel immune modulator 7-thia-8-oxoguanosine, *J. Biol. Response Modif.* **9:**24–32.

Smee, D. F., Alaghamandan, H. A., Gilbert, J., Burger, R. A., Jin, A., Sharma, B. S., Ramasamy, K., Revankar, G. R., and Cottam, H. B., 1991, Immunoenhancing properties and antiviral activity of 7-deazaguanosine in mice, *Antimicrob. Agents Chemother.* **35:**1.

Soike, K. F., Czarniecki, C. W., Baskin, G., Blanchard, J., and Liggitt, D., 1989, Enhancement of simian varicella virus infection in African green monkeys by recombinant human tumor necrosis factor alpha, *J. Infect. Dis.* **159:**331–335.

Sosa, S., Saha, A., Hadden, E. M., and Hadden, J., 1994, Immunological profile of methyl inosine monophosphate, in: *Immunotherapy of Infections* (K. N. Masihi, ed.), Dekker, New York, pp. 107–113.

Sredni, B., Rosenthal-Galili, Z., Michlin, H., Sobelman, D., Seger, Y., Blagerman, S., Kalechman, Y., and

Rager-Zisman, B., 1994, Restoration of murine cytomegalovirus (MCMV) induced myelosuppression by AS101, *Immunol. Lett.* **43**:159–165.

Starnes, H. F., Pearce, M. K., Tewari, A., Yim, J. H., Zou, J. C., and Abrams, J. S., 1990, Anti-IL-6 monoclonal antibodies protect against lethal Escherichia coli infection and lethal tumor necrosis factor-alpha challenge in mice, *J. Immunol.* **145**:4185–4191.

Stellato, T. A., Townsend, M. C., Gordon, N., Danziger, L. H., Galloway, P., Hawkins, N. L., and Fry, D. E., 1988, Effects of muramyl dipeptide and core body temperature on peritoneal bacterial clearance, *Arch. Surg.* **123**:465–469.

Strube, W., Kretzdorn, D., Grunmach, J., Bergle, R. D., and Thein, P., 1989, The effectiveness of the paramunity inducer Baypamun (PIND-ORF) for the prevention and metaphylaxis of an experimental infection with infectious bovine rhinotracheitis virus in cattle, *Tierarztliche Praxis.* **17**:267–272.

Subauste, C. S., and Remington, J. S., 1991, Role of gamma interferon in Toxoplasma gondii infection, *Eur. J. Clin. Microbiol. Infect. Dis.* **10**:58–67.

Sullivan, R., Fredette, J. P., Leavitt, J. L., Gadenne, A. S., Griffin, J. D., and Simons, E. R., 1989, Effects of recombinant human GM-CSF on transmembrane potentials in granulocytes: Relationship between enhancement of ligand-mediated depolarization and augmentation of superoxide anion production, *J. Cell. Physiol.* **139**:361–369.

Suzuki, K., Lee, W. J., Hashimoto, T., Tanaka, E., Murayama, T., Amitani, R., Yamamoto, K., and Kuze, F., 1994, Recombinant granulocyte-macrophage colony stimulating factor (GM-CSF) or tumor necrosis factor-alpha (TNF-alpha) activate human alveolar macrophages to inhibit growth of *Mycobacterium avium complex, Clin. Exp. Immunol.* **98**:169–173.

Suzuki, Y., Joh, K., and Kobayashi, A., 1991, Tumor necrosis factor-independent protective effect of recombinant IFN-gamma against acute toxoplasmosis in T cell-deficient mice, *J. Immunol.* **147**:2728–2733.

Sypek, J. P., Chung, C. L., Mayor, S. H. E., Subramanyam, J. M., Goldman, S. J., Sieburth, D. S., Wolf, S. F., and Schaub, R. G., 1993, Resolution of cutaneous leishmaniasis: Interleukin 12 initiates a protective T helper type immune response, *J. Exp. Med.* **177**:1797–1802.

Takeda, Y., Yoshikai, Y., Ohga, S., and Nomoto, K., 1990, Augmentation of host defense against bacterial infection pretreated intraperitoneally with an alpha-glucan RBS in mice, *Immunopharmacol. Immunotoxicol.* **12**:457–477.

Tamura, M., Yoo, Y. C., Yoshimatsu, K., Yoshida, R., Oka, T., Ohkuma, K., Arikawa, J., and Azuma, I., 1995, Effects of muramyl dipeptide derivatives as adjuvants on the induction of antibody response to recombinant hepatitis B surface antigen, *Vaccine* **13**:77–82.

Tanaka, M., Hori, Y., Sakai, F., Ueda, H., Goto, T., Okuhara, M., Tsuda, Y., and Okada, Y., 1993, WS1279, a novel lipopeptide isolated from Streptomyces willmorei. Biological activities, *J. Antibiot.* **46**:1699–1706.

Taverne, J., Tavernier, J., Fiers, W., and Playfair, J. H., 1987, Rccombinant tumour necrosis factor inhibits malaria parasite in vivo but not in vitro, *Clin. Exp. Immunol.* **67**:1–4.

Ten Hagen, T. L. M., Van Vianen, W., and Bakker-Woudenberg, I. A. J. M., 1995, Modulation of nonspecific antimicrobial resistance of mice to *Klebsiella pneumoniae* septicemia by liposome-encapsulated muramyl tripeptide phosphatidylethanolamine and interferon-gamma alone or combined, *J. Infect. Dis.* **171**:385–392.

Thorel, T., Joseph, M., Capron, A., Vorng, H., and Pascal, M., 1988, In vitro and in vivo immunomodulation by LF 1695 of human and rat macrophages and platelets in schistosomiasis, *Int. J. Immunopharmacol.* **10**:739–746.

Titus, R. G., Sherry, B., and Cerami, A., 1989, Tumor necrosis factor plays a protective role in experimental cutaneous leishmaniasis, *J. Exp. Med.* **170**:2097–2105.

Todd, B., Pope, J. H., and Georghiou, P., 1991, Interleukin-2 enhances production in 24 hours of infectious human immunodeficiency virus type 1 in vitro by naturally infected mononuclear cells from seropositive donors, *Arch. Virol.* **121**:227–232.

Tomioka, H., Sato, K., and Saito, H., 1990, Effect of ofloxacin combined with Lactobacillus casei against Mycobacterium fortuitum infection induced in mice, *Antimicrob. Agents Chemother.* **34**:632–636.

Tripp, C. S., Wolf, S. F., and Unanue, E. R., 1993, Interleukin 12 and tumor necrosis factor alpha are costimulators of interferon-gamma production by natural killer cells in severe combined immunodeficiency mice with listeriosis, and interleukin 10 is a physiologic antagonist, *Proc. Natl. Acad. Sci. USA* **90**:3725–3729.

Trizio, D., Isetta, A. M., Doria, G. F., Fornasiero, M. C., Ferrari, M., Ferreccio, R., Carminati, P., and Roncucci, R., 1990, Immunopharmacology of a class of synthetics with therapeutic potential in infections and other types of diseases, in: *Immunotherapeutic Prospects of Infectious Diseases* (K. N. Masihi and W. Lange, eds.), Springer-Verlag, Berlin, pp. 3–8.

Turnek, J., Toman, M., Novak, J., Krchnak, V., and Horavova, P., 1994, Adjuvant effect of liposomes and adamantylamide dipeptide on antigenicity of entrapped synthetic peptide derived from HIV-1 transmembrane region glycoprotein gp41, *Immunol. Lett.* **39**:157–161.

Tursz, T., Morin, A., Deschamps de Paillette, E., and Johnson, A. G., 1990, Poly A-Poly U: An updated review, in: *Immunotherapeutic Prospects of Infectious Diseases* (K. N. Masihi and W. Lange, eds.), Springer-Verlag, Berlin, pp. 263–272.

Uchiya, K., and Sugihara, H., 1989, Enhancing effect of Salmonella enteritidis SPA on nonspecific resistance, *Kansenshogaku Zasshi* **63**:463–470.

Uehling, D. T., Hopkins, W. J., and Balish, E., 1990, Decreased immunologic responsiveness following intensified vaginal immunization against urinary tract infection, *J. Urol.* **143**:143–145.

Ungar, B. L., Kao, T. C., Burris, J. A., and Finkelman, F. D., 1991, Cryptosporidium infection in an adult mouse model. Independent roles for IFN-gamma and CD4+ T lymphocytes in protective immunity, *J. Immunol.* **147**:1014–1022.

Urban, J. F., Madden, K. B., Svetic, A., Cheever, A., Trotta, P. P., Gause, W. C., Katona, I. M., and Finkelman, F. D., 1992, The importance of Th2 cytokines in protective immunity to nematodes, *Immunol. Rev.* **127**:205–220.

Van der Meer, J. W. M., Barza, M., Wolff, S. M., and Dinarello, C. A., 1988, A low dose of recombinant interleukin 1 protects granulocytopenic mice from lethal gram-negative infection, *Proc. Natl. Acad. Sci. USA* **85**:1620–1623.

Van der Meer, J. W., Helle, M., and Aarden, L., 1989, Comparison of the effects of recombinant interleukin 6 and recombinant interleukin 1 on nonspecific resistance to infection, *Eur. J. Immunol.* **19**:413–416.

van der Poll, T., Janse, J., van Leenen, D., von der Moehlen, M., Levi, M., and ten Cate, H., 1993, Release of soluble receptors for tumor necrosis factor in clinical sepsis and experimental endotoxemia, *J. Infect. Dis.* **168**:955–960.

Vanham, G. L., Kestens, L., van Hoof, J., Penne, G., Colebunders, R., Goilav, C., Vandenbruaene, M., Habib, R. E., and Gigase, P., 1993, Immunological parameters during treatment with ditiocarb (Imuthiol), *AIDS* **7**:525–530.

Verini, M. A., and Ungheri, D., 1989, Activity of FCE 20696, a new synthetic immunomodulator, in models of viral and bacterial pathology, *Immunopharmacology* **17**:157–165.

Villarrubia, V. G., Valladolid, J. M., Elorza, F. L., Sada, G., Vilchez, J. G., Jimenez, M., and Herrerias, J. M., 1992, Therapeutic response of chronic active hepatitis B (CAHB) to a new immunomodulator: AM3. Immunohematological effects, *Immunopharmacol. Immunotoxicol.* **14**:141–164.

Vogels, M. T. E., Mensink, E. J. B. M., Ye, K., Boerman, O. C., Verschueren, C. M. M., Dinarello, C. A., and Van der Meer, J. W. M., 1994, Differential gene expression for IL-1 receptor antagonist, IL-1, and TNF receptors and IL-1 and TNF synthesis may explain IL-1-induced resistance to infection, *J. Immunol.* **153**:5772–5781.

Vyakarnam, A., McKeating, J., Meager, A., and Beverley, P., 1990, Tumor necrosis factors (alpha, beta) induced by HIV-1 in peripheral blood mononuclear cells potentiate virus replication, *AIDS* **4**:21–27.

Wang, M., Friedman, H., and Djeu, J. Y., 1989, Enhancement of human monocyte function against Candida albicans by colony-stimulating factors (CSF): IL-3, granulocyte-macrophage-CSF, and macrophage-CSF, *J. Immunol.* **143**:671–677.

Weinberg, A., and Merigan, T. C., 1988, Recombinant interleukin 2 as an adjuvant for vaccine-induced protection. Immunization of guinea pigs with herpes simplex virus subunit vaccines, *J. Immunol.* **140**:294–299.

Weiser, W. Y., Van Niel, A., Clark, S. C., David, J. R., and Remold, H. G., 1987, Recombinant human granulocyte/macrophage colony-stimulating factor activates intracellular killing of Leishmania donovani by human monocyte-derived macrophages, *J. Exp. Med.* **166**:1436–1446.

Williams, D. M., Byrne, G. I., Grubbs, B., Marshal, T. J., and Schachter, J., 1988, Role in vivo for gamma interferon in control of pneumonia caused by Chlamydia trachomatis, *Infect. Immun.* **56**:3004–3006.

Williams, D. L., Yaeger, R. G., Pretus, H. A., Browder, I. W., McNamee, R. B., and Jones, E. L., 1989, Immunization against Trypanosoma cruzi, adjuvant effect of glucan, *Int. J. Immunopharmacol.* **11**:403–410.

Wong, G. H. W., and Goeddel, D. V., 1986, Tumor necrosis factors α and β inhibit virus replication and synergize with interferons, *Nature* **323**:819–822.

Wong, G., Krowka, J., and Stites, D. P., 1988, In vitro anti human immunodeficiency virus activities of tumor necrosis factor alpha and interferon gamma, *J. Immunol.* **140**:120–124.

Wyde, P. R., Six, H. R., Ambrose, M. W., and Throop, B. J., 1990, Muramyl dipeptides and polyinosinic-polycytidylic acid given to mice prior to influenza virus challenge reduces pulmonary disease and mortality, *J. Biol. Response Modif.* **9**:98–102.

Yamamoto, N., Fukushima, M., Tsurumi, T., Maeno, K., and Nishiyama, Y., 1987, Mechanism of inhibition of herpes simplex virus replication by prostaglandin A1 and prostaglandin J2, *Biochem. Biophys. Res. Commun.* **146**:1425–1431.

Yoshida, O., Nakashima, H., Yoshida, T., Kaneko, Y., Yamamoto, I., Matsuzaki, K., Uryu, T., and Yamamoto, N., 1989, Sulfation strategy for antivirals to human immunodeficiency virus (HIV), *Biochem. Pharmacol.* **37**:2887–2891.

Yoshida, R., Sato, K., Yoo, Y. C., Yoshimatsu, K., Tamura, M., Ishihara, C., Arikawa, J., and Azuma, I., 1994, Effect of the synthetic lipid A-related compound, DT-5461, on resistance to Sendai virus infection in mice, *Immunopharmacology* **28**:153–161.

Zhan, Y. F., Stanley, E. R., and Cheers, C., 1991, Prophylaxis or treatment of experimental brucellosis with interleukin-1, *Infect. Immun.* **59**:1790–1794.

PART IV

ALLERGY IMMUNOPHARMACOLOGY

CHAPTER 7

BASOPHILS AND MAST CELLS
Basic Biology and Clinical Significance

JOHN J. COSTA and STEPHEN J. GALLI

1. INTRODUCTION

Basophils and mast cells are thought to represent critical effector cells in IgE-dependent host responses to parasites and allergic diseases, and may also have important functions in a variety of other immunological, pathological, and perhaps physiological processes. Ehrlich identified mast cells in human connective tissues on the basis of the metachromatic staining properties of their prominent cytoplasmic granules (Ehrlich, 1878). Metachromasia refers to the change in color of some basic dyes that occurs when they bind to certain highly charged molecules, including some of the constituents of mast cell cytoplasmic granules. Ehrlich also described the basophil, a circulating leukocyte that contains cytoplasmic granules with staining properties similar to those of the mast cell (Ehrlich, 1879). Mast cells and basophils share several notable features besides staining properties (summarized in Table I). Both cell types are derived from bonc marrow progenitor cells and both mast cells and basophils represent a major source of histamine and other potent chemical mediators which have been implicated in a wide variety of inflammatory and immunologic processes, including allergic disorders with components of immediate hypersensitivity (reviewed in Galli and Lichtenstein, 1988; Holgate *et al.*, 1993; Metcalfe *et al.*,

---

JOHN J. COSTA • Departments of Pathology and Medicine, Beth Israel Hospital and Harvard Medical School, and Division of Experimental Pathology, Beth Israel Hospital, Boston, Massachusetts 02215. STEPHEN J. GALLI • Department of Pathology, Beth Israel Hospital and Harvard Medical School, and Division of Experimental Pathology, Beth Israel Hospital, Boston, Massachusetts 02215.

Immunopharmacology Reviews, Volume 2, edited by John W. Hadden and Andor Szentivanyi. Plenum Press, New York, 1996.

TABLE I
Natural History, Major Mediators, and Surface Membrane Structures of Human Mast Cells and Basophils[a]

Characteristic	Basophils	Mast cells
Natural history		
Origin of precursor cells	Bone marrow	Bone marrow
Site of maturation	Bone marrow	Connective tissues (a few in the bone marrow)
Mature cells in the circulation	Yes (usually <1% of blood leukocytes)	No
Mature cells recruited into tissues from circulation	Yes (during immunologic, inflammatory responses)	No
Mature cells normally residing in connective tissues	No (not detectable by microscopy)	Yes
Proliferative ability of morphologically mature cells	None reported	Yes (under certain circumstances)
Life span	Days (like other granulocytes)	Weeks to months (based on studies in rodents)
Mediators		
Major mediators stored preformed in cytoplasmic granules	Histamine, chrondroitin sulfates, neutral protease with bradykinin-generating activity, β-glucuronidase, elastase, cathepsin G-like enzyme, major basic protein, Charcot–Leyden crystal protein	Histamine, heparin and/or chrondroitin sulfates, neutral proteases (chymase and/or tryptase), many acid hydrolases, cathepsin G, carboxypeptidase
Major lipid mediators produced on appropriate activation	Leukotriene C_4 (LTC_4)	Prostaglandin D_2, LTC_4, platelet-activating factor
Cytokines released on appropriate activation	IL-4	Tumor necrosis factor-α (mouse mast cells produce many more; see text)
Surface structures		
Ig receptor	$Fc_{\epsilon}RI$, $Fc_{\gamma}RII$(CDw32)	$Fc_{\epsilon}RI$
Cytokine/growth factor receptors for:	IL-2(CD25), IL-3, IL-4, IL-5, IL-8, stem cell factor (SCF) (some basophils express low numbers of c-kit receptors)	SCF (c-*kit* receptor)
Cell adhesion structures	LFA-1[b] α chain (CD11a), C43bi receptor (CD11b), gp150/95 (CD11c), LFA-1β chain (CD18), ICAM-1 (CD54), and CD44	ICAM-1[c] (CD54), CD44

[a]Reproduced with permission from Galli, S.J., 1993, *N. Engl. J. Med.* **328**:257.
[b]LFA, lymphocyte function-associated antigen.
[c]ICAM, intercellular adhesion molecule.

1981; Schwartz and Huff, 1993; Galli, 1990, 1993). And in all mammalian species yet analyzed, both mast cells and basophils express plasma membrane receptors ($Fc_εRI$) that specifically bind, with high affinity, the Fc portion of IgE antibody (Beaven and Metzger,, 1993; Kinet, 1990; Ishizaka, 1988; Benhamou and Siraganian, 1992).

Because of their many similarities, it once was believed that basophils might represent the circulating precursor of mast cells, or that mast cells were "tissue basophils." However, current evidence greatly favors the view that mature basophils represent terminally differentiated granulocytes, and not circulating mast cell precursors. The latter position is supported by the following observations: (1) no actual evidence has been presented, in any species, indicating that mature circulating basophils are capable either of mitosis or of differentiation into mast cells; (2) the rare reports of patients with hereditary or acquired abnormalities affecting basophil numbers or morphology indicate that eosinophils may also be affected in these disorders but not mast cells (Juhlin and Michaelsson, 1977; Tracey and Smith, 1978; Mitchell *et al.*, 1983); (3) morphologically identifiable human tissue mast cells can exhibit mitotic activity (Dvorak *et al.*, 1976), indicating that this cell lineage is capable of replication independent of a stage resembling that of circulating basophils; and (4) human basophils are not enriched for cells that represent precursors of mast cells (Agis *et al.*, 1993). Thus, basophils are circulating granulocytes that can infiltrate tissues or appear in exudates during a variety of inflammatory or immunologic processes. By contrast, morphologically identifiable mast cells do not normally circulate, but reside in virtually all normal vascularized tissues.

Moreover, it is now appreciated that mature basophils and mast cells differ in many aspects of morphology, natural history, tissue distribution, mediator production, cell surface phenotype, growth factor requirements, and response to drugs (Table I). Nevertheless, mast cells and basophils share important functional characteristics. After sensitization with IgE, exposure to specific multivalent antigen triggers both cell types to undergo an integrated, noncytolytic series of biochemical (Beaven and Metzger, 1993; Kinet, 1990; Ishizaka, 1988; Benhamou and Siraganian, 1992) and ultrastructural (Dvorak *et al.*, 1983a; Galli *et al.*, 1984; Dvorak, 1991; Selye, 1965) alterations, often referred to as *anaphylactic degranulation* or *exocytosis*, that results in the exposure of the matrices of the cytoplasmic granules to the external medium. These events are associated with the release of the preformed mediators which are stored in the cytoplasmic granules (such as histamine, heparin or other sulfated proteoglycans, and certain proteases), the *de novo* synthesis and release of such lipid mediators as prostaglandin D_2 and/or leukotriene C_4, and the release of multifunctional cytokines. A similar sequence of events may be initiated by antibodies to IgE or to the $Fc_εRI$ itself. On the other hand, mast cells and basophils differ in their responsiveness to other potential activators of secretion, and also in the specific pattern of mediators that are released by the activated cells.

In this chapter, we will summarize current understanding of the basic biology of mast cells and basophils, review the cells' patterns of activation and mediator production, and discuss the potential contributions of these cells to health and disease.

2. DEVELOPMENT AND DISTRIBUTION

2.1. Mast Cells

2.1.1. Distribution and Heterogeneity

Mast cells are ordinarily distributed throughout normal connective tissues, where they are often situated adjacent to blood and lymphatic vessels, near or within nerves, and beneath epithelial surfaces, such as those of the respiratory and gastrointestinal systems and the skin, that are exposed to the external environment (Metcalfe *et al.*, 1981; Schwartz and Huff, 1993; Galli, 1990, 1993; Galli *et al.*, 1984; Dvorak, 1991; Selye, 1965). In some species, mast cells are also abundant in the fibrous capsules of internal organs and in physiologic transudates, such as peritoneal fluid. Mast cells are also a normal, if numerically minor, component of the bone marrow and lymphoid tissues. However, unlike mature basophils, mature mast cells do not circulate in the blood.

In humans and many other mammalian species, mast cell numbers in normal tissues exhibit considerable variation according to anatomical sites (Schwartz and Huff, 1993; Galli, 1990). However, mast cell distribution can change during perturbations of homeostasis. For example, mast cells can appear within the respiratory or gastrointestinal epithelium, and in secretions at these sites, in association with certain inflammatory or immunologic reactions (Enerbäck *et al.*, 1989). The numbers of mast cells at sites of chronic inflammation due to a variety of different causes can often be many times higher than in the corresponding normal tissues (Metcalfe *et al.*, 1981; Dvorak, 1991; Selye, 1965; Enerbäck *et al.*, 1989; Bienenstock *et al.*, 1989). In most cases, the extent to which such changes in mast cell number reflect proliferation of resident mast cell populations, as opposed to the recruitment and differentiation of mast cell precursors, remains to be determined.

Human basophils and mast cells exhibit several differences in morphology. Indeed, morphologic distinctions between mature basophils and mast cells have been appreciated in all mammalian species that have been carefully studied (Dvorak, 1991; Dvorak *et al.*, 1983b). Although typical human basophils and mast cells can be discriminated from each other in appropriately fixed and processed light microscopic sections, the differences between these two cell types are particularly evident by transmission electron microscopy. The ultrastructural features of human basophils and mast cells are summarized in Table II. Figure 1 is an electron micrograph showing a human basophil adjacent to a human mast cell in the same tissue.

The concept of mast cell heterogeneity is based on evidence derived from studies in humans and experimental animals indicating that mast cells can vary in multiple aspects of phenotype, including morphology, histochemistry, mediator content, and response to drugs and stimuli of activation (Schwartz and Huff, 1993; Galli, 1990; Maximow, 1905; Enerbäck, 1986; Kitamura, 1989; Miller *et al.*, 1989; Bienenstock *et al.*, 1986). These findings raise the possibility that mast cells of different phenotype might have different roles in health and disease and might respond differently to drugs

TABLE II
Morphologic Features of Mature Basophils and Mast Cells in Humans[a]

Characteristic	Basophils	Mast cells
Size	5–7 μm	6–12 μm
Surface	Irregular, short, thick processes	Numerous, rather uniformly distributed, elongated thin processes
Nucleus	Segmented	Nonsegmented (usually round to oval in electron micrographs)
Nuclear chromatin condensation	Marked	Moderate
Cytoplasmic granules	Fewer and larger than in mast cells; contain predominantly electron-dense particulate material with occasional membranous whorls	Smaller, more numerous, and generally more variable in appearance than in basophils; contain scroll-like structures, particles, or crystals, alone or in combination
Aggregates of cytoplasmic glycogen	Present	Absent
Cytoplasmic lipid bodies	Rare	Common (but not present in all cells)
Granule–granule fusion during "anaphylactic" degranulation	Rare (granule membranes usually fuse individually with plasma membrane)	Common

[a]Reproduced with permission from Galli, S.J., and Lichtenstein, L.M., In: *Allergy: Principles and Practice*, 3rd ed. (E. Middleton, Jr., C.E. Reed, E.F. Ellis, J.F. Adkinson, Jr., and J.W. Yunginger, eds.), Mosby, St. Louis, p. 106.

used in clinical settings. Cells within a given population can be said to exhibit heterogeneity once a certain minimal (but generally undefined) level of variation in one or more of their characteristics has been demonstrated. Thus, this is a purely descriptive term. For example, a particular cell type can be said to exhibit heterogeneity with respect to size, ultrastructural appearance, mediator content, and/or other characteristics taken alone or in combination.

The distinction between rodent connective tissue-type mast cell (CTMCs) and mucosal-type mast cell (MMCs) subsets is the classic example of mast cell heterogeneity. As pointed out by Enerbäck (Enerbäck, 1986) and others, these terms are least confusing when used to refer to the mature mast cell phenotype typical of a particular anatomical site, e.g., the rat or mouse small intestinal mucosa (for MMCs); the rat or mouse peritoneal cavity or skin (for "serosal" or CTMCs). Nevertheless, one occasionally finds the term "MMCs" used to refer to populations of mast cells that share characteristics of true MMCs, but that are derived from nonmucosal sites (e.g., certain growth factor-dependent mast cells generated *in vitro*, discussed below). Populations of rat or mouse MMCs expand remarkably during T-cell-dependent immune responses to certain intestinal parasites (Galli, 1990; Enerbäck, 1986; Kitamura, 1989; Miller *et al.*, 1989; Bienenstock *et al.*, 1986). By contrast, CTMCs exhibit little or no "T cell dependence," and occur in athymic nude mice or rats in numbers similar to

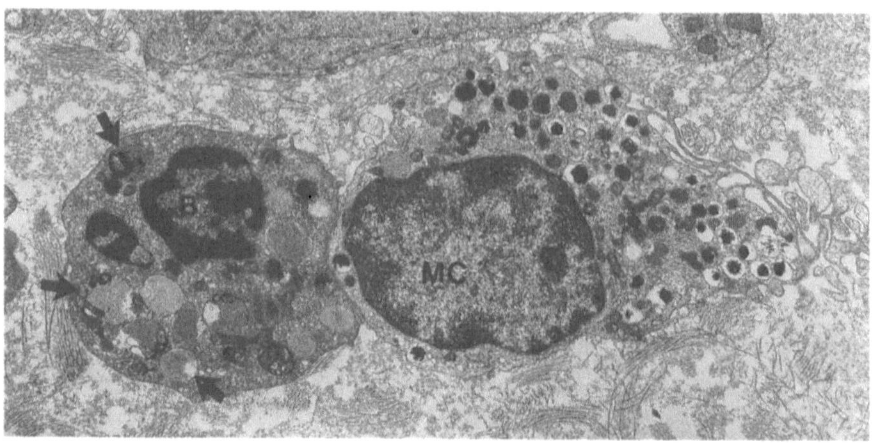

FIGURE 1. A basophil (*B*) adjacent to a mst cell (*MC*) in the ileal submucosa of a patient with Crohn's disease. The basophil exhibits a bilobed nucleus, whose chromatin is strikingly condensed beneath the nuclear membrane. The basophil surface is relatively smooth with a few blunt processes. The mast cell nucleus is larger and its chromatin less condensed than that of the basophil. The mast cell's granules are smaller, more numerous, and more variable in shape and content that those of the basophil (arrows). The mast cell surface has numerous elongated, thin folds. (Original magnification, ×9000.) (Reproduced with permission from Dvorak, A. M., Monahan, R. A., Osage, J. E., and Dickersin, G. R., 1980, *Hum. Pathol.* **11**:606.)

those present in normal animals (Galli, 1990; Enerbäck, 1986; Kitamura, 1989; Miller *et al.*, 1989; Bienenstock *et al.*, 1986).

The initial appreciation that rodent mast cells were not homogeneous was based on histochemical differences. It was later shown that rat CTMCs and MMCs also could be distinguished on the basis of their predominant cytoplasmic granule-associated chymotryptic protease (Lagunoff and Benditt, 1963; Woodbury *et al.*, 1978; Woodbury and Neurath, 1980), termed rat mast cell protease I (RMCP I) and RMCP II, respectively. In the mouse, a similar heterogeneity of mucosal and connective tissue-type mast cells has been observed (Miller *et al.*, 1989; Reynolds *et al.*, 1990). However, different populations of mouse mast cells exhibit even more variation in cytoplasmic granule-associated protease content than do rat mast cells (Reynolds *et al.*, 1990).

Human mast cells also exhibit variation in phenotype. Human pulmonary mast cells vary in cytoplasmic granule ultrastructure, size, and response to stimuli of degranulation, and human intestinal mast cells exhibit variation in histochemistry (e.g., in the sensitivity of their staining to formalin fixation) (Schwartz and Huff, 1993; Dvorak, 1991; Bienenstock *et al.*, 1986). It should be noted, however, that the separation of mast cell populations into distinct mucosal and connective tissue subclasses is not as clear in humans as it is in mice and rats. For example, most anatomical sites in humans contain some mast cells (MC_T) that express immunoreactivity for tryptase (localized to scroll-containing cytoplasmic granules), but no detectable chymase (<0.04 pg/cell), and other mast cells (MC_{TC}) that contain immunoreactivity for both tryptase and chymase (localized to crystal-containing cytoplasmic granules) (Schwartz and Huff, 1993; Irani *et al.*, 1986). It is not yet clear whether MC_T entirely lack chymase or have small amounts that are undetectable with current techniques. However, it is possible to classify human mast cells in multiple anatomical sites on the basis of their predominant protease content as MC_T or MC_{TC} (Schwartz and Huff, 1993; Irani *et al.*, 1986). Thus, MC_T predominate in lung and small intestinal mucosa and MC_{TC} predominate in skin and small intestinal submucosa (Schwartz and Huff, 1993; Irani *et al.*, 1986).

Numbers of intestinal mucosal and submucosal MC_T, but not MC_{TC}, are reduced in patients with either congenital combined immunodeficiency disease or the acquired immunodeficiency syndrome, consistent with a T cell-dependent requirement for generation and/or maintenance of normal populations of MC_T (Irani *et al.*, 1987). In this respect, MC_T seem similar to rat or mouse MMC, and MC_{TC} resemble murine CTMC. However, other properties of MC_T or MC_{TC} are not predictable based on the properties of rat MMCs and CTMCs. For example, in the rat, $RMCPI^+$ CTMC are much more sensitive than RMCP II^+ MMC to stimulation with basic compounds such as substance P and in their susceptibility to inhibition by disodium chromoglycate (DSCG; reviewed in Bienenstock *et al.*, 1989; Pearce, 1986). By contrast, Church *et al.* (1989) reported that partially purified preparations of human skin mast cells (>85% MC_{TC}) were very sensitive to stimulation by substance P and other basic secretagogues, but not to inhibition by DSCG, whereas mast cells isolated from lung (<10% MC_{TC}) and from colon mucosa or muscle (60% MC_{TC}) were insensitive to substance P stimulation but sensitive to inhibition of histamine release by DSCG.

As discussed in detail elsewhere (Galli, 1990), mast cell phenotypic variation theoretically might reflect the following mechanisms, acting alone or in combination: (1) the existence of distinct mast cell lineages, (2) the process of cellular maturation/differentiation, (3) the functional status of the cell, and (4) the influence of microenvironmental factors. While it is not yet certain whether distinct mast cell lineages occur in humans or, for that matter, in any other species, it is clear that each of the other three potential mechanisms can account for some examples of mast cell heterogeneity. Moreover, many examples of mast cell heterogeneity probably reflect the operation of complex regulatory mechanisms, particularly the effect of cytokine and other microenvironmental factors which can influence mast cell proliferation, maturation/differentiation, and/or function (Galli, 1990, 1993; Kitamura, 1989).

2.1.2. Mast Cell Development in Mice and Rats

Culture of normal mouse hematopoietic cells in media containing IL-3 yields an essentially homogeneous population of growth factor-dependent immature mast cells (Galli, 1990; Reynolds *et al.*, 1990). When they have been derived from mouse bone marrow cells, such mast cells will be designated herein as IL-3-derived, bone marrow-derived cultured mast cells (IL-3-derived BMCMCs). Table III compares some of the phenotypic characteristics of IL-3-derived BMCMCs with those of mouse CTMCs and MMCs.

While IL-3-derived BMCMCs shared some phenotype characteristics with mouse MMCs, both *in vivo* and *in vitro* studies indicate that, in appropriate circumstances, these cells can acquire phenotype features that are more similar to those of CTMCs. The first demonstration of this point was achieved using genetically mast cell-deficient mice. Mutations at *W*, the dominant white-spotting locus on mouse chromosome 5, or *Sl*, the steel locus on mouse chromosome 10, affect several important developmental programs, including gametogenesis, pigmentation, hematopoiesis, and mast cell development. Thus, many *W* or *Sl* mutations render the homozygous mutant animals sterile, devoid of coat pigmentation, anemic, and profoundly mast cell deficient (Kitamura, 1989; Galli and Kitamura, 1987; Kitamura *et al.*, 1989; Galli *et al.*, 1994).

TABLE III
Phenotypic Characteristics of Mast Cell Populations in the Mouse

Characteristic	Connective tissue or serosal (peritoneal) mast cells	Mucosal mast cells	Growth factor-dependent, bone marrow-derived cultured mast cells (BMCMCs)[a]
Cytoplasmic granule ultrastructure	Uniformly electron-dense	Variably electron-dense	Variably electron-dense
T cell dependence	No	Yes	Yes
Major granule-associated proteoglycan	Heparin	Chondroitin sulfates	Chondroitin sulfates
Staining with the heparin-binding dye, berberine sulfate	Yes	No	No
Staining with alcian blue	Yes	Yes	Yes
Staining with safranin	Yes	No	No
Histamine content	High	Low (by histochemistry)	Low
Serotinin content	Variable	Low (by histochemistry)	High
Surface expression of globopentaosylceramide	High	Not determined	Low
High-affinity surface receptors for IgE	Yes	Yes	Yes
Sensitivity to stimulation with compound 48/80	High	Low	Low

[a]The characteristics listed are those for BMCMCs that have been generated in IL-3-containing medium. The phenotypic characteristics of these cells can become more like those of CTMCs when they are maintained in the presence of mouse 3T3 fibroblasts or soluble rrSCF *in vitro*, or after they have been transferred to certain tissues of W/W^v mast cell-deficient mice *in vivo* (see text).

The *W* or *Sl* mutant mice most commonly used in studies of mast cell development and function are WBB6F$_1$-*W/W*^{v} (*W/W*^{v}) or WCB6F$_1$-*Sl/Sl*^{d} (*Sl/Sl*^{d}) mice (reviewed in Galli, 1990; Kitamura, 1989; Galli and Kitamura, 1987; Kitamura *et al.*, 1989; Galli *et al.*, 1994). *W/W*^{v} and *Sl/Sl*^{d} mice are virtually devoid of mature, morphologically identifiable mast cells in all organs and anatomical sites examined (reviewed in Galli, 1990; Kitamura, 1989; Galli and Kitamura, 1987; Kitamura *et al.*, 1989; Galli *et al.*, 1994). However, transplantation of congenic +/+ bone marrow cells can repair the anemia and the mast cell deficiency of *W/W*^{v} mice (Kitamura *et al.*, 1978). By contrast, the anemia and the mast cell deficiency of *Sl/Sl*^{d} mice are refractory to bone marrow transplantation from the congenic +/+ mice. Moreover, transplantation of bone marrow cells from *Sl/Sl*^{d} mice can repair the mast cell deficiency of *W/W*^{v} animals (Kitamura and Go, 1979). Thus, the mast cell deficiency of *W/W*^{v} mice reflects a defect intrinsic to cells in the mast cell lineage, whereas the mast cell deficiency of the *Sl/Sl*^{d} mouse reflects a problem in the microenvironments necessary for normal mast cell development.

Since the *W/W*^{v} mouse provides an environment suitable for the development, from pluripotent bone marrow-derived precursors, of both CTMCs and MMCs (Galli, 1990; Kitamura, 1989; Galli and Kitamura, 1987; Kitamura *et al.*, 1989; Galli *et al.*, 1994), this experimental system was used to determine whether IL-3-derived BMCMCs could give rise to CTMCs and MMCs *in vivo*. Analysis of the phenotype of the mast cells that developed in *W/W*^{v} mice after systemic or local injection of IL-3-derived BMCMCs expanded *in vitro* showed that these BMCMCs gave rise to at least two phenotypically distinct populations of mast cells in the *W/W*^{v} recipients (Nakano *et al.*, 1985; Otsu *et al.*, 1987). In anatomic sites that in +/+ mice ordinarily contain berberine sulfate-positive (heparin-rich) mast cells (dermis, peritoneal cavity, muscularis propria of the stomach), the adoptively transferred mast cells were berberine sulfate-positive and expressed other morphological, histochemical, and biochemical characteristics of CTMCs. But in anatomic sites populated in +/+ mice by berberine sulfate-negative MMCs (e.g., the gastric mucosa), the adoptively transferred mast cells in the *W/W*^{v} recipients were also berberine sulfate-negative. Moreover, populations enriched for peritoneal mast cells (a type of CTMC) (Nakano *et al.*, 1985), or even single peritoneal mast cells (Sonoda *et al.*, 1986), on injection into *W/W*^{v} mice, can give rise to progeny with the morphologic and histochemical features of either MMCs or CTMCs, as appropriate for the site (e.g., MMCs in the gastric mucosa, CTMCs in the gastric muscularis propria). Finally, combined *in vitro* and *in vivo* studies showed that single clonal populations of mouse mast cells derived from peritoneal mast cells can express biochemical, morphological, and histochemical characteristics similar to those of either CTMCs or MMCs, and that these features exhibited bidirectional and reversible alteration, depending on the specific conditions that are experienced by the population *in vitro* or *in vivo* (Kanakura *et al.*, 1988).

In vitro work showed that fibroblasts represent one source of factors that can promote IL-3-derived BMCMCs to develop features of CTMCs (Levi-Schaffer *et al.*, 1986). Subsequent work, discussed below, indicated that stem cell factor (SCF) represents a major fibroblast-derived factor that can induce BMCMCs to acquire phenotypic characteristics of CTMCs. However, a number of other cytokines can also influence mast cell development and/or proliferation in the mouse. For example, IL-4 (Lee *et al.*, 1986; Mosmann *et al.*, 1986), IL-9 (Hultner *et al.*, 1989; Hultner *et al.*, 1990; Renauld *et al.*, 1990), or IL-10 (Thompson-Snipes *et al.*, 1990), when combined with IL-3, can enhance the proliferation of IL-3-derived BMCMCs. By contrast, when used as the only exogenous growth factor, these cytokines have little or no ability to induce BMCMC proliferation. The combination of IL-3 and IL-4 also has been shown to trigger the proliferation of purified mouse peritoneal mast cells ("serosal" mast cells or CTMCs) grown in methylcellulose (Tsujii *et al.*, 1990). By contrast, it has been reported that either granulocyte/macrophage colony-stimulating factor (GM-CSF) (Bressler *et al.*, 1989) or transforming growth factor (TGF)-β1 (Broide *et al.*, 1989) can inhibit mouse BMCMC proliferation in response to IL-3.

2.1.3. Stem Cell Factor and *c-kit*

It is now known that the mast cell deficiency and other phenotypic abnormalities expressed by *W* or *Sl* mutant mice reflect the consequences of these mutations on the production and/or function of the stem cell factor receptor (SCFR), which is encoded by the c-*kit* protooncogene that is allelic with the *W* locus in the mouse, or the production or function of SCF, the ligand for this receptor, which is encoded at the *Sl* locus in the mouse (reviewed in Galli *et al.*, 1994; Williams *et al.*, 1992; Besmer, 1991).

The extracellular domain of the SCFR has homology with members of the immunoglobulin superfamily while the receptor's intracellular amino acid sequence displays extensive homology with the tyrosine protein kinase receptor superfamily, particularly with the transmembrane receptors for colony-stimulating factor-1 (CSF-1R) and platelet-derived growth factor (PDGFR) (Galli *et al.*, 1994; Williams *et al.*, 1992; Besmer, 1991). The SCFR is expressed on mast cells, melanocytes, germ cells and on early hematopoietic progenitor cells. In general, SCFR expression diminishes with the progressive maturation of lymphohematopoietic lineages (Galli *et al.*, 1994; Williams *et al.*, 1992; Besmer, 1991). The mast cell represents an interesting exception to this rule, in that mature mast cells continue to express high levels of the SCFR (Galli *et al.*, 1994; Williams *et al.*, 1992; Besmer, 1991). By contrast, studies of human basophils indicate that these cells express few or no SCFRs (Lerner *et al.*, 1991; Columbo *et al.*, 1992).

Although the tissues of *W/W*^{v} mice express normal levels of c-*kit* mRNA, which is normal in size (Nocka *et al.*, 1989), the SCFR that is expressed in *W/W*^{v} tissues retains little, if any, kinase activity as a result of the structural alteration of the gene product. Specifically, the *W*^{v} mutation results in an amino acid substitution in the kinase domain, which dramatically reduces the kinase activity (Nocka *et al.*, 1990a), while *W* comprises a deletion of the region of c-*kit* which encodes the transmembrane part of the SCFR, thus preventing cell surface expression of the receptor (Hayashi *et al.*, 1991).

Identification of the SCFR as the *W* gene product greatly assisted in the identification of the c-kit ligand, a novel growth factor that is the product of the *Sl* locus (reviewed in Galli *et al.*, 1994; Williams *et al.*, 1992; Besmer, 1991). Although several names have been proposed for this c-kit ligand, including stem cell factor (SCF), kit ligand (KL), mast cell growth factor (MGF), and Steel factor, we will use the designation SCF (Galli *et al.*, 1994). The *Sl* mutation represents a deletion of all SCF coding sequences while the Sl^d allele encodes an abundant, smaller-than-normal SCF transcript (Flanagan *et al.*, 1991). Northern analyses have shown that mouse 3T3 cells (Huang *et al.*, 1990) and bone marrow-derived stromal cell lines (Anderson *et al.*, 1990) express an abundant 6-kb SCF transcript as well as two smaller alternative transcripts, which are about 5 and 3 kb in size. Two forms of the SCF protein have been identified: a soluble factor comprising the first 164 or 165 amino acids of the extracellular domain and a transmembrane form comprising the full-length translation product (Galli *et al.*, 1994; Williams *et al.*, 1992; Besmer, 1991). The soluble form of SCF is derived from the larger cell-associated precursor by proteolysis, in a fashion analogous to the processing of the secreted forms of CSF-1 and TGF-α from their membrane-associated precursors (Galli *et al.*, 1994; Williams *et al.*, 1992; Besmer, 1991). The probable site of proteolytic cleavage in SCF is encoded by the exon that is missing from the shorter of the two SCF cDNAs (Flanagan *et al.*, 1991).

In general, the most dramatic effects of SCF in hematopoiesis reflect its actions as a survival factor for early hematopoietic progenitors and its ability to synergize with other growth factors to regulate the proliferation and differentiation of cells in multiple hematopoietic lineages (Galli *et al.*, 1994; Williams *et al.*, 1992; Besmer, 1991). However, the effects of SCF on mast cell development are notable for both their diversity and their importance in the natural history of this particular hematopoietic lineage. Repeated injection of recombinant rat SCF into the skin of $WCB6F_1$-Sl/Sl^d mice resulted in the local development of a large number of mast cells with phenotypic characteristics of CTMCs (Zsebo *et al.*, 1990; Tsai *et al.*, 1991a), and many of the mast cells in these sites were undergoing proliferation (Tsai *et al.*, 1991a). Sl/Sl^d mouse skin ordinarily contains no detectable mast cell precursors (Kitamura, 1989; Kitamura *et al.*, 1989). Thus, these experiments showed that SCF influenced the recruitment, retention and/or survival of mast cell precursors at the injection sites, as well as promoted the proliferation and maturation of these cells (Zsebo *et al.*, 1990; Tsai *et al.*, 1991a). The effects on recruitment of mast cell precursors probably reflected the ability of these cells to recognize the extracellular domain of SCF, which can be assessed as mast cell adherence (Flanagan and Leder, 1990) or chemotaxis (Meininger *et al.*, 1992) *in vitro*, whereas the effects on the survival of the mast cell lineage at these sites probably reflected the ability of SCF to suppress mast cell apoptosis, which can be demonstrated either *in vitro* (Mekori *et al.*, 1993; Iemura *et al.*, 1994) or *in vivo* (Iemura *et al.*, 1994).

SCF represents the only cytokine that can induce significant proliferation of immature mouse mast cells and/or mature mouse CTMCs (Zsebo *et al.*, 1990; Tsai *et al.*, 1991a,b; Nocka *et al.*, 1990b) as well as the only cytokine that can induce IL-3-derived BMCMCs to acquire multiple phenotypic characteristics of CTMCs [including a substantially higher histamine content (Tsai *et al.*, 1991b), significant ability to synthesize and store heparin (Tsai *et al.*, 1991b), and a CTMC-like protease phenotype (Gurish *et al.*, 1991)]. On the other hand, IL-3-derived BMCMCs maintained in SCF do not acquire phenotypic characteristics identical to those of freshly isolated peritoneal mast cells (PMCs), and PMCs maintained in SCF have a substantially lower histamine content and, as a population, exhibit less mature histochemical characteristics than do freshly isolated PMCs (Tsai *et al.*, 1991b). These findings might reflect the lack of an additional factor or factors that, together with SCF, can induce or maintain full CTMC maturation *in vitro*. Alternatively, the observation that BMCMCs or PMCs maintained in SCF differ in phenotype from freshly isolated PMCs also may reflect, at least in part, consequence of the active proliferation of mast cell populations that are maintained in SCF. In addition to its effects on mast cell proliferation and maturation, under certain circumstances SCF can directly induce mouse mast cell degranulation and mediator release (Wershil *et al.*, 1992; Coleman *et al.*, 1993) and can enhance the mast cell mediator release that is observed on IgE-dependent activation of the cells (Coleman *et al.*, 1993).

Because mast cells, like other cell types, can be influenced by many different cytokines, *in vivo* studies are particularly important for characterizing the relative importance of various growth factors during the cell's natural history. In mice, the lack of mast cells in W/W^v (*c-kit/SCFR* mutant) and Sl/Sl^d (*SCF* mutant) mice clearly demonstrates that SCF and its receptor are essential for normal mast cell development. However, both *in vivo* (Tsai *et al.*, 1991a) and *in vitro* (Haig *et al.*, 1994) studies in rats, and *in vitro* studies in mice (Gurish *et al.*, 1991), indicate that the phenotypic characteristics of the mast cells that develop in the presence of SCF can be significantly influenced by other factors in the cells' microenvironment, particularly IL-3 (Gurish *et al.*, 1991; Haig *et al.*, 1994). Similarly, even though short-term *in vivo* studies (Wershil *et al.*, 1992), as well as *in vitro* experiments (Coleman *et al.*, 1993), indicate that SCF can promote mast cell degranulation, whether by itself or in conjunction with IgE and antigen (Coleman *et al.*, 1993), the long-term administration of SCF to mice *in vivo* can *diminish* the mast cell's responsiveness to stimulation by IgE and antigen, and can also *decrease* the severity of IgE-dependent passive anaphylaxis (Ando *et al.*, 1993). While the explanation for these *in vivo* findings remains to be determined, the results certainly indicate that the effects of SCF on mast cell function may be quite complex.

In vivo studies have also shown that the long-term administration of recombinant SCF can induce significant mast cell hyperplasia in primates (Galli *et al.*, 1993), as well as in mice and rats (Tsai *et al.*, 1991a). Baboons (*Papio* species) or cynomolgus monkey (*Macaca fascicularis*) treated subcutaneously with recombinant human SCF (rhSCF) for 28 or 21 days, respectively, developed mast cell hyperplasia in many anatomical sites (Galli *et al.*, 1993). However, the magnitude of the effect varied considerably according to anatomical site. In cynomolgus monkeys, treatment with rhSCF at 6.0 mg/kg per day resulted in increased numbers of mast cells at all sites examined except the CNS, with increases ranging from 3-fold, in the heart, to 1500-

fold, in the spleen. When rhSCF was given at 100 μg/kg per day, significant elevations of mast cell numbers occurred in the skin at the injection sites, bone marrow, mesenteric lymph node, liver, and spleen. Remarkably, in monkeys treated with rhSCF for 21 days and then maintained without the growth factor for an additional 15 days, mast cell numbers in most sites were statistically indistinguishable from the baseline numbers observed in vehicle-treated control monkeys (Galli *et al.*, 1993). Moreover, the rhSCF-treated monkeys appeared to be clinically well, not only throughout the course of treatment, but also during the period when mast cell populations were declining precipitously to normal levels (Galli *et al.*, 1993).

2.1.4. Mast Cell Development in Humans

In contrast to murine mast cells and human basophils, human mast cells have been difficult to culture from blood or bone marrow in sufficient numbers for studying mast cell growth and differentiation. Human mononuclear cells separated by density sedimentation from adult peripheral blood, umbilical cord blood, or bone marrow, and then grown in short-term liquid suspension cultures with IL-3, give rise to cultures rich in basophils rather than mast cells (Tadokoro *et al.*, 1983; Ishizaka *et al.*, 1985; Otsuka *et al.*, 1986). Similarly, single lineage and mixed CFUs containing basophils but not mast cells were observed when mononuclear cells were cultured in methylcellulose in the presence of IL-3 (Leary *et al.*, 1986). Small numbers of mast cells (1 to 3% of cultured cells) have been identified by histochemistry in cultures of human bone marrow-derived mononuclear cells suspended over agar or agarose in the presence of rhIL-3 (Kirshenbaum *et al.*, 1989a,b). Based on experiments employing immunomagnetic selection approaches, the bone marrow progenitor for human mast cells resides in the $CD34^+$ population of hematopoietic progenitor cells (Kirshenbaum *et al.*, 1991).

Mast cells that express phenotypic characteristics of mature human mast cells can be derived by culturing appropriate progenitor cells together with mouse 3T3 fibroblasts (Furitsu *et al.*, 1989). According to immunogold labeling, these mast cells coexpress cell surface IgE receptors and cytoplasmic granules that contain tryptase. By ultrastructure, these mast cells may express a variety of cytoplasmic granule morphologies including the scroll, mixed, reticular, dense core, or homogeneous patterns found in the mature human mast cells that occur within normal tissues (Dvorak *et al.*, 1993a).

The ability of mouse 3T3 fibroblasts to promote human mast cell development *in vitro*, and the fact that the human SCFR can bind mouse SCF (Zsebo *et al.*, 1990), suggesting that SCF may promote mast cell development in humans, as it does in murine rodents and experimental primates. When $CD34^+$ human bone marrow cells were cultured *in vitro* rhSCF plus IL-3, both mast cells and many other hematopoietic lineages developed (Kirshenbaum *et al.*, 1992). As a result, the cultures did not exhibit a net enrichment for mast cells. By contrast, rhSCF used as the only exogenous cytokine favored the development of mast cells from populations of human bone marrow or peripheral blood mononuclear cells (Valent *et al.*, 1992), human umbilical cord blood mononuclear cells (Mitsui *et al.*, 1993), or human fetal liver cells (Irani *et al.*, 1992). However, the human mast cells that develop in cultures supplemented with soluble rhSCF appear to represent only a subset of the human mast cell phenotypes that are observed *in vivo*. For example, these rhSCF-derived human mast cells express little or no cytoplasmic granule-associated chymase (Mitsui *et al.*, 1993; Irani *et al.*, 1992). Whether membrane-associated forms of SCF might differ from soluble SCF in promoting human mast cell development remains to be determined.

Recently, Costa *et al.* (1993a) quantified mast cell numbers in skin biopsies obtained from patients enrolled in a Phase I study of rhSCF. Treatment of these subjects with rhSCF at 5 to 50 μg/kg per day for 14 days resulted in an ~70% increase in the number of dermal mast cells in skin distant from the SCF injection sites. These represent the first data indicating that rhSCF can induce mast cell hyperplasia *in vivo* in humans.

The systemic expansion of mast cell numbers in mice, rats, monkeys, or humans receiving *exogenous* SCF suggests that changes in the level of expression of *endogenous* SCF may explain, at least in part, some of the striking alterations in mast cell numbers that have been noted in association with a variety of reparative responses, immunological reactions, and disease processes (Galli *et al.*, 1993, 1994). Moreover, it is likely that the wide variation in the numbers of mast cells that ordinarily are present in different normal tissues may reflect, in large part, differences in the levels of endogenous SCF bioactivity which are expressed at the various anatomical sites (Galli *et al.*, 1993, 1994).

2.2. Basophils

Like other granulocytes, basophils differentiate and mature in the bone marrow and then circulate in the blood. Basophils are not normally found in connective tissues. In humans, the basophil is the least common blood granulocyte, with a prevalence of approximately 0.5% of total leukocytes and approximately 0.3% of nucleated marrow cells (Juhlin, 1963; Galli and Dvorak, 1995). Because the normal frequency of blood and bone marrow basophils is so low, accurate basophil determinations ordinarily require absolute counting methods (Gilbert and Ornstein, 1975). The basophil's prominent, metachromatic cytoplasmic granules permit it to be identified easily in Wright–Giemsa-stained preparations of peripheral blood or bone marrow cells. Both cytogenetic evidence (Shohet and Blum, 1968) and *in vitro* studies (Denburg *et al.*, 1983; Dvorak *et al.*, 1985a; Ogawa *et al.*, 1983) indicate that basophils share a common precursor with other granulocytes and monocytes. Specifically, in humans, basophils are derived from pluripotent $CD34^+$ hematopoietic progenitor cells (Kirshenbaum *et al.*, 1991). Human basophils appear to exhibit kinetics of production and peripheral circulation similar to that of eosinophils (Osgood, 1937; Murakami *et al.*, 1969). However, unlike the eosinophil, the basophil ordinarily does not occur in peripheral tissues in significant numbers. Basophils can infiltrate sites of many immunologic or inflammatory processes (often in association with eosinophils) and participate in the reactions to some tumors (Galli *et al.*, 1984; Galli and Askenase, 1986). In such cases, the basophils are readily distinguishable from mast cells residing in the same tissues (Dvorak *et al.*, 1983b). The ultrastructural features of human basophils are summarized in Table II and are illustrated in Fig. 1.

Mouse peripheral blood basophils have not yet been highly purified, but these cells appear to exhibit light (Urbina *et al.*, 1981) and electron (Dvorak *et al.*, 1982) microscopic features that are similar to those of the basophils of other mammalian species. Genetically mast cell-deficient WBB6F$_1$-*W/W*^{v} mice and the congenic normal (+/+) mice have similar numbers of circulating basophils. Moreover, the number of circulating basophils in mice [approximately 20 to 3×10^3 nucleated cells (Jacoby *et al.*, 1984)] is substantially greater than the apparent number of circulating mast cell precursors (Kitamura *et al.*, 1989).

Culture of human bone marrow cells or umbilical cord blood cells in suspension in the presence of IL-3 generates populations that are highly enriched in basophils (25% or more), with the remaining cells consisting of neutrophils, eosinophils, monocytes, and rare mast cells (Kirshenbaum *et al.*, 1989a; Aglietta *et al.*, 1981; Valent *et al.*, 1989a). Moreover, high-affinity binding sites for IL-3 have been identified on the human basophil surface (Valent *et al.*, 1989b), and basophil numbers are slightly increased in the blood of patients who are treated with rhIL-3 (Ganser *et al.*, 1990). While these findings indicate that IL-3 is an important growth factor for human basophils, other cytokines can also contribute to the development of this lineage. Granulocyte–macrophage colony-stimulating factor (GM-CSF), but not G- or M-CSF, can enhance the growth of basophils from peripheral blood (Hutt-Taylor *et al.*, 1988). IL-5 and nerve growth factor (NGF) may also synergize with other growth factors to enhance basophil development *in vitro* (Tsuda *et al.*, 1991). Although basophils also express receptors for several other cytokines, including IL-2 (CD25), IL-4, and IL-8, neither these cytokines, IL-1, nor IL-6 appear to promote significant basophil differentiation (Denburg, 1990; Valent and Bettelheim, 1990).

3. MEDIATORS

Basophils and mast cells contain, or elaborate on appropriate stimulation, a diverse array of potent, biologically active mediators (Galli and Lichtenstein, 1988; Holgate *et al.*, 1993; Metcalfe *et al.*, 1981; Schwartz and Huff, 1993). Some of these products are stored performed in the cells' cytoplasmic granules (e.g., proteoglycans, proteases, histamine); others are synthesized on activation of the cell by IgE and antigen or other stimuli (e.g., products of arachidonic acid oxidation through the cyclooxygenase or lipooxygenase pathways, and, in some cells, PAF). Cytokines represent the most recently identified group of mast cell and basophil mediators, at least one of which (TNF-α) can be both preformed and stored, as well as newly synthesized by activated cells (Gordon *et al.*, 1990; Costa *et al.*, 1992). These agents can mediate a diverse array of effects in inflammation, immunity, and tissue remodeling, and can also influence the clotting, fibrinolytic, complement, and kinin systems.

3.1. Preformed Mediators

Mediators that are stored preformed in the cytoplasmic granules include histamine, proteoglycans, serine proteases, carboxypeptidase A, and small amounts of sulfatases and exoglycosidases. Mast cells and basophils form histamine by the decarboxylation of histidine, and store histamine as an ionic complex with the highly charged carboxyl and/or sulfate groups of the glycosaminoglycan side chains of the proteoglycans which constitute much of the matrix of the secretory granules. Mast cells isolated from human lung, skin, lymphoid tissue, or small intestine contain about 3–8 pg of histamine per cell whereas human basophils contain about 1–2 pg/cell (Galli and Lichtenstein, 1988; Schwartz and Huff, 1993). Studies in genetically mast cell-deficient and congenic normal mice indicate that mast cells represent the source of virtually all of the histamine stored in normal tissues, with the notable exceptions of the glandular stomach (where enterochromaffin cells account for ~50% of the histamine) and the central nervous system (where, with the exception of the meninges, neural sources account for most of the histamine; Yamatodani *et al.*, 1982). Basophils are the source of most of the histamine present in normal human blood (Porter and Mitchell, 1972). Mouse and rat mast cells contain significant quantities of serotonin, but this amine has not been detected in populations of human mast cells or basophils (Holgate *et al.*, 1993; Metcalfe *et al.*, 1981).

Human mast cell populations contain variable mixtures of heparin (~60 kDa) and chondroitin sulfate proteoglycans (Stevens *et al.*, 1988; Thompson *et al.*, 1988). Although the sulfated glycosaminoglycans of normal human blood basophils have not been characterized, chondroitin sulfates account for the majority of the proteoglycans in the basophils of patients with myelogenous leukemia (Metcalfe *et al.*, 1984). Proteoglycans are composed of a central protein core with extended unbranched carbohydrate side chains (glycosaminoglycans) of repeating disaccharide subunits (Kjellen and Lindahl, 1991). The central protein core of heparin has numerous serine-glycine repeating residues which, besides conferring protease resistance to the proteoglycan, form the attachment points for glycosaminoglycans. It is now known that, within individual species, the protein cores of all mast cell proteoglycans are encoded by the same gene; hence, the different proteoglycans are generated by posttranslational steps which add different side chains to each molecule (Tantravahi *et al.*, 1986). Each disaccharide of the glycosaminoglycans has between zero and, in the case of heparin, three sulfate groups, whose high charge contributes to many of the characteristic physicochemical properties of these molecules (Schwartz and Huff, 1993; Kjellen and Lindahl, 1991).

Mast cell and basophil proteoglycans probably express multiple biological functions, both within and outside of the cells. By ionic interactions, they bind histamine, neutral proteases, and carboxypeptidases, and may contribute to the packaging and storage of these molecules within the secretory granules. When the granule matrices are exposed to physiological conditions of pH and ionic strength during the process of degranulation, the various mediators associated with the proteoglycans dissociate at different rates, histamine very rapidly but tryptase and chymase much more slowly (Schwartz and Huff, 1993). In addition to regulating the kinetics of release of mediators from the granule matrices, proteoglycans can also regulate the activity of some of the associated mediators. For example, heparin stabilizes tryptase in a configuration that is required for its normal enzymatic activity (Schwartz and Huff, 1993; Schwartz and Bradford, 1986).

In addition to these roles, heparin and other mast cell- or basophil-derived proteoglycans may have a number of other functions. Heparin can bind and protect from degradation many growth factors, such as bFGF and certain hematopoietic factors (Rusolahti and Yamaguchi, 1991), can bind to (and alter the activity of) leukocyte products such as eosinophil major basic protein (Kjellen and Lindahl, 1991), can influence the biological properties of extracellular matrix proteins such as laminin, fibronectin, and vitronectin (Kjellen and Lindahl, 1991; Ruoslahti and Yamaguchi, 1991), and, through its ability to bind to antithrombin III, can function as an anticoagulant (Metcalfe *et al.*, 1981; Kjellen and Lindahl, 1991). However, the extent to which each of these functions is actually expressed at sites of mast cell activation probably depends on many factors, including the processes that regulate the dissociation of proteoglycans from the other constituents of the cytoplasmic granule matrix.

Neutral proteases represent the major protein component of mast cell secretory granules. Both basophils and mast cells contain enzymes with TAME-esterase activity, which can be used as a marker of mast cell or basophil activation *in vivo*. By weight, tryptase is the major enzyme stored in the cytoplasmic granules of human mast cells, and this neutral protease has been detected in all human mast cell populations that have been examined (Schwartz and Huff, 1993). Human mast cell tryptase is a serine endopeptidase that exists in the granule in active form as a tetramer of 134 kDa containing subunits of 31 to 35 kDa, each of which contains an active site (Irani *et al.*, 1986). Negligible amounts of tryptase have been identified in normal human basophils by immunoassay, and furthermore, it is not clear whether this activity represents the same enzyme that is present in the mast cell (Irani *et al.*, 1986). Because the enzyme is at least highly concentrated in, and may be unique to, the human mast cell, measurements of the levels of mast cell tryptase in biologic fluids such as plasma, serum, or inflammatory exudates have been used to assess mast cell activation in these settings (Schwartz *et al.*, 1987). Tryptase is stored in the mast cell's cytoplasmic granules in the active form bound to heparin, and is released on degranulation as a complex with this proteoglycan. The active tetrameric form of tryptase is stabilized by its association with heparin and perhaps other proteoglycans within the mast cell granule (Schwartz and Bradford, 1986). Although the function of mast cell tryptase *in vivo* is unknown, tryptase can selectively cleave human C3 to its component peptides, C3b and C3a, and, while complexed with heparin, can degrade C3 to inactive peptides. Mast cell chymase is also a serine protease that is stored in active form in the mast cell granule, but as a monomer with a molecular mass of 30 kDa (Schechter *et al.*, 1983; Johnson *et al.*, 1986). Human mast cell chymase is present in 85% of the mast cells of the skin and intestinal submucosa, but some mast cells present within the intestinal mucosa and lung do not stain with monoclonal antibodies directed against the protease (Irani *et al.*, 1986). Other components of the mast cell granule stored in complex with proteoglycans are the carboxypeptidases A and B, the former in rodent mast cells and the latter in human mast cells (McClure *et al.*, 1964; Everitt and Neurath, 1980). Human basophils, like eosinophils, can form Charcot–Leyden crystals and contain Charcot–Leyden crystal protein (lysophospholipase) in quantities similar to that of eosinophils (Ackerman *et al.*, 1982, 1993). This protein has been localized ultrastructurally to the major cytoplasmic granule population of basophils (Dvorak and Ackerman, 1989).

3.2. Newly Synthesized Lipid Mediators

The activation of mast cells with appropriate stimuli not only causes the secretion of preformed granule-associated mediators, but also can initiate the *de novo* synthesis of certain lipid-derived substances. Of particular importance are the cyclooxygenase and lipooxygenase metabolites of arachidonic acid, which possess potent inflammatory activities and which may also play a role in modulating the release process itself (Valone *et al.*, 1993). The major cyclooxygenase product of mast cells is prostaglandin D_2 (PGD_2), whereas the major lipoxygenase products derived from mast cells and basophils are the sulfidopeptide leukotrienes (LT): LTC_4, LTD_4, and LTE_4 (Valone *et al.*, 1993). The substrate for the formation of both prostaglandins and leukotrienes, as well as for the third class of lipid mediator, platelet-activating factor (PAF), is arachidonic acid, which is released from the phospholipids constituting the membranes and, in some cells, lipid bodies, of mast cells and basophils by various phospholipase A2 enzymes (Dvorak, 1991; Valone *et al.*, 1993; Dvorak *et al.*, 1983c). However, the specific products of arachidonic acid metabolism which are produced by different populations of mast cells or by blood basophils vary considerably (Galli and Lichtenstein, 1988; Holgate *et al.*, 1993; Valone *et al.*, 1993). For example, mast cells isolated from a variety of different human tissues release both LTC_4 and PGD_2, whereas peripheral blood basophils release LTC_4 but no detectable PGD_2.

PGD_2, the primary prostaglandin synthesized by murine or human mast cells, is generated very rapidly after IgE-dependent mast cell activation (Galli and Lichtenstein, 1988; Schwartz and Huff, 1993; Valone *et al.*, 1993). PGD_2 enhances venular permeability, leukocyte adherence to vascular endothelial cells, and pulmonary vasoconstriction, and also acts as a peripheral vasodilator (Galli and Lichtenstein, 1988; Schwartz and Huff, 1993; Valone *et al.*, 1993). PGD_2 is also a potent inhibitor of platelet aggregation; it is chemokinetic for human neutrophils and, in conjunction with LTD_4, it can induce the accumulation of neutrophils in human skin (Galli and Lichtenstein, 1988; Schwartz and Huff, 1993; Valone *et al.*, 1993). High levels of PGD_2 metabolites have been detected in the urine of patients with mastocytosis, and PGD_2 is believed to contribute to hypotension is such patients (Roberts *et al.*, 1980).

The primary products of the 5-lipooxygenase pathway of arachidonic acid metabolism which are generated by mast cells and basophils are the sulfidopeptide leukotrienes. Studies with purified cells show that basophils and mast cells produce only LTC_4; however, in mixed cell preparations and certain *in vivo*, LTC_4 is rapidly metabolized to LTD_4 and LTE_4 (Galli and Lichtenstein, 1988; Valone *et al.*, 1993). Through interactions with their receptors on smooth muscle cells, these products, formerly known as "slow-reacting substance of anaphylaxis" (SRS-A), induce a prolonged cutaneous wheal and flare reaction and, in the respiratory system, prolonged bronchoconstriction (Galli and Lichtenstein, 1988; Valone *et al.*, 1993). These products also can enhance venular permeability, enhance bronchial mucous secretion, and induce constriction of arterial, arteriolar, and intestinal smooth muscle (Galli and Lichtenstein, 1988; Valone *et al.*, 1993). Accordingly, the sulfidopeptide leukotrienes are regarded as important mediators of some of the pathophysiological hallmarks of late-phase reactions (see below), both in the airways in patients with asthma, as well as in other sites.

Human mast cells, but not human basophils, also can product LTB_4, albeit in much smaller quantities than PGD_2 or the sulfidopeptide leukotrienes (Galli and Lichtenstein, 1988; Metcalfe *et al.*, 1981; Valone *et al.*, 1993). At low concentrations, LTB_4 expresses neutrophil chemotactic activity and, at higher concentrations, LTB_4 can induce neutrophil secretion (Schwartz and Huff, 1993; Valone *et al.*, 1993). On injection into human skin, LTB_4 can induce a wheal and flare followed several hours later by an indurated lesion containing interstitial fibrin and neutrophils, effects that are enhanced by the simultaneous administration of PGD_2 (Soter *et al.*, 1983).

Human lung or gut mast cells produce PGD_2 in amounts that are roughly equivalent to their production of LTC_4. The skin mast cell also makes PGD_2, but produces relatively little LTC_4, on average ~60 ng of LTC_4 per 10^6 cells. By contrast, human lung mast cells produce from one to many hundreds of nanograms per 10^6 cells (Galli and Lichtenstein, 1988). Among human basophils, cells from individuals who are the most sensitive to IgE-dependent activation produce far more LTC_4 than do the cells of other individuals (MacGlashan and Lichtenstein, 1986). Thus, there are three patterns of release of products of arachidonic acid metabolism by human mast cells and basophils: (1) gut or lung mast cells produce similar amounts of LTC_4 and PGD_2; (2) skin mast cells produce largely PGD_2; and (3) basophils generate only LTC_4.

PAF [more recently designated PAF-acether or alkylglyceryletherphosphorylcholine (AGEPC)] has been detected in mouse bone marrow-derived mast cells, rabbit basophils, and human mast cells, but not following activation of human basophils (Galli and Lichtenstein, 1988; Valone *et al.*, 1993). PAF can aggregate and degranulate platelets, induce wheal and flare reactions on injection into human skin, increase lung resistance, and lead to systemic hypotension, suggesting a potential role for this mediator in systemic anaphylaxis (Galli and Lichtenstein, 1988; Valone *et al.*, 1993). PAF is produced in large quantities by lung mast cells (as well as many other cells, including human neutrophils) but, in the case of the mast cell, the mediator is not significantly released by these cells *in vitro* (Lichtenstein *et al.*, 1984). However, PAF and its inactive derivative, lyso-PAF, appear in biologic fluids after antigen challenge (Miadonna *et al.*, 1989). While the cellular source of the PAF that is detected in such settings has not yet been identified, this mediator may contribute to the prolonged increase in human bronchial reactivity that is observed on antigen challenge in asthmatic subjects (Cass *et al.*, 1986).

3.3. Cytokines

The recent demonstration of cytokine production by mast cells and basophils has greatly expanded the possible mechanisms by which these cells might contribute to the pathophysiology of allergic and immunological diseases or host defense (reviewed in Gordon *et al.*, 1990; Costa *et al.*, 1992). Studies with virus-transformed mouse mast cell lines revealed that these cells expressed mRNA and/or bioactivity for GM-CSF, IL-4, and IL-3 (Chung *et al.*, 1986; Brown *et al.*, 1987; Humphries *et al.*, 1988). Subsequent studies, reported independently by three groups at about the same time, showed that IL-3-dependent *in vitro*-derived mouse mast cells or mast cell lines that had been activated via the $Fc_{\varepsilon}RI$ contained increased levels of mRNA for many cytokines (IL-1α, 3, 4, 5, and 6, and GM-CSF, as well as the chemokines MIP-1α and β, JE, and TCA3), and also released the corresponding bioactivities for some of these cytokines (IL-1, 3, 4, and 6, GM-CSF) (Plaut *et al.*, 1989; Wodnar-Filipowicz *et al.*, 1989; Burd *et al.*, 1989).

The first cytokine bioactivity to be clearly associated with normal mast cells was TNF-α/cachectin (Young *et al.*, 1987; Gordon and Galli, 1990). Gordon and Galli demonstrated that unstimulated mouse peritoneal mast cells constitutively contain approximately twice as much TNF-α bioactivity as do LPS-stimulated mouse peritoneal macrophages (Gordon and Galli, 1990), and that the TNF-α that is released from mouse mast cells on appropriate stimulation reflects cytokine that is rapidly released from these preformed stores, as well as even larger amounts of newly synthesized TNF-α, which is released over a period of hours after cell activation (Gordon and Galli, 1990, 1991). Thus, the biological effects of mast cell-derived TNF-α can be expressed immediately after IgE-dependent activation of these cells, and can be sustained for long intervals thereafter.

Table IV summarizes the key concepts that have been derived from these and other studies of nonhuman mast cells. Currently, little information is available regarding the mechanism(s) of cytokine gene induction in mast cells. A requirement for prolonged receptor cross-linkage and extracellular calcium has been demonstrated (Plaut *et al.*, 1990), and a major component of the IL-3 and GM-CSF inductional response has been shown to reflect posttranscriptional stabilization of mRNA (Wodnar-Filipowicz and Moroni, 1990).

Human mast cells and basophils also elaborate cytokines. Mast cells from a variety of anatomic sites including the bone marrow (Steffen *et al.*, 1989), skin (Klein *et al.*, 1989; Walsh *et al.*, 1991), and lung (Ohkawara *et al.*, 1992) have all been shown to contain TNF-α mRNA and immunoreactive or bioactive protein product, and enhanced production of TNF-α has been demonstrated after $Fc_{\varepsilon}RI$ cross-linking (Benyon *et al.*, 1991). Moreover, in skin organ culture systems, IgE-dependent activation of human skin mast cells results in the expression of the adherence

TABLE IV
Features of Mast Cell Cytokine Production[a]

1. Mast cells can transcribe and translate many different cytokines, including IL-1, 3, 4, 5, and 6, GM-CSF, TNF-α, IFN-γ, TGF-β, and the chemokines MIP-1α, MIP-1β, TCA3, and JE.
2. Mast cell cytokine genes can be differentially regulated, in that different signals can have distinct effects on the species, amounts, and kinetics of cytokine production.
3. In response to cellular activation (e.g., through the $Fc_{\epsilon}RI$), mast cells can release at least one cytokine, TNF-α, from both preformed and stored, as well as newly synthesized pools.
4. It is not yet clear whether all subpopulations of mast cells can produce the same spectrum of cytokines.
5. The pattern of mast cell cytokine production can vary depending on the stimulus used to activate the cells and can be regulated by cytokines and other microenvironmental factors which can influence mast cell phenotype.
6. Induction of cytokine mRNA in mast cells is not always accompanied by release of detectable cytokine bioactivity.
7. Under some circumstances, induction and/or release of mast cell cytokines can occur in response to stimuli that do not induce detectable release of histamine.
8. Release of some cytokines (e.g., TNF-α) can continue for hours after initial $Fc_{\epsilon}RI$-dependent mast cell activation.
9. Mast cell cytokine mRNA expression and/or cytokine release can be inhibited by cyclosporin A or dexamethasone.

[a]Most of these points so far have been established primarily by analyses of various mouse mast cell populations (see text).

molecule E-selectin (ELAM-1) on adjacent vascular endothelial cells, and this expression can be partially blocked by antibodies to TNF-α (Klein *et al.*, 1989) or to TNF-α and IL-1 (Leung *et al.*, 1991).

IL-4 has been demonstrated in human skin and lung mast cells by immunohistochemistry, and these cells release both histamine and IL-4 bioactivity into culture supernatants after anti-IgE challenge (Bradding *et al.*, 1992). Immunohistochemical analysis has revealed that some mast cells in nasal turbinate specimens from patients with allergic rhinitis or from nonatopic volunteers display immunoreactivity for IL-4, 5 and/or 6 (Bradding *et al.*, 1993).

Several lines of evidence indicate that mouse basophils can produce IL-4 on stimulation through the $Fc_{\epsilon}RI$ (Seder *et al.*, 1991; Dvorak *et al.*, 1993b). More recently, mature human basophils isolated from peripheral blood have been shown to release IL-4 in response to $Fc_{\epsilon}RI$-dependent activation (Brunner *et al.*, 1993; Arock *et al.*, 1993); and such release can be enhanced in basophils that have been exposed to IL-3, but not to IL-5, GM-CSF, or nerve growth factor (Brunner *et al.*, 1993; Arock *et al.*, 1993).

3.4. Mast Cell–Leukocyte Cytokine Cascades

When one considers the diversity of multifunctional cytokines that have been detected in different mast cell populations, the broad spectrum of biological responses that can be influenced by these cytokines, and the possibility that the expression of cytokine bioactivity by mast cell populations can be differentially regulated by various stimuli of mast cell activation (reviewed in Gordon *et al.*, 1990; Costa *et al.*, 1992; Galli *et al.*, 1991a), one might reasonably propose an enormous number of *potential* roles for mast cell cytokines in adaptive or pathological responses. Consideration of all of the biological effects of each mast cell-associated cytokine would require a separate review for each molecule. However, the known effects of these agents include regulation of IgE production (IL-4, IFN-γ), regulation of mast cell proliferation, phenotype, and function (IL-3 and 4, GM-CSF, IFN-γ, TGF-β), modulation of leukocyte (basophil, eosinophil, neutrophil, and monocyte) effector function (IL-3, 4, and 5, GM-CSF, IFN-γ, chemokines, TNF-α), and numerous actions in inflammation, clotting, angiogenesis, wound repair, tissue remodeling, and the development of pathological fibrosis (reviewed in Gordon *et al.*, 1990; Costa *et al.*, 1992; Galli *et al.*, 1991a). As reviewed elsewhere (Galli and Lichtenstein, 1988; Holgate *et al.*, 1993; Metcalfe *et al.*, 1981; Schwartz and Huff, 1993; Galli, 1990, 1993; Selye, 1965; Gordon *et al.*, 1990; Costa *et al.*, 1992; Galli *et al.*, 1991a), mast cells have been implicated in many of the same responses.

We have proposed that the expression of many IgE-dependent reactions, as well as other responses in which mast cells play an important role, reflect the activities of a "mast cell–leukocyte cytokine cascade" (Galli, 1993; Gordon *et al.*, 1990; Galli *et al.*, 1991a). In this hypothesis, mast cell activation has an essential or important role in the initiation of the response in part through the release of TNF-α and other cytokines which can directly or indirectly influence the recruitment and/or function of additional effector cells (neutrophils, eosinophils, basophils, lymphocytes, monocytes, and platelets). These recruited cells then importantly influence the progression of the response by providing additional sources of certain cytokines also produced by mast cells (e.g., TNF-α), and new sources of some cytokines (e.g., eosinophil-derived TGF-α; Wong *et al.*, 1990; Liu *et al.*, 1992) that are not produced by the mast cell. As the reactions progress further, cytokines from mast cells and other resident cells, and from recruited (leukocyte) sources, exert complex effects on resident cells such as vascular endothelial cells, fibroblasts, epithelial cells, nerves, and mast cells. These contribute to the vascular and epithelial changes, as well as to the tissue remodeling, angiogenesis and fibrosis, which are so prominent in many disorders associated with mast cell activation and leukocyte infiltration. At certain points in the natural history of these processes, mast cell- or eosinophil-derived cytokines may also contribute to the downregulation of the response.

4. MECHANISMS OF ACTIVATION

4.1. $Fc_{\varepsilon}RI$

The best-understood cellular event that underlies expression of basophil or mast cell function is the process of degranulation, a stereotyped constellation of stimulus-activated biochemical and morphological events that result in the fusion of the cytoplasmic granule membranes with the plasma membrane (with external release of granule-associated mediators), associated with the generation and release of products of arachidonic acid oxidation and the release of stored and/or newly generated cytokines. Although a variety of agents can initiate basophil or mast cell degranulation, the best-studied pathway of stimulation is that transduced through $Fc_{\varepsilon}RI$ expressed on the basophil or mast cell surface (Beaven and Metzger, 1993; Kinet, 1990; Ishizaka, 1988; Benhamou and Siraganian, 1992). Human basophils generated *in vitro* express about 2.7×10^5 $Fc_{\varepsilon}RI$ per cell, which bind monovalent IgE with a K_A of 2.8×10^9 moles/liter (Ogawa *et al.*, 1983). Similar values have been obtained for the $Fc_{\varepsilon}RI$ of rat and mouse mast cells (Ishizaka, 1988). The $Fc_{\varepsilon}RI$ consists of one α, one β, and two identical disulfide-linked γ chains, all components of which have been cloned and sequenced (Beaven and Metzger, 1993; Kinet, 1990). When adjacent $Fc_{\varepsilon}RIs$ are bridged, either by bivalent or multivalent antigen interacting with receptor-bound IgE, or by antibodies directed against either receptor-bound IgE or the receptor itself, the cells are rapidly activated for the release of stored and newly generated mediators. This process is energy- and temperature-dependent, requires the mobilization of calcium, resulting in increased levels of free calcium in the cytosol, and occurs without evidence of toxicity to the responding cell. It has been shown that the bridging of only a few hundred pairs of IgE molecules is necessary to trigger human basophil histamine release (Dembo *et al.*, 1979). Moreover, the number of IgE–IgE bridges necessary to trigger release in the basophils of individual subjects apparently is not normally distributed; a subset of donors appears to be exceedingly sensitive to this stimulus (MacGlashan and Lichtenstein, 1986). Because so few of a basophil's or mast cell's $Fc_{\varepsilon}RI$ must be bridged to initiate the degranulation response, these cells may be sensitized simultaneously with IgE antibodies of many different specificities, and therefore can react to stimulation by many different antigens.

IgE- and antigen-dependent activation represents the basis for the immunologically specific expression of mast and basophil function in IgE-dependent immune responses and allergic disorders. At the ultrastructural level, stimulation of appropriately sensitized human basophils with specific antigen provokes fusion of the membranes enveloping individual cytoplasmic granules with the plasma membrane (Dvorak *et al.*, 1980). As a result, the granules' contents, including stored mediators, are released via multiple narrow communications between single granules and the cell surface. IgE-dependent degranulation of human lung mast cells (Dvorak *et al.*, 1984) also results in the fusion of granule membranes with the plasma membrane. However, in this cell type, the first ultrastructural changes that are detectable in the stimulated cells are granule swelling and reduced electron density of the granule matrix (Dvorak *et al.*, 1984, 1985b). Individual cytoplasmic granules then fuse, forming interconnecting chains of swollen granules filled with altered fibrillar matrix. These progressively expand, appearing as multiple tortuous cytoplasmic channels. Histamine release is initiated by the opening of these channels to the exterior through multiple narrow points of fusion with the plasma membrane.

The degranulation that is initiated by bridging of $Fc_{\varepsilon}RIs$ is associated with phosphorylation of Tyr and Ser residues on the β chain and Tyr and Thr residues on the γ chains of the $Fc_{\varepsilon}RI$ (Beaven and Metzger, 1993; Kinet, 1990; Benhamou and Siraganian, 1992), the activation of membrane-associated serine proteases and GTP-binding proteins, the activation of serine-threonine and tyrosine kinases, including mitogen-activated protein kinases (MAP kinases), 90kDa-S6 kinases ($pp90^{rsk}$), and pp70-S6 kinases (Beaven and Metzger, 1993; Kinet, 1990; Benhamou and Siraganian, 1992; Tsai *et al.*, 1993), the activation of phospholipase C, methyltransferase, and adenylate cyclase, the stimulation of phosphatidylinositol turnover, and the generation of diacylglycerol and activation of protein kinase C and phospholipase(s) A_2 (Beaven and Metzger, 1993; Kinet, 1990; Benhamou and Siraganian, 1992). In addition, a large body of evidence indicates that mobilization of calcium, from either extracellular sources or intracellular stores, is necessary for a fully developed release process (Beaven and Metzger, 1993; Kinet, 1990; Benhamou and Siraganian, 1992). The finding that calcium ionophores by themselves can induce basophil or mast cell mediator release suggests that calcium transfer across cell membranes represents at least one mechanism by which activation for mediator release can be initiated (Beaven and Metzger, 1993; Kinet, 1990; Benhamou and Siraganian, 1992). However, the precise coordination of the various biochemical and morphological events that are associated with $Fc_{\varepsilon}RI$-mediated basophil and mast cell activation remain to be fully elucidated.

4.2. Nonimmunologic Direct Activation

In addition to IgE and specific antigen, a variety of biologic substances (including products of complement activation and certain cytokines), chemical agents, and physical stimuli can elicit release of basophil or mast cell mediators (see Table V). However, the responsiveness of human basophils and different populations of human mast cells to individual stimuli varies. For example, cutaneous mast cells appear to be much more sensitive to stimulation by neuropeptides than are pulmonary mast cells (Galli and Lichtenstein, 1988; Church *et al.*, 1989). Moreover, these stimuli can induce a pattern of mediator release that differs from that associated with IgE-dependent mast cell activation. For example, human cutaneous mast cells activated by substance P release about the same amounts of preformed mediators as do mast cells stimulated through the $Fc_{\varepsilon}RI$, but produce smaller amounts of lipid mediators (Galli and Lichtenstein, 1988; Church *et al.*, 1989). And work in the mouse indicates that substance P-activated mast cells also may produce lower levels of TNF-α than do cells activated through the $Fc_{\varepsilon}RI$ (Wershil *et al.*, 1994).

In addition to neuropeptides, several other classes of small peptides of potential biologic significance can induce basophil and/or mast cell mediator release. The best studied are the anaphylatoxins, products of complement activation, and the bacterial peptides, f-Met-Leu-Phe and its congeners (Grant *et al.*, 1975; Hook *et al.*, 1976). Both C5a and f-Met peptides release histamine from human basophils. However, f-Met-Leu-Phe is a more complete secretagogue, in that it induces release of both histamine

TABLE V
Stimuli of Human Basophil or Mast Cell Histamine Release

	Basophils		Mast cells	
Stimulus	Direct release	Enhance IgE-mediated release	Direct release	Enhance IgE-mediated release
C5a	+	ND[a]	+[b]	ND
f-Met Leu Phe	+	ND	+[b]	ND
Mannitol (hyperosmolar)	+	ND	+	ND
Substance P	−	ND	+[b]	ND
Morphine	−	ND	+[b]	ND
IL-1	±[c]	+	±	+
IL-3	+	+	−	ND
IL-5	−	+	−	ND
GM-CSF	+	+	−	ND
Stem cell factor (SCF)	±	+	+	+
MCAF	+	+	ND	ND
MIP-1α	+	ND	+	ND
RANTES	+	ND	ND	ND
NAP-1	+	ND	ND	ND
CTAP-III	+	ND	ND	ND

[a]ND, not determined.
[b]Cutaneous mast cells are much more sensitive to these stimuli than are mast cells derived from other sites.
[c]Some studies yes, some no.

and leukotrienes, whereas C5a produces a response that is largely limited to histamine release. Nevertheless, C5a-derived peptides provoke a sequence of ultrastructural changes in basophils that are similar to those induced by anti-IgE and specific antigen (Dvorak *et al.*, 1981). Neither of these peptides is effective in causing mediator release from human lung or gut mast cells, but C5a and f-Met-Leu-Phe can induce histamine release from human skin mast cells (Lawrence *et al.*, 1987).

Morphine and other narcotics represent examples of pharmacological agents that can induce mast cell mediator release, but predominantly from skin mast cells (Lawrence *et al.*, 1987; Tharp *et al.*, 1987). In this respect, the agents are similar to neuropeptides, which can trigger mediator release from human skin mast cells but not significantly from human basophils or gut or lung mast cells (see above). It is therefore of some interest that the intravenous infusion of large doses of morphine regularly causes an increase in plasma histamine levels and often results in shock (Galli and Lichtenstein, 1988). Since the only mast cell in the body that seems to respond to morphine, including those from the heart, is the skin mast cell, these findings indicate that the rather selective activation of cutaneous mast cells may be sufficient to induce clinically significant systemic responses. The human skin mast cell also differs from other human mast cells or basophils is exhibiting responsiveness to the classic secretagogue of rat peritoneal mast cells, compound 48/80 (Lawrence *et al.*, 1987).

4.3. Induction or Modulation of Basophil or Mast Cell Mediator Release by Cytokines

A considerable body of evidence now indicates that cytokines can directly release and/or augment IgE-stimulated mediator release in mast cells and basophils, but often with markedly different responses in each cell type. Among these agents, members of the chemokine cytokine superfamily and stem cell factor appear to be particularly important. Chemokines, which can be produced by T cells, B cells, macrophages, mast cells, and eosinophils, as well as other cell types, are basic heparin-binding polypeptides which share significant structural similarities and have potent proinflammatory biological activities (Wolpe and Cerami, 1989; Oppenheim *et al.*, 1991). Members of both the C-C branch of this family [including macrophage inflammatory protein (MIP)-1α and β, monocyte chemotactic and activating factor (MCAF), RANTES, and I-309], as well as the C-X-C branch of this group [including connective tissue-activating peptide (CTAP)-III, and its derivative, neutrophil activating peptide (NAP)-2] are potent basophil secretagogues (Dahinden *et al.*, 1989; Reddigari *et al.*, 1992; Kuna *et al.*, 1992; Bischoff *et al.*, 1992; Alam *et al.*, 1992a,b). MCAF,MIP-1α, CTAP-III, and NAP-2 all cause direct, dose-dependent histamine release from basophils (Dahinden *et al.*, 1989; Reddigari *et al.*, 1992; Kuna *et al.*, 1992; Bischoff *et al.*, 1992a; Alam *et al.*, 1992a,b), and some of them also enhance anti-IgE induced basophil mediator release. MIP-1α also has been reported to induce histamine release from mouse mast cells, but only in certain mouse strains (Alam *et al.*, 1992b).

Recently, MCAF, RANTES, and IL-3 have been demonstrated to be the predominant constituents of mononuclear cell supernatants which exhibit histamine-releasing activity for basophils, suggesting that chemokines may account for a significant fraction of the bioactivities which previously have been attributed to uncharacterized "histamine-releasing factors" (Kuna *et al.*, 1993). Interestingly, another member of the C-X-C group, IL-8, can *inhibit* the release of histamine from basophils in response to certain stimuli (Kuna *et al.*, 1991).

IL-1, 3, 5, or GM-CSF also have been shown to cause basophil histamine release directly, or to enhance the basophil histamine release that is observed in response to other stimuli. IL-3 or GM-CSF can directly induce the release of histamine and LTC_4 from basophils, as well as increase the response of basophils to anti-IgE, FMLP, calcium ionophores, or C3a (Haak-Frendscho *et al.*, 1988; Hirai *et al.*, 1988; MacDonald *et al.*, 1989; Alam *et al.*, 1989; Bischoff *et al.*, 1990a). Although it does not directly induce release, IL-5 can prime basophils for enhanced release of histamine and LTC_4 in response to other agonists (Hirai *et al.*, 1990; Bischoff *et al.*, 1990b). The *in vivo* relevance of these observations is not clear. For example, in clinical trails of IL-3 or GM-CSF, no adverse events that might be attributable to excessive histamine release or augmented basophil releasability have been reported, with the possible exception of facial flushing seen in two patients who received recombinant IL-3 (Ganser *et al.*, 1991; Antman, 1990). IL-1 has been reported to induce the release of histamine from human adenoidal mast cells, although the magnitude of the response was small (< 10%) (Subramanian and Bray, 1987). Preincubation of purified human lung mast cells with IL-1α can prime these cells for enhanced IgE-dependent release of LTC_4 and prostaglandin D_2 (Salari and Chan-Yeung, 1989).

SCF, perhaps the most important regulator of mast cell development *in vivo*, also can induce mediator release from some populations of mouse mast cells (Coleman *et al.*, 1993; Galli *et al.* 1991b) or rat mast cells (Nakajima *et al.*, 1992) *in vitro*, can augment the magnitude of mouse peritoneal mast cell mediator release in response to IgE-dependent activation *in vitro* (Coleman *et al.*, 1993), and can trigger mast cell activation, and a mast cell-dependent inflammatory response, when injected intradermally in mice *in vivo* (Wershil *et al.*, 1992). SCF also can influence human mast cell and basophil mediator release. *In vitro* studies of isolated human mast cells indicate that concentrations of rhSCF which are similar to the levels of endogenous SCF in the serum of normal subjects (~3 ng/ml) can induce low levels of histamine or PGD_2 release from skin (Columbo *et al.*, 1992) but perhaps not from lung (Bischoff and Dahinden, 1992) mast cells, and that brief (10 min to 1 hr) preincubation of skin or lung mast cells with even lower concentrations of rhSCF can significantly enhance the ability of these cells to release mediators in response to $Fc_{\varepsilon}RI$-dependent stimulation (Columbo *et al.*, 1992; Bischoff and Dahinden, 1992). In human basophils, rhSCF induces little or no mediator release directly, but short-term exposure of basophils to high concentrations of rhSCF can augment IgE-dependent mediator release from these cells (Columbo *et al.*, 1992).

In mice, activation of dermal mast cells by SCF *in vivo* is c-*kit* dependent and occurs at doses of cytokine as low as 140 fmole/site (Wershil *et al.*, 1992). We recently reported preliminary data suggesting that administration of rhSCF to humans *in vivo* may produce similar effects. In phase I trials, daily subcutaneous administration of rhSCF (10–50 μg/kg per day) for 14 days resulted in an ~50% increase in urine methylhistamine concentrations, but little or no change in circulating levels of mast cell tryptase (Costa *et al.*, 1993a). However, wheal and flare reactions commonly occurred at rhSCF injection sites (Demetri *et al.*, 1993; Costa *et al.*, 1994), and electron microscopic evaluation revealed extensive anaphylactic degranulation of cutaneous mast cells at these sites (Costa *et al.*, 1994). Other adverse events suggestive of mast cell activation and mediator release included upper airway symptoms such as cough, hoarseness or laryngeal spasm, and, in one patient, transient hypotension (Demetri *et al.*, 1993).

As noted above, the effects of endogenous SCF (or of long-term administration of rrSCF) on mast cell function may be quite complex. Indeed, we have shown that long-term administration of rrSCF to mice *in vivo* is associated with significantly *diminished* responsiveness of mast cells at rrSCF injection sites to IgE-dependent activation and *reduced* severity of IgE-dependent passive anaphylaxis (Ando *et al.*,

1993). We have suggested that levels of endogenous SCF may contribute to the regulation of the mast cell's responsiveness to activation of IgE and antigen, substance P (Wershil *et al.*, 1994), and perhaps other stimuli (Galli *et al.*, 1994) and/or may regulate the expression of mast cell cytokines, some of which may have autocrine effects on this cell type (Wershil *et al.*, 1992). Finally, there has been a long history of speculation that one "physiological" role of the mast cell is to release constitutively, perhaps by a process of vesicular transport, low levels of the same mediators which, when produced rapidly in larger quantities, result in the development of an inflammatory response (reviewed in Galli *et al.*, 1984). We have speculated that endogenous SCF may be able to regulate such mast cell secretory activity, and thus may influence the "physiological" function of this cell (Wershil *et al.*, 1992), as well as modulate its activity in IgE-dependent immune responses and allergic reactions.

5. THE ROLES OF BASOPHILS AND MAST CELLS IN HEALTH AND DISEASE

The actual roles of basophils and mast cells in health, disease, and host defense have been remarkably difficult to ascertain. In part, this reflects the rarity of "experiments of nature" affecting these populations. Few individuals lacking basophils have been reported, and such persons usually also have other abnormalities that potentially affect immune or inflammatory responses (Juhlin and Michaelsson, 1977; Tracey and Smith, 1978; Mitchell *et al.*, 1983). Thus, the role of the basophil defect in any clinical problems expressed by those patients is uncertain. We are not aware of reports of humans with a profound mast cell deficiency.

In the absence of information derived from patients with isolated abnormalities of basophil or mast cell numbers or function, concepts of the roles of these cells in human health and disease have been developed based on more indirect lines of evidence, including animal experiments. This work indicates that the major roles of basophils and mast cells in host defense are in the orchestration of local immunologic and inflammatory reactions, and that their major role in disease is to represent an important source of the mediators responsible for many reactions of immediate hypersensitivity and related disorders (Galli and Lichtenstein, 1988; Holgate *et al.*, 1993; Metcalfe *et al.*, 1981; Schwartz and Huff, 1993; Galli, 1990, 1993). The roles of basophils and mast cells are expressed primarily by the release to the exterior of preformed, cytoplasmic, granule-associated, cytokines or newly generated (lipid) mediators. Although the limited ability of basophils or mast cells to phagocytose bacteria and other particles has been reported, little evidence suggests that this represents an important aspect of their contribution to host defense or pathology. Similarly, although mast cells have been shown to have an activation-dependent respiratory burst akin to that of neutrophils, this is not believed to play a role in mast cell-mediated pathology at the present time.

Several studies indicate that basophils and mast cells can internalize and store in their granules certain products of other cell types, including eosinophil peroxidase (Dvorak *et al.*, 1985a,c). This mechanism may contribute to the limitation of the toxicity or other biologic activities of the internalized compounds, or alternatively may place the expression of the compounds' biologic activity under the regulation of signals that elicit basophil or mast cell degranulation.

5.1. Animal Models to Analyze Mast Cell Function

There are several reasons why proof of the importance of mast cells in specific immunological or pathological responses has been difficult to obtain (Galli *et al.*, 1992). Many "mast cell-associated" mediators are also produced by other cell types. As a result, even convincing evidence that one of these mediators has a critical role in a particular biological response is not, by itself, sufficient evidence that the mast cell is important in that response. Even pharmacological experiments employing antagonists of individual mast cell-associated mediators, or inhibitors of mast cell activation are limited by the strength of the evidence documenting that the effects of the drugs used are selective for the mast cell. Analysis of mast cell function *in vivo* is further complicated by the fact that mast cell activation usually results in the elaboration of multiple mediators, which may have diverse, and sometimes even opposing, biological effects. The *net* biological consequences of the combined activities of all of these mediators may be difficult to predict. Finally, the phenotypic heterogeneity of mast cell populations with regard to morphology, mediator content, and response to drugs and secretagogues suggests that phenotypically distinct mast cells may have different roles in health and disease (Galli, 1990).

Accordingly, we propose that the most direct approach for identifying and quantifying the specific roles of mast cells in biological responses *in vivo* is to search for differences in the expression of biological responses in anatomical sites that differ only in that one site contains mast cells and the other does not (Galli and Kitamura, 1987; Nakano *et al.*, 1985; Galli *et al.*, 1992). This general approach is summarized in Table VI. Briefly, if W/W^v and Sl/Sl^d mice express a particular biological response differently than do the congenic normal (+/+) mice, this may reflect the virtual absence of mature mast cells in the mutants or some other effect of their *W* or *Sl* mutations. Since adoptively transferred mast cell populations gradually acquire multiple phenotypic characteristics of the native mast cell populations present in the same anatomical sites in normal mice (Galli and Kitamura, 1987; Nakano *et al.*, 1985; Galli *et al.*, 1992), W/W^v mice selectively repaired of their mast cell deficiency by the injection of cultured, growth factor-dependent mast cells (i.e., BMCMCs) derived from congenic +/+ mouse bone marrow cells are especially valuable models for the investigation of mast cell function *in vivo*. This approach is particularly useful when the expression of biological responses can be evaluated in paired anatomical sites in the same mice, one site containing adoptively transferred mast cell populations and the other virtually devoid of mast cells.

Studies employing mast cell-reconstituted W/W^v mice have identified three

TABLE VI
General Scheme for Investigating Mouse Mast Cell Function *in Vivo*[a]

1. Search for quantitative differences in the expression of biological responses in genetically mast cell-deficient WBB6F$_1$-*W/W*^{v} and WCB6F$_1$-*Sl/Sl*^{d} mice and the congenic normal (+/+) mice.
2. Compare the responses in *W/W*^{v} mice and in *W/W*^{v} mice that have received bone marrow transplantation from congenic +/+ mice.
   Note: This determines whether the response that is abnormally expressed in *W/W*^{v} mice is influenced by mast cells and/or other cells derived from hematopoietic precursors.
3. Analyze the response in *W/W*^{v} mice that have been *selectively* reconstituted with mast cells ("mast cell knock-in mice").
   Note: This determines whether the response that is abnormally expressed in *W/W*^{v} mice has a mast cell-dependent component.
4. Define the mechanism(s) by which mast cells contribute to the response.

[a]Modified with permission from Galli, S.J., 1990, *Lab. Invest.* **62**:5.

patterns of mast cell involvement in biological responses (Galli *et al.*, 1992). In some reactions, mast cells appear to have an essential role, in that the responses are not detectably expressed in the absence of the mast cell. In other responses, mast cells appear to regulate the intensity and/or kinetics of the response, but the reactions can be detectably expressed in the absence of mature mast cells. In yet other responses, no specific mast cell-dependent contribution has been identified. For example, this approach has established that virtually all of the inflammation associated with IgE-dependent reactions elicited in mouse skin (Wershil *et al.*, 1987, 1991a) or stomach (Wershil *et al.*, 1991b) is mast cell-dependent, that immune resistance to the cutaneous feeding of larval *Haemaphysalis longicornis* ticks in mice requires IgE and mast cells (Matsuda *et al.*, 1990), and that mast cells are responsible for the bronchial hyper-responsiveness to methacholine observed after anti-IgE challenge in mice (Martin *et al.*, 1993a). Essentially all of the inflammation produced by intradermal injection of substance P also is mast cell dependent (Matsuda *et al.*, 1989; Yano *et al.*, 1989), whereas mast cells can significantly augment, but are not essential for, the inflammation induced by PMA (Wershil *et al.*, 1988) or immune complexes (Ramos *et al.*, 1990). By contrast, most analyses have detected no impairment of the expression of T cell-mediated contact hypersensitivity reactions in the skin of mast cell-deficient mice (Galli and Hammel, 1984; Mekori *et al.*, 1987).

5.2. Immediate Hypersensitivity

The immediate hypersensitivity reaction is the pathophysiologic hallmark of allergic rhinitis, allergic asthma, and anaphylaxis, and the central role of the mast cell in the pathogenesis of these disorders is widely accepted. To avoid confusion between immunologic mechanisms and clinical syndromes in the discussion of these disorders, we begin by defining some key terms.

5.2.1. Type I Hypersensitivity Reaction

As originally described by Gell and Coombs, this refers to a pathologic immune response that is initiated by the interaction of antigen-specific IgE molecules located on the surface of mast cells and/or basophils with the relevant multivalent antigen. The physiologic effects of Type I reactions (synonyms: allergic reaction, immediate hypersensitivity) are the result of the biologic responses of target cells (e.g., vascular endothelial cells, smooth muscle, glands, leukocytes) to mediators released by activated mast cells and/or basophils. The term "Type I immediate hypersensitivity reaction" describes an immunopathologic *mechanism*, and conveys no information as the degree (mild versus severe) or distribution (local versus systemic) of the reaction. In addition, because a population of mast cells/basophils that possess surface-bound antigen-specific IgE is required for the expression of a response to that antigen, *prior exposure* to that antigen (or to another molecule possessing an immunologically identical epitope) resulting in the development of IgE-secreting plasma cells must precede the occurrence of a true Type I reaction.

5.2.2. Immediate or Early Phase Responses

The signs and symptoms that develop at the site of antigen exposure within the first few minutes of a Type I reaction reflect the biological activities of the mast cell or basophil-derived mediators which are released immediately after the activation of these cells. In sites that do not contain basophils, such as normal skin, these mediators are derived largely, perhaps exclusively, from mast cells. Thus, in most allergic patients, intradermal challenge with specific antigen or anti-IgE induces an immediate wheal and flare reaction, accompanied by intense pruritis, which reaches a maximum 15–30 min later (Galli and Lichtenstein, 1988; Schwartz and Huff, 1993; Atkins, 1989; Lemanske and Kaliner, 1993). Such immediate allergic reactions are usually accompanied by an increase in local levels of LTC_4 and PGD_2, as well as the liberation of histamine and tryptase (Schwartz and Huff, 1993; Atkins, 1989; Lemanske and Kaliner, 1993). Although there are several possible cellular sources for some of these mediators, tryptase is thought to be strictly mast cell-derived, providing the strongest biochemical evidence implicating mast cells in these responses in humans. Human Langerhans cells also express $Fc_{\varepsilon}RI$ (Bieber *et al.*, 1992; Wang *et al.*, 1992), but it is not clear whether these cells represent a significant source of the mediators that orchestrate the development of cutaneous IgE-dependent early phase responses.

The symptoms associated with the early phase reactions that occur at other locations reflect local and sometimes unique anatomic responses to this same panel of mediators (Naclerio *et al.*, 1985). Thus, nasal reactions are characterized by sneezing, rhinorhea, congestion, and pruritis, while pulmonary responses may be limited to bronchospasm and possibly bronchorrhea.

Studies in "mast cell knock-in mice" showed that essentially all of the augmented vascular permeability, tissue swelling, and deposition of cross-linked ^{125}I-labeled fibrin associated with IgE-dependent passive cutaneous anaphylaxis reactions (Wershil *et al.*, 1987), or IgE-dependent reactions in the stomach wall (Wershil and Galli, 1989), were mast cell-dependent. In humans, mast cell participation in the immediate phase of Type I reactions in multiple anatomical sites has been clearly established by several lines of evidence, including studies that have demonstrated release of both histamine and tryptase, with a strong correlation between levels of these two mediators, in the nasal secretions or skin blister fluids that were induced by exposure to allergen (Alter and Schwartz, 1989). Such findings support the concept that mast cells may be essential for the expression of IgE-dependent immediate phase responses in humans, as well as in mice.

5.2.3. Anaphylaxis

Traditionally, this term has been used to describe an antigen-specific, IgE-mediated reaction that is both severe (life-threatening) and systemic (several organ systems involved) (Marquardt and Wasserman, 1993). In this context, anaphylaxis could be considered to represent a severe, systemic Type I immediate hypersensitivity reaction. However, because degranulation of mast cells and/or basophils may occur via *non*-IgE-dependent mechanisms, and because the biological effects of the liberated mast cell and/or basophil mediators are the same regardless of the mechanism by which they are released, the term *anaphylaxis* preferably should be used to describe a *clinical syndrome* that is severe, abrupt, and manifest by cutaneous (urticaria/angioedema), respiratory (asthma, laryngeal edema), cardiovascular (hypotension, cardiovascular collapse), and/or gastrointestinal (nausea, vomiting, diarrhea, cramping) signs and symptoms occurring singly or in combination (Marquardt and Wasserman, 1993). When used in this fashion, the term does not imply any particular pathologic mechanism. The older term, *anaphylactoid*, which has been used to describe reactions with the *clinical* features of anaphylaxis (as above), but which are thought to be mediated independently of IgE, can be confusing and therefore its use is to be discouraged.

Several lines of evidence indicate that systemic anaphylaxis in humans can be associated with extensive mast cell activation. For example, increased levels of mast cell tryptase were detected in the serum samples obtained 1–4 hr after the onset of anaphylactic symptoms in six patients (9–75 ng/ml) (Schwartz *et al.*, 1987). By contrast, little or no tryptase (<5 ng/ml) was detected in serum from normal controls (Enander *et al.*, 1991) or from patients with myocardial disease or sepsis, including some with profound hypotension or shock. These findings, and other studies of serum tryptase levels during anaphylaxis (Schwartz *et al.*, 1989; van der Linden *et al.*, 1992), leave little doubt that mast cells are activated during systemic anaphylaxis in humans. However, the histamine that is detected in the plasma of patients with anaphylaxis may be derived from both mast cells and basophils. Studies in genetically mast cell-deficient mice indicate that mast cells are required for some forms of IgE-dependent anaphylaxis, whereas other examples of fatal systemic anaphylaxis can occur independently of this cell type (reviewed in Takeishi *et al.*, 1991; Martin *et al.*, 1993b). It is not yet clear, however, to what extent basophils contribute to the latter responses.

5.2.4. Late-Phase Responses

In many allergic patients, the immediate reaction to cutaneous antigenic challenge is followed 4–8 hr later by a period of persistent swelling and leukocyte infiltration termed the *late-phase reaction* (LPR) (Atkins, 1989; Lemanske and Kaliner, 1993). It is now clear that an LPR may develop following IgE-dependent reactions in the respiratory tract, nose, and other anatomical locations, as well as in the skin. Moreover, many of the clinically significant consequences of IgE-dependent reactions, both in the respiratory tract and in the skin, are now thought to reflect the actions of the leukocytes that are recruited to these sites during LPRs, rather than the direct effects of the mediators released by mast cells at early intervals after antigen challenge (Galli and Lichtenstein, 1988; Galli, 1993; Atkins, 1989; Lemanske and Kaliner, 1993).

On the other hand, several lines of evidence, derived from both clinical and animal studies, suggest that the leukocyte infiltration associated with LPRs occurs as a result of mast cell degranulation. Thus, studies in mast cell knock-in mice have demonstrated that both the early phase of tissue swelling associated with IgE-dependent cutaneous reactions, as well as the subsequent influx of leukocytes at these sites (which reached maximal levels 6–12 hr after antigen challenge), are essentially entirely mast cell-dependent (Wershil *et al.*, 1991a). Furthermore, the injection of rabbit anti-TNF-α antisera at sites of IgE-dependent cutaneous mast cell activation diminished the leukocyte infiltration observed at the reactions by ~50% (Wershil *et al.*, 1991a). This study thus provided rather compelling evidence indicating that mast cell production of a cytokine, in this case, TNF-α, can importantly contribute to the expression of a mast cell-dependent biological response.

In humans, the leukocytes that are recruited to sites of LPRs include basophils, eosinophils, neutrophils, and macrophages; all of these cells may influence the reactions by providing additional proinflammatory mediators and cytokines. The recruitment of basophils to LPRs provides these responses with an $FC_{\varepsilon}RI^{+}$ cell type, in addition to the mast cell, which can release biologically active mediators in response to the antigen present at these sites. Increased numbers of basophils can be observed several hours after allergen challenge of nasal secretions of patients with allergic rhinitis, the bronchoalveolar lavage fluid of patients with asthma, or in skin windows or skin test sites in patients with atopic dermatitis (Mitchell and Askenase, 1983; Bascom *et al.*, 1988; Liu *et al.*, 1991; Guo *et al.*, 1994). In many of these settings, analysis of fluids obtained several hours after antigen challenge demonstrates elevations in histamine, TAME-esterase activity, and LTC_4,but not PGD_2 or tryptase; such findings provide further evidence for the involvement of basophils in these LPRs (Naclerio *et al.*, 1985; Liu *et al.*, 1991; Guo *et al.*, 1994). Moreover, the extent of basophil recruitment into nasal secretions during experimental antigen-induced nasal

LPRs is proportional to the intensity of the symptoms that are associated with these reactions (Bascom *et al.*, 1988).

Basophil recruitment into sites of tissue inflammation is thought to reflect the actions of chemotactic factors (such as C5a or cytokines of the chemokine group; see Section 4.4 and Lett-Brown *et al.*, 1976; Ward *et al.*, 1975), as well as interactions between complementary adhesion molecules expressed on the surface of the basophil (e.g., VLA-4, CD11/18, and glycoproteins that contain the sialyl-Lewis^{X} moiety) and vascular endothelial cells [e.g., VCAM-1, ICAM-1, and E-selectin (ELAM-1)]. The expression of these molecules is subject to complex regulatory mechanisms *in vivo*, which probably include effects of cytokines (e.g., TNF-α, IL-1) and other products derived from activated mast cells. For example, treatment of human umbilical vein endothelial cells (HUVEC) with either TNF-α or IL-1 increases their ability to bind basophils (Bochner *et al.*, 1988). Stimulation of basophils with anti-IgE or antigen also results in increased basophil adherence to HUVEC, increased basophil expression of CD11b and CD11c, and decreased basophil expression of Leu-8 antigen (Bochner *et al.*, 1989; Bochner and Sterbinsky, 1991). Notably, shedding of Leu-8 has been proposed as the mechanism by which basophils, after their attachment to vascular endothelium, are subsequently released to migrate through the vascular wall and into the interstitium (Bochner and Sterbinsky, 1991). Finally, IL-3 treatment of basophils, but not neutrophils, leads to a rapid and sustained increase in cell surface expression of CD11b (Mac 1) (Bochner *et al.*, 1990), suggesting that the local production of IL-3 during allergic reactions may contribute to the basophil recruitment that occurs at these sites.

5.2.5. Chronic Allergic Inflammation

In patients with chronic atopic disease, including allergic asthma, allergic rhinitis, and atopic dermatitis, the sites of pathology contain complex inflammatory infiltrates which include T cells (particularly those that produce the "TH_2"-type pattern of cytokines that can promote allergic responses; Kay, 1992; Romagnani, 1991), monocytes/macrophages, eosinophils, and neutrophils, as well as mast cells and basophils. It is likely that all of these participants significantly influence the course of these disorders and, in aggregate, contribute to the local development of the pathology associated with these conditions. While the recruitment and function of some of these leukocytes may be regulated by mechanisms that are largely independent of the activity of mast cells and basophils, recent findings suggest that mast cell and basophil products may play a larger role in the chronic manifestations of allergic inflammation than previously had been supposed.

As noted above, IgE-dependent activation induces mouse mast cells to release TNF-α and a broad panel of other multifunctional cytokines (Gordon *et al.*, 1990a; Costa *et al.*, 1992), and human mast cells also can produce TNF-α (Steffen *et al.*, 1989; Klein *et al.*, 1989; Walsh *et al.*, 1991; Ohkawara *et al.*, 1992; Benyon *et al.*, 1991) and perhaps many other cytokines (Bradding *et al.*, 1992, 1993). On appropriate activation, human basophils can produce IL-4 (Brunner *et al.*, 1993; Arock *et al.*, 1993). In aggregate, such cytokines can influence many aspects of the pathophysiology at sites of allergic diseases, including some of the chronic changes (e.g., fibrosis) associated with these disorders (reviewed in Galli, 1993; Gordon *et al.*, 1990a; Costa *et al.*, 1992; Galli *et al.*, 1991a). Furthermore, given that mast cell degranulation results in the local release of proteoglycans that can bind a variety of growth factors (Ruoslahti and Yamaguchi, 1991), $Fc_{\varepsilon}RI$-mediated mast cell activation may also regulate the function, concentration, and spatial distribution of cytokines and growth factors (whether derived from mast cells or other sources) within the tissue microenvironment. In other words, the traditional concept of the "self-limited allergic reaction," which was thought to reflect the release of mast cell mediators whose biological half-lives were measured in minutes or hours, must now be recognized as incomplete. Indeed, the complex and temporally prolonged consequences of cytokine expression, when considered together with the potential long-term effects of some of the cells' other mediators, suggest that mast cell activation may importantly contribute to many of the chronic features of allergic diseases and other disorders that are associated with mast cell activation. Many other factors probably also contribute to the chronicity of allergic inflammation, including prolonged or repeated exposure to relevant allergens and perhaps the diminished threshold for mast cell activation which can be observed *in vivo* after even a single antigenic challenge.

5.3. Asthma

Approximately 80–90% of individuals who develop asthma prior to 30 years of age have an allergic etiology for their disease. Several lines of evidence indicate that mast cells importantly contribute to the initiation and maintenance of the pathology of allergic asthma. Studies in genetically mast cell-deficient and congenic normal mice indicate that some IgE-mediated responses that produce changes in pulmonary function similar to those observed in allergic asthma are entirely mast cell-dependent (Ando *et al.*, 1993; Takeishi *et al.*, 1991), and tests in mast cell knock-in mice show that the enhanced bronchial reactivity to methacholine that is observed after anti-IgE challenge in mice is also completely mast cell-dependent (Martin *et al.*, 1993a).

In patients with allergic asthma, evidence of mast cell degranulation is provided by elevated levels of histamine and tryptase in the BAL fluid of patients with moderately symptomatic asthma (Broide *et al.*, 1991) and in BAL fluids after endobronchial allergen challenge (Wenzel *et al.*, 1988). Moreover, a recent study of 17 children with mild to moderate chronic asthma showed a strong correlation between bronchial hyperresponsiveness to histamine and levels of mast cell tryptase in their BAL fluid (Ferguson *et al.*, 1992). However, in contrast to earlier reports, recent studies with highly specific monoclonal antibodies have *not* demonstrated any significant differences in the numbers of MC_T or MC_{TC} mast cells in the airway mucosa of atopic asthmatics, atopic nonasthmatics, or healthy control subjects (Bradley *et al.*, 1991). This finding indicates that significant mast cell hyperplasia is unlikely to have an important role in the etiology of allergic asthma.

In light of the extended time course of release observed for some mast cell-derived cytokines, the potent proinflammatory properties of these products, and the amplification and prolongation of the response that is achieved by the recruitment of additional effector cell types, each of them capable of contributing additional mediators to the ongoing inflammatory response, there is growing agreement that the local elaboration of multiple cytokines, by many different cell types, importantly contributes to the pathophysiology of asthma. Indeed, we have proposed that much of the cytokine production in such settings may reflect the long-term consequences of ongoing or repeated IgE-dependent mast cell activation, through the effects of mast cell–leukocyte cytokine cascades (Galli, 1993; Gordon *et al.*, 1990; Galli *et al.*, 1991a). TNF-α may be especially important in these reactions, since this cytokine can be produced by both mast cells and eosinophils (Costa *et al.*, 1993b), and can enhance nonspecific bronchial hyperresponsiveness (Kips *et al.*, 1992), as well as mediate many proinflammatory effects. This hypothesis is supported by studies in a nonhuman primate model of asthma, which demonstrated that a monoclonal antibody to ICAM-1, a leukocyte adherence structure whose expression on the surface of vascular endothelial cells can be augmented by IL-1 or TNF-α, attenuated both airway eosinophilia and airway hyperresponsiveness (Wegner *et al.*, 1990). In a subsequent study, inhalation allergen challenge of nonhuman primates induced rapid expression of E-selectin exclusively on vascular endothelial cells, an event that was correlated with the influx of neutrophils into the lungs and the onset of late-phase airway obstruction. Moreover, a monoclonal antibody to E-selectin, but not a monoclonal antibody to ICAM-1, blocked both neutrophil influx and the pulmonary LPR (Gundel *et al.*, 1991).

Clearly, however, cells other than mast cells also represent potentially important sources of cytokines in the chronic allergic inflammation that is characteristic of allergic asthma. One such alternative source of cytokines is the eosinophil, which can produce TGF-α (Wong *et al.*, 1990; Liu *et al.*, 1992), TGF-β (Wong *et al.*, 1991), IL-1 (del Pozo *et al.*, 1990; Weller *et al.*, 1993), IL-3 (Kita *et al.*, 1991), IL-5 (Desreumaux *et al.*, 1992; Broide *et al.*, 1992), IL-6 (Hamid *et al.*, 1992), GM-CSF (Kita *et al.*, 1991; Moqbel *et al.*, 1991; Broide *et al.*, 1992), TNF-α (Costa *et al.*, 1993b), and MIP-1α (Costa *et al.*, 1993b); another is the lymphocyte. For example, BAL fluid cells from mild atopic asthmatics show increased expression of IL-2, 3, 4, and 5 and GM-CSF mRNA by ISH compared with nonatopic controls, and T lymphocytes appear to represent the predominant type of IL-4 or IL-5-positive cells (Robinson *et al.*, 1992). Moreover, the frequency of allergen-specific T lymphocytes is elevated in the peripheral blood of asthmatics with or without late-phase pulmonary responses, and these levels are directly correlated with allergen PC_{15} values in bronchoprovocation studies (Burastero *et al.*, 1993).

Although the discovery that activated mast cells and basophils can elaborate multifunctional cytokines, and the emerging appreciation of the potential importance of these molecules in allergic inflammation, have captured center stage, it should be kept in mind that the other mast cell and basophil mediators may importantly influence disease pathophysiology. In this regard, recent preclinical studies of a

TABLE VII
Conditions Associated with Basophilopenia or Basophilia[a]

Condition	Effect on blood basophil levels
Anaphylaxis, urticaria (certain cases)	↓
Severe acute illnesses (myocardial infarction, pneumonia, bleeding peptic ulcer)	↓ (acute phases) ↑ (during recovery)
Administration of ACTH or corticosteroids	↓
Administration of thyroid hormone, thyrotoxicosis	↓
Ovulation	↓
Lipemia	↓
Chronic myeloid leukemia (and basophilic leukemia)	Markedly ↑, especially terminally
Other myeloproliferative disorders (myeloid metaplasia, polycythemia vera)	Moderately ↑
Systemic mast cell disease	↑ (in a minority of patients)
Drug allergies	Slightly ↑ (chronic phase)
Ulcerative colitis	Slightly ↑
Juvenile rheumatoid arthritis	Slightly ↑
Myxedema	Slightly ↑

[a]Reproduced with permission from Galli, S.J., and Goetzl, E.J., 1995, In: *Blood: Principles and Practice of Hematology* (R.I. Handin, S.E. Lux, and T.P. Stossel, eds.), Lippincott, Philadelphia, in press.

selective 5-lipoxygenase inhibitor (BI-L-239) demonstrated dose-dependent inhibition of inhaled allergen-induced LTC_4 release into BAL fluid, as well as reductions in late-phase bronchoconstriction, neutrophil infiltration, and airway hyperresponsiveness (Wegner *et al.*, 1993). It should also be emphasized that while recent studies support a central role for mast cell-derived products in allergen-induced asthma, mast cells may not be important participants in asthma resulting from other etiologies. For example, analysis of BAL fluid obtained from patients with exercise-induced asthma 1 or 24 hr after exercise challenge revealed no changes in the numbers or types of cells in BAL fluids, or in the levels of BAL fluid histamine or tryptase (Jarjour *et al.*, 1992).

5.4. Parasitic Diseases

Several lines of evidence indicate that mast cells or basophils participate in adaptive immunological responses against parasites. Infection with helminthic parasites is associated with increased levels of parasite-specific IgE and nonspecific IgE, as well as mast cell hyperplasia (Jarrett and Miller, 1982; Askenase, 1980). Moreover, the ability of worm antigens to cause degranulation of mast cells obtained from parasite-infected animals, as well as the toxic properties of some mast cell mediators on these parasites, are well documented (Jarrett and Miller, 1982; Askenase, 1980). Finally, some mast cell- or basophil-derived mediators, including histamine and serotonin, have physiological effects on vascular permeability, intestinal ion and mucus secretion, and/or gut motility, which might enhance local expressions of host defense against parasites (Jarrett and Miller, 1982; Askenase, 1980). Accordingly, it has been hypothesized that mast cell and basophil sensitization by parasite-specific IgE, followed by mast cell and basophil degranulation in response to exposure to parasite antigens, promotes the expulsion of the parasites (Jarrett and Miller, 1982; Askenase, 1980).

In accord with this hypothesis, studies of *Trichinella spiralis* or *Strongyloides ratti* infections, as well as some experiments with the roundworm *Nippostrongylus brasiliensis*, showed that the duration of these experimental parasite infections was prolonged in mast cell-deficient mice when compared to the results in normal animals (reviewed in Reed, 1989). However, the impairment of immunity in mast cell-deficient mice was never as severe as in athymic nude mice, and, in each instance, the mast cell-deficient mice eventually were able to resolve the infection (Reed, 1989). Moreover, the successful elimination of parasites in the absence (or virtual absence) or a specific IgE response has also been reported (Jacobson *et al.*, 1977; Watanabe *et al.*, 1988). Thus, several lines of evidence indicate that mucosal mast cell hyperplasia and activation may contribute to host defense against certain helminthic infections, but, in most cases, mast cells may not represent an essential component of these immune responses.

The most compelling evidence for a role for mast cells or basophils in defense against parasites is in immune responses to ectoparasites such as ticks. However, the relative importance of basophils or mast cells as effectors in these reactions to ticks may vary according to the species of host and the species of tick. Studies utilizing mast cell knock-in mice have demonstrated that IgE and mast cells are essential for the expression of immune resistance to the cutaneous feeding of larval *Haemaphysalis longicornis* ticks (Matsuda *et al.*, 1990). In contrast, basophils may be more important than mast cells in immune resistance to the feeding of a different tick species (*Dermacentor variabilis*) in mice (Steeves and Allen, 1990), and both basophils and eosinophils appear to be required for immune resistance to the feeding of larval *Amblyomma americanum* ticks in guinea pigs (Brown *et al.*, 1982). Finally, there has been a single report of a patient who lacked basophils and eosinophils (and expressed an IgA deficiency) and who suffered from severe scabies (Juhlin and Michaelsson, 1977). These and other findings support the concept that resident mast cells and recruited basophils may have similar, overlapping, or complementary functions in immune responses to ectoparasites, worms, and perhaps other parasites, with the relative contributions of each cell type varying according to the type of parasite, species of host animal, or other factors (Galli and Askenase, 1986).

5.5. Arthritis

Mast cells are present in normal human synovium, but their numbers can be increased one- to tenfold in a variety of arthritides, including those associated with syphilis or tuberculosis, juvenile rheumatoid arthritis, adult rheumatoid arthritis, systemic lupus erythematosus, mixed connective tissue disease, osteoarthritis, psoriatic arthritis, post-intestinal bypass arthropathy, and chronic villonodular synovitis (Bromley *et al.*, 1984; Okada, 1973; Crisp *et al.*, 1984; Godfrey *et al.*, 1984; Woolley *et al.*, 1989; Gruber *et al.*, 1989). Mast cells are also present in the synovial fluid during some of these conditions (Freemont and Denton, 1985; Malone *et al.*, 1986, 1987). Malone examined synovial tissue from 20 patients with rheumatoid arthritis and demonstrated positive correlations between the number of mast cells and either the extent of lymphocytic infiltration or the number of synovial T helper/inducer lymphocytes (Malone *et al.*, 1987). The intra-articular injection of corticosteroids in some of these patients resulted in 67–96% decrease in the number of identifiable synovial mast cells (Malone *et al.*, 1987).

Based on the biological effects of mast cell-derived mediators, it has been suggested that mast cells might contribute to the inflammation and tissue remodeling that is observed in these disorders (Woolley *et al.*, 1989; Gruber *et al.*, 1989). Indeed, Malone and Metcalfe have recently demonstrated that mast cells may participate in the development of experimental arthritis in rats via an IgE-dependent mechanism (Malone and Metcalfe, 1988). On the other hand, the relative importance of mast cells, as opposed to other cell types, in the pathogenesis of rheumatoid arthritis or other naturally occurring arthridites remains to be determined.

5.6. Nerve–Mast Cell Interactions

The biological significance of potential interactions between nerves and mast cells has been the subject of considerable speculation (Bienenstock *et al.*, 1989; Stead *et al.*, 1989b; Arizono *et al.*, 1990). Morphological studies have documented a very close anatomical association between mast cells and nonmyelinated nerves, particularly in the gastrointestinal tract; in many instances, such nerves contain substance P, CGRP, and/or other neuropeptides (reviewed in Bienenstock *et al.*, 1989; Arizono *et al.*, 1990; Stead *et al.*, 1987, 1989b). And several lines of evidence indicate that the close anatomical relationship between mast cells and certain nerves may be functionally significant. Antidromic electrical stimulation (ES) of sensory nerves in the rat induces dilatation and augmented permeability of cutaneous blood vessels, and also results in degranulation of cutaneous mast cells (Kiernan, 1977). Direct neural stimulation can result in degranulation of mucosal mast cells in rat glandular stomach (Cho *et al.*, 1985) or ileum (Bani-Sacchi *et al.*, 1986), and systemic release of MMCP II, an indicator of activation of rat gastrointestinal mast cells (Woodbury *et al.*, 1989), can be elicited in appropriately sensitized animals after Pavlovian conditioning (MacQueen *et al.*, 1989). Such findings have supported the concept that some of the psychological factors which can result in the exacerbation of allergic asthma and other atopic disorders may reflect, at least in part, the effects of neural activity on mast cell function (Bienenstock *et al.*, 1989; Stead *et al.*, 1989b; MacQueen *et al.*, 1989).

To evaluate whether nerve–mast cell interactions might significantly influence physiologic responses in the gastrointestinal tract, Perdue *et al.* (1991) studied epithelial Cl^- secretion *ex vivo* in intestinal tissue from genetically mast cell-deficient W/W^v

mice, the congenic normal (+/+) mice, and *W/W*^{v} mice that had undergone repair of their gastrointestinal mast cell deficiency by adoptive transfer of bone marrow cells from the congenic +/+ mice. This study showed that ~50% of the Cl^- response to transmural electrical activation of jejunal tissues, as opposed to ~70% of the Cl^- response to antigen stimulation, was mast cell-dependent. This work thus directly supported the hypothesis that physiological responses in the gastrointestinal tract can be regulated by nerve–mast cell interactions.

Several different neuropeptides that can induce alterations in vascular tone and/or permeability when injected *in vivo* also can stimulate degranulation of a variety of human and rodent mast cell populations *in vitro* or *in vivo* (reviewed in Yano *et al.*, 1989). Cutaneous mast cells are particularly sensitive to stimulation by substance P, which can induce a wheal and flare response when injected into human skin in doses as low as 10 pmole. Pharmacological studies indicate that this flare response is largely mediated by histamine, suggesting that such effects may reflect neuropeptide-dependent mast cell degranulation. However, the more prolonged wheal component of the reaction occurs through a combination of histamine-dependent and histamine-independent mechanisms (reviewed in Foreman and Jordan, 1983; Foreman, 1987). Studies in genetically mast cell-deficient *W/W*^{v} mice, the congenic normal (+/+) mice, and *W/W*^{v} mice locally and selectively repaired of their cutaneous mast cell deficiency by the adoptive transfer of *in vitro*-derived mast cells of +/+ origin indicate that all of the augmented vascular permeability, tissue swelling, fibrin deposition, and leukocyte infiltration associated with the intradermal injection of substance P is mast cell-dependent (Matsuda *et al.*, 1989; Yano *et al.*, 1989). Since the tissue swelling and induration perceived clinically as a wheal probably largely reflects the local extravasation of fibrinogen and the subsequent development of a fibrin gel at the reaction site, the demonstration that mast cells are required for essentially all of the fibrinogen extravasation and fibrin deposition at sites of i.d. substance P injection in mice suggests that, in humans, mast cell products other than histamine may contribute to the development of the wheal at sites of i.d. injection of substance P.

Several lines of evidence now indicate that mast cell products also might downregulate certain vascular changes induced by release of neuropeptides. The rat CTMC protease RMCP I can effectively hydrolyze a variety of polypeptides *in vitro*, including neurotensin (Le Trong *et al.*, 1987). Although RMCP I does not effectively degrade substance P (Le Trong *et al.*, 1987), proteases isolated from dog mastocytoma cells can hydrolyze this peptide (Caughey *et al.*, 1988). Moreover, hydrolysis of polypeptides by RMCP I is particularly resistant to inhibition by rat serum or α1-antitrypsin when the protease remains associated with the mast cell granules, as it would under physiologic conditions *in vivo* (Le Trong *et al.*, 1987). *In vivo* studies indicate that degranulated rat cutaneous mast cells may be able to degrade the potent vasodilator calcitonin gene-related peptide (CGRP) (Brian and Williams, 1988), which can occur together with substance P in the same nerves (Gibbins *et al.*, 1985; Lundberg *et al.*, 1985). Moreover, the duration of vasodilation which follows injection of CGRP into rat or human skin is markedly diminished when substance P is injected at the same time, suggesting that substance P-induced mast cell degranulation can result in attenuation of CGRP-induced vasodilation (Brain and Williams, 1988).

These examples by no means exhaust the potentially important interactions between neuropeptides, mast cells, and the nervous system (Stead *et al.*, 1989b; Goetzl *et al.*, 1989). Indeed, certain populations of mast cells may themselves be able to generate molecules similar to neuropeptides (Goetzl *et al.*, 1989; Wershil *et al.*, 1993). Nor do we wish to imply that all aspects of "neurogenic inflammation" are mast cell-dependent, as this is very unlikely (Kowalski and Kaliner, 1988). However, the available evidence does illustrate how particular phenotypic characteristics of individual populations of mast cells may permit them to participate in both the augmentation and the subsequent downregulation of certain manifestations of neuropeptide-induced inflammation.

5.7. Roles in Other Pathological Responses

While the reactivity of basophils and certain mast cell populations to activation by f-Met-Leu-Phe or anaphylatoxins suggests that these cells may contribute to host responses to bacteria or to reactions associated with complement activation, the clinical significance of these potential roles for basophils and mast cells is uncertain. Studies in genetically mast cell-deficient and congenic normal mice indicate that mast cells are not required for the expression of gastrointestinal smooth muscle contraction in response to C3a or C5a (Stimler-Gerard and Galli, 1987). Nor are mast cells required for the inflammation associated with cutaneous reactions associated with local complement activation; however, mast cells can augment the magnitude of the inflammation associated with these responses (Ramos *et al.*, 1990). In light of these studies, we would suggest that the relative importance of mast cells and basophils as sources of mediators during pathologic reactions associated with complement activation may vary considerably depending on the specific characteristics of the response. For example, it is unclear whether human basophils and mast cells represent important sources of mediators during the IgE-independent anaphylaxis that is associated with immune complex formation.

Mast cells or basophils or their products have been implicated in a bewildering variety of diseases (e.g., scleroderma, pulmonary fibrosis of diverse etiology, inflammatory bowel disease, and peptic ulcer disease), adaptive immune responses, responses to toxic agents, and reparative responses, such as wound healing (reviewed in Galli and Lichtenstein, 1988; Holgate *et al.*, 1993; Metcalfe *et al.*, 1981; Schwartz and Huff, 1993; Galli, 1990; Selye, 1965; Bienenstock *et al.*, 1986; Wershil and Galli, 1992). However, few of these roles have been evaluated using mast cell knock-in mice. Accordingly, the importance of the mast cell or the basophil in these reactions, if any, remains to be determined.

ACKNOWLEDGMENTS. We thank Ann M. Dvorak, M.D., for providing the electron micrograph. Some of the work reviewed herein was supported by United States Public

Health Service grants AI 22674, AI 23990, AI 31982, AI 33372, and HL 02240, by AMGEN, Inc., and by the Beth Israel Hospital Pathology Foundation.

REFERENCES

Ackerman, S. J., Weil, G. J., and Gleich, G. W., 1982, Formation of Charcot–Leyden crystals by human eosinophils, *J. Exp. Med.* **155:**1609.

Ackerman, S. J., Corrette, S. E., Rosenberg, H. F., Bennett, J. C., Mastrianni, D. M., Nicholson-Weller, A., Weller, P. F., Chin, D. T., and Tenen, D. G., 1993, Molecular cloning and characterization of human eosinophil Charcot–Leyden crystal protein (lysophospholipase). Similarities to IgE binding proteins and the S-type animal lectin superfamily, *J. Immunol.* **150:**456.

Agis, H., Willheim, M., Sperr, W. R., Wilfing, A., Kromer, E., Kabrna, E., Spanblochl, E., Strobl, H., Geissler, K., Spitler, A., Boltz-Nitulescu, G., Majdic, O., Lechner, K., and Valent, P., 1993, Human blood monocytes do not make mast cells when cultured in the presence of SCF: Characterization of the circulating mast cell progenitor cell, *J. Immunol.* **151:**4221.

Aglietta, M., Camussi, G., and Piacibello, W., 1981, Detection of basophils growing in semisolid agar culture, *Exp. Hematol.* **9:**95.

Alam, R., Welter, J. B., Forsythe, P. A., Lett-Brown, M. A., and Grant, J. A., 1989, Comparative effect of recombinant IL-1, -2, -3, -4 and -6, IFN-γ, granulocyte–macrophage-colony-stimulating factor, tumor necrosis factor-α, and histamine-releasing factors on the secretion of histamine from basophils, *J. Immunol.* **142:**3431.

Alam, R., Lett-Brown, M. A., Forsythe, P. A., Anderson-Walters, D. J., Kenamore, C., Kormos, C., and Grant, J. A., 1992a, Monocyte chemotactic and activating factor is a potent histamine-releasing factor for basophils, *J. Clin. Invest.* **89:**723.

Alam, R., Forsythe, P. A., Stafford, S., Lett-Brown, M. A., and Grant, J. A., 1992b, Macrophage inflammatory protein-1α activates basophils and mast cells, *J. Exp. Med.* **176:**781.

Alter, S. C., and Schwartz, L. B., 1989, Tryptase: An indicator of mast cell-mediated allergic reactions, *Prov. Chall. Proc.* **167:**183.

Anderson, D. M., Lyman, D. S., Baird, A., Wignall, J. M., Eisenman, J., Rauch, C., March, C. J., Boswell, H. S., Grimpel, S. D., and Cosman, D., 1990, Molecular cloning of mast cell growth factor, a hematopoietin that is active in both membrane bound and soluble forms, *Cell* **63:**235.

Ando, A., Martin, T. R., and Galli, S. J., 1993, Effects of chronic treatment with the c-kit ligand, stem cell factor, on immunoglobulin E-dependent anaphylaxis in mice: Genetically mast cell-deficient Sl/Sl^d mice acquire anaphylactic responsiveness, but the congenic normal mice do not exhibit augmented responses, *J. Clin. Invest.* **92:**1639.

Antman, K. H., 1990, G-CSF and GM-CSF in clinical trials, *Yale J. Biol. Med.* **63:**387.

Arizono, N., Matsuda, S., Hattori, T., Kojima, Y., Maeda, T., and Galli, S. J., 1990, Anatomical variation in mast cell nerve associations in the rat small intestine, heart, lung, and skin. Similarities of distances between neural processes and mast cells, eosinophils, or plasma cells in the jejunal lamina propria, *Lab. Invest.* **62:**626.

Arock, M., Merle-Beral, H., Dugas, B., Ouaaz, F., Le Goff, L., Vouldoukis, I., Mencia-Huerta, J.-M., Schmitt, C., Leblond-Missenard, V., Debre, P., and Mosslayi, M. D., 1993, IL-4 release by human leukemic and activated normal basophils, *J. Immunol.* **151:**1441.

Askenase, P. W., 1980, Immunopathology of parasitic diseases: Involvement of basophils and mast cells, *Springer Semin. Immunopathol.* **2:**417.

Atkins, P. C., 1989, Cutaneous late phase responses—An allergic inflammatory response, *Allergy Proc.* **10:**417.

Bani-Sacchi, T., Barattini, M., Bianchi, S., Blandina, P., Brunelleschi, S., Fantozzi, R., Mannaioni, P. F., and Masini, E., 1986, The release of histamine by parasympathetic stimulation in guinea-pig auricle and rat ileum, *J. Physiol (London)* **371:**29.

Bascom, R., Wachs, M., Naclerio, R. M., Pipkorn, U., Galli, S. J., and Lichtenstein, L. M., 1988, Basophil influx occurs after nasal antigen challenge: Effects of topical corticosteroid pretreatment, *J. Allergy Clin. Immunol.* **81:**580.

Beaven, M. A., and Metzger, H., 1993, Signal transduction by Fc receptors: The Fc epsilon RI case, *Immunol. Today* **14:**222.

Benhamou, M., and Siraganian, R. P., 1992, Protein-tyrosine phosphorylation: An essential component of Fc RI signalling, *Immunol. Today* **13:**195.

Benyon, R. C., Bissonette, E. Y., and Befus, A. D., 1991, Tumor necrosis factor-α dependent cytotoxicity of human skin mast cells is enhanced by anti-Ige antibiotics, *J. Immunol.* **147:**2253.

Besmer, P., 1991, The kit ligand encoded at the murine Steel locus: A pleiotropic growth and differentiation factor, *Curr. Opin. Cell Biol.* **3:**939.

Bieber, T., de la Salle, H., Wollenberg, A., Hakimi, J., Chizzonite, R., Ring, J., Hanau, D., and de la Salle, C., 1992, Human epidermal Langerhans' cells express the high affinity receptor for immunoglobulin E (Fc RI), *J. Exp. Med.* **175:**1285.

Bienenstock, J., Befus, A. D., and Denburg, J. A., 1986, Mast cell heterogeneity: Basic questions and clinical applications, in: *Mast Cell Differentiation and Heterogeneity* (A. D. Befus, J. Bienenstock, and J. A. Denburg, eds.), Raven Press, New York, pp. 391–402.

Bienenstock, J., Blennerhassett, M., Kakuta, Y., MacQueen, G., Marshall, J., Perdue, M., Siegel, S., Tsuda, T., Denburg, J., and Stead, R., 1989, Evidence for central and peripheral nervous system interaction with mast cells, in: *Mast Cell and Basophil Differentiation and Function in Health and Disease* (S. J. Galli and K. F. Austen, eds.), Raven Press, New York, pp. 275–284.

Bischoff, S. C., and Dahinden, C. A., 1992, c-kit ligand, a unique potentiator of mediator release by human lung mast cells, *J. Exp. Med.* **175:**237.

Bischoff, S. C., de Weck, A. L., and Dahinden, C. A., 1990a, Interleukin 3 and granulocyte-colony-stimulating factor render human basophils responsive to low concentrations of complement component C5a, *Proc. Natl. Acad. Sci. USA* **87:**6813.

Bischoff, S. C., Brunner, T., de Weck, A. L., and Dahinden, C. A., 1990b, Interleukin 5 modifies histamine release and leukotriene generation by human basophils in response to diverse agonists, *J. Exp. Med.* **172:**1577.

Bischoff, S. C., Krieger, M., Brunner, T., and Dahinden, C. A., 1992, Monocyte chemotactic protein 1 is a potent activator of human basophils, *J. Exp. Med.* **175:**1271.

Bochner, B. S., and Sterbinsky, S. A., 1991, Altered expression of CD11 and Leu 8 during human basophil degranulation, *J. Allergy Clin. Immunol.* **87:**302, #649 (abstract).

Bochner, B. S., Peachell, P. T., Brown, K. E., and Schleimer, R. P., 1988, Adherence of human basophils to cultured umbilical vein vascular endothelial cells, *J. Clin. Invest.* **81:**1355.

Bochner, B. S., MacGlashan, D. W., Marcotte, G. V., and Schleimer, R. P., 1989, IgE-dependent regulation of human basophil adherence to vascular endothelium, *J. Immunol.* **142:**3180.

Bochner, B. S., McKelvey, A. A., Sterbinsky, S. A., Hildreth, J. E., Derse, C. P., Klunk, D. A., Lichtenstein, L. M., and Schleimer, R. P., 1990, IL-3 augments adhesiveness for endothelium and CD11b expression in human basophils not neutrophils, *J. Immunol.* **145:**1832.

Bradding, P., Feather, I. H., Howarth, P. H., Mueller, R., Roberts, J. A., Britten, K., Bews, J. P. A., Hunt, T. C., Okayama, Y., Heusser, C. H., Bullock, G. R., Church, M. K., and Holgate, S. T., 1992, Interleukin 4 is localized to and released by human mast cells, *J. Exp. Med.* **176:**1381.

Bradding, P., Feather, I. H., Wilson, S., Bardin, P. G., Heusser, C. H., Holgate, S. T., and Howarth, P. H., 1993, Immunolocalization of cytokines in the nasal mucosa of normal and perennial rhinitis subjects, *J. Immunol.* **151:**3855.

Bradley, B. L., Azzawi, M., Jacobson, M., Assoufi, B., Collins, J. V., Irani, A.-M.A., Schwartz, L. B., Durham, S. R., Jeffery, P. K., and Kay, A. B., 1991, Eosinophils, T-lymphocytes, mast cells, neutrophils, and macrophages in bronchial biopsy specimens from atopic subjects with asthma: Comparison with biopsy specimens from atopic subjects without asthma and normal control subjects and relationship to bronchial hyperresponsiveness, *J. Allergy Clin. Immunol.* **88:**661.

Brain, S. D., and Williams, T. J., 1988, Substance P regulates the vasodilator activity of calcitonin gene-related peptide, *Nature* **335:**73.

Bressler, R. B., Thompson, H. L., Keffer, J. M., and Metcalfe, D. D., 1989, Inhibition of the growth of IL-3-dependent mast cells from murine bone marrow by recombinant granulocyte–macrophage-colony-stimulating factor, *J. Immunol.* **143:**135.

Broide, D. H., Wasserman, S. I., Alvaro-Garcia, J., Zvaifler, N. I., and Firestein, G. S., 1989, Transforming growth factor-b1 selectively inhibits IL-3-dependent mast cell proliferation without affecting mast cell function or differentiation, *J. Immunol.* **143:**1591.

Broide, D. H., Gleich, G. J., Cuomo, A. J., Coburn, D. A., Federman, E. C., Schwartz, L. B., and Wasserman, S. I., 1991, Evidence of ongoing mast cell and eosinophil degranulation in symptomatic asthma airway, *J. Allergy Clin. Immunol.* **88:**637.

Broide, D. H., Paine, M. M., and Firestein, G. S., 1992, Eosinophils express interleukin 5 and granulocyte macrophage-colony-stimulating factor mRNA at sites of allergic inflammation in asthmatics, *J. Clin. Invest.* **90:**1414.

Bromley, M., Fisher, W. D., and Woolley, D. E., 1984, Mast cells at sites of cartilage erosion in the rheumatoid joint, *Ann. Rheum. Dis.* **43:**76.

Brown, M. A., Pierce, J. H., Watson, C. J., Falco, J., Ihu, J. N., and Paul, W. E., 1987, B cell stimulatory factor-l/interleukin-4 mRNA is expressed by normal and transformed mast cells, *Cell* **50:**809.

Brown, S. J., Galli, S. J., Gleich, G. J., and Askenase, P. W., 1982, Ablation of immunity to Amblyomma americanum by anti-basophil serum: Cooperation between basophils and eosinophils in expression of immunity to extoparasites (ticks) in guinea pigs, *J. Immunol.* **129:**790.

Brunner, T., Heusser, C. H., and Dahinden, C. A., 1993, Human peripheral blood basophils primed by interleukin 3 (IL-3) produce IL-4 in response to immunoglobulin E receptor stimulation, *J. Exp. Med.* **177:**605.

Burastero, S. E., Fenoglio, D., Crimi, E., Brusasco, V., and Rossi, G. A., 1993, Frequency of allergen-specific T lymphocytes in blood and bronchial response to allergen in asthma, *J. Allergy Clin. Immunol.* **91:**1075.

Burd, P. R., Rogers, H. W., Gordon, J. R., Martin, C. A., Jayaraman, S., Wilson, S. D., Dvorak, A. M., Galli, S. J., and Dorf, M. E., 1989, Interleukin-3-dependent and -independent mast cells stimulated with IgE and antigen express multiple cytokines, *J. Exp. Med.* **170:**245.

Cass, F. M., Dixon, C. M., and Barnes, P. J., 1986, Inhaled platelet-activating factor causes bronchoconstriction and increased bronchial reactivity in man, *Am. Rev. Respir. Dis.* **133:**A212.

Caughey, G. H., Leidig, F., Viro, N. F., and Nadel, J. A., 1988, Substance P and vasoactive intestinal peptide degranulation by mast cell tryptase and chymase, *J. Pharmacol. Exp. Ther.* **244:**133.

Cho, C. H., Hung, K. M., and Ogle, C. W., 1985, The aetiology of gastric ulceration induced by electrical vagal stimulation in rats, *Eur. J. Pharmacol.* **110:**211.

Chung, S. W., Wong, P. M. C., Shen-Ong, G., Pruscetti, S., Ishizaka, T., and Eaves, C. J., 1968, Production of granulocyte–macrophage colony-stimulating factor by Abelson virus-induced tumorigenic mast cell lines, *Blood* **68:**1074.

Church, M. K., Benyon, R. C., Rees, P. H., Lowman, M. A., Campbell, A. M., Robinson, C., and Holgate, S. T., 1989, Functional heterogeneity of human mast cells, in: *Mast Cell and Basophil Differentiation and Function in Health and Disease* (S. J. Galli and K. F. Austen, eds.), Raven Press, New York, pp. 161–170.

Coleman, J. W., Holliday, M. R., Kimber, I., Zsebo, K. M., and Galli, S. J., 1993, Regulation of mouse peritoneal mast cell secretory function by stem cell factor, IL-3 or IL-4, *J. Immunol.* **150:**556.

Columbo, M., Horowitz, E. M., Botana, L. M., MacGlashan, D. W., Jr., Bochner, B. S., Gillis, S., Zsebo, K. M., Galli, S., and Lichtenstein, L. M., 1992, The recombinant human c-kit receptor ligand, rhSCF, induces mediator release from human cutaneous mast cells and enhances IgE-dependent mediator release from both skin mast cells and peripheral blood basophils, *J. Immunol.* **149:**599.

Costa, J. J., Burd, R. P., and Metcalfe, D. D., 1992, Mast cell cytokines, in: *The Role of the Mast Cell in Health and Disease* (M. A. Kaliner and D. D. Metcalfe, eds.), Dekker, New York, pp. 443–466.

Costa, J. J., Demetri, G. D., Hayes, D. F., Merica, E. A., Menchaca, D. M., and Galli, S. J., 1993a, Increased skin mast cells and urine methyl histamine in patients receiving recombinant methionyl human stem cell factor, *Proc. Am. Assoc. Cancer Res.* **34:**211 (abstract).

Costa, J. J., Matossian, K., Resnick, M. B., Beil, W. J., Wong, D. T. W., Gordon, J. R., Dvorak, A. M., Weller, P. F., and Galli, S. J., 1993b, Human eosinophils can express the cytokines tumor necrosis factor-α and macrophage inflammatory protein-1α, *J. Clin. Invest.* **91:**2673.

Costa, J. J., Demetri, G. D. Harris, T. J., Dvorak, A. M., Hayes, D. F., Merica, E. A., Menchaca, D. M., Gringeri, A. J., and Galli, S. J., 1994, Recombinant human stem cell factor (rhSCF) induces cutaneous mast cell activation and hyperplasia, and hyperpigmentation in human in vivo, *J. Allergy Clin. Immunol.* **93:**225a.

Crisp, A. J., Chapman, C. M., Kirkham, S. E., Schiller, A. L., and Krane, S. M., 1984, Articular mastocytosis in rheumatoid arthritis, *Arthritis Rheum.* **27:**845.

Dahinden, C., Kurimoto, Y., de Weck, A. L., Lindley, I., Dewald, B., and Baggiolini, M., 1989, The neutrophil-activating peptide NAF/NAP-1 induces histamine and leukotriene release by interleukin-3 primed basophils, *J. Exp. Med.* **170:**1787.

del Pozo, V., de Andres, B., Martin, E., Maruri, N., Zubeldia, J. M., Palomino, P., and Lahoz, C., 1990, Murine eosinophils and IL-1: αIL-1 mRNA detection by in situ hybridization: Production and release of IL-1 from peritoneal eosinophils, *J. Immunol.* **144:** 3117.

Dembo, M., Goldstein, B., Sobotka, A. K., and Lichtenstein, L. M., 1979, Degranulation of human basophils: Quantitative analysis of histamine release and desensitization, due to a bivalent penicilloyl hapten, *J. Immunol.* **123:**1864.

Demetri, G., Costa, J., Hayes, D., Sledge, G., Galli, S., Hoffman, R., Merica, E., Rich, W., Harkins, B., McGuire, B., and Gordon, M., 1993, A phase I trial of recombinant methionyl human stem cell factor (SCF) in patients with advanced breast carcinoma pre- and post-chemotherapy (CHEMO) with cyclophosphamide (C) and doxorubicin (A), *Proc. Am. Soc. Clin. Oncol.* **12:**A367 (abstract).

Denburg, J. A., 1990, Cytokine-induced human basophil/mast cell growth and differentiation in vitro, *Springer Semin. Immunopathol.* **12:**401.

Denburg, J. A., Richardson, M., Telizyn, S., and Bienenstock, J., 1983, Basophil/mast cell precursors in human peripheral blood, *Blood* **61:**775.

Desreumaux, P., Janin, A., Colombel, J. F., Prin, L., Plumans, J., Emilie, D., Torpier, G., and Capron, M., 1992, Interleukin-5 messenger RNA expression by eosinophils in the intestinal mucosa of patients with coeliac disease, *J. Exp. Med.* **175:**293.

Dvorak, A. M., 1991, *Basophil and Mast Cell Degranulation and Recovery*, Volume 4, Plenum Press, New York.

Dvorak, A. M., and Ackerman, S. J., 1989, Ultrastructural localization of the Charcot–Leyden crystal protein (lysophospholipase) to granules and intragranular crystals in mature human basophils, *Lab. Invest.* **60:**557.

Dvorak, A. M., Mihm, M. C., Jr., and Dvorak, H. F., 1976, Morphology of delayed-type hypersensitivity reactions in man. II. Ultrastructural alterations affecting the microvasculature and the tissue mast cells, *Lab. Invest.* **34:**179.

Dvorak, A. M., Newball, H. H., Dvorak, H. F., and Lichtenstein, L. M., 1980, Antigen-induced IgE-mediated degranulation of human basophils, *Lab. Invest.* **43:**126.

Dvorak, A. M., Lett-Brown, M., Thueson, D., and Grant, J. A., 1981, Complement-induced degranulation of human basophils, *J. Immunol.* **126:**523.

Dvorak, A. M., Nabel, G., Pyne, K., Cantor, H., Dvorak, H. F., and Galli, S. J., 1982, Ultrastructural identification of the mouse basophil, *Blood* **59:**1279.

Dvorak, A. M., Galli, S. J., Schulman, E. S., Lichtenstein, L. M., and Dvorak, H. F., 1983a, Basophil and mast cell degranulation: Ultrastructural analysis of mechanisms of mediator release, *Fed. Proc.* **42:**2510.

Dvorak, A. M., Dvorak, H. F., and Galli, S. J., 1983b, Ultrastructural criteria for identification of mast cells and basophils in humans, guinea pigs, and mice, *Am. Rev. Respir. Dis.* **128:**S49.

Dvorak, A. M., Dvorak, H. F., Peters, S. P., Schulman, E. S., MacGlashan, D. W., Jr., Pyne, K., Harvey, V. S., Galli, S. J., and Lichtenstein, L. M., 1983c, Lipid bodies: Cytoplasmic organelles important to arachidonate metabolism in macrophages and mast cells, *J. Immunol.* **131:**2965.

Dvorak, A. M., Hammel, I., Schulman, E. S., Peters, S. P., MacGlashan, D. W., Jr., Schleimer, R. P., *et al.*,

1984, Differences in the behavior of cytoplasmic granules and lipid bodies during human lung mast cell degranulation, *J. Cell Biol.* **99:**1678.

Dvorak, A. M., Ishizaka, T., and Galli, S. J., 1985a, Ultrastructure of human basophils developing in vitro. Evidence for the acquisition of peroxidase by basophils, and for different effects of human and murine growth factors on human basophil and eosinophil maturation, *Lab. Invest.* **53:**57.

Dvorak, A. M., Schulmann, E. S., Peters, S. P., MacGlashan, D. W., Jr., Newball, H. H., Schleimer, R. P., and Lichtenstein, L. M., 1985b, Immunoglobulin E-mediated degranulation of isolated human lung mast cells, *Lab. Invest.* **53:**45.

Dvorak, A. M., Klebanoff, S. J., Henderson, W. R., Monahan, R. A., Pyne, K., and Galli, S. J., 1985c, Vesicular uptake of eosinophil peroxidase by guinea pig basophils and by cloned mouse mast cells and granule-containing lymphoid cells, *Am. J. Pathol.* **118:**425.

Dvorak, A. M., Furitsu, T., and Ishizaka, T., 1993a, Ultrastructural morphology of human mast cell progenitors in sequential cocultures of cord blood cells and fibroblasts, *Int. Arch. Allergy Immunol.* **100:**219.

Dvorak, A. M., Seder, R. A., Paul, W. E., Kissell-Rainville, S., Plaut, M., and Galli, S. J., 1993b, Ultrastructural characteristics of Fc R-positive basophils in the spleen and bone marrow of mice immunized with goat anti-mouse IgD antibody, *Lab. Invest.* **68:**708.

Ehrlich, P., 1878, Beitrage zur Theorie und Praxis der histologischen Farbung, Leipzig, Thesis.

Ehrlich, P., 1879, Uber die spezifischen Granulationen de Blutes, *Arch. Anat. Physiol. Abt.* 571.

Enander, I., Matsson, P., Nystrand, J., Andersson, A. S., Eklund, E., Bradford, T. R., and Schwartz, L. B., 1991, A new radioimmunoassay for human mast cell tryptase using monoclonal antibodies, *J. Immunol. Methods* **138:**39.

Enerbäck, L., 1986, Mast cell heterogeneity: The evolution of the concept of a specific mucosal mast cell, in: *Mast Cell Differentiation and Heterogeneity* (A. D. Befus, J. Bienenstock, and J. A. Denburg, eds.), Raven Press, New York, pp. 1–26.

Enerbäck, L., Pipkom, U., Aldenborg, F., and Wingren, U., 1989, Mast cell heterogeneity in man: Properties and function of human mucosal mast cells, in: *Mast Cell and Basophil Differentiation and Function in Health and Diseases* (S. J. Galli and K. F. Austen, eds.), Raven Press, New York, pp. 27–37.

Everitt, M., and Neurath, H., 1980, Rat peritoneal mast cell carboxypeptidase: Localization, purification, and enzymatic properties, *FEBS Lett.* **110:**292.

Ferguson, A. C., Whitelaw, M., and Brown, H., 1992, Correlation of bronchial eosinophil and mast cell activation with bronchial hyperresponsiveness in children with asthma, *J. Allergy Clin. Immunol.* **90:**609.

Flanagan, J. G., and Leder, P., 1990, The kit ligand: A cell surface molecule altered in Steel mutant fibroblasts, *Cell* **62:**185.

Flanagan, J. G., Chan, D. C., and Leder, P., 1991, Transmembrane form of the kit ligand growth factor is determined by alternative splicing and is missing in the Sl^d mutant, *Cell* **64:**1025.

Foreman, J. C., 1987, Substance P and calcitonin gene-related peptide: Effects on mast cells and in human skin, *Int. Arch. Allergy Appl. Immunol.* **82:**366.

Foreman, J. C., and Jordan, C. C., 1983, Histamine release and vascular changes induced by neuropeptides, *Agents Actions* **13:**105.

Freemont, A. J., and Denton, J., 1985, Disease distribution of synovial fluid mast cells cytophagocytic mononuclear cells in inflammatory arthritis, *Ann. Rheum. Dis.* **44:**312.

Furitsu, T., Saito, H., Dvorak, A. M., Schwartz, L. B., Irani, A. M. A., Burdick, J. F., Ishizaka, K., and Ishizaka, T., 1989, Development of human mast cells in vitro, *Proc. Natl. Acad. Sci. USA* **86:**10039.

Galli, S. J., 1990, New insights into the "riddle of mast cells": Microenvironmental regulation of mast cell development and phenotypic heterogeneity, *Lab. Invest.* **62:**5.

Galli, S. J., 1993, New concepts about the mast cell, *N. Engl. J. Med.* **328:**257.

Galli, S. J., and Askenase, P. W., 1986, Cutaneous basophil hypersensitivity, in: *The Reticuloendothelial System: A Comprehensive Treatise* (P. Abramoff, S. M. Phillips, and M. R. Escobar, eds.), Plenum Press, New York, pp. 321–369.

Galli, S. J., and Dvorak, A. M., 1995, Production, biochemistry, and function of basophils and mast cells, in:

Williams Hematology, 5th ed. (E. Beutler, M. A. Lichtman, B. S. Coller, and T. J. Kipps, eds.), McGraw–Hill, New York, pp. 805–810.

Galli, S. J., and Hammel, I., 1984, Unequivocal delayed hypersensitivity in mast cell-deficient and beige mice, *Science* **226:**710.

Galli, S. J., and Kitamura, Y., 1987, Animal model of human disease. Genetically mast cell-deficient W/W^v and S/Sl^d mice: Their value for the analysis of the roles of mast cells in biological responses in vivo, *Am. J. Pathol.* **127:**191.

Galli, S. J., and Lichtenstein, L. M., 1988, Biology of mast cells and basophils, in: *Allergy: Principles and Practice*, 3rd ed. (E. Middleton, Jr., C. E. Reed, E. F. Ellis, N. F. Adkinson, Jr., and J. W. Yunginger, eds.), Mosby, St. Louis, pp. 106–134.

Galli, S. J., Dvorak, A. M., and Dvorak, H. F., 1984, Basophils and mast cells: Morphologic insights into their biology, secretory patterns, and functions, *Prog. Allergy* **34:**1.

Galli, S. J., Gordon, J. R., and Wershil, B. K., 1991a, Cytokine production by mast cells and basophils, *Curr. Opin. Immunol.* **3:**865.

Galli, S. J., Tsai, M., Langley, K. E., Zsebo, K. M., and Geissler, E. N., 1991b, Stem cell factor (SCF), a ligand for c-kit, induces mediator release from some populations of mouse mast cells, *FASEB J.* **5:**A1092.

Galli, S. J., Geissler, E. N., Wershil, B. K., Gordon, J. A., Tsai, M., and Hammel, I., 1992, Insights into mast cell development and function derived from analyses of mice carrying mutations at beige, W.c-kit or Sl/SCF (c-kit ligand) loci, in: *The Role of the Mast Cell in Health and Disease* (M. A. Kalinger and D. D. Metcalfe, eds.), Dekker, New York, pp. 129–202.

Galli, S. J., Iemura, A., Garlick, D. S., Gamba-Vitalo, C., Zsebo, K. M., and Andrews, R. G., 1993, Reversible expansion of primate mast cell populations in vivo by stem cell factor, *J. Clin. Invest.* **91:**148.

Galli, S. J., Zsebo, K. M., and Geissler, E. N., 1994, The kit ligand, stem cell factor, *Adv. Immunol.* **55:**1.

Ganser, A., Lindemann, A., Seipelt, G., Ottmann, O. G., Herrmann, F., Eder, M., Frisch, J., Schulz, G., Mertelsmann, R., and Hoelzer, D., 1990, Effects of recombinant human interleukin-3 in patients with normal hematopoiesis and in patients with bone marrow failure, *Blood* **76:**666.

Ganser, A., Lindemann, A., Seipelt, G., Ottmann, O. G., Herrmann, F., Eder, M., Frisch, J., Schulz, G., Mertelsmann, R., and Hoelzer, D., 1991, Clinical effects of recombinant human interleukin-3, *Am. J. Clin. Oncol.* **14:**S51.

Gibbins, I. L., Furness, J. B., Costa, M., MacIntyre, I., Hillyard, C. J., and Girigis, S., 1985, Co-localization of calcitonin gene-related peptide-like immunoreactivity with substance P in cutaneous, vascular, and visceral sensory neurons of guinea pigs, *Neurosci. Lett.* **57:**125.

Gilbert, H. S., and Ornstein, L., 1975, Basophil counting with a new staining method using alcian blue, *Blood* **46:**279.

Godfrey, H. P., Ilardi, C., Engber, W., and Graziano, F. U., 1984, Quantitation of human synovial mast cells in rheumatoid arthritis and other rheumatic diseases, *Arthritis Rheum.* **27:**852.

Goetzl, E. J., Finch, R. J., Peterson, K. E., Turck, C. W., and Sneedharan, S. P., 1989, Mast cell and basophil mediation of lymphocytic functions, in: *Mast Cell and Basophil Differentiation and Function in Health and Disease* (S. J. Galli and K. F. Austen, eds.), Raven Press, New York, pp. 247–254.

Gordon, J. R., and Galli, S. J., 1990, Mast cells as a source of both preformed and immunologically inducible TNF-α-cachectin, *Nature* **346:**274.

Gordon, J. R., and Galli, S. J., 1991, Release of both preformed and newly synthesized tumor necrosis factor α (TNF-α)/cachectin by mouse mast cells stimulated by the Fc RI. A mechanism for the sustained action of mast cell-derived TNF-α during IgE-dependent biological responses, *J. Exp. Med.* **174:**103.

Gordon, J. R., Burd, P. R., and Galli, S. J., 1990, Mast cells as a source of multifunctional cytokines, *Immunol. Today* **11:**458.

Grant, J. A., Dupree, E., Goldman, A. S., Schultz, D. R., and Jackson, A. L., 1975, Complement-mediated release of histamine from human leukocytes, *J. Immunol.* **114:**1101.

Gruber, B. L., Marchese, M. J., Suzuji, K., Schwartz, L. B., Okada, Y., Nagase, H., and Ramamurthy, N. S., 1989, Synovial procollagenase activation by human mast cell tryptase dependence upon matrix metalloproteinase 3 activation, *J. Clin. Invest.* **84:**1657.

Gundel, R. H., Wegner, C. D., Torcellini, C. A., *et al.*, 1991, Endothelial leukocyte adhesion molecule-1 mediates antigen-induced acute airway inflammation and late phase airway obstruction in monkeys, *J. Clin. Invest.* **88:**1407.

Guo, C.-B., Liu, M. C., Galli, S. J., Bochner, B. S., Kagey-Sobotka, A., and Lichtenstein, L. M., 1994, Identification of Ige bearing cells in the late phase response to antigen in the lung as basophils, *Am. J. Respir. Cell Mol. Biol.* **10:**384.

Gurish, M. F., Ghildyal, N., Arm, J., Austen, K. F., Avraham, S., Reynolds, D., and Stevens, R. L., 1991, Cytokine mRNA are preferentially increased relative to secretory granule protein mRNA in mouse bone marrow-derived mast cells that have undergone IgE-mediated activation and degranulation, *J. Immunol.* **146:**1527.

Haak-Frendscho, M., Arai, N., Arai, K.-I., Baeza, M. L., Finn, A., and Kaplan, A. P., 1988, Human recombinant granulocyte–macrophage colony-stimulating factor and interleukin 3 cause basophil histamine release, *J. Clin. Invest.* **82:**17.

Haig, D. M., Huntley, J. F., MacKellar, A., Newlands, G. F. J., Inglis, L., Sangha, R., Cohen, D., Hapel, A., Galli, S. J., and Miller, H. R. P., 1994, Effects of stem cell factor (kit-ligand) and interleukin-3 on the growth and serine proteinase expression of rat bone marrow-derived or serosal mast cells, *Blood* **83:**72.

Hamid, Q., Barkans, J., Meng, Q., Ying, S., Abrams, J. S., Kay, A. B., and Moqbel, R., 1992, Human eosinophils synthesize and secrete interleukin-6, in vitro, *Blood* **80:**1496–1501.

Hayashi, S.-I., Kunisada, T., Ogawa, M., Yamaguchi, K., and Nishikawa, S.-I., 1991, Exon skipping by mutation of an authentic splice site of c-kit gene in W/W mouse, *Nucleic Acids Res.* **19:**1267.

Hirai, K., Morita, Y., Misaki, Y., Ohta, K., Takaishi, T., Suzuki, S., Motoyoshi, K., and Miyamoto, T., 1988, Modulation of human basophil histamine release by hemopoietic growth factors, *J. Immunol.* **141:**3958.

Hirai, K., Yamaguchi, M., Misaki, Y., Takaishi, T., Ohta, K., Morita, K., Ito, K., and Miyamoto, T., 1990, Enhancement of human basophil histamine release by interleukin 5, *J. Exp. Med.* **172:**1525.

Holgate, S. T., Robinson, C., and Church, M. K., 1993, Mediators of immediate hypersensitivity, in: *Allergy, Principles and Practice*, 4th ed. (E. Middleton, Jr., C. E. Reed, E. F. Ellis, N. F. Adkinson, Jr., J. W. Yunginger, and W. W. Burrs, eds.), Mobsy, St. Louis, pp. 267–301.

Hook, W. A., Schiffman, E., Aswaniklemar, S., and Siraganian, R. P., 1976, Histamine release by chemotactic formyl methionine-containing peptides, *J. Immunol.* **117:**594.

Huang, E., Nocka, K., Beier, D. R., Chu, T. Y., Buck, J., Lahm, H. W., Wellner, D., Leder, P., and Besmer, P., 1990, The hematopoietic growth factor KL is encoded at the Sl locus and is the ligand of the c-kit receptor, the gene product of the W locus, *Cell* **63:**225.

Hultner, L., Moeller, J., Schmitt, E., Jager, G., Reisbach, G., Ring, J., and Dormer, P., 1989, Thiol-sensitive mast cell lines derived from mouse bone marrow respond to a mast cell growth-enhancing activity different from both IL-3 and IL-4, *J. Immunol.* **142**:3440.

Hultner, L., Druez, C., Moeller, J., Uyttenhove, C., Schmitt, E., Ruce, E., Dormer, P., and Van Snick, J., 1990, Mast cell growth enhancing activity (MEA) is structurally related and functionally identical to the novel mouse T cell growth factor P40/TCGF III, *Eur. J. Immunol.* **20:**1413.

Humphries, R. K., Abraham, S., Krystal, G., Lansdorp, P., Lemolne, F., and Eaves, C. J., 1988, Activation of multiple hemopoietic growth factor genes in Abelson virus-transformed myeloid cells, *Exp. Hematol.* **16:**774.

Hutt-Taylor, S. R., Harnish, D., Richardson, M., Ishizaka, T., and Denburg, J. A., 1988, Sodium butyrate and a T-lymphocyte cell line-derived differentiation factor induce basophilic differentiation of the human promyelocytic leukemia cell line HL-60, *Blood* **71:**209.

Iemura, A., Tsai, M., Ando, A., Wershil, B. K., and Galli, S. J., 1994, The c-kit ligand, stem cell factor, promotes mast cell survival by suppressing apoptosis, *Am. J. Pathol.* **83:**72.

Irani, A. A., Schechter, N. M., Craig, S. S., DeBlois, G., and Schuartz, L. B., 1986, Two human mast cell subsets with distinct neutral protease compositions, *Proc. Natl. Acad. Sci. USA* **83:**4464.

Irani, A. A., Craig, S. S., DeBlois, G., Elson, C. O., Schechter, N. M., and Schwartz, L. B., 1987, Deficiency of the tryptase-positive, chymase-negative mast cell type in gastrointestinal mucosa of patients with defective T lymphocyte function, *J. Immunol.* **138:**4386.

Irani, A.-M. A., Nilsson, G., Mettinen, U., Craig, S. S., Ashman, L. K., Ishizaka, T., Zsebo, K. M., and Schwartz, L. B., 1992, Recombinant human stem cell factor stimulates differentiation of mast cells from dispersed fetal liver cells, *Blood* **80:**3009.

Ishizaka, T., 1988, Mechanisms of IgE-mediated hypersensitivity, in: *Allergy: Principles and Practice*, 3rd ed. (E. Middleton, Jr., C. E. Reed, E. F. Ellis, N. F. Adkinson, Jr., and J. W. Yunginger, eds.), Mosby, St. Louis, pp. 71–93.

Ishizaka, T., Dvorak, A. M., Conrad, D. H., Niebyl, J. R., Marquetti, J. P., and Ishizaka, K., 1985, Morphologic and immunologic characterization of human basophils developed in cultures of cord blood mononuclear cells, *J. Immunol.* **134:**532.

Jacobson, R. H., Reed, N. D., and Manning, D. D., 1977, Expulsion of Nippostrongylus, brasiliensis from mice lacking antibody production potential, *Immunology* **32:**867.

Jacoby, W., Cammarata, P. V., Findley, S., and Pincus, S. H., 1984, Anaphylaxis in mast cell-deficient mice, *J. Invest. Dermatol.* **83:**302.

Jarjour, N. N., Calhoun, W. J., Stevens, C. A., and Salisbury, S. M., 1992, Exercise-induced asthma is not associated with mast cell activation or airway inflammation, *J. Allergy Clin. Immunol.* **89:**60.

Jarrett, E. E. E., and Miller, H. R. P., 1982, Production and activities of IgE in helminth infections, *Prog. Allergy* **31:**178.

Johnson, L. A., Moon, K. E., and Eisenberg, M., 1968, Purification to homogeneity of the human skin chymotryptic proteinase "chymase," *Ann. Biochem.* **155:**358.

Juhlin, L., 1963, Basophil leukocyte differential in blood and bone marrow, *Acta Haematol.* **29:**89.

Juhlin, L., and Michaelsson, G., 1977, A new syndrome characterized by absence of eosinophils and basophils, *Lancet* **1:**1233.

Kanakura, Y., Thompson, H., Nakano, T., Yamamura, T., Asai, H., Kitamura, Y., Metcalfe, D. D., and Gaui, S. J., 1988, Multiple bidirectional alterations of phenotype and changes in proliferative potential during the in vitro and in vivo passage of clonal mast cell populations derived from mouse peritoneal mast cell, *Blood* **72:**877.

Kay, A. B., 1992, "Helper" (CD4+) T cells and eosinophils in allergy and asthma, *Am. Rev. Respir. Dis.* **145:**S22.

Kiernan, J. A., 1977, Study of chemically induced acute inflammation in the skin of the rat, *Q. J. Exp. Physiol.* **62:**151.

Kinet, J.-P., 1990, The high-affinity receptor for IgE, *Curr. Opin. Immunol.* **2:**499.

Kips, J. C., Tavernier, J., and Pauwels, R. A., 1992, Tumor necrosis factor causes bronchial hyperresponsiveness in rats, *Am. Rev. Respir. Dis.* **145:**332.

Kirschenbaum, A. S., Goff, J. P., Dreskin, S. C., Irani, A.-M., Schwartz, L. B., and Metcalfe, D. D., 1989a, Interleukin-3-dependent growth of basophil-like and mast-like cells from human bone marrow, *J. Immunol.* **42:**2424.

Kirshenbaum, A. S., Dreskin, S. C., and Metcalfe, D. D., 1989b, A staphylococcal protein A rosetting assay for the demonstration of high affinity IgE receptors on rIL-3-dependent human basophil-like cells grown in mixed culture, *J. Immunol.* **123:**55.

Kirshenbaum, A. S., Kessler, S. W., Goff, J. P., and Metcalfe, D. D., 1991, Demonstration of the origin of human mast cells from CD34+ bone marrow progenitor cells, *J. Immunol.* **146:**1410.

Kirshenbaum, A. S., Goff, J. P., Kessler, S. W., Mican, J. M., Zsebo, K. M., and Metcalfe, D. D., 1992, Effect of IL-3 and stem cell factor on the appearance of human basophil and mast cells from CD34+ pluripotent progenitor cells, *J. Immunol.* **148:**772.

Kita, H., Ohnishi, T., Okubo, Y., Weller, D., Abrams, J. S., and Gleich, G. J., 1991, Granulocyte/macrophage colony-stimulating factor and interleukin 3 release from human peripheral blood eosinophils and neutrophils, *J. Exp. Med.* **174:**745.

Kitamura, Y., 1989, Heterogeneity of mast cells and phenotypic changes between subpopulations, *Annu. Rev. Immunol.* **7:**59.

Kitamura, Y., and Go, S., 1979, Decreased production of mast cells in Sl/Sl^d mice, *Blood* **53:**492.

Kitamura, Y., Go, S., and Hatanaka, S., 1978, Decrease of mast cells in W/W^v mice and their increase by bone marrow transplantation, *Blood* **52:**447.

Kitamura, Y., Nakayama, H., and Fujita, J., 1989, Mechanisms of mast cell deficiency in mutant mice of W/W^v and S/Sl^d genotype, in: *Mast Cell and Basophil Differentiation and Function in Health and Disease* (S. J. Galli and K. F. Austen, eds.), Raven Press, New York, pp. 15–25.

Kjellen, L., and Lindahl, U., 1991, Proteoglycans: Structures and interactions, *Annu. Rev. Biochem.* **60:**443.

Klein, L. M., Lavker, R. M., Matis, W. L., and Murphy, G. F., 1989, Degranulation of human mast cells induces an endothelial antigen central to leukocyte adhesion, *Proc. Natl. Acad. Sci. USA* **86:**8972.

Kowalski, M. L., and Kaliner, M. A., 1988, Neurogenic inflammation, vascular permeability, and mast cells, *J. Immunol.* **140:**3905.

Kuna, P., Reddigari, S. R., Kornfield, D., and Kaplan, A. P., 1991, IL-8 inhibits histamine release from human basophils induced by histamine releasing factors, connective tissue activating peptide III, and IL-3, *J. Immunol.* **147:**1920.

Kuna, P., Reddigari, S. R., Rucinski, D., Oppenheim, J. J., and Kaplan, A. P., 1992, Monocyte chemotactic and activating factor is a potent histamine-releasing factor for human basophils, *J. Exp. Med.* **175:**489.

Kuna, P., Reddigari, S. R., Schall, T. J., Rucinski, D., Sadlick, M., and Kaplan, A. P., 1993, Characterization of the human basophil response to cytokines, growth factors, and histamine releasing factors of the intercrine/chemokine family, *J. Immunol.* **150:**1932.

Lagunoff, D., and Benditt, E. P., 1963, Proteolytic enzymes of mast cells, *Ann. N.Y. Acad. Sci.* **103:**185.

Lawrence, I. D., Warner, J. A., Cohan, V. L., Hubbard, W. C., Kagey-Sobotka, A., and Lichtenstein, L. M., 1987, Purification and characterization of human skin mast cells: Evidence for human mast cell heterogeneity, *J. Immunol.* **139:**3062.

Leary, A. G., Ikebuchi, K., Hirai, Y., Wong, A. A., Yang, Y. C., Clark, S. C., and Ogawa, M., 1988, Synergism between interleukin-6 and interleukin-3 in supporting proliferation of human hematopoietic stem cells: comparison with interleukin-1α, *Blood* **71:**1759.

Lee, F., Yokota, T., Otsuka, T., Meyerson, P., Villaret, D., Coffman, R., Mosmann, T., Rennick, D., Roehm, N., Smith, C., *et al.*, 1986, Isolation and characterization of a mouse interleukin cDNA clone that expresses B cell stimulatory factor 1 activities and T cell and mast cell stimulating activities, *Proc. Natl. Acad. Sci. USA* **83:**2061.

Lemanske, R. F., Jr., and Kaliner, M. A., 1993, Late phase allergic reactions, in: *Allergy: Principles and Practice*, 4th ed. (E. Middleton, Jr., C. E. Reed, E. F. Ellis, N. F. Adkinson, Jr., J. W. Yunginger, and W. W. Busse, eds.), Mosby, St. Louis, pp. 320–361.

Lerner, N. B., Nocka, K. H., Cole, S. R., Qui, F. H., Strife, A., Ashman, L. K., and Besmer, P., 1991, Monoclonal antibody YB5.B8 identifies the human c-kit protein product, *Blood* **77:**1876.

Le Trong, H., Neurath, H., and Woodbury, R. G., 1987, Substrate specificity of the chymotrypsin-like protease in secretory granules isolated from rat mast cells, *Proc. Natl. Acad. Sci. USA* **84:**364.

Lett-Brown, M. A., Boetcher, D. A., and Leonard, E. J., 1976, Chemotactic responses of normal human basophil to C5a and 5 lymphocyte-derived chemotactic factor, *J. Immunol.* **117:**246.

Leung, D. Y. M., Pober, J. S., and Cotrans, R. S., 1991, Expression of endothelial–leukocyte adhesion molecule-1 in elicited late phase allergic reactions, *J. Clin. Invest.* **87:**1805.

Levi-Schaffer, F., Austen, K. F., Gravallese, P. M., and Stevens, R. L., 1986, Co-culture of interleukin 3-dependent mouse mast cells with fibroblasts results in a phenotypic change of the mast cells, *Proc. Natl. Acad. Sci. USA* **83:**6485.

Lichtenstein, L. M., Schleimer, R. P., MacGlashan, D. W., Jr., *et al.*, 1984, In vitro and in vivo studies of mediator release from human mast cells, in: *Asthma III: Physiology, Immunopharmacology, and Treatment* (A. B. Kay, K. F. Austen, and L. M. Lichtenstein, eds.), Academic Press, New York, pp. 1–23.

Liu, M. C., Hubbard, W. C., Proud, D., Stealey, B. A., Galli, S. J., Kagey-Sobotka, A., Bleeker, E. R., and Lichtenstein, L. M., 1991, Immediate and late inflammatory responses to ragweed antigen challenge of the peripheral airways in allergic asthmatics: Cellular, mediator and permeability changes, *Am. Rev. Respir. Dis.* **144:**51.

Liu, M. C., Matossian, K., Wong, D. T. W., Weller, P. F., and Galli, S. J., 1992, Expression of mRNA for transforming growth factor-α (TGF-α) by eosinophils at sites of segmental airway challenge with antigen in allergic asthmatic subjects, *Am. Rev. Respir. Dis.* **145:**A452 (abstract).

Lundberg, J. M., Franco-Cereceda, A., Hua, X., Hokfeit, T., and Fischer, J. A., 1985, Co-existence of substance P and calcitonin gene-related peptide-like immunoreactivities in sensory nerves in relation to cardiovascular and bronchoconstrictor effects of capsaicin, *Eur. J. Pharmacol.* **108:**315.

McClure, W. O., Neurath, H., and Walsh, K. A., 1964, The reaction of carboxypeptidase A with hippuryl-DL-b-phenyl lactate, *Biochemistry* **3:**1897.

MacDonald, S. M., Schleimer, R. P., Kagey-Sobotka, A., Gillis, S., and Lichtenstein, L. M., 1989, Recombinant IL-3 induces histamine release from human basophils, *J. Immunol.* **142:**3527.

MacGlashan, D. W., Jr., and Lichtenstein, L. M., 1986, Characteristics of human basophil sulfidopeptide leukotriene release: Releasability defined as the ability of the basophil to respond to dimeric cross-links, *J. Immunol.* **136:**2231.

MacQueen, G., Marshall, J., Perdue, M., Siegal, S., and Bienenstock, J., 1989, Pavlovian conditioning of rat mucosal mast cells to secrete rat mast cell protease II, *Science* **243:**83.

Malone, D. G., and Metcalfe, D. D., 1988, Demonstration and characterization of transient arthritis in rats following sensitization of synovial mast cells with antigen-specific IgE and parenteral challenge with specific antigen, *Arthritis Rheum.* **31:**1063.

Malone, D. G., Irani, A.-M., Schwartz, L. B., Barrett, K. E., and Metcalfe, D. D., 1986, Mast cell numbers and histamine levels in synovial fluids from patients with diverse arthritides, *Arthritis Rheum.* **29:**956.

Malone, D. G., Wilder, R. L., Saavedra-Delgado, A. M., and Metcalfe, D. D., 1987, Mast cell numbers in rheumatoid synovial tissues. Correlations with quantitative measures of lymphocyte infiltration and modulation by anti-inflammatory therapy, *Arthritis Rheum.* **30:**130.

Marquardt, D. L., and Wasserman, S. I., 1993, Anaphylaxis, in: *Allergy: Principles and Practice*, 4th ed. (E. Middleton, Jr., C. E. Reed, E. F. Ellis, N. F. Adkinson, Jr., J. W. Yunginger, and W. W. Busse, eds.), Mosby, St. Louis, pp. 1525–1536.

Martin, T. R., Takeishi, T., Katz, H. R., Austen, K. F., Drazen, J. M., and Galli, S. J., 1993a, Mast cell activation enhances airway responsiveness to methacholine in the mouse, *J. Clin. Invest.* **9:**1176.

Martin, T. R., Ando, A., Takeishi, T., Katona, I. M., Drazen, J. M., and Galli, S. J., 1993b, Mast cells contribute to the changes in heart rate, but not hypotension or death associated with active anaphylaxis in mice, *J. Immunol.* **151:**367.

Matsuda, H., Kawakita, K., Kiso, Y., Nakano, T., and Kitamura, Y., 1989, Substance P induces granulocyte infiltration through degranulation of mast cells, *J. Immunol.* **142:**927.

Matsuda, H., Watanabe, N., Kiso, Y., Hirota, S., Ushio, H., Kannan, Y., Azuma, M., Koyama, H., and Kitamua, Y., 1990, Necessity of IgE antibodies and mast cells for manifestation of resistance against larval Haemaphysalis longicornis ticks in mice, *J. Immunol.* **144:**259.

Maximow, A., 1905, Uber dic Zellformen des lockeren Bindegewebes, *Arch. Mikrosk. Anat. Entwick lungsmech.* **67:**680.

Meininger, C. J., Yano, H., Rottapel, R., Bernstein, A., Zsebo, K. M., and Zetter, B. R., 1992, The c-kit receptor ligand functions as a mast cell chemoattractant, *Blood* **79:**958.

Mekori, Y. A., Chang, J. C. C., Wershil, B. K., and Galli, S. J., 1987, Studies of the role of mast cells in contact sensitivity responses. Passive transfer of the reaction into mast cell-deficient mice locally reconstituted with cultured mast cells: Effect of reserpine on transfer of the reaction with DNP-specific cloned T cells, *Cell. Immunol.* **109:**39.

Mekori, Y. A., Oh, C. K., and Metcalfe, D. D., 1993, IL-3-dependent murine mast cells undergo apoptosis on removal of IL-3, *J. Immunol.* **151:**3775.

Metcalfe, D. D., Kaliner, M., and Donlon, M. A., 1981, The mast cell, *CRC Crit. Rev. Immunol.* **2:**23.

Metcalfe, D. D., Bland, C. E., and Wasserman, S. I., 1984, Biochemical and functional characterization of proteoglycans isolated from basophils of patients with chronic myelogenous leukemia, *J. Immunol.* **132:**1943.

Miadonna, A., Tedeschi, A., Arnoux, B., Sala, A., Zanussi, C., and Benveniste, J., 1989, Evidence of PAF-acether metabolic pathway activation in antigen challenge of upper respiratory airways, *Am. Rev. Respir. Dis.* **140:**142.

Miller, H. R. P., Huntley, J. F., Newlands, G. F. J., Mackellar, A., Irvine, J., Haig, D. M., MacDonald, A., Lammas, A. D., Wakelin, D., and Woodbury, R. G., 1989, Mast cell granule proteases in mouse and rat:

A guide to mast cell heterogeneity and activation in the gastrointestinal tract, in: *Mast Cell and Basophil Differentiation and Function in Health and Disease* (S. J. Galli and K. F. Austen, eds.), Raven Press, New York, pp. 81–91.

Mitchell, E. B., and Askenase, P. W., 1983, Basophils in human disease, *Clin. Rev. Allergy* **1**:427.

Mitchell, E. B., Platts-Mills, T. A. E., Pereira, R. S., *et al.*, 1983, Basophil and eosinophil deficiency in a patient with hypogammaglobulinemia associated with thymoma, in: *Primary Immunodeficiency Diseases, Birth Defects*, Vol. 19 (R. J. Wedgewood, F. S. Rosen, and N. W. Paul, eds.), Liss, New York, pp.331–357.

Mitsui, H., Furitsu, T., Dvorak, A. M., Irani, A. M., Schwartz, L. B., Inagaki, N., Takei, M., Ishizaka, K., Zsebo, R. M., Gillis, S., *et al.*, 1993, Development of human mast cells from umbilical cord blood cells by recombinant human and murine c-kit ligand, *Proc. Natl. Acad. Sci. USA* **90**:735.

Moqbel, R., Hamid, Q., Ying, S., Barkans, J., Hartnell, A., Tsicopoulos, A., Wardlaw, A. J., and Kay, A. B., 1991, Expression of mRNA and immunoreactivity for the granulocyte-macrophage colony-stimulating factor in activated human eosinophils, *J. Exp. Med.* **174**:749.

Mosmann, T. R., Bond, M. W., Coffman, R. L., Ohara, J., and Paul, W. E., 1986, T-cell and mast cell lines respond to B-cell stimulatory factor-1, *Proc. Natl. Acad. Sci. USA* **83**:5654.

Murakami, I. Ogawa, M., Amo, H., and Ota, K., 1969, Studies on kinetics of human leukocytes in vivo with ^{3}H-thymidine autoradiography. II. Eosinophils and basophils, *Nippon Ketsueki Gakkai Zasshi* **32**:384.

Naclerio, R. M., Proud, D., Togias, A. G., Adkinson, N. F. Jr., Meyers, D. A., Kagey-Sobotka, A., Plant, M., Norman, D. S., and Lichtenstein, L. M., 1985, Inflammatory mediators in late antigen-induced rhinitis, *N. Engl. J. Med.* **313**:65.

Nakajima, K., Hirai, K., Yamaguchi, M., Takaishi, T., Ohta, K., Morita, Y., and Ito, K., 1992, Stem cell factor has histamine releasing activity in rat connective tissue-type mast cells, *Biochem. Biophys. Res. Commun.* **183**:1076.

Nakano, T., Sonoda, T., Hayashi, C., Yamatodani, A., Kanayama, Y., Yamamura, T., Asai, H., Yonezawa, T., Kitamura, Y., and Galli, S. J., 1985, Fate of bone marrow-derived cultured mast cells after intracutaneous, intraperitoneal and intravenous transfer into genetically mast cell-deficient W/W^{v} mice. Evidence that cultured mast cells can give rise to both connective tissue-type and mucosal mast cells, *J. Exp. Med.* **162**:1025.

Nocka, K., Majunder, S., Chabot, B., Ray, P., Cervone, M., Bernstein, A., and Besmer, P., 1989, Expression of the c-kit protooncogene in known cellular targets of W mutations in normal and W mutant mice: Evidence for an impaired c-kit kinase in mutant mice, *Genes Dev.* **3**:816.

Nocka, K., Tan, J. C., Chiu, E., Chu, T. Y., Ray, P., Traktman, P., and Besmer, P., 1990a, Molecular bases of dominant negative and loss of function mutations at the murine c-kit/white spotting locus: W37, W^{v}, W41 and W, *EMBO J.* **9**:1805.

Nocka, K., Buck, J., Levi, E., and Besmer, P., 1990b, Candidate ligand for the c-kit transmembrane kinase receptor: KL, a fibroblast derived growth factor stimulates mast cells and erythroid progenitors, *EMBO J.* **9**:3287.

Ogawa, M., Nakahata, T., Leary, A. G., Sterk, A. R., Ishizaka, K., and Ishizaka, T., 1983, Suspension culture of human mast cells/basophils from umbilical cord blood mononuclear cells, *Proc. Natl. Acad. Sci. USA* **80**:4494.

Ohkawara, Y., Yamaguchi, K., Tanno, Y., Tamura, G., Ohtani, H., Nagura, H., Ohkuda, K., and Takishima, T., 1992, Human lung mast cells and pulmonary macrophages produce tumor necrosis factor-α in sensitized lung tissue after IgE receptor triggering, *Am. J. Respir. Cell Mol. Biol.* **7**:385.

Okada, Y., 1973, The mast cell in synovial membrane of patients with joint disease, *Jpn. J. Orthop. Surg.* **47**:657.

Oppenheim, J. J., Zachariae, C. O. C., Mukaida, N., and Matsushima, K., 1991, Properties of the novel proinflammatory supergene "intercrine" cytokine family, *Annu. Rev. Immunol.* **9**:617.

Osgood, E. E., 1937, Culture of human marrow: Length of life of the neutrophil, eosinophils, and basophils of normal blood as determined by comparative culture of blood and sternal marrow from healthy persons, *J. Am. Med. Assoc.* **109**:933.

Otsu, K., Nakano, T., and Kanakura, Y., 1987, Phenotypic changes of bone marrow-derived mast cells after intraperitoneal transfer into W/W^v mice that are genetically deficient in mast cells, *J. Exp. Med.* **165:**615.

Otsuka, H., Dolovich, J., Befus, A. D., Telizyn, S., Bienenstock, J., and Denburg, J. A., 1986, Basophilic cell progenitors, nasal, metachromatic cells, and peripheral blood basophils in ragweed allergic patients, *J. Allergy Clin. Immunol.* **78:**365.

Pearce, F. L., 1986, Functional differences between mast cells from various locations, in: *Mast Cell Differentiation and Heterogeneity* (A. D. Befus, J. Bienenstock, and J. A. Denburg, eds.), Raven Press, New York, pp. 215–222.

Perdue, M. H., Masson, S., Wershil, B. K., and Galli, S. J., 1991, Role of mast cells in ion transport abnormalities associated with intestinal anaphylaxis. Correction of the diminished secretory response in genetically mast cell-deficient W/W^v mice by bone marrow transplantation, *J. Clin. Invest.* **87:**687.

Plaut, M., Pierce, H. J., Watson, C. J., Hanley-Hyde, J., Nordan, R. P., and Paul, W. E., 1989, Mast cell lines produce lymphokines in response to cross-linkage of Fc RI or to calcium ionophores, *Nature* **339:**64.

Plaut, M., Kagey-Sobotka, A., Niv, Y., Pierce, J. H., and Paul, W. E., 1990, Regulation of mast cell lymphokine production, *FASEB J.* **4:**A1705 (abstract).

Porter, J. F., and Mitchell, R. G. L., 1972, Distribution of histamine in human blood, *Physiol. Rev.* **52:**361.

Ramos, B. F., Qureshi, R., Olsen, K. M., and Jakschik, B. A., 1990, The importance of mast cells for the neutrophil influx in immune complex-induced peritonitis in mice, *J. Immunol.* **145:**1868.

Reddigari, S. R., Kuna, P., Miragliotta, G. F., Kornfield, D., Baeza, M. L., Castor, C. W., and Kaplan, A. P., 1992, Connective tissue-activating peptide-III and its derivative, neutrophil-activating peptide-2, release histamine from human basophils, *J. Allergy Clin. Immunol.* **89:**666.

Reed, N. D., 1989, *Mast Cell and Basophil Differentiation and Function in Health and Disease* (S. J. Galli and K. F. Austen, eds.), Raven Press, New York, pp. 205–215.

Renauld, J.-C., Goethals, A., Houssiau, D., Merz, H., Van Roost, E., and Van Snick, J., 1990, Human P40/IL-9. Expression in activated DC4+ T cells, genomic organization, and comparison with the mouse gene, *J. Immunol.* **144:**4235.

Reynolds, D. S., Stevens, R. L., Lane, W. S., Carr, M. H., Austen, K. F., and Serafin, W. E., 1990, Different mouse mast cell populations express various combinations of at least six distinct mast cell serine proteases, *Proc. Natl. Acad. Sci. USA* **87:**3230.

Roberts, L J., II, Sweetman, B. J., Lewis, R. A., Austen, K. F., and Oates, J. A., 1980, Increased production of prostaglandin D2 in patients with systemic mastocytosis, *N. Engl. J. Med.* **303:**1400.

Robinson, D. S., Hamid, Q., Ying, S., Tsicopoulous, A., Barkans, J., Bentley, A. M., Corrigan, C., Durham, S. R., and Kay, A. B., 1992, Predominant TH2-like bronchoalveolar T-lymphocyte population in atopic asthma, *N. Engl. J. Med.* **326:**298.

Romagnani, S., 1991, Human TH1 and TH2 subsets: Doubt no more, *Immunol. Today* **12:**256.

Ruoslahti, E., and Yamaguchi, Y., 1991, Proteoglycans as modulators of growth factor activities, *Cell* **64:**867.

Salari, H., and Chan-Yeung, M., 1989, Interleukin-1 potentiates antigen-mediated arachidonic acid metabolite formation in mast cells, *Clin. Exp. Allergy* **19:**637.

Schechter, N. M., Franki, J. E., Geesin, J. C., and Lazarus, G. S., 1983, Human skin chymotryptic proteinase. I. Isolation and relation to cathepsin G and rat mast cell protease, *J. Biol. Chem.* **258:**2973.

Schwartz, L. B., and Bradford, T. M., 1986, Regulation of tryptase from human lung mast cells by heparin stabilization of the active tetramer, *J. Biol. Chem.* **261:**7372.

Schwartz, L. B., and Huff, T., 1993, Biology of mast cells and basophils, in: *Allergy: Principles and Practice*, 4th ed. (E. Middleton, Jr., C. E. Reed,. E. F. Ellis, N. F. Adkinson, Jr., J. W. Yunginger, and W. W. Busse, eds.), Mosby, St. Louis, pp. 135–168.

Schwartz, L. B., Metcalfe, D. D., Miller, J. S., Earl, H., and Sullivan, T., 1987, Tryptase levels as an indicator of mast cell activation in systemic anaphylaxis and mastocytosis, *N. Engl. J. Med.* **316:**1622.

Schwartz, L. B., Yuninger, J. W., Miller, J., Bokhari, R., and Dull, D., 1989, Time course of appearance and disappearance of human mast cell tryptase in the circulation after anaphylaxis, *J. Clin. Invest.* **83:**1551.

Seder, R. A., Paul, W. E., Dvorak, A. M., Sharkis, S. J., Kagey-Sobotka, A., Niv, Y., Finkleman, F. D., Barbieri, S. A., Galli, S. J., and Plaut, M., 1991, Mouse splenic and bone marrow cell populations that express high-affinity Fc receptors and produce interleukin-4 are highly enriched in basophils, *Proc. Natl. Acad. Sci. USA* **88:**2835.

Selye, A. M., 1965, *The Mast Cells*, Butterworths, London.

Shohet, S. B., and Blum, S. F., 1968, Coincident basophil chronic myelogenous leukemia and pulmonary tuberculosis, *Cancer* **22:**173.

Sonoda, S., Sonoda, T., Nakano, T., Kanayama, Y., Kanakura, Y., Asai, H., Yonezawa, T., and Kitamura, Y., 1986, Development of mucosal mast cells after injection of a single connective tissue-type mast cell in the stomach mucosa of genetically mast cell-deficient W/W^v mice, *J. Immunol.* **137:**1319.

Soter, N. A., Lewis, R. A., Corey, E. J., and Austen, M. F., 1983, Local effects of synthetic leukotrienes (LTC_4, LTD_4, LTE_4 and LTB_4) in human skin, *J. Invest. Dermatol.* **80:**115.

Stead, R. H., Tomioka, M., Quinonez, G., Simon, G. T., Felten, S. Y., and Bienenstock, J., 1987, Intestinal mucosal mast cells in normal and nematode-infected rat intestines are in intimate contact with peptidergic nerves, *Proc. Natl. Acad. Sci. USA* **84:**2975.

Stead, R. H., Dixon, M. F., Bramwell, N. H., Riddell, R. H., and Bienenstock, J., 1989a, Mast cells are closely apposed to nerves in the human gastrointestinal mucosa, *Gastroenterology* **97:**575.

Stead, R. H., Perdue, M. H., Blennerhassett, M. G., Kakuta, Y., Sestini, P., and Bienenstock, J., 1989b, The innervention of mast cells, in: *The Neuroendocrine–Immune Network* (S. Freier, ed.), CRC Press, Boca Raton, FL, pp. 19–37.

Steeves, E. B., and Allen, J. R., 1990, Basophils in skin reactions of mast cell-deficient mice infected with Dermacentor variabilis, *Int. J. Parasitol.* **20:**655.

Steffen, M., Abboud, M., Potter, G. K., Yung, Y. P., and Moore, M. A., 1989, Presence of tumour necrosis factor or a related factor in human basophil/mast cells, *Immunology* **66:**445.

Stevens, R. L., Fox, C. C., Lichtenstein, L. M., and Austen, K. F., 1988, Identification of chondroitin sulfate E proteoglycans and heparin proteoglycans in the secretory granules of human lung mast cells, *Proc. Natl. Acad. Sci. USA* **85:**2284.

Stimler-Gerard, N. P., and Galli, S. J., 1987, Mast cells are not required for anaphylatoxin-induced ileal smooth muscle contraction, *J. Immunol.* **138:**1908.

Subramanian, N., and Bray, M. A., 1987, Interleukin 1 releases histamine from human basophils and mast cells in vitro, *J. Immunol.* **138:**271.

Tadokoro, K., Stadler, B. M., and de Weck, A. L., 1983, Factor dependent in vitro growth of normal bone marrow derived basophil-like cells, *J. Exp. Med.* **158:**857.

Takeishi, T., Martin, T. R., Katona, I. M., Finkelman, F. D., and Galli, S. J., 1991, Differences in the expression of the cardiopulmonary alterations associated with anti-immunoglobulin E-induced or active anaphylaxis in mast cell-deficient and normal mice. Mast cells are not required for the cardiopulmonary changes associated with certain fatal anaphylactic responses, *J. Clin. Invest.* **88:**598.

Tantravahi, R. V., Stevens, R. L., Austen, K. F., and Weis, J. H., 1986, A single gene in mast cells encodes the core peptides of heparin and chondroitin sulfate proteoglycans, *Proc. Natl. Acad. Sci. USA* **83:**9207.

Tharp, M. D., Kagey-Sobotka, A., Fox, C. C., Marone, G., Lichtenstein, L. M., and Sullivan, T. J., 1987, Function heterogeneity of human mast cells from different anatomical sites: In vitro responses to morphine sulfate, *J. Allergy Clin. Immunol.* **79:**646.

Thompson, H. L., Schulmann, E. S., and Metcalfe, D. D., 1988, Identification of chondroitin sulfate E in human lung mast cells, *J. Immunol.* **140:**2708.

Thompson-Snipes, L., Dhar, V., O'Garra, A., Moore, K., Bond, M., and Rennick, D., 1990, Cytokine synthesis inhibitory factor is a potent co-factor for mast cell growth, *FASEB J.* **4:**A1705 (abstract).

Tracey, R., and Smith, H., 1978, An inherited anomaly of human eosinophils and basophils, *Blood Cells* **4:**291.

Tsai, M., and Shih, L., Newlands, G. F. J., Takeishi, T., Langley, K. E., Zsebo, K. M., Miler, H. R., Geissler, E. N., and Galli, S. J., 1991a, The rat c-kit ligand, stem cell factor, induces the development of connective tissue-type and mucosal mast cells in vivo. Analysis by anatomical distribution, histochemistry, and protease phenotype, *J. Exp. Med.* **174:**125.

Tsai, M., Takeishi, T., Thompson, H. L., Langley, K. E., Zsebo, K. M., Metcalfe, D. D., Geissler, E. N., and

Galli, S. J., 1991b, Induction of mast cell proliferation, maturation, and heparin synthesis by the rat c-kit ligand, stem cell factor, *Proc. Natl. Acad. Sci. USA* **88:**6382.

Tsai, M., Chen, R.-H., Tam, S.-Y., Blenis, J., and Galli, S. J., 1993, Activation of MAP kinases, pp90[rsk] and pp70-S6 kinases in mouse mast cells by signalling through the c-kit receptor tyrosine kinase or Fc RI: Rapamycin inhibits activation of pp70-S6 kinase and proliferation in mouse mast cells, *Eur. J. Immunol.* **23:**3286–3291.

Tsuda, T., Wong, D. A., Dolovich, J., Bienenstock, J., and Denburg, J. A., 1991, Synergistic effects of nerve growth factor and granulocyte–macrophage colony-stimulating factor on human basophilic cell differentiation, *Blood* **77:**971.

Tsuji, K., Nakahata, T., Takagi, M., Kobayashi, T., Ishiguro, A., Kikuchi, T., Naganuma, K., Koike, K., Miyajuma, A., Arai, K., *et al.*, 1990, Effects of interleukin-3 and interleukin-4 on the development of "connective tissue-type" mast cells: Interleukin-3 supports their survival and interleukin-4 triggers and supports their proliferation synergistically with interleukin-3, *Blood* **75:**421.

Urbina, C., Ortiz, C., and Hurtado, I., 1981, A new look at basophils in mice, *Int. Arch. Allergy Appl. Immunol.* **66:**158.

Valent, P., and Bettelheim, P., 1990, The human basophil, *Crit. Rev. Oncol. Hematol.* **10:**327.

Valent, P., Schmidt, G., Besemer, J., Mayer, P., Zenke, G., Liehl, E., Hinterberger, W., Lechner, K., Maurer, D., and Bettelheim, P., 1989a, Interleukin-3 is a differentiation factor for human basophils, *Blood* **73:**1763.

Valent, P., Besemer, J., Muhm, M., Majdic, O., Lechner, K., and Bettelheim, P., 1989b, Interleukin-3 activates human blood basophils via high affinity binding sites, *Proc. Natl. Acad. Sci. USA* **86:**5542.

Valent, P., Spanblochl, E., Sperr, W. R., Sillaber, C., Zsebo, K. M., Agis, H., Strobl, H., Geissler, K., Bettelheim, P., and Lechner, K., 1992, Induction of differentiation of human mast cells from bone marrow and peripheral blood mononuclear cells by recombinant human stem cell factor/kit-ligand in long-term culture, *Blood* **80:**2237.

Valone, F. H., Boggs, J. M., and Goetzl, E. J., 1993, Lipid mediators of hypersensitivity and inflammation, in: *Allergy: Principles and Practice*, 4th ed. (E. Middleton, Jr., C. E. Reed, E. F. Ellis, N. F. Adkinson, Jr., J. W. Yunginger, and W. W. Busse, eds.), Mosby, St. Louis, pp. 302–319.

van der Linden, P.-W. G., Hack, C. E., Poorman, J., Vivie-Kipp, Y. C., Struyvenberg, A., and van der Zwan, J. K., 1992, Inset-sting challenge in 138 patients: Relation between clinical severity of anaphylaxis and mast cell activation, *J. Allergy Clin. Immunol.* **90:**110.

Walsh, L. J., Trinchieri, G., Waldorf, H. A., Whitaker, D., and Murphy, G. F., 1991, Human dermal mast cells contain and release tumor necrosis factor α which induces endothelial leukocyte adhesion molecule-1, *Proc. Natl. Acad. Sci. USA* **88:**4220.

Wang, B., Rieger, A., Kilgus, O., Ochiai, K., Maurer, D., Fodinger, D., Kinet, J.-P., and Stingl, G., 1992, Epidermal Langerhans' cells from normal human skin bind monomeric IgE via Fc RI, *J. Exp. Med.* **175:**1353.

Ward, P. A., Dvorak, H. F., Cohen, S., Yoshida, T., Data, R., and Selvaggio, D., 1975, Chemotaxis of basophils by lymphocyte-dependent and lymphocyte-independent mechanisms, *J. Immunol.* **4:**1523.

Watanabe, N., Katakura, K., Kobayashi, A., *et al.*, 1988, Protective immunity and eosinophilia in IgE-deficient SJA/9 mice infected with Nippostrongylus brasiliensis and Trinchinella spiralis, *Proc. Natl. Acad. Sci. USA* **85:**4460.

Wegner, C. D., Gundel, R. H., Reilly, P., Haynes, N., Letts, L. G., and Rothlein, R., 1990, Intracellular adhesion molecule-1 (ICAM-1) in the pathogenesis of asthma, *Science* **247:**456.

Wegner, C. D., Gundel, R. H., Abraham, W. M., Schulman, E. S., Kontny, M. J., Lazer, E. S., Homon, C. A., Graham, A. G., Torcellini, C. A., Clarke, C. C., Jager, P., Wolyniec, W. W., Letts, L. G., and Farina, P. R., 1993, The role of 5-lipoxygenase products in preclinical models of asthma, *J. Allergy Clin. Immunol.* **91:**917.

Weller, P. F., Rand, T. H., Barrett, T., Elovic, A., Wong, D. T. W., and Finberg, R. W. 1993, Accessory cell function of human eosinophils. HLA-DR-dependent, MHC-restricted antigen-presentation and IL-1α expression, *J. Immunol.* **150:**2554.

Wenzel, S. E., Fowler, A. A., III, and Schwartz, L. B., 1988, Activation of pulmonary mast cells by bronchoalveolar allergen challenge. In vivo release of histamine and tryptase in atopic subjects with and without asthma, *Am. Rev. Respir. Dis.* **137**:1002.

Wershil, B. K., and Galli, S. J., 1989, ^{125}I-fibrin deposition of IgE-dependent gastric reactions in the mouse: The role of mast cells (MCs), *FASEB J.* **3**:A789 (abstract).

Wershil, B. K., and Galli, S. J., 1992, An approach for analyzing the role of mast cells in immunotoxicologic processes and other biologic responses, in: *Clinical Immunotoxicology* (D. S. Newcombe, N. R. Rose, and J. C. Bloom, eds.), Raven Press, New York, pp. 49–82.

Wershil, B. K., Mekori, Y. A., Murakami, T., and Galli, S. J., 1987, ^{125}I-fibrin deposition in IgE-dependent immediate hypersensitivity reactions in mouse skin. Demonstration of the role of mast cells using genetically mast cell-deficient mice locally reconstituted with cultured mast cells, *J. Immunol.* **139**:2605.

Wershil, B. K., Murakami, T., and Galli, S. J., 1988, Mast cell-dependent amplification of an immunologically nonspecific inflammatory response. Mast cells are required for the full expression of cutaneous acute inflammation induced by phorbol 12-myristate 13-acetate, *J. Immunol.* **140**:2356.

Wershil, B. K., Wang, Z.-S., Gordon, J. R., and Galli, S. J., 1991a, Recruitment of neutrophils during IgE-dependent cutaneous late phase responses in the mouse is mast cell dependent: Partial inhibition of the reaction with antiserum against tumor necrosis factor-alpha, *J. Clin. Invest.* **87**:446.

Wershil, B. K., Wang, Z.-S., and Galli, S. J., 1991b, Evidence of mast cell-dependent neutrophil infiltration during IgE-dependent gastric inflammation in the mouse: Does this represent a gastric late phase reaction (LRP)? *Gastroenterology* **100**:A625 (abstract).

Wershil, B. K., Tsai, M., Geissler, E. N., Zsebo, K. M., and Galli, S. J., 1992, The rat c-kit ligand, stem cell factor, induces c-kit receptor-dependent mouse mast cell activation in vivo. Evidence that signaling through the c-kit receptor can induce expression of cellular function, *J. Exp. Med.* **175**:245.

Wershil, B. K., Turck, C. W., Sreedharan, S. P., Yang, J., An, S., Galli, S. J., and Goetzl, E. J., 1993, Variants of vasoactive intestinal peptide in mouse mast cells and rat basophilic leukemia cells, *Cell Immunol.* **151**:369.

Wershil, B. K., Lavigne, J. A., and Galli, S. J., 1994, Stem cell factor (SCF) can influence neuroimmune interactions: Bone marrow-derived mast cells (BMDMC) maintained in SCF acquire the ability to release histamine and tumor necrosis factor-alpha (TNF-α) in response to substance P (SP), *FASEB J.* **8**:A742.

Williams, D. E., de Vries, P., Namen, A. E., Widmer, M. B., and Lyman, S. D., 1992, The Steel factor, *Dev. Biol.* **151**:368.

Woodnar-Filipowicz, A., and Moroni, C., 1990, Regulation of interleukin 3 mRNA expression in mast cells occurs at the posttranscriptional level and is mediated by calcium ions, *Proc. Natl. Acad. Sci. USA* **87**:777.

Wodnar-Filipowicz, A., Heusser, C. H., and Moroni, C., 1989, Production of the haemopoietic growth factors GM-CSF and interleukin-3 by mast cells in response to IgE receptor-mediated activation, *Nature* **339**:150.

Wolpe, S. D., and Cerami, A., 1989, Macrophage inflammatory proteins 1 and 2: Members of a novel superfamily of cytokines, *FASEB J.* **3**:2565.

Wong, D. T. W., Weller, P. F., Galli, S. J., Elovic, A., Rand, T. H., Gallagher, G. T., Chiang, T., Chou, M. Y., Matossian, K., McBride, J., and Todd, R., 1990, Human eosinophils express transforming growth factor-alpha, *J. Exp. Med.* **172**:673.

Wong, D. T. W., Elovic, A., Matossian, K., Nagura, N., McBride, J., Chou, M. Y., Gordon, J. R., Rand, T. H., Galli, S. J., and Weller, P. F., 1991, Eosinophils from patients with blood eosinophilia express transforming growth factor β1, *Blood* **78**:2702.

Woodbury, R. G., and Neurath, H., 1980, Structure, specificity, and localization of the serine proteases of connective tissue, *FEBS Lett.* **114**:189.

Woodbury, R. G., Everitt, M., Sanada, Y., Katanuma, N., Lagunoff, D., and Neurath, H., 1978, A major serine protease in skeletal muscle. Evidence for its mast cell origin, *Proc. Natl. Acad. Sci. USA* **75**:5311.

Woodbury, R. G., Le Trong, H., Cole, K., Neurath, H., and Miller, H. R. P., 1989, Rat mast cell proteases, in:

Mast Cell and Basophil Differentiation and Function in Health and Disease (S. J. Galli and K. F. Austen, eds.), Raven Press, New York, pp. 71–79.

Woolley, D. E., Bartholomew, J. S., Taylor, D. J., and Evanson, J. M., 1989, Mast cells and rheumatoid arthritis, in: *Mast Cell and Basophil Differentiation and Function in Health and Disease* (S. J. Galli and K. F. Austen, eds.), Raven Press, New York, pp. 183–193.

Yamatodani, A., Maeyama, K., Watanabe, T., Wada, H., and Kitamura, Y., 1982, Tissue distribution of histamine in a mutant mouse deficient in mast cells: Clear evidence for the presence of non-mast cell histamine, *Biochem. Pharmacol.* **31:**305.

Yano, H., Wershil, B. K., Arizono, N., and Galli, S. J., 1989, Substance P-induced augmentation of cutaneous vascular permeability and granulocyte infiltration in mice is mast cell dependent, *J. Clin. Invest.* **84:**1276.

Young, J. D.-E., Liu, C.-C., Butler, G., Cohn, Z. A., and Galli, S. J., 1987, Identification, purification, and characterization of a mast cell-associated cytolytic factor related to tumor necrosis factor, *Proc. Natl. Acad. Sci. USA* **84:**9175.

Zsebo, K. M., Williams, D. A., Geissler, E. N., Broudy, V. C., Martin, F. H., Atkins, H. L., Hsu, R. Y., Birkett, N. C., Okino, K. H., Murdock, D. C., *et al.*, 1990, Stem cell factor (SCF) is encoded at the Sl locus of the mouse and is the ligand for the c-kit tyrosine kinase receptor, *Cell* **63:**213.

CHAPTER 8

HISTAMINE

ROSS E. ROCKLIN and DENNIS J. BEER

1. INTRODUCTION

Histamine has long been recognized as a mediator of acute allergic reactions in humans and was one of the first chemical substances shown to be associated with mast cells. β-Imidazolylethylamine was first synthesized in 1907 (Shore *et al.*, 1959) and was given the name *histamine* (Greek, *histos*) because of its ubiquitous presence in animal tissues. Analyzing the effects in animals of intravenously administered histamine, Dale and Laidlaw (1910) first demonstrated the potent bronchospastic and vasodilator activity of this mediator. Later, in the same laboratory, it was noted that many of the symptoms of antigen injection into a sensitized animal could be reproduced by histamine, leading to the conclusion that it was a humoral mediator of the acute allergic response (Best *et al.*, 1927). Lewis's (1927) description of the wheal-and-flare response in human skin further expanded on the vascular actions of histamine. The latter observation suggested that this mediator could be released from cellular stores within the skin on appropriate stimulation. It was not until 1953, however, that histamine present in human skin was localized to mast cells of the dermis (Riley and West, 1953).

Traditionally, histamine has been considered a mediator whose release in certain tissues results in either the production of the symptoms of allergic disease, gastric acid, or neurotransmission. It has only been in the past 20 years that the role of histamine as a modulator of the immune response has been appreciated. The latter has come about primarily through the observation that receptors for histamine are also present on immunocompetent lymphoid cells (T and B lymphocytes) and leukocytes

ROSS E. ROCKLIN • Clinical Research, Astra USA, Inc., Westborough, Massachusetts 01581. DENNIS J. BEER • Pulmonary Medicine, Newton–Wellesley Hospital, Newton, Massachusetts 02162.

Immunopharmacology Reviews, Volume 2, edited by John W. Hadden and Andor Szentivanyi. Plenum Press, New York, 1996.

(neutrophils, eosinophils, basophils, and monocytes/macrophages). Thus, the release of histamine within the local milieu of an emerging immune/inflammatory response may potentially modify, in either a positive or a negative way, the development of that reaction. The outcome of such reactions is determined to some extent by the type of histamine receptors present on the tissues or cells involved. In general, stimulation of histamine type I (H_1) receptors leads to enhanced proinflammatory events, while stimulation of histamine type II (H_2) receptors is associated with downregulation of immune/inflammatory responses.

In this chapter the general functions of histamine will be briefly reviewed as well as its role as a modulator of immune and inflammatory cell function.

2. BIOCHEMISTRY

2.1. Structure

Histamine is 2-(4-imidazolyl) ethylamine (or β-aminoethylimidazole). It is a hydrophilic molecule comprised of an imidazole ring and an amino group connected by two methylene groups. The pharmacologically active form at both H_1 and H_2 receptors is the monocationic Ng-H tautomer, that is, the charged form of the species depicted in Fig. 1. However, different chemical properties of this monocation may be involved at these two different receptor sites (Ganellin and Parsons, 1982).

There are many drugs with histaminelike properties, and most contain the following fragment:

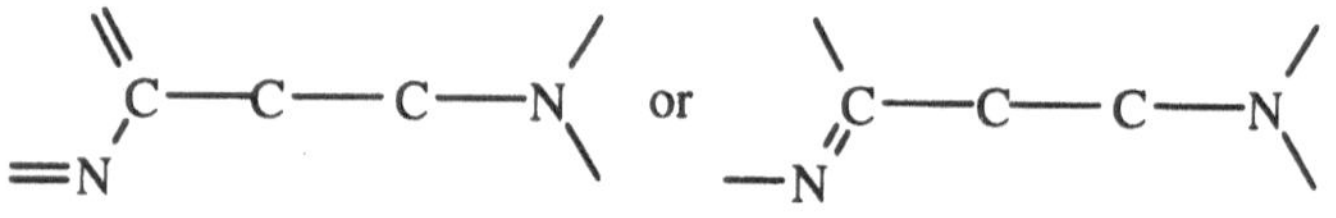

It should be noted that there are a number of exceptions to the above statement. Some compounds with appreciable histaminelike activity consist of small nitrogen-containing heterocyclic rings to which there are attached 2-aminoethyl side chains. Among such agonists there is a striking lack of correlation between their action on gastric secretion and their other histaminelike actions. This reflects the existence of two subclasses of receptor for histamine termed H_1 and H_2 that show different

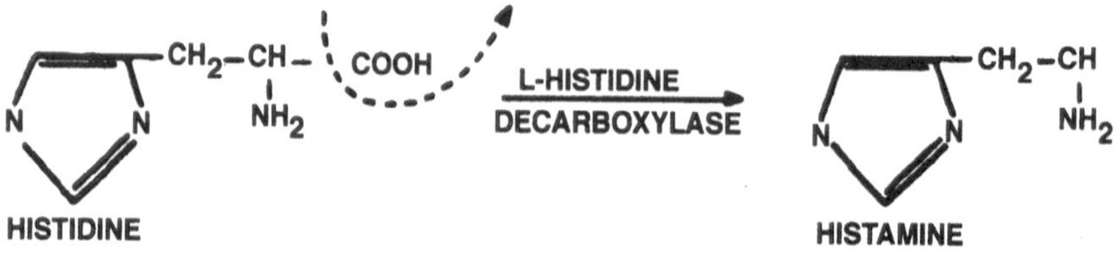

FIGURE 1. Structure of histamine.

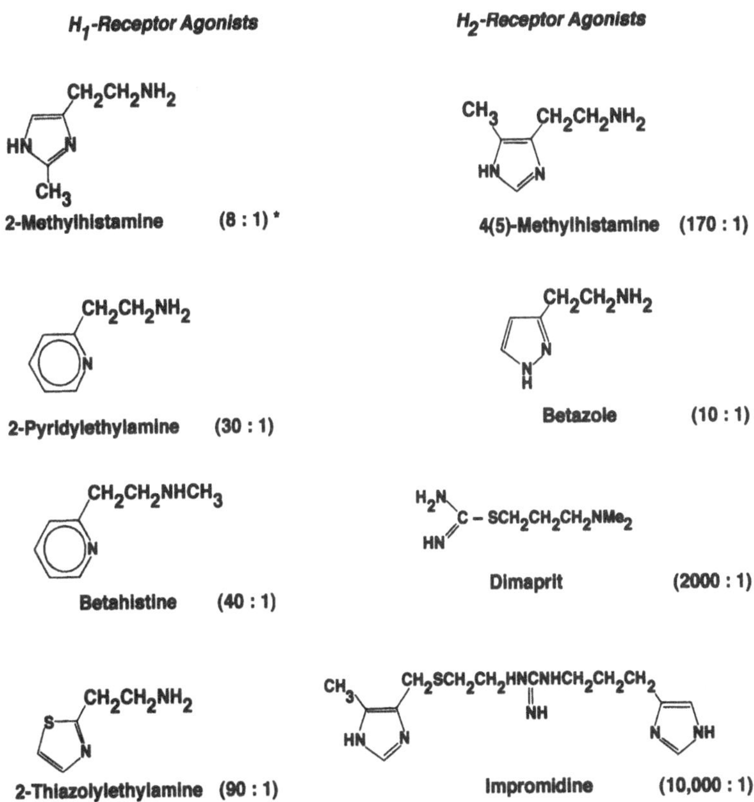

FIGURE 2. Structures of some H_1 and H_2 agonists. Ratios in parentheses indicate the approximate relative activities of the compounds at H_1 and H_2 receptor types (H_1:H_2 for the H_1 agonists and H_2:H_1 for the H_2 agonists).

structural requirements for both binding and activation. Some H_1 and H_2 agonists are shown in Fig. 2.

2.2. Synthesis

Histamine is formed from L-histidine by enzymatic decarboxylation catalyzed by the pyridoxyl 5′-phosphate-dependent enzyme L-histidine decarboxylase (Fig. 1) (Watanabe *et al.*, 1979; Tran and Snyder, 1981). This enzyme is specific for histidine and can be distinguished from the nonspecific aromatic amino acid decarboxylase (DOPA decarboxylase) by its susceptibility to inhibition by α-methylhistidine but not by α-methyl DOPA, as well as by its K_m for histidine (Weissbach *et al.*, 1961; Fukui *et al.*, 1980). Two different isozymes have been isolated from brain and fetal tissues (Watanabe *et al.*, 1982). Stomach tissue contains both isozymes. Each isozyme has a similar K_m for histidine and may represent mast-cell- and non-mast-cell-derived enzymes.

Histidine decarboxylase unassociated with mast cells is an inducible enzyme subject to environmental regulation (Schayer, 1966, 1968). In mouse lung, a variety of stimuli including epinephrine (Graham *et al.*, 1964), dopa and dopamine (Graham *et al.*, 1964), endotoxin (Schayer and Reilly, 1972), Freund's complete adjuvant (Schayer and Reilly, 1972), and exercise (Graham *et al.*, 1964) have been demonstrated to induce histidine decarboxylase activity. Prednisone had no effect on histidine decarboxylase activity in rat or guinea pig lung (Schayer, 1968). Pretreatment of animals with protein synthesis inhibitors, but not mRNA synthesis inhibitors, generally blocks induction of histidine decarboxylase. Many of the stimuli that induce enzyme activity in mouse lung decreased histidine decarboxylase activity in rat lung, demonstrating the species dependency of histidine decarboxylase induction. It is important to understand that induction of the enzyme does not simply reflect an increase in mast cells as was demonstrated in mouse lung following repeated injection of the histamine-releasing agent compound 48/80 (Schayer, 1968).

The uptake of L-histidine into the mast cell occurs via energy-independent, sodium-independent transport (Lagunoff and Bauza, 1982), possibly coupled to histidine decarboxylase activity, and is unaffected by extracellular histamine. Some cellular reincorporation of [^{3}H]histamine can be demonstrated in culture (Weill and Renoux, 1982); however, the high K_m for uptake for histamine in relation to histidine favors regranulation by synthesis rather than uptake. The K_m for histidine uptake is roughly equal to plasma levels, and thus dietary histidine may influence uptake and regranulation.

Uptake of intracellularly synthesized histamine into mast cell granules is ATP-dependent and favored by a pH gradient across the granule membrane resulting in ion trapping (Lagunoff and Bauza, 1982). The mast cell granule, composed of approximately 60% protein, 30% heparin, 10% histamine, 1 to 2% phospholipid, and less than 0.2% ATP (Uvnas, 1974), functions as a cationic exchanger with histamine binding to carboxylic acid groups. Analysis by dye binding indicates that histamine may also complex with the *N*-sulfate or the uronic carboxylic group of heparin (Lagunoff, 1974).

2.3. Metabolism

Histamine is stored in secretory granules, where it is concentrated and ionically bound to carboxyl groups on proteoglycan and/or protein at the acid pH of the secretory granule. With activation and degranulation of mast cells and basophils, secreted histamine is readily solubilized from other granule components at the physiological pH and ionic strength in the extracellular milieu. Extracellular histamine is rapidly and sequentially metabolized to methylhistamine by *N*-methyltransferase and to methylimidazole acetic acid by monamine oxidase, or to imidazole acetic acid by diamine oxidase, and to riboside-*N*-3-imidazole acetic acid by imidazole acetate phosphoribosyl transferase and phosphoribotidylimidazole acetyl phosphatase (Schayer, 1959; Kapeller-Adler, 1965; Snyder and Axelrod, 1965). Approximately 90% of the histamine is destroyed in one pass through the circulation. Thus, evaluations of plasma histamine that occur during an acute allergic reaction are transient. Measurements of urinary histamine reflect plasma levels over the collection period but may vary in the same subject because only a small fraction of unmetabolized plasma histamine is excreted.

Measurements of histamine's metabolites in brain (tele-methylhistamine and tele-methylimidazoleacetic acid) have been used to evaluate histamine turnover in animals, and the same measurements in cerebrospinal fluid (CSF) have been used to determine histaminergic activity in human brains (Prell and Green, 1994). Studies of human CSF suggest that brain histaminergic activity increases with age and is higher in females than in males.

2.4. Assay

The classical method of measuring histamine in biologic samples relied on its capacity to contract isolated guinea pig ileum pretreated with atropine (Austen, 1976). Although still used, bioassay of histamine has largely been replaced by a chemical assay involving condensation of *O*-phthalaldehyde with histamine resulting in a product that may be detected and quantified fluorometrically (Shore *et al.*, 1959). The fluorometric assay for histamine has been greatly refined but is still limited in sensitivity to 1 to 5 ng/ml. Since histamine concentrations in biologic fluids are frequently lower than this, other assay techniques have had to be developed. These include various forms of a radioenzymatic transfer assay in which a radiolabeled methyl group from *S*-adenosylmethionine is transferred to the imidazole ring of histamine in the presence of histamine *N*-methyltransferase, an enzyme extracted from guinea pig brain or rat kidney. Increased specificity and sensitivity of the assay has been gained by utilizing a thin-layer chromatography step to separate the radiolabeled condensation product from contaminants and by incorporation of a second radiolabel to correct for losses during the extraction and separation procedures (Brown *et al.*, 1982). The radioenzymatic transfer assay for histamine is sufficiently sensitive to detect concentrations in biologic samples as low as 100 pg/ml.

2.5. Histamine Receptor Subtypes (H_1, H_2, H_3)

The classical pharmacologic effects described for histamine are primarily mediated by two receptor subtypes, H_1 and H_2. A recently described H_3 receptor is also present. Radioligand binding studies and more recently molecular biological studies have shown that they all belong to the superfamily of G-protein-coupled receptors (Gantz *et al.*, 1991; Arrang, 1994).

Histamine has effects on smooth muscles such as those of the bronchi and gut, but markedly relaxes others, including those of small blood vessels. It is also a very potent stimulus to gastric acid production. Effects attributable to those actions dominate the overall response to the drug; however, there are several others, of which edema formation and stimulation of sensory nerve endings are perhaps more familiar. Some of these effects, such as bronchoconstriction and contraction of the gut, are mediated by one type of histamine receptor, the H_1 receptor (Ash and Schild, 1966), which are readily blocked by pyrilamine and other such classical antihistamines, now designated as histamine H_1-receptor blocking drugs or simply H_1 blockers. Other effects, most notably gastric secretion, are completely refractory to such antagonists, involve activation of H_2 receptors, and are susceptible to inhibition by histamine H_2-receptor blocking drugs (Black *et al.*, 1972). Most of the effects of histamine on leukocyte and immune cell function are mediated via H_2 receptors. Still others, such as the hypotension resulting from vascular dilatation, are evidently mediated by receptors of both H_1 and H_2 types, since they are abrogated only by a combination of H_1 and H_2 blockers.

A third type of histamine receptor (H_3) has been described in the central nervous system (Schwartz, 1979; Arrang *et al.*, 1983). Presynaptic H_3 receptors occur on histaminergic neurons of the CNS (autoreceptors) and on nonhistaminergic neurons of the central and autonomic nervous system (heteroreceptors). H_3 heteroreceptors have been identified on postganglionic sympathetic nerve fibers innervating the resistance vessels and the heart (Arrang, 1994). In addition, H_3 heteroreceptors are found on the sympathetic neurons supplying the human saphenous vein and the vasculature of the pig retina and on the serotoninergic, dopaminergic, and noradrenergic neurons of the brain of various mammalian (including man) species (Schlicker *et al.*, 1994).

The two classical types of histamine receptors (H_1 and H_2) can be distinguished by their differential responses to various histaminelike agonists. Thus, 2-methylhistamine preferentially elicits responses mediated by H_1 receptors, whereas 4-methylhistamine has a correspondingly preferential effect mediated through H_2 receptors (Black *et al.*, 1972). These compounds are representatives of two classes of histaminelike drugs, the H_1- and H_2-receptor agonists. The structures of some are shown in Fig. 2. The availability of these H_1 and H_2 agonists and of the corresponding antagonists has greatly enriched understanding of the pharmacology and physiology of histamine and has allowed new therapeutic approaches (Busse, 1994; Nash *et al.*, 1994).

The pharmacologic effects of H_3 receptor ligands (*R*-[−]-α-methylhistamine, imetit) and antagonists (thioperamide, clobenpropit) have been investigated to help define the receptor specificity and signal transduction mechanisms (Schlicker *et al.*, 1994).

2.6. Signal Transduction Mechanisms

Histamine has been shown to induce a rise in intracellular levels of cyclic AMP via stimulation of H_2 receptors in a variety of tissues including T lymphocytes and gastric parietal cells (Bourne *et al.*, 1974; Bearer *et al.*, 1981). Furthermore, elevation of intracellular cyclic AMP following the addition of histamine to cultures of human keratinocytes *in vitro* is associated with reduced mitosis by these cells. This latter effect can be reproduced by the addition of the H_2 antagonist 4-methylhistamine. In several other tissues, such as mouse fibroblasts and lymphocytes, elevations in intracellular cyclic AMP have also been shown to inhibit cellular proliferation. In addition, histamine receptor stimulation may also induce an elevation in intracellular cyclic 3′,5′-guanosine monophosphate (GMP) levels in these tissues. Elevation in cyclic GMP levels induces a stimulation of DNA synthesis in these cells (Hadden *et al.*, 1972; Friedman, 1976). Histamine was shown to generate optimal amounts of intracellular cyclic AMP at concentrations of 10^{-4} M, whereas maximal levels of cyclic GMP production were induced at 10^{-3} M. It was concluded that histamine-stimulated increases in intracellular cyclic AMP resulted in inhibition of cell growth, while histamine-mediated increases in cyclic GMP partially antagonized this inhibition.

In addition to cAMP elevations, evidence obtained in mast cells suggests that stimulation of the histamine receptor leads to an early methylation of membrane phospholipids. Rat peritoneal mast cells incubated with L-[methyl-^{3}H]-methionine and then exposed to histamine (10^{-6} M) undergo a rapid but transient increase in phospholipid methylation. The latter may lead to a localized increase in membrane fluidity in the region surrounding the receptor. The response was thought to be related to stimulation of the H_2 receptor as a result of employing selective H_1 and H_2 antagonists and agonists. It was suggested that histamine stimulation of adenylate cyclase could result from localized changes in the lipid structure (increased fluidity in the membrane which permits increased coupling of the receptor to regulatory proteins) and/or by increased binding of calcium to the regulatory unit of the enzyme.

Histamine stimulation of the H_1 receptor also appears to be linked to phosphatidylinositol turnover and the generation of a calcium signal. Incubation of guinea pig brain slices with 10^{-4} M histamine resulted in an increase in [^{3}H]inositol 1-phosphate levels (Berridge, 1975). This response was blocked by the antagonists mepyramine (H_1) in equimolar concentrations, but not by cimetidine (H_2). Furthermore, dimaprit (H_2 agonist) did not evoke this response, but addition of 2-thio-ethylamine (H_1 agonist) to the brain slices did result in an increase in [^{3}H]inositol 1-phosphate accumulation. There was a very good correlation between [^{3}H]inositol 1-phosphate accumulation and H_1 receptor density in various portions of the brain (Berridge, 1975). In rabbit aorta, both histamine and 2-amino-ethylthiazole (H_1 agonist) induced a dose-dependent increase in phosphatidylinositol labeling, but this did not occur with incubation with impromidine (H_2 agonist). The histamine effect could be inhibited by selective antagonists in the following order: mepyramine > pyrilamine > cimetidine. In addition, H_1 receptors have recently been shown to potentiate phospholipase C activity (Dickenson and Hill, 1993).

3. PHARMACOLOGY

3.1. Cardiovascular

Histamine has a variety of potent effects on the cardiovascular system, which vary remarkably between species (Owen, 1977; Altura and Halery, 1978). On isolated heart preparations, histamine generally has a positive ionotropic (H_1 and H_2) and chronotropic (H_2) effect. Similar effects can be observed *in vivo* but are complicated by varying effects of the anesthesia and reflux responses elicited by histamine's stimulatory effects on sympathetic nerves. A positive chronotropic effect can readily be demonstrated in humans (Weiss *et al.*, 1932).

The most characteristic effects of histamine are on the microvasculature. Histamine causes marked hypotension by a combined action on H_1 and H_2 receptors, causing relaxation of arterioles and precapillary sphincters. The endothelial cells of the postcapillary venules constrict to histamine, resulting in cellular separation and an increase in permeability across the exposed basement membrane (Majno *et al.*, 1969; Northover, 1975). These actions of histamine combine to produce a phenomenon referred to as the triple response (Lewis, 1927). intradermal injection of histamine causes the immediate formation of a red spot, localized to the site of injection, resulting from microvessel vasodilation. This area is surrounded by a brighter red flare of irregular outline, resulting indirectly from a histamine-induced reflex vasodilation. In 1–2 min the original red spot blanches and fills with edema as a result of the increased vascular permeability. The pain and itch associated with the formation of the wheel and flare may in part result from histamine's ability to stimulate afferent nerve ending (Keele and Armstrong, 1964). The modulatory effects of H_2 receptor antagonists on the cardiovascular system have recently been reviewed (Bertaccini *et al.*, 1993).

3.2. Pulmonary

Histamine has potent and species-specific effects on the smooth musculature of the bronchial tree. Generally, histamine causes constriction of isolated airway tissue through H_1 receptors. In sheep bronchi, however, only H_2 receptors are evident, which when stimulated produce bronchodilation (Eyre, 1973). In cat trachea, activation of both H_1 and H_2 receptors causes relaxation (Maengwyn-Davies, 1968; Eyre, 1973). Even in guinea pig tracheal tissue, which is exquisitely sensitive to the contractile effects of histamine, evidence has been presented for functionally opposed histamine H_1 and H_2 receptors (Okpako *et al.*, 1978). However, it is believed that H_2 receptors have no *in vivo* or *in vitro* physiologic significance in guinea pig airways (Brink *et al.*, 1982).

Similar discordant results are observed in humans. For example, it has been observed that in normal subjects great differences existed in the sensitivity to histamine and in the effects of H_2 receptor blockade on histamine responses (Michoud *et al.*, 1981). In very sensitive subjects cimetidine (H_2 receptor antagonist) decreased responsiveness to histamine, while in only modestly sensitive subjects cimetidine enhanced airway reactivity. Thus, the nature of the sample population with respect to its sensitivity to histamine may relate to the role of H_2 receptors in individual responsiveness. In asthmatics, who are generally very sensitive to histamine, cimetidine had little effect on baseline pulmonary functions and was without effect on bronchial reactivity to aerosol histamine challenge (Nogrady and Bevan, 1981). The role of antihistamines in allergic diseases has recently been reviewed (Busse, 1994).

3.3. Gastric Exocrine Glands

Histamine is a remarkably powerful gastric secretagogue and evokes a copious secretion of gastric juice of high acidity in doses below those that influence the blood pressure. Its effect on the composition of gastric juice varies somewhat with species and dose, but in humans the output of pepsin and intrinsic factor of Castle is increased along with that of acid. The principal effect, to increase the production of acidic gastric juice, is well sustained during a prolonged infusion of histamine. It results from a direct stimulant effect on the parietal cells where, acting on H_2 receptors that are linked to adenylate cyclase, histamine drives a membrane pump (H^+,K^+-ATPase) that extrudes protons. The potent secretagogue activity of histamine reflects the dominant function of this autacoid in the physiological stimulation of gastric acid production (see below). Physiological stimulation also involves acetylcholine released by vagal activity and the hormonal secretagogue, gastrin. There are important, mutually supportive interactions between the three secretagogues, and some of these appear to operate at the level of the parietal cell. For example, reduction in vagal influence, by vagotomy or administration of atropine, depresses the effect of histamine. In addition, blockade of H_2 receptors not only inhibits acid production in response to histamine but also reduces the effect of gastrin or vagal stimulation (Code, 1965; Soll and Grossman, 1981; Berglindh, 1984). Recent evidence suggests that H_3 receptors are also involved in the control of gastric acid secretion (Lewin *et al.*, 1992). H_2 receptor antagonists are used prophylactically to treat peptic ulcer disease (Nash *et al.*, 1994).

3.4. Nerve Endings

Histamine can stimulate various nerve endings. Thus, when introduced into the epidermis, it causes itch; when delivered more deeply into the dermis, it evokes pain, sometimes accompanied by itching. Stimulant actions on one or another type of nerve ending, including autonomic afferents and efferents, have been mentioned above as factors that contribute to the "flare" component of the triple response and to indirect effects of histamine on the heart, bronchi, and other organs. The neuronal receptors for histamine are generally of the H_1 type (Rocha e Silva, 1966).

3.5. Adrenal Medulla and Ganglia

Histamine stimulates ganglion cells and chromaffin cells when it is administered in large amounts or by close arterial injection, but not when conventional doses are given intravenously. Nevertheless, a secondary rise in blood pressure attributable to adrenal medullary stimulation is seen in experimental animals given large doses of histamine intravenously and in patients with pheochromocytoma given modest doses.

3.6. Central Nervous System

Histamine does not penetrate the blood–brain barrier to any significant degree, and effects on the central nervous system (CNS) are not usually evident in response to parenteral injections of the autacoid. However, when injected directly into the cerebral ventricles or given by iontophoretic application into certain regions of the brain, histamine may elicit behavioral responses, elevate blood pressure, increase heart rate, lower body temperature, increase secretion of antidiuretic hormone, cause arousal or emesis, increase or decrease firing of neurons, and stimulate or inhibit the secretion of several adenohypophyseal hormones (Schwartz, 1979). These central effects seem to involve H_1, H_2 and H_3 receptors, and at least some effects may reflect the existence of central histaminergic nerves and neuroendocrine mechanisms. Recent studies also show that histamine may be involved in producing circadian rhythmicity (Nowak, 1994).

4. IMMUNOPHARMACOLOGIC EFFECTS OF HISTAMINE

4.1. Leukocytes

4.1.1. Basophils

Evidence that histamine might exert an influence on inflammatory events was first shown by Bourne *et al.* (1971), who observed that the exogenous addition of histamine to cultures of human basophils inhibited the subsequent antigen-stimulated release of histamine (Table I). The concentration of histamine causing 50% inhibition of release was 10^{-7} to 10^{-6} M. The inhibitory effect of histamine on mediator release was localized to the activation phase and not to the release phase. Maximum suppression (80–90%) of histamine release occurred when histamine was added simultaneously with antigen but was reduced to 20–40% when added as little as 2 min after the addition of antigen. These results were interpreted to mean that histamine interferes with an intracellular event occurring during activation that is not dependent on extracellular calcium or magnesium.

The type of histamine receptor involved in this reaction was investigated by Lichtenstein and Gillespie (1973). They found that the inhibition of histamine release by exogenously added histamine was antagonized by the H_2 antagonist burimamide (10^{-5} M) but not by H_1 antagonists such as chlorpheniramine, pyrilamine, and promethazine (up to 10^{-4} M). The binding characteristics of these reactions occurred maximally with 10^{-5} to 10^{-6} M concentrations of antagonists, and they therefore appeared to act through receptor blockade and not through a mechanism that suggested an alteration in histamine metabolism.

TABLE I
Histamine Modulation of Polymorphonuclear Leukocyte Function

Cell type	Assay	Effect of histamine	Receptor specificity	
			H_1	H_2
Basophil (human)	Histamine release	↓	−	+
	Chemotactic response (C5a)	↓	−	+
	Cyclic AMP	↑	−	+
	Histidine uptake	↑	+	−
Lung mast cell (human)	Histamine release	0		
Skin mast cell (human)	Histamine release	↓	−	+
Eosinophil (human)	Chemotactic response (C5a)	↑	+	−
	Chemotactic response (C5a)	↓	−	+
	Chemotaxis (histamine)	↑	+	+
	Cyclic AMP	↑	−	+
	Complement receptors (C3b and C4)	↑	+	−
Neutrophils (human)	Chemokinesis	0		
	Chemokinesis (f-Met-Leu-Phe, casein)	↑	−	+
	Chemotaxis (f-Met-Leu-Phe, casein)	↓	−	+
	Lysosomal enzyme release (activated serum)	↓	−	+
	Cyclic AMP	↑	−	+
	Adherence (C5a)	↓	−	+
	Membrane potential (f-Met-Leu-Phe)	↓	−	+
	Superoxide anion production (f-Met-Leu-Phe)	↓	−	+
	Peroxide formation (f-Met-Leu-Phe)	↓	−	+

It is known that agents that raise intracellular levels of cAMP inhibit histamine release (Lichtenstein, 1975). Changes in intracellular levels of cAMP were measured in studies in which histamine was employed (Lichtenstein and Gillespie, 1973). The addition of histamine to cultures of basophils was associated with a significant rise in intracellular levels of cAMP (Table I). A direct correlation between the inhibition of mediator release caused by exogenously added histamine and a rise in intracellular levels of cAMP was shown to be mediated through the H_2 receptor.

The ability of histamine to inhibit basophil and mast cell secretion may vary depending on the releasing stimuli and the cell source. For example, basophil secretion induced by antigen is inhibitable by histamine, whereas that induced by the calcium ionophore A23187 is not suppressed by histamine or other cAMP-elevating agents (Lichtenstein, 1975). Moreover, histamine inhibited secretion by human basophils and skin mast cells (Ting *et al.*, 1980) but did not alter secretion by human lung mast cells challenged by antigen (Kaliner, 1978).

In addition to affecting the secretion of mediators by basophils, histamine has also been shown to influence the migration of these cells. Experiments (Lett-Brown *et al.*, 1976; Lett-Brown and Leonard, 1977) demonstrated that histamine inhibited the chemotactic response of basophils to C5a but not a lymphokine-derived chemotactic factor or the bacterial peptide, *N*-formylmethionylleucylphenylalanine (f-Met-Leu-Phe). The IC_{50} of this reaction occurred at 10^{-8} M histamine. Histamine itself did not influence the motility of basophils.

4.1.2. Eosinophils

Histamine effects on eosinophil function include the regulation of cell migration, the appearance of complement receptors, and an elevation in intracellular cyclic nucleotide levels (Table I). Histamine appears to be directly chemotactic for eosinophils (Clark *et al.*, 1975). The chemotactic effect of histamine on eosinophils can be blocked only by the combination of H_1 plus H_2 antagonists and not by either alone, leading investigators to speculate that a third type of histamine receptor might be involved (Clark *et al.*, 1977; Bryant and Kay, 1977). In addition to its direct effects on eosinophil migration, histamine has also been reported to inhibit the directed movement of eosinophils in response to endotoxin-activated serum or kallikrein, at concentrations greater than 10^{-5} M. Concentrations below 10^{-6} M histamine increased the eosinophil chemotactic response to endotoxin-activated serum. Facilitation of directed movement appeared to be mediated via H_1 receptors, since only H_1 antagonists, but not H_2 antagonists, block this response (Clark *et al.*, 1977).

The expression of certain receptors present on human eosinophils influenced by histamine has also been studied (Anwar and Kay, 1977, 1978). The exogenous addition of histamine increased the appearance of C3b and C4 receptors on these cells. Enhancement of C3b receptors by histamine could be blocked by H_1 antagonists such as chlorpheniramine and mepyramine at concentrations of 5×10^{-5} M but not by similar concentrations of burimamide or metiamide. Increased expression of C3b receptors resulted in the facilitation of eosinophil-dependent killing of certain parasites such as schistosomula and trichinella. The increased killing induced by histamine was again mediated through the H_1 receptor, since H_1 antagonists, but not H_2 antagonists, abrogated this effect. Since parasitism is associated with high levels of IgE, part of which is directed against the parasite, sensitization of mast cells with IgE may lead to antigen-induced degranulation and subsequent histamine release. It has been suggested that the released histamine recruits eosinophils to the site of the reaction and potentiates their ability to destroy the parasite.

4.1.3. Neutrophils

A considerable body of evidence has accumulated to indicate that histamine is capable of altering a number of functions of neutrophils including enzyme release, chemotaxis and chemokinesis, adherence, superoxide anion production, and hydrogen peroxide formation (Table I).

Selective release of inflammatory mediators from leukocyte lysosomes has been shown to be reduced by compounds that increase intracellular cAMP levels and augmented by agents that increase intracellular cGMP (Weissman *et al.*, 1971). Histamine, in a dose-dependent fashion (10^{-8}–10^{-5} M), as well as other adenylate cyclase-active agents such as isoproterenol, PGE_1, and cholera enterotoxin, all inhibited the secretion of lysosomal enzymes from cytochalasin B-treated human neutrophils in response to zymosan-activated serum (Busse and Sosman, 1976). The H_2 antihistamine, metiamide, prevented the histamine-induced inhibition of lysosomal enzyme release as well as the parallel increase in intracellular cAMP levels of granulocyte lysosomal enzyme release.

The effects of histamine on neutrophil chemotaxis and chemokinesis induced by f-Met-Leu-Phe have been analyzed (Seligman *et al.*, 1983). Chemotaxis stimulated by f-Met-Leu-Phe was inhibited by histamine (10^{-4} M). However, chemokinesis induced by this agent was enhanced by histamine. In these studies, histamine alone had no effect o random nonstimulated neutrophil migration. In related experiments, it was shown that both H_1 and H_2 agonists enhanced f-Met-Leu-Phe-stimulated chemokinesis and inhibited chemotaxis, while only the H_2 antagonist cimetidine reversed the effects of histamine and its other analogues. The H_1 antagonist pyrilamine stimulated chemokinesis and inhibited chemotaxis at high concentrations. The simultaneous addition of both H_1 and H_2 agonists, each at less than saturating concentrations, produced additive but not synergistic inhibition of chemotaxis, which suggested that a single receptor for histamine mediated both stimulation of chemokinesis and inhibition of chemotaxis. Taken together, these studies raise questions as to the specific histamine receptor subtype(s) involved in modulation of neutrophil motility.

Histamine and both H_1 and H_2 agonists, in a dose-dependent fashion, have also been shown to inhibit the f-Met-Leu- Phe-stimulated changes in membrane potential, superoxide anion production, and hydrogen peroxide formation without blocking the binding or internalization of [^{3}H]f-Met-Leu-Phe (Seligman *et al.*, 1983). These effects could be blocked by cimetidine (H_2). Histamine was unable to influence these same neutrophil functions induced by phorbol myristic acid or the calcium ionophore A23187. Taken collectively, these data suggested that a single site with specificity for both H_1 and H_2 analogue structures modulated the various f-Met-Leu-Phe-stimulated functions studied. It was suggested that a single receptor for histamine could enhance chemokinesis while inhibiting chemotaxis by any of at least several mechanisms. Histamine could have multiple independent effects on steps early in neutrophil activation. Alternatively, if histamine selectively inhibited the detection of a gradient of chemotactic factor without inhibiting the stimulation of motility by a chemoattractant, then enhanced chemokinesis and inhibited chemotaxis could result. In addition, the inhibition by histamine of superoxide anion or hydrogen peroxide production could disrupt regulation of the chemoattractant gradient by the myeloperoxidase/halide/peroxide system with subsequent differential effects on chemotaxis and chemokinesis (Clark *et al.*, 1977).

4.2. T Lymphocytes

4.2.1. Cell-Mediated Cytotoxicity

Following sensitization either *in vivo* or *in vitro*, T lymphocytes can exhibit a cytotoxic response that is directed against the sensitizing antigens. The first effect described of histamine on T-lymphocyte function was that for cytotoxicity (Bourne *et al.*, 1974). In the mouse system employed, 7 days is required to develop fully differentiated effector cytotoxic cells when allogeneic tissue is used to sensitize. This cytotoxic response can be inhibited by agents that increase intracellular levels of cAMP. Histamine has a similar effect to these latter agents, presumably by its ability to increase intracellular levels of cAMP. The inhibitory effect of histamine on cytotoxicity appears to be mediated through the H_2 receptor, since burimamide, metiamide, and cimetidine can block the effect of histamine but not H_1 antagonists such as diphenhydramine or mepyramine (Plaut *et al.*, 1975; Plaut and Roszkowski, 1979). That these antagonists are operating to block the H_2 receptor and not by other mechanisms was shown by experiments in which the dose response to histamine was shifted to the right using an agonist-log dose–response curve. That is, orders of magnitude more histamine were required to obtain the same levels of inhibition in the presence of the antagonist. In addition, H_2 agonists such as 4-methylhistamine and dimaprit can mimic the effects of histamine by inhibiting cytotoxicity but not an H_1 agonist such as 2-methylhistamine. (See Table II for summary of the effects of histamine on lymphocyte function.)

Human blood lymphocytes precultured with histamine for 24 hr have a significant decrease in their natural killer (NK) and antibody-dependent cellular cytotoxic activities (Nair and Schwartz, 1983). In addition, when lymphocytes were incubated with histamine, washed, and then combined in coculture with autologous cytotoxic lymphocytes, there was inhibition of the cytotoxic response. Culture supernatants of lymphocytes stimulated with 10^{-8} to 10^{-3} M histamine were shown to contain a soluble suppressor factor, designated *histamine-induced soluble suppressor factor* (HISSF), that significantly inhibited the NK function of allogeneic lymphocytes. Production of HISSF was specifically blocked by the H_2 receptor antagonist cimetidine, but not by the H_1 receptor antagonist clemastine. A monoclonal antibody directed against HISSF was capable of abrogating its suppressive activities (Schwartz and Nair, 1990). In addition, inhibition of NK activity by HISSF was reversed completely by treating effector lymphocytes with IFN-α for a short period of time or culturing them with IL-2 for 36 hr.

4.2.2. Production of Lymphokines

T lymphocytes, when activated *in vitro* by specific antigens or nonspecifically by mitogens, produce a number of proteins having effects on a variety of cells. They are involved in various aspects of the expression of cell-mediated and humoral immunity. The effects of histamine on lymphokine production are either inhibitory, or in some

TABLE II
Histamine Modulation of Lymphocyte Function

Cell type	Assay	Effect of histamine	Receptor specificity	
			H_1	H_2
In vivo primed cytotoxic T lymphocytes (mouse)	Cytolytic activity	↓	−	+
	cAMP	↑	−	+
In vitro primed cytotoxic T lymphocytes (mouse)	Cytolytic activity	0		
In vitro induction of cytotoxic T lymphocytes (mouse)	Induction of cytotoxicity	↓	−	+
NK cells (mouse, human)	Cytolytic activity	↓	?	?
Antibody-dependent cellular cytotoxicity (human)	Cytolytic activity	↓	?	?
Lymphokine-producing cells (guinea pig, human)	MIF, LIF, interferon, IL-2	↓	−	+
Proliferating T lymphocytes (mouse, guinea pig, human)	[^{3}H]-TdR uptake	↓	−	+
Con-A-induced suppressor cells (mouse)	Inhibition of cytolytic activity	↑	−	+
Suppressor T lymphocytes (mouse, guinea pig, human)	Inhibition of blastogenesis, lymphokine production, and antibody production	↑	−	+
Contrasuppressor cells (mouse)	Generation of hapten self-cytotoxic T cells	↑	+	−
T lymphocytes (human)	Induction of chemoattractant lymphokines			
	LCF	↑	−	+
	$LyMIF_{35K}$	↑	+	−
	$LyMIF_{75K}$	↑	+	−
Thymic cells (mouse)	Thy-I antigen expression	↑	−	+
T lymphocytes (human)	E-rosette formation	↓	+(?)	+(?)
	RFc γ expression	↑	−	+
T helper cells (human)	Ia/DR antigen expression	↓	−	+
B lymphocytes (mouse)	IgG response (SRBC)	↓	?	?
	Antibody production	↓	?	?
B lymphocytes (human)	Pokeweed-induced IgG production	↓	+(?)	+(?)
	IgG, IgM, IgA, PFC	↓	−	+

instances facilitate their production. For example, the elaboration of macrophage migration inhibitory factor (MIF) is decreased when histamine is added *in vitro* in culture. Histamine inhibits MIF production in a dose-dependent fashion (10^{-3}–10^{-5} M) and these effects can be abrogated through the use of H_2 receptor antagonists such as burimamide and metiamide (Rocklin, 1976, 1977). The mechanism by which histamine inhibits MIF production appears to be indirectly through the activation of suppressor cells (see below). Agents that raise intracellular levels of cAMP may also inhibit MIF production. It is not clear, however, that histamine-induced inhibition of MIF production is through the latter mechanism. *In vitro* production of other lymphokines including leukocyte inhibitory factor (LIF), interferon, and IL-2 is also decreased by the addition of histamine (Bourne *et al.*, 1974; Rigal *et al.*, 1979; Huchet and Grandjon, 1988).

4.2.3. Proliferation

The ability of lymphocytes to undergo increased DNA synthesis and mitosis in response to a specific stimulus has been termed *lymphocyte proliferation* and reflects an expansion of an immunoreactive clone of cells. This event can occur in response to a specific antigen or nonspecifically if plant lectins are used such as phytohemagglutinin, concanavalin A (Con A), or pokeweed. Histamine has been shown to modulate lymphocyte proliferation in a number of species. In the mouse, histamine (10^{-4} and 10^{-5} M) has been shown to decrease Con A-induced proliferation (Plaut *et al.*, 1975; Plaut and Roszkowski, 1979). The effects of histamine were only seen when suboptimal concentration of mitogen was used and not when optimal concentrations were employed. The latter suppression of proliferation was shown to be mediated through the H_2 receptor. Histamine also decreased the proliferative response to allogeneic stimuli (Schwartz *et al.*, 1977). Concentrations of 10^{-7}–10^{-4} M histamine were required to decrease a mixed lymphocyte culture reaction. It is of interest that the proliferative response to lipopolysaccharide is not altered by histamine. The latter response is thought to be specific for B cells, whereas the above mitogens and antigens are primarily T-cell responses.

Guinea pig lymphocytes are also susceptible to the pharmacological effects of histamine. Antigen-induced proliferation is inhibited by 10^{-6}–10^{-3} M of the drug (Rocklin, 1976). The latter response is mediated through the H_2 receptor, since burimamide blocks the inhibitory effects of histamine, but not diphenhydramine.

Studies in normal subjects as well as patients indicate that histamine also modulates the proliferative response of human lymphocytes. For example, the Con A-induced proliferative response is inhibited by histamine in a dose-dependent fashion (Plaut *et al.*, 1975). Substantial inhibition is achieved using suboptimal concentrations of mitogen and this effect is mediated via the H_2 receptor. Mixed lymphocyte culture proliferative responses can also be inhibited by histamine (Ballett and Merler, 1976). It also appears that genetic factors determine the response of individuals to histamine. Patients having the HLA haplotype HLA-B12 have a decreased response to histamine and PGE_2 using culture conditions similar to those described above (Staszak *et al.*, 1980). That is, lymphocytes from these individuals are not inhibited to the same extent by histamine as cells from individuals not possessing that HLA type. The fact that their response to PGE_2 as well as histamine is altered suggests that the defect may reside at a point beyond the histamine receptor and not with the expression of the receptor itself.

4.2.4. Suppressor Cell Activity

T-suppressor cells can regulate a variety of immunological responses including other T-cell reactions such as proliferation, lymphokine production and cytotoxicity, as well as B-cell functions related to antibody production. Suppressor cells can be activated *in vitro* over a 24- to 48-hr period by various stimuli including specific antigens, mitogens, and histamine. This process requires the participation of macrophages (as well be discussed below), T-inducer cells, and suppressor cell precursors. The effects of histamine on suppressor cell activity have been twofold. On the one hand, agents that raise cAMP (including histamine) decrease the induction of antigen-induced suppressor cells that regulate antibody production (Mozes *et al.*, 1974). This latter effect can be blocked by H_1 antagonists such as diphenhydramine. In addition, under certain experimental conditions, histamine can inhibit the production of suppressor cells in mice that are modulating cytotoxic T-lymphocyte functions (Schwartz *et al.*, 1980). The results from other experiments indicate that histamine can provide a positive signal to suppressor cells that leads to their activation. T cells activated in this manner have been shown to suppress lymphocyte proliferation, lymphokine production, and IgG production (Rocklin, 1977; Lima and Rocklin, 1981).

The mechanism by which histamine leads to suppression of certain lymphocyte functions has been determined. Histamine, in a dose-dependent manner, induces the production by lymphocytes of a soluble factor with immunosuppressive properties (Rocklin, 1977). This latter factor, termed *histamine-induced suppressor factor* (HSF), can inhibit lymphocyte proliferation and lymphokine production in the absence of histamine. The production of HSF requires stimulation of the H_2 receptor, since burimamide and metiamide can block its production while diphenhydramine has no effect. The cell that produces HSF is a T cell (B cells and macrophages do not produce an HSF-like material), is contained within the population of cells that possess Fc receptors for IgG (Tγ), is within the population identified as having CD8$^+$, as well as adhering to Sepharose beads containing insolubilized histamine (Rocklin, 1977; Rocklin *et al.*, 1980).

Soluble immune response suppressor (SIRS) is an immunosuppressive protein that inhibits plaque-forming cell responses (antibody production) and tumor cell division *in vitro* and plaque-forming cell and delayed-type hypersensitivity response *in vitro* (Schapner and Aune, 1986). Because histamine had been reported to activate human suppressor cells, the potential role for histamine in SIRS production was investigated (Schapner *et al.*, 1987). Human mononuclear cells incubated with 10^{-4} or 10^{-5} M histamine released a soluble suppressor factor capable of inhibiting an *in vitro* polyclonal IgM plague-forming cell assay. This factor was functionally, physicochemically, and antigenically similar to previously described human SIRS. The T-lymphocyte subset activated by histamine to produce SIRS was contained within the CD8$^+$, but not the CD4$^+$, population of cells. Cimetidine and ranitidine, two structurally distinct H_2 receptor antagonists, inhibited histamine induction of CD8$^+$ T-cell production of SIRS. The relationship of the previously described histamine-induced suppressor activities, HSF and HISSF, to the SIRS pathway remains to be defined.

4.3. B Lymphocytes

Immunoglobulin Production and Antibody Secretion *in Vitro*

It was first demonstrated in mice that the addition of histamine (10^{-4} M) and agents that raise intracellular levels of cAMP decrease the number of plaque-forming cells (PFC) by splenic lymphocytes *in vitro* (Melmon *et al.*, 1974). The nature of the histamine receptor involved in this reaction was considered to be the H_1 receptor because diphenhydramine blocked the inhibitory effect of histamine and not an H_2 antagonist. These studies have been extended to an investigation of antibody-secreting cells and IgG production by human lymphocytes. In the latter studies (Lima and Rocklin, 1981), the addition of histamine directly to cultures of blood mononuclear cells had little effect on the spontaneous production of IgG but significantly suppressed pokeweed mitogen-induced IgG production in a dose-dependent fashion (10^{-4}–10^{-6} M). The kinetics of histamine-induced suppression indicated that pokeweed mitogen-induced IgG production was reduced if histamine was added up to 72 hr after the addition of the mitogen. Thereafter, adding histamine to the cultures had little effect on IgG production.

The histamine-responsive suppressor cell in the above system was found to be a T cell that was sensitive to irradiation at 2000 R (Lima and Rocklin, 1981). In addition, the histamine-inducible suppressor cell was identified by a monoclonal antibody directed against OKT8 ($CD8^+$). The addition of anti-OKT8 plus complement abolished the suppression caused by histamine. Evidence was also presented in these studies that both H_1 and H_2 receptors may be involved in suppression using H_1 and H_2 agonists and antagonists.

Employing an *in vitro* system that detects antibody-secreting cells, the ability of a histamine-induced suppressor factor to modulate the numbers of plaque-forming cells (PFC) secreting IgG, IgM, or IgA was investigated (Garovoy *et al.*, 1983). T-cell activation and generation of T-helper cells was accomplished during a mixed lymphocyte culture (MLC). The addition of the suppressor factor was made on day 0 to the cultures and the plaques were measured on day 6. The suppressor factor reproducibly reduced the number of PFC/10^6 cells by 60–80%. The factor was active at a dilution of 1/1000 and suppressed IgG, IgM, and IgA isotypes equivalently. The mechanism of action on one aspect of this reaction that related to the helper cell component was investigated. Purified T lymphocytes were activated in a unidirectional MLC and subsequently combined with unprimed B cells in the absence of exogenous antigen to induce a polyclonal PFC response. The factor present only during the generation phase of the activated T cells was added at the time of the coculture to activated T cells plus unprimed B cells, and inhibited the total PFC response by 80%. To further study the effect of the factor on T-cell activation, the expression of Ia and DR antigens on activated T cells was monitored. Ia/DR antigens are normally detected on 50–60% of activated T cells generated by day 6 during a MLC. The factor reproducibly reduced by 50% the presence of detectable Ia/DR antigens. These studies suggest that the factor inhibits the MLC-induced polyclonal B-cell response by suppressing the generation and function of T-helper cells. The reduced expression of Ia/DR antigens may serve to limit T–B cooperation required for the PFC response.

4.4. Macrophages

The appearance of histamine receptors on macrophages is not well documented, although a few direct effects of histamine on macrophage function have been observed (Table III). Histamine does not alter the response of macrophages to a preformed lymphokine such as MIF, does not interfere with antigen binding to macrophages or the presentation of macrophage-bound antigen to lymphocytes, does not inhibit lymphocyte–macrophage interactions (rosetting) that lead to T-cell activation, does not activate adenylate cyclase, does not augment the appearance of C3b receptors, and is not directly chemotactic for macrophages or interfere with the chemotactic response to C5a (Rocklin, 1976, 1977). The fact that histamine does not activate macrophages or monocytes and does not stimulate increased levels of cAMP in macrophages as well as not directly affecting a number of macrophage functions argues strongly against the presence of histamine receptors on macrophages. Alternatively, if such receptors are present, they may not be functionally coupled to adenylate cyclase.

Certain functional responses of macrophages to histamine have been reported. Studies with alveolar macrophages have suggested that histamine increases the respiratory burst of these cells (Diaz *et al.*, 1979) and this effect is H_1 receptor-dependent. In addition, the production of C2 by human monocytes was decreased by histamine (Lapping *et al.*, 1980). This effect was specific for histamine in that histidine and imidazole acetic acid had no effect on C2 production. In further studies, histamine decreased the appearance of C4, C3, factor B, and B1H. The ability of histamine to modulate complement production may result in negative-feed regulation and prevent further cleavage of C3 and C5 by limiting the formation of C3 and C5 convertases. The latter effects of histamine may have important implications for complement-mediated phenomena occurring during IgE-mediated and antigen–antibody complex reactions.

5. PATHOPHYSIOLOGY

5.1. Atopy

There is evidence that immunoregulation in allergic patients is abnormal and involved T cells bearing histamine receptors. Mononuclear cells from atopic patients generate less histamine-induced suppressor activity than those from nonatopic con-

TABLE III
Effect of Histamine on Macrophage Function

Cell function	Histamine receptor	
	H_1	H_2
1. Response to MIF	–	–
2. Antigen binding	–	–
3. Antigen presentation	–	–
4. Lymphocyte–macrophage rosette function	–	–
5. Generation of adenylate cyclase	–	–
6. C3b receptors	–	–
7. Chemotaxis (C5a)	–	–
8. Increased respiratory burst	+	–
9. Inhibits complement component synthesis	–	+

trol subjects (Abdou *et al.*, 1979; Beer *et al.*, 1982). This defect in suppressor cell response was not global and appeared to be specific for histamine because their response to another suppressor signal, Con A, was apparently normal. In the process of investigating the mechanism for this diminished response to histamine, it was found that the number of H_2 receptor-bearing T lymphocytes (but not H_1 receptor-bearing T cells) was decreased in these atopic patients. One explanation for the reduced functional suppressor response to histamine, as well as the reduced phenotypic expression of H_2 receptors in the atopic population, was that they represent secondary changes resulting from chronic *in vivo* exposure of their lymphocytes to circulating histamine, rather than a primary abnormality. This question was addressed when nonatopic patients with systemic mastocytosis, a disease characterized by elevated levels of circulating histamine, had their histamine-responsive suppressor cells evaluated (Beer *et al.*, 1982). In the latter group of patients, the suppressor cell response to histamine was normal as was the expression of H_1 and H_2 receptors on their T lymphocytes. This observation mitigates against the observed abnormalities in atopics as representing secondary changes from *in vitro* "desensitization" or receptor "downregulation." Rather, the suppressor cell abnormalities observed in allergic subjects may represent a primary defect inherent to the atopic diathesis.

5.2. Immunodeficiency

Four patients with chronic mucocutaneous candidiasis, cutaneous anergy, and abnormal *in vitro* lymphocyte function were administered cimetidine. The administration of cimetidine to these four patients resulted in a positive conversion of their delayed hypersensitivity skin tests (Jorizzo *et al.*, 1980). This included reactivity to monilia and streptokinase streptodornase. In addition, their *in vitro* lymphokine production to these antigens also became positive. When the drug was withdrawn from the patients, they relapsed into an anergic state. Further administration of the drug again resulted in a conversion to a positive state. This study clearly demonstrated that cimetidine could modulate immune function in these anergic patients but thus far had not resulted in a clinical improvement of their disease.

Patients with the common variable form of hypogammaglobulinemia may exhibit a variety of immunologic defects including decreased helper T-cell function, increased suppressor cell function, and effective B-cell function (White and Ballow, 1984). In three of the five adult patients with this disease treated with cimetidine, enhanced suppressor cell function was diminished. The patients were treated for 1 month with cimetidine, and their T- and B-cell function was monitored. Three patients with enhanced suppressor cell function had a reduction in suppressor cell activity function as well as a reduction in the number of $T8^+$ cells. Of particular interest, one of the three patients had a marked increase in both *in vitro* and *in vivo* immunoglobulin secretion and serum immunoglobulin concentration. When the drug was stopped, there was a reversion in the three patients to their pretreatment findings. When the drug was readministered, the decreased suppressor activity and increased immunoglobulin concentration was once again observed in the same patient. These changes were not observed in the two patients who did not exhibit enhanced suppressor cell activity. Presumably, the enhanced effect on immunoglobulin production by cimetidine was related to blockade of H_2 receptors on suppressor cells. These exciting findings indicated that certain immunosuppressed patients may be treated pharmacologically when there is evidence of enhanced suppressor cell function.

H_2-receptor antagonists may ameliorate part of the immunodeficiency associated with human immunodeficiency virus (HIV) infection. Cimetidine was administered to 33 patients with HIV and AIDS-related complex (ARC) (Brockmeyer *et al.*, 1988). Preliminary data showed improvement in performance status, subjective health status, body weight, fever, lymphnode size, immunoglobulin level, the number of helper T lymphocytes, and the lymphocyte proliferative response. There were no side effects, and the benefit lasted as long as the drug was continued.

5.3. Malignancy

The activity of cell-mediated defense systems is stimulated by consecutive formation of interleukin-1 β (IL-1β), IL-2, and interferon-γ (IFN-γ). The system is inhibited by IL-4 and also by prostaglandin E_2 (PGE_2) and histamine, which are released when the immune system is activated. The inhibition is strong in cancer patients, because PGE_2 is formed in many cancer cells and its formation is stimulated by IL-1β. The release of histamine is also stimulated by IL-1β. Thus, PGE_2 and histamine are feedback inhibitors of cell-mediated immunity. This inhibition can be abolished by inhibitors of the cyclooxygenase (e.g., indomethacin) and H_2 receptor antagonists (e.g., cimetidine). This may offer a new option to stimulate the immune system to kill cancer cells (Uotila, 1993).

The participation of histamine receptor-bearing cells has been evaluated in patients with abnormal immune function caused by malignancy. Thus, patients with Hodgkin's disease and anergy have decreased allogeneic-induced cytotoxic responses; passage of their lymphocytes over histamine columns resulted in improved responses (Zarling *et al.*, 1980). In another study (Osband *et al.*, 1981), patients with histiocytosis X and abnormal lymphocyte function were found to have decreased H_2 receptor-bearing T cells. The addition of a thymic extract *in vitro* reversed the phenotypic abnormality in their lymphocytes. Subsequently, the patients were administered thymosin *in vivo* and had a clinical improvement of their disease. This was also associated with an increase in the number of H_2 receptor-bearing cells.

Cimetidine and ranitidine (H_2 antagonists) can increase IL-2 and immunoglobulin production in normal volunteers (Aweeka *et al.*, 1989) and cimetidine has restored IL-2 production during chemotherapy for ovarian cancer (Kikuchi *et al.*, 1988). Cimetidine may also restore NK cell activity in cancer patients by reducing histamine-induced suppressor factor production (Calvieri *et al.*, 1988). No harmful effect of cimetidine or ranitidine on the immune system of cancer patients has been described, and most preclinical evaluations showed no effect of ranitidine on the immune system of normal subjects.

Kaposi's sarcoma (KS) may respond to cimetidine. KS most commonly occurs in immunodeficient patients, such as posttransplant patients or patients treated with steroids, and may regress if the immunosuppressive drugs or steroids are stopped. In addition, KS has become the most common malignancy in patients with AIDS. Two patients with classic but rapidly progressive KS were treated with cimetidine, 200 mg intravenously every 12 hr; both had dramatic improvement of the KS (Calvieri and Fattorossi, 1985). A remarkable side effect was that pretreatment immunosuppression improved, with near normalization of the ratio of helper to suppressor T lymphocytes, and improved blastogenic response of lymphocytes. NK cell activity returned to normal with cimetidine therapy (Calvieri *et al.*, 1988).

A single agent, cimetidine or ranitidine in routine doses has been reported to have occasional beneficial effects in patients with lung cancer (Armitage and Sidner, 1979), melanoma (Morton *et al.*, 1987), mycosis fungoides (Mamus *et al.*, 1984), gastric lymphoma (Strauchen *et al.*, 1987), and classic KS (Calvieri and Fattorossi, 1985). Cimetidine may or may not enhance the response of melanoma to interferon if the interferon is injected intratumorally or systemically; the highest response rate (five of eight) was observed in patients with subcutaneous nodules who received intratumoral injections of human leukocyte interferon in conjunction with cimetidine (Flodgren *et al.*, 1983).

REFERENCES

Abdou, N., Martinez, J. C., Santos, J., and Stechschulte, D. J., 1979, Nonspecific suppressor cell function in atopic subjects, *J. Allergy Clin. Immunol.* **64**:485–490.

Altura, B. M., and Halery, S., 1978, Cardiovascular actions of histamine, in: *Handbook of Experimental Pharmacology* (M. Rocha e Silva, ed.), Springer, Berlin, pp. 1–39.

Anwar, A. R. E., and Kay, A. B., 1977, The ECF-A tetrapeptide and histamine selectively enhance human eosinophil complement receptors, *Nature* **269**:522–524.

Anwar, A. R. E., and Kay, A. B., 1978, Enhancement of human eosinophil complement receptors by pharmacologic mediators, *J. Immunol.* **121**:1245–1250.

Armitage, J. O., and Sidner, R. D., 1979, Antitumor effect of cimetidine? *Lancet* **1**:882–883.

Arrang, J. M., 1994, Pharmacological properties of histamine receptor subtypes, *Cell. Mol. Biol.* **40**:475–281.

Arrang, J. M., Garbag, M., and Schwartz, J., 1983, Autoinhibition of brain histamine release mediated by a novel class (H_3) of histamine receptor, *Nature* **302**:832.

Ash, A. S. F., and Schild, H. O., 1966, Receptors mediating some actions of histamine, *Br. J. Pharmacol.* **27**:427–439.

Austen, K. F., 1976, Biologic assay of histamine, in: *Methods in Immunology and Immunochemistry* (C. A. Williams, and M. W. Chase, eds.), Academic Press, New York, Volume 5, p. 126.

Aweeka, F., Lizak, P., Garovoy, M., McTavish, J., and Reddish, M., 1989, Interleukin-2 and immunoglobin increases with H_2-antagonists in humans, *Transplant Proc.* **21**:1718–1721.

Ballet, J. J., and Merler, E., 1976, The separation and reactivity in vitro of a subpopulation of human lymphocytes which binds histamine. Correlation of histamine reactivity with cellular maturation, *Cell. Immunol.* **24**:250–269.

Bearer, C., Chang, L., Rosenfeld, G., and Thompson, W., 1981, Histamine stimulation of rat gastic parietal adenyl-cyclase: Modulation by guanine nucleosides, *Arch. Biochem. Biophys.* **207**:325.

Beer, D., Osband, M., McCaffrey, R., Soter, N., and Rocklin, R. E., 1982, Abnormal histamine activated suppressor cell activity in atopic subjects, *N. Engl. J. Med.* **306**:454–458.

Berglindh, T., 1984, The mammalian gastric parietal cell in vitro, *Annu. Rev. Physiol.* **46**:377–392.

Berridge, M. J., 1975, The interaction of cyclic nucleotides and calcium in the control of cellular activity, *Adv. Cyclic Nucleotide Res.* **6**:1–98.

Bertaccini, G., Poli, E., and Coruzzi, G., 1993, Histamine H_2 receptor antagonists and the cardiovascular system, *Pharmacol. Res.* **28**:301–316.

Best, C. H., Dale, H. H., Dudley, H. W., and Thorpe, W. V., 1927, The nature of vasodilator constituents of certain tissue extracts, *J. Physiol. (London)* **62**:397.

Black, J. W., Duncan, W. A. M., Durant, C. J., Ganellin, C. R., and Parsons, E. M., 1972, Definition and antagonism of histamine H2-receptors, *Nature* **236**:385–390.

Bourne, H. R., Melmon, K. L., and Lichtenstein, L. M., 1971, Histamine augments leukocyte cyclic AMP and blocks antigenic histamine release, *Science* **173**:743–745.

Bourne, H. R., Lichtenstein, L. M., Henney, C. S., Melmon, K. L., Weinstein, Y., and Shearer, G. M., 1974, Modulation of inflammation and immunity by cyclic AMP, *Science* **184**:19–28.

Brink, C., Douglas, J. S., and Duncan, P. G., 1982, Changes in the response of guinea pig airways in vivo and in vitro to cimetidine and propranolol during development, *Br. J. Pharmacol.* **75**:531.

Brockmeyer, N. H., Krenzfelde, E., and Kirch, W., 1988, Immunomodulatory properties of cinetidine in ARC patients, *Clin. Immunol. Immunopathol.* **48**:500.

Brown, M. J., Ind., P. W., Causon, R., and Lee, T. H., 1982, A novel double isotope technique for the enzymatic assay of plasma histamine: Application to estimation of mast cell activation assessed by antigen challenge in asthmatics, *J. Allergy Clin. Immunol.* **69**:20.

Bryant, D. H., and Kay, A. B., 1977, Cutaneous eosinophil accumulation in atopic and non-atopic individuals: The effects of an ECF-A tetrapeptide and histamine, *Clin. Allergy* **211**:2127.

Busse, W. W., 1994, Role of antihistamines in allergic disease, *Ann. Allergy* **72**:371–375.

Busse, W. W., and Sosman, J., 1976, Histamine inhibition of neutrophil lysosomal enzyme release: An H_2 histamine receptor response, *Science* **194**:737–738.

Calvieri, S., and Fattorossi, A., 1985, Cimetidine for Kaposi's sarcoma, *Clin. Exp. Dermatol.* **10**:499–501.

Calvieri, S., Gianelli, V., and Zampetti, M., 1988, Cimetidine and natural killer cell activity, *Clin. Exp. Dermatol.* **13**:282.

Clark, R. A. F., Gallin, J. I., and Kaplan, A. P., 1975, The selective eosinophil chemotactic activity of histamine, *J. Exp. Med.* **142**:1462–1476.

Clark, R. A. F., Sandler, J. A., Gallin, J. I., and Kaplan, A. P., 1977, Histamine modulation of eosinophil migration, *J. Immunol.* **118:**137–145.

Code, C. F., 1965, Histamine and gastric secretion: A later look, 1955–1965, *Fed. Proc.* **24:**1311–1325.

Dale, H. H., and Laidlaw, P. P., 1910, The physiologic action of beta-imidazolethylamine, *J. Physiol. (London)* **41:**318.

Diaz, P., Jones, D. G., and Kay, A. B., 1979, Histamine-coated particles generate superoxide (O_2) and chemiluminescence in alveolar macrophages, *Nature* **278:**454–456.

Dickenson, J. M., and Hill, S. J., 1993, Coupling of histamine H1 and adenosine A1 receptors to phospholipase C in DDT1MF-2 cells: Synergistic interactions and regulation by cyclic AMP, *Biochem. Soc. Trans.* **21:**1124–1129.

Eyre, P., 1973, Histamine H2-receptors in the sheep bronchus and cat trachea: The actions of burimamide, *Br. J. Pharmacol.* **48:**321.

Flodgren, P., Borgstrom, S., Jonsson, P. E., Lindström, C., and Sjögren, H. O., 1983, Metastatic malignant melanoma: Regression induced by combined treatment with interferon [HuIFN–alpha (Le)] and cimetidine, *Int. J. Cancer* **32:**657–665.

Friedman, D. L., 1976, Role of cyclic nucleotides in cell growth and differentiation, *Physiol. Rev.* **56:**652.

Fukui, H., Watanabe, T., and Wada, H., 1980, Immunochemical cross reactivity of the antibody elicited against L-histidine decarboxylase purified from the whole bodies of fetal rats with the enzyme from rat brain, *Biochem. Biophys. Res. Commun.* **93:**333.

Ganellin, C. R., and Parsons, M. E., 1982, *Pharmacology of Histamine Receptors*, Wright/PSG, Bristol.

Gantz, I., Schaffer, M., DelValle, J., Logsdon, C., Campbell, V., Uhler, M., and Yamade, T., 1991, Molecular cloning of a gene encoding the histamine H2 receptor, *Proc. Natl. Acad. Sci. USA* **88:**429–433.

Garovoy, M., Reddish, M., and Rocklin, R. E., 1982, Inhibition of helper T cell function and expression of "Ia" by histamine-induced suppressor factor, *J. Immunol.* **130:**357–361.

Graham, P., Kahlson, G., and Rosengren, E., 1964, Histamine formation in physical exercise, anoxia, and under the influence of adrenaline and related substances, *J. Physiol. (London)* **172:**174.

Hadden, J. W., Hadden, E. M., Haddox, M. K., and Goldberg, N. D., 1972, Guanosine 3′-5′ cyclic monophosphate: A possible intracellular mediator of mitogenic influences in lymphocytes, *Proc. Natl. Acad. Sci. USA* **69:**3024.

Huchet, R., and Grandjon, D., 1988, Histamine-induced regulation of IL-2 synthesis in men: Characterization of two pathways of inhibition, *Ann. Inst. Pasteur Immunol.* **139:**485.

Jorizzo, J. L., Sams, W. M., Jr., Jegasothy, V. V., and Olamsky, A. J., 1980, Cimetidine as an immunomodulator: Chronic mucocutaneous candidiasis as a model, *Ann. Intern. Med.* **92:**192–195.

Kaliner, M., 1978, Human lung tissue and anaphylaxis: The effects of histamine on the immunologic release of mediators *Am. Rev. Resp. Dis.* **118:**1015–1022.

Kapeller-Adler, R., 1965, Histamine catabolism in vitro and in vivo, *Fed. Proc.* **24:**757.

Keele, C. A., and Armstrong, D., 1964, *Substances Producing Pain and Itch*, Williams & Wilkins, Baltimore.

Kikuchi, Y., Kizawa, I., and Oomori, K., 1988, Effects of cimetidine on interleukin-2 production by peripheral blood lymphocytes in advanced ovarian cancer, *Eur. J. Cancer Clin. Oncol.* **24:**1185–1190.

Lagunoff, D., 1974, Analysis of dye binding sites in mast cell granules, *Biochemistry* **13:**3982.

Lagunoff, D., and Bauza, M., 1982, The formation and storage of histamine in the mast cell, in: *Advances in the Biosciences*, Volume 23 (B. Uvnas and K. Tasaka, eds.), Pergamon Press, New York, pp. 29–38.

Lappin, D., Moseley, H. L., and Whaley, K., 1980, Effect of histamine on monocyte complement production, *Clin. Exp. Immunol.* **42:**515–522.

Lett-Brown, M. A., and Leonard, E. J., 1977, Histamine-induced inhibition of normal basophil chemotaxis to C5a, *J. Immunol.* **118:**815–818.

Lett-Brown, M. A., Boetcher, D. A., and Leonard, E. J., 1976, Chemotactic response of normal human basophils to C5a and to lymphocyte-derived chemotactic factor, *J. Immunol.* **117:**246–252.

Lewin, M. J., Bado, A., Cherifi, Y., and Reyl-Desmars, F., 1992, The gastric H3 receptor, *Yale J. Biol. Med.* **65:**607–611.

Lewis, T., 1927, *The Blood Vessels of the Human Skin and Their Responses*, Shaw, London.

Lichtenstein, L. M., 1975, The mechanisms of basophil histamine release induced by antigen and by the calcium ionophore A23187, *J. Immunol.* **114**:1692–1699.

Lichtenstein, L. M., and Gillespie, E., 1973, Inhibition of histamine release by histamine is controlled by an H-2 receptor, *Nature* **244**:287–288.

Lima, M., and Rocklin, R. E., 1981, Histamine modulates in vitro IgG production by human mononuclear cells, *Cell. Immunol.* **64**:324–336.

Maengwyn-Davies, G. D., 1968, The dual mode of action of histamine in the cat isolated tracheal chain, *J. Pharm. Pharmacol.* **20**:572.

Majno, G., Shea, S. M., and Leventhal, M., 1969, Endothelial contraction induced by histamine-type mediators, *J. Cell Biol.* **42**:647.

Mamus, S. W., Mladenovic, J., Hurdinsky, M. K., Dahl, M. V., and Kay, N. E., 1984, Cimetidine-induced remission of mycosis fungoides, *Lancet* **2**:409.

Melmon, K. L., Bourne, H. R., Weinstein, V., Shearer, G. M., Kram, J., and Bauminger, S., 1974, Hemolytic plaque formation by leukocytes in vitro. Control by vasoactive hormones, *J. Clin. Invest.* **53**:13–21.

Michoud, M. D., Lelorier, J., and Amyot, B., 1981, Factors modulating the interindividual variability of airway responsiveness to histamine. The influence of H_1 and H_2 receptors, *Clin. Respir. Physiol.* **17**:807.

Morton, R. F., Creagen, E. T., Cullinan, S. A., Mailliard, J. A., Ebbert, L., Vedder, M. H., and Chang, M., 1987, Phase II studies of single agent cimetidine and the combination N-phosphonacetyl-L-aspartate (NSC-224131) plus L-alanosine (NSC-153353) in advanced malignant melanoma, *J. Clin. Oncol.* **5**:1078.

Mozes, E., Weinstein, Y., Bourne, H. R., Melmon, K. L., and Shearer, G. M., 1974, In vitro correction of antigen-induced immune suppression: Effect of histamine, dibutyryl cyclic AMP and cholera enterotoxin, *Cell. Immunol.* **11**:57–63.

Nair, M. P. N., and Schwartz, S. A., 1983, Effect of histamine antagonists on natural and antibody-dependent cellular cytotoxicity of human lymphocytes in vitro, *Cell. Immunol.* **81**:45.

Nash, J., Lambert, L., and Deakin, M., 1994, Histamine H_2-receptor antagonists in peptic ulcer disease. Evidence for a prophylactic use, *Drugs* **47**:862–871.

Nogrady, S. G., and Bevan, C., 1981, H_2 receptor blockade and bronchial hyperreactivity to histamine in asthma, *Thorax* **36**:268.

Northover, A. M., 1975, Action of histamine on endothelial cells of guinea-pig isolated hepatic portal vein and its modification by indomethacin or removal of calcium, *Br. J. Exp. Pathol.* **56**:52.

Nowak, J. A., 1994, Histamine in the central nervous system: Its role in circadian rhythmicity, *Acta Neurobiol. Exp.* **54**:65–82.

Okpako, D. T., Chand, N., and Eyre, P., 1978, The presence of inhibitory histamine H_2-receptors in guinea pig tracheobronchial muscle, *J. Pharm. Pharmacol.* **30**:181.

Osband, M., Lipton, J. M., Lavin, P., Levy, R., Vawter, G., Greenberger, J., McCaffrey, R., and Parkman, R., 1981, Histiocytosis X: Demonstration of abnormal immunity, T-cell histamine H-2 receptor deficiency and successful treatment with thymic extract, *N. Engl. J. Med.* **304**:146–153.

Owen, D. A. A., 1977, Histamine receptors in the cardiovascular system, *Gen. Pharmacol.* **8**:141.

Plaut, M., and Roszkowski, W., 1979, Lymphocyte subpopulations bearing histamine receptors, in: *Histamine Receptors* (T. O. Yellin, ed.), Spectrum Publications, Holliswood, NY, pp. 361–376.

Plaut, M., Lichtenstein, L. M., and Henney, C. S., 1975, Properties of a subpopulation of T-cells bearing histamine receptors, *J. Clin. Invest.* **55**:856–874.

Prell, G. D., and Green, J. P., 1994, Measurements of histamine metabolites in brain and cerebrospinal fluid provides insights into histaminergic activity, *Agents Actions* **41**:C5–C8.

Rigal, D., Monier, J. C., and Souweine, G., 1979, Effect of histamine on leukocyte migration test in man, *Cell. Immunol.* **46**:360–372.

Riley, J. F., and West, G. B., 1953, The presence of histamine in tissue mast cells, *J. Physiol. (London)* **120**:528.

Rocha e Silva, M., ed., 1966, *Histamine: Its Chemistry, Metabolism and Physiological and Pharmacological Actions, Handbuch der Experimentellen Pharmakologie*, Volume 18, Part 1, Springer-Verlag, Berlin.

Rocklin, R. E., 1976, Modulation of cellular-immune responses in vivo and in vitro by histamine receptor-bearing lymphocytes, *J. Clin. Invest.* **57:**1051–1058.

Rocklin, R. E., 1977, Histamine-induced suppressor factor (HSF): Effect on migration inhibitory factor (MIF) production and proliferation, *J. Immunol.* **118:**1734.

Rocklin, R. E., Beard, J., Gupta, S., Good, R. A., and Melmon, K. L., 1980, Characterizations of the human blood lymphocytes that produce a histamine-induced suppressor factor (HSF), *Cell. Immunol.* **51:**226–237.

Schayer, R. W., 1959, Catabolism of physiologic quantities of histamine *in vivo*, *Physiol. Rev.* **39:**116.

Schayer, R. W., 1966, Enzymatic formation of histamine from histadine, in: *Handbook of Experimental Pharmacology* (O. Eichler and A. Farah, eds.), Springer, Berlin.

Schayer, R. W., 1968, Histidine decarboxylase in mast cells, *Ann. N.Y. Acad. Sci.* **103:**164.

Schayer, R. W., and Reilly, M. A., 1972, Studies on the mechanism of activation and deactivation of histadine decarboxylase, *Eur. J. Pharmacol.* **20:**271.

Schlicker, E., Malinowska, B., Kathmann, M., and Gothert, M., 1994, Modulation of neurotransmitter release via histamine H3 receptors, *Fundam. Clin. Pharmacol.* **8:**128–137.

Schnaper, H. W., and Aune, T. M., 1986, Suppression of immune response to sheep erythrocytes by the lymphokine soluble immune response suppressor (SIRS) in vivo, *J. Immunol.* **137:**863–867.

Schnaper, H. W., Aune, T. M., and Roby, R. K., 1987, A role for histamine type II (H-2) receptor binding in production of the lymphokine, soluble immune response suppressor (SIRS), *J. Immunol.* **139:**1185–1190.

Schwartz, A., Askenase, P. W., and Gershon, R. K., 1977, The effect of locally injected vasoactive amines on the elicitation of delayed-type hypersensitivity, *J. Immunol.* **118:**159–165.

Schwartz, A., Askenase, P. W., and Gershon, R. K., 1980, Histamine inhibition of the in vitro induction of cytotoxic T-cell responses, *Immunopharmacology* **2:**179–190.

Schwartz, J. C., 1979, Histamine receptors in brain, *Life Sci.* **25:**895–912.

Schwartz, S. A., and Nair, M. P. N., 1990, Histamine in the immunoregulation of cellular cytotoxicity, in: *Histamine and H2 Antagonists in Inflammation and Immunodeficiency* (R. E. Rocklin, ed.), Dekker, New York, pp. 65–79.

Seligman, B. E., Fletcher, M. P., and Gallin, J. I., 1983, Histamine modulation of human neutrophil oxidative, metabolism, locomotion, degranulation and membrane potential changes, *J. Immunol.* **130:**1902.

Shore, P. A., Burkhalter, A., and Cohn, V. H., 1959, A method for fluorimetric assay of histamine in tissue, *J. Pharmacol. Exp. Ther.* **127:**182.

Snyder, S. H., and Axelrod, J., 1965, Tissue metabolism of histamine-^{14}C in vivo, *Fed. Proc.* **24:**774.

Sol, A. H., and Grossman, M. I., 1981, The interaction of stimulants on the function of isolated canine parietal cells, *Philos. Trans. R. Soc. London Ser. B* **296:**5–15.

Staszak, C., Goodwin, J. S., Troup, G. M., Pahtak, D. R., and Williams, R. C., Jr., 1980, Decreased sensitivity to prostaglandin and histamine in lymphocytes from normal HLA-B12 individuals: A possible role in autoimmunity, *J. Immunol.* **125:**181–185.

Strauchen, J. A., Moran, C., Goldsmith, M., and Greenberg, M., 1987, Spontaneous regression of gastric lymphoma, *Cancer* **60:**1872–1875.

Ting, S., Dunsky, E. H., and Zweiman, B., 1980, Histamine suppression of eosinophilotaxis and histamine release in vivo, *J. Allergy Clin. Immunol.* **65:**196–197.

Tran, V. T., and Snyder, S. H., 1981, Histidine decarboxylase. Purification from fetal rat liver, immunologic properties, and histochemical localization in brain and stomach, *J. Biol. Chem.* **256:**680.

Uotila, P., 1993, Inhibition of prostaglandin E2 formation and histamine action in cancer immunotherapy, *Cancer Immunol. Immunother.* **37:**251–254.

Uvnas, B., 1974, Histamine storage and release, *Fed. Proc.* **33:**2172.

Watanabe, T., Nakamura, H., Liang, L. Y., Yamatodani, A., and Wada, H., 1979, Partial purification and characterization of L-histidine decarboxylase from fetal rats, *Biochem. Pharmacol.* **28:**1149.

Watanabe, T., *et al.*, 1982, Purification and properties of histidine decarboxylase isozymes and their pharmacological significance, in: *Advances in the Biosciences* (B. Uvnas and K. Tasaka, eds.), Pergamon Press, New York.

Weill, B. J., and Renoux, M. S., 1982, Study of granule reappearance and histamine synthesis in rat mast cells maintained in short term cultures, *Cell. Immunol.* **68**:220.

Weiss, S., Robb, G. P., and Ellis, L. B., 1932, The systemic effects of histamine in man, *Arch. Intern. Med.* **49**:360.

Weissbach, H., Lovenberg, W., and Udenfriend, S., 1961, Characteristics of mammalian histidine decarboxylating enzymes, *Biochim. Biophys. Acta* **50**:177.

Weissman, N. G., Zurier, R. B., Spieler, P. J., Goldstein, I. M., 1971, Mechanisms of lysosomal enzyme release from leukocytes exposed to immune complexes and other particles, *J. Exp. Med.* **134/3**:149S.

White, W. B., and Ballow, M., 1984, Cimetidine modulates suppressor cell activity in common variable hypogammaglobuineinia, *Clin. Res.* **32**:362A.

Zarling, J., Berman, C., and Raich, P. C., 1980, Depressed cytotoxic T-cell responses in previously treated Hodgkins' and non-Hodgkins' lymphoma patients. Evidence for histamine receptor bearing suppressor cells, *Cancer Immuno. Immunother.* **7**:243–249.

PART V

AUTOIMMUNITY

CHAPTER 9

BIOLOGIC INTERVENTIONS IN AUTOIMMUNE DISEASES

VIBEKE STRAND and NORMAN TALAL

1. INTRODUCTION

Biologic therapeutics are diverse and therefore hard to define as a group. Often they are molecules that occur naturally in humans or mimic such molecules in form or function. Biologic interventions are well-intended guesses but nevertheless based on our still imperfect understanding of complex and interlocking physiologic and pathologic mechanisms. They are aimed at specifically altering biologic processes presumed to contribute to the pathogenesis of a variety of autoimmune diseases.

Several types of biologic agents have been investigated in the treatment of autoimmune disease. The majority of the studies involve patients with rheumatoid arthritis (RA) or multiple sclerosis (MS), although pilot studies have been performed in diabetes, psoriasis, inflammatory bowel disease, systemic lupus erythematosus (SLE), and systemic sclerosis (SSc). This chapter will review the data from these initial studies. Results from clinical trials in RA and MS will be summarized, which offer instructive lessons for future therapeutic interventions.

VIBEKE STRAND • Division of Immunology, Stanford University, Stanford, California 94305. NORMAN TALAL • Clinical Immunology Section, Audie L. Murphy Memorial Veterans Hospital, and Department of Medicine, The University of Texas Health Science Center at San Antonio, San Antonio, Texas 78284.

Immunopharmacology Reviews, Volume 2, edited by John W. Hadden and Andor Szentivanyi. Plenum Press, New York, 1996.

2. CURRENT POTENTIAL THERAPIES

2.1. Monoclonal Antibodies and Immunotoxins

2.1.1. Pan-T Cell

2.1.1a. OKT3. With the rapid advances in recombinant and hybridoma technology, monoclonal antibodies (mAbs) have emerged as new approaches for the treatment of autoimmune diseases. Much evidence suggests that autoimmune processes resemble normal immune responses in being antigen-driven and T cell-dependent. Because the T cell has been implicated in pathogenesis, mAbs were developed to target surface CD antigens expressed by T-cell populations. The first clinical attempt to modulate immune function utilized a murine IgG1 mAb against the pan-T-cell antigen CD3 (OKT3) for the treatment of acute renal allograft rejection (Cosimi *et al.*, 1981; Fung *et al.*, 1987a,b). Its use has been limited by the treatment-associated toxicities (including fever, hypotension, pulmonary and pedal edema) (Chatenoud *et al.*, 1988; Thistlethwaite *et al.*, 1988), the immunogenicity (Goldstein *et al.*, 1986; Hirsch *et al.*, 1989; Abramowicz *et al.*, 1992) and short serum half-life of the murine mAb, and the increased incidence of secondary lymphomas (Zutter *et al.*, 1988; Penn, 1990; Swinnen *et al.*, 1990; Emery and Lake, 1991) related in part to the underlying immune status of the host.

Murine mAbs were first developed because of the stability of producing rat and mouse myeloma lines in long-term tissue culture. Although murine IgG2a and IgG3 isotypes activate murine complement, they are not effective in mediating complement-dependent cytolysis (CDC) in humans, nor antibody-dependent cellular cytotoxicity (ADCC). Rodent antibodies do induce a host antiglobulin response which leads to rapid clearance of the mAb from circulation, and can interfere with binding of mAb to the target antigen. The immunogenicity of a variety of mAbs in patients with cancer or graft-versus-host disease, accompanied by profound immunosuppression, appeared to be low. However, in patients with autoimmune diseases, immune responses to administered mAbs have been routinely observed (Dillman, 1990; Wilks *et al.*, 1990; Horneff *et al.*, 1991c). In an attempt to make murine mAbs more effective in eliminating their target cell population, toxin conjugates were designed to facilitate cytolysis of cells expressing the targeted surface antigen. Fusion proteins of the Pseudomonas exotoxin and conjugates to the yttrium 90 isotope (Waldmann *et al.*, 1992) or ribosomal inhibiting proteins such as ricin (Byers *et al.*, 1990) were used. This potential for increased efficacy was, unfortunately, countered by the immunogenicity of the toxin molecules themselves.

Employing a variety of techniques, chimeric and subsequently humanized mAbs were developed to increase efficacy, decrease immunogenicity, and prolong serum half-life (Morrison and Oi, 1989; Waldmann, 1991). *In vitro*, several of these IgG1 humanized mAbs mediate ADCC with human mononuclear cells (Hale *et al.*, 1988; Junghans *et al.*, 1990). Studies in primates and clinical trials in humans have demonstrated these mAbs to be less immunogenic, eliciting predominantly an antiidiotype response, with serum half-lives three to four times longer than murine versions (Hakimi *et al.*, 1991; Isaacs *et al.*, 1992; Moreland *et al.*, 1993b).

2.1.1b. CD5 Immunoconjugate. An immunoconjugate of murine IgG1 mAb against the pan-T-cell surface antigen CD5, linked to ricin A chain (a ribosomal inhibitory protein), CD5 Plus, was developed for the treatment of acute graft-versus-host disease following bone marrow transplantation. An open label evaluation in 76 patients with RA, with and without concomitant MTX therapy, suggested benefit (Strand *et al.*, 1993). Although acute decrease in the T and $CD5^+$ B-cell populations was observed after administration of this agent, normalization to ≥50% of pretreatment values occurred within 30–45 days of treatment (Fishwild and Strand, 1993), suggesting that redistribution and not depletion accounted for the majority of the decrease in peripheral T-cell counts. Clinical effects were observed lasting ≥6 months in some patients, and were not related to the biologic effect of this agent. Antiimmunoconjugate responses were observed in all but one patient. Nonetheless, 15 patients received a second course of therapy, with evidence of biologic and clinical effect.

Subsequent data have suggested that CD5 is a coactivation antigen on the T-cell surface; mAbs to this antigen may have effect by modulating peripheral and/or synovial T-cell activation (Verwilghen *et al.*, 1992). A multicenter, randomized controlled trial in RA patients, comparing placebo to several dose levels of CD5 Plus, and examining regular retreatment, has been completed but the results are not yet known.

The administration of CD5 Plus was evaluated in two open label pilot studies of patients with lupus nephritis and/or thrombocytopenia, refractory to treatment with steroids and cyclophosphamide (Wacholtz and Lipsky, 1992). In the first series benefit was reported in four of six patients with objective improvement in renal function of ≥5 months' duration in three patients. A second pilot study conducted at the NIH also reported improvement in two of four patients with biopsy-proven nephritis of 4 and >6 months' duration, but no clinical responses in two patients with thrombocytopenia (Stafford *et al.*, 1993).

2.1.1c. CAMPATH 1H. Another pan-T-cell mAb, CAMPATH 1, targets the CD52 antigen expressed on the majority of human peripheral lymphocytes and monocytes. Developed for the treatment of graft rejection and lymphoma (Riechmann *et al.*, 1988), the humanized form, CAMPATH 1H, has recently been studied in several open label protocols in patients with RA and/or vasculitis, following IV or SQ dosing (Mathieson *et al.*, 1990; Kyle *et al.*, 1991; Isaacs *et al.*, 1992; Johnston and Spreen, 1994). Rapid and profound depletion of the peripheral T-cell population was observed, with more delayed reconstitution of the CD4 T-cell population compared to CD8 cells. Lymphopenia has persisted for longer than a year in some patients. Treatment-associated infections have been reported in 11% of patients (12/106), presumably secondary to the induced cytopenia. Two deaths have been ascribed to infectious complications.

Clinical benefit was evident early in the trials but was of short duration. Although a dose–response correlation was not observed, responses of more than 1 month's duration occurred only in those patients receiving >30 mg. Again, a correlation between the biologic effect, absolute CD4 lymphopenia, and clinical response was not observed. Fever, chills, and hypotension have been prominent treatment-associated symptoms, attributed to lympholysis. Antiidiotypic antibody responses are noted in 90% of patients. Despite evidence of *in vitro* blocking activity, biologic and therapeutic responses have been observed with retreatment.

2.1.2. Anti-CD4 mAbs

Targeting the helper/inducer T-cell subset, administration of rat anti-mouse L3T4 (analogous to the human CD4) mAbs caused improvement in the underlying disease process in a variety of animal models including murine models of SLE (NZB/W; Wofsy, 1987), collagen-induced arthritis (Rauges *et al.*, 1985), myasthenia gravis (Christadoss and Dauphmee, 1986), experimental allergic encephalitis (Waldor *et al.*, 1985), type I diabetes (Koike *et al.*, 1987), thyroiditis (Nabozny *et al.*, 1991), and uveitis (Atalla *et al.*, 1990). Based on these experimental findings, murine and chimeric anti-CD4 mAbs have been administered to patients with RA, SLE, and MS. Anecdotal reports of their use in Crohn disease, uveitis, and psoriasis have suggested benefit.

The majority of the studies reported to date in RA have been open label evaluations. Benefit has been observed following administration of murine anti-CD4 mAbs of differing isotypes (IgG1 and IgG2a) and with different epitope specificities (Herzog *et al.*, 1987, 1989; Walker *et al.*, 1989; Goldberg *et al.*, 1991; Horneff *et al.*, 1991a, 1992; Reiter *et al.*, 1991; Wendling *et al.*, 1991, 1992; Racadot *et al.*, 1992; Burmester and Emmrich, 1993). Patients with long-standing disease (approximately 50–60% had refractory disease) received daily intravenous doses of 10–100 mg for 5–7 days, equaling total doses of 70–700 mg per treatment course. Acute depletion of the CD4 T-cell population resulted; reconstitution of peripheral counts varied according to the mAb utilized. With most of the mAbs, CD4 lymphocyte counts returned toward pretreatment levels within 24 hr after an initial dose: decreases to 17% of baseline (MT-151 = IgG2a), 50% (BL4 = IgG2a), 25% (BF5 = IgG1), and 90% (MAX 16H5 = IgG1) were reported. However, sustained depletion to 50% of pretreatment levels for as long as several months was observed following treatment with MAX 16H5, in contrast to BF5 where CD4 levels normalized rapidly. Measured serum half-lives varied according to the murine antibody, as well as the isotype. Antibody responses to the various murine mAbs were reported in approximately 33–66% of patients, generally measured 15 to 30 days after treatment.

In general, improvement has been observed in 60–75% of patients within days to weeks after treatment and has been short-lived, on the order of 3–6 months. Acute-phase reactants (ESR and CRP) were decreased only after the administration of the IgG1 murine mAb BF5. Retreatment has been successful with evidence of biologic and clinical effects.

Further refinement of this therapy to a chimeric IgG1 form proved to be very effective in mediating depletion of the CD4 T-cell and monocyte population (Choy *et al.*, 1992; Choy and Kingsley, 1993a; Moreland *et al.*, 1993b,c; van der Lubbe *et al.*, 1993). Depletion to 30% of baseline levels was evident within an hour of administration, and CD4 levels remained below 50% for as long as several months thereafter. Long-term (⩾30 months) CD4 T-cell cytopenia occurred after repetitive doses of the chimeric mAb; however, clinical benefit lasted only as long as 6 months, and did not appear to be related to the biologic effect of this agent. No change in acute-phase reactants was observed. A randomized, controlled multicenter trial of the chimeric anti-CD4 mAb in RA patients on stable doses of MTX, comparing placebo to three monthly doses of 5, 10, or 50 mg in patients, was recently completed in the United States. Defining efficacy as ⩾50% improvement in either tender or swollen joint counts at the end of 3 months, no statistically significant differences were noted among the pretreatment groups (Moreland *et al.*, 1993).

Anecdotal reports in patients with SLE have indicated short-term benefit following administration of murine anti-CD4 mAbs. A trial utilizing the chimeric anti-CD4 mAb is currently under way in patients with lupus nephritis.

2.1.3. DAB IL-2

Another group of agents have been designed to be more selective, targeting the activated T-cell (and a portion of the B-cell) population. A fusion toxin, DAB IL-2, is a recombinant construct of truncated diphtheria toxin and IL-2 that binds to the high-affinity IL-2. It has shown benefit in initial open label and subsequent placebo-controlled trials in patients with refractory RA (Sewell *et al.*, 1993; Woodworth, 1993). A second product, DAB_{389} IL-2, is believed to be more potent and better tolerated than its predecessor, and is undergoing evaluation in patients with RA.

Both products have been evaluated in relation to placebo in short-term studies of patients with active RA and long-standing disease. Patients were randomized to receive either drug or placebo for the first course of treatment, with subsequent courses utilizing the active agent. In the DAB_{486} IL-2 protocol, no responses were observed in the placebo cohort following the blinded first course, in comparison to the significant number of responders in the active group. Subsequent open label treatment courses resulted in a progressive increase in responders, such that 33% of all enrolled patients demonstrated ⩾25% improvement in both tender and swollen joint counts (+ two of four other parameters: patient assessment, physician assessment, grip strength, 50-ft walking time) (Moreland *et al.*, 1993d). These data suggest that a subset of patients, with refractory disease, were responders, and that successive treatment courses offered progressive benefit. Transient depletion of CD4/CD25 and CD8/CD25 peripheral T cells was observed during the treatment course, without apparent relationship to clinical improvement. Elevated liver transaminase levels (up to three times the normal levels) occur in approximately 50% of patients in a dose-related manner and appear to be less pronounced with repetitive treatment. Antibodies to the diphtheria toxin are measured in 40–60% of patients before treatment; 100% after.

Anti-IL-2 antibodies are present in approximately 10–20% of patients at baseline and in 90% after administration of DAB IL-2.

The 486 product has been administered to patients with Type I diabetes, with recent onset of disease (within 16 weeks) in an open label protocol (Woodworth, 1993). Following treatment with DAB IL-2, maintenance therapy with cyclosporin (Cy-A) was initiated, at 5 mg/kg per day. Approximately 25% of the patients enrolled in the study have received Cy-A for ≥12 months and remain off insulin. These are intriguing data since this is longer than would be expected for a typical period of responsiveness following first encounter with any other therapeutic agent.

2.1.4. Anti-Tac

A second agent, the anti-Tac mAb, binds to the same CD25 surface antigen on activated T (and B) cells. Recently, the humanized form has been under evaluation for the treatment of transplant rejection. It is expected to be introduced into clinical trials in autoimmune diseases soon.

2.2. Cytokines

The interferons were the first recombinant cytokines to be studied as therapeutic agents. Three interferons—IFN-α, -β, and γ—are distinguished by molecular as well as antigenic characteristics. Type I IFNs (IFN-α and -β) share homology, utilize a common receptor, and appear to exert their effects by similar mechanisms. IFN-γ is a type II interferon, which differs in amino acid sequence and binds to a different receptor.

2.2.1. IFN-γ

IFN-γ was the first biologic agent to be studied in the treatment of RA. Although it may have both immunostimulatory as well as immunosuppressive effects *in vivo*, it was postulated that pharmacologic doses administered frequently could result in downregulation of the cytokine receptor, thus decreasing antigen presentation and T-cell activation. However, plasma levels of IFN-γ are not detectable after subcutaneous administration; necessitating the use of a biologic marker (such as serum β_2-microglobulin or neopterin) to ensure successful delivery of the product. Initial open label trials, performed in the mid-1980s, suggested benefit in approximately two-thirds of RA patients, utilizing subcutaneous self-administration, dosing regimens ranged from daily to weekly and from 10 to 200 g/week. The specific biologic activity of the different IFN-γ preparations varied, as they were usually administered according to protein content rather than specific activity. Also, no biologic markers were utilized to monitor delivery of the agent or treatment-associated effects (Schindler and Faller, 1990).

Subsequently, six placebo-controlled trials have evaluated the efficacy of IFN-γ.

Adverse effects were in general mild. Twenty-nine to fifty percent of the treated groups showed improvement. In two of the six studies, this was statistically significant compared to placebo (Fox, 1991). Both toxicity and clinical effect were judged to be mild. Perhaps more importantly, these studies documented the high placebo responses following parenteral administration of a drug (Weinblatt *et al.*, 1990). At the present time, IFN-γ has been approved for use in Germany but elsewhere its use in the treatment of RA has met with little enthusiasm.

Based on preclinical data indicating its efficacy in inhibiting fibroblast collagen production, IFN-γ has been evaluated in the treatment of systemic sclerosis (SSc). Three uncontrolled trials have been reported, all showing benefit in skin thickness score, and amelioration in internal organ involvement in some patients (Kahan *et al.*, 1989; Freundlich *et al.*, 1992; Hein *et al.*, 1992). Of interest, in one protocol requiring <12 months' duration of disease 3 of 18 patients developed renal crisis. To determine whether this was disease-related or a potential treatment effect will require a larger, randomized controlled trial.

2.2.2. IFN-β

IFNs (which have antiviral effects) were investigated as potential therapeutics in the treatment of multiple sclerosis (MS) based on the belief that an underlying viral infection led to the development of disease. Subsequent observations have substantiated the rationale for this type of intervention: administration of IFN-β, either systemically or intrathecally, suppressed or prevented clinical manifestations of disease in the experimental allergic encephalomyelitis (EAE) model and abrogated passive transfer of disease by infusion of sensitized lymphocytes from affected animals (Jacobs *et al.*, 1994).

Initial open label studies utilizing intrathecal administration of naturally produced IFN-β (nIFN-β) were confirmed by a randomized, double-blind, placebo-controlled multicenter trial. Following 6 months of treatment, evaluation at 18 months indicated a significant decrease in number of disease flares in the treated group versus controls with a trend toward less clinical deterioration by the Kurtske or EDSS scale. When it was demonstrated that systemic administration of IFN-β, in higher doses, produced direct effects within the CNS, intramuscular administration of the less expensive recombinant form was substituted. A blinded pilot study against placebo determined the dose and dosing interval of rIFN-β to be 6×10^6 IU once a week (Jacobs *et al.*, 1994).

The MS Collaborative Research Group (MSCRG) designed a multicenter, randomized, double-blind, placebo-controlled protocol, under NIH auspices, to evaluate the efficacy of IM administration of rIFN-β in 312 patients with relapsing MS. Enrollment criteria required an EDSS score of 1.0–3.5. Outcome was chosen to be increase in disability, e.g., the time to the onset of sustained progression, rather than exacerbation rate. Treatment failure was defined as deterioration in the EDSS score from baseline by $\geqslant 1.0$ point, persistent for 6 months. Outcomes included progression of disease by EDSS scores, three measures of disease exacerbation (time to first exacerbation, total number of on-study exacerbations, and number of ACTH or methylprednisolone treatments administered), patient, family, and physician global assessments, and serial gadolinium-enhanced MRI examinations of the brain (Jacobs *et al.*, 1994).

Enrollment and evaluation will be completed in 1994, and the results of this detailed and carefully planned protocol are eagerly awaited. Many of the decisions regarding study design and selection of outcome measures serve as an excellent prototype for multicenter, randomized, placebo-controlled evaluations of therapies in other autoimmune diseases.

In parallel, another IFN-β product (Betaseron) was studied in the treatment of MS, utilizing disease exacerbations as primary outcome parameter. The data demonstrated a decrease in number of disease flares in the treatment groups as well as prolongation in the time to first disease exacerbation, which, as discussed above, should correlate with function. An FDA advisory panel therefore recommended approval of this product in 1993 (FDA, 1993).

2.3. Cytokine Antagonists

Cytokine antagonists may be of two types: (1) receptor antagonist proteins which bind to the receptor on target cells and (2) soluble receptor molecules which may bind and effectively neutralize the cytokine within the circulation. Receptor antagonist proteins must bind >90% of the receptors on a cell surface to have effect. They are thus very selective but inefficient, and to be effective require administration in large doses. In contrast, circulating receptor molecules may competitively block endogenous cytokines from binding and activating cells expressing membrane receptors. The effect requires much lower doses, but more prolonged time in the circulation (Arend and Dayer, 1990).

2.3.1. IL-1Ra

The IL-1 receptor antagonist (IL-1Ra) is naturally produced by monocytes and represents the negative effector arm of an IL-1 regulatory circuit. IL-1Ra as a recombinant protein has been studied in the treatment of RA, psoriasis, inflammatory bowel disease, and sepsis (Thompson, 1993).

IL-1Ra was self-administered subcutaneously by 20 patients with active RA for 7 days, followed by a 2-week washout and 28 days' further treatment in 15. Clinical benefit was seen during the treatment phase, with loss of effect during the washout period. The maximum tolerated dose was defined to be 4 mg/kg per day. In general, IL-1Ra was well tolerated; 3 patients withdrew from treatment and 14 noted skin reactions sporadically. Pharmacokinetic data revealed measurable serum levels up to 24 hr after subcutaneous injection. Open label, long-term administration was continued in 11. No biologic effects or host immune responses to administered product were detected (Lebsack *et al.*, 1991). A randomized, blinded, controlled study of 175 patients comparing nine dosing regimens was recently completed in the United States (Lebsack *et al.*, 1993). During 7 weeks of treatment, short-term improvement, defined as ⩾ 50% decrease in number of tender/and or swollen joints, was observed. Administration of IL-1Ra was associated with localized skin reactions in 58% and serious infections in 5%.

2.3.2. sIL-R

The soluble IL-1 receptor (sIL-1R) is a truncated form of the IL-1 receptor, which retains binding affinity for IL-1 indistinguishable from the full-length membrane-bound receptor. Administration of this product has proved beneficial in both the EAE and antigen-induced arthritis (AIA) models (Jacobs, 1991). In an initial clinical study, sIL-1R was administered to patients with delayed cutaneous allergic responses. Fifteen patients were evaluated in a blinded controlled fashion for the effect of sIL-1R on the late-phase response, the area of induration following an immediate wheal-and-flare reaction to injected allergen. Following allergen testing to determine the appropriate dose for inducing a late-phase response, and a single subcutaneous injection of IL-1R for safety, patients received injections of relevant antigen in both forearms and two sites on the upper back. Positive controls of histamine and negative controls of saline were placed adjacent to the antigen injection sites. Patients then received injections of sIL-1R at three of the four sites; on both forearms and in one site on the back, in doses of 1 to 100 μg. The area of induration at each site was assessed over 24 hr, accompanied by biopsy. At the lowest doses of 1 and 10 μg, a statistically significant decrease in induration was observed compared to the placebo site. At doses ⩾ 25 μg a systemic effect was seen; induration was reduced at all four sites. No adverse events were noted, nor was an immune response to administered sIL-1R detected (Mullarkey *et al.*, 1993). This is an elegant demonstration of a dose response.

This agent is currently under evaluation for the treatment of RA (Sanders and Jacobs, 1994). A Phase I placebo-controlled study of intraarticular administration of sIL-1R in 16 patients with active RA was recently completed. Four doses were evaluated: 25, 100, 250, and 500 μg; at each dose level 1 patient received injection of diluent and 3, active agent. A dose-related reduction in the injected knee circumference was observed at 48 hr which was statistically significant at the 250-μg dose compared to placebo (Drevlow *et al.*, 1993).

2.3.3. Anti-TNF-α mAb

A chimeric IgG1 anti-TNF mAb has been developed, which binds human TNF with high affinity and neutralizes its cytotoxic effects in a human TNF transgenic murine model. This mAb was studied in an open label pilot protocol in 20 patients with RA, treated with a total of 20 mg/kg over 2 weeks. All patients demonstrated benefit, accompanied by improvement in pain by visual analog scale and the acute-phase reactant CRP. Median duration of response was stated to be 4 months. The mAb had a long serum half-life; it was detectable up to 40 days after administration. Adverse events were mild; no cytokine release syndrome was noted. Nine patients received a second course of treatment with apparent benefit; pruritis and urticaria were noted in three. A host immune response was observed in 8 (40%) (Elliott *et al.*, 1993; Maini *et al.*, 1993).

2.3.4. sTNF-R

A fusion protein of two type I TNF receptors on an IgG1 backbone has been developed for the treatment of inflammatory and autoimmune conditions. This soluble TNF receptor (sTNF-R) has been demonstrated to be effective in the collagen II-induced arthritis model and is currently under evaluation for the treatment of RA.

2.4. Adhesion Molecule Antagonists

Several mAbs are under development that target the adhesion molecules involved in leukocyte adhesion to endothelial cells and subsequent trafficking to sites of inflammation. Extensive work in a variety of animal models has suggested this approach may offer therapeutic benefit in arthritis, transplant rejection, asthma, reperfusion injury, and stroke.

2.4.1. Anti-ICAM-1 mAb

LFA-1 (CD11a/CD18) on the surface of T cells plays a prominent role in transendothelial migration and activation of T cells. Its ligand, ICAM-1 (CD54), is present on the surface of endothelial cells, synovial lining cells, and leukocytes. High levels of ICAM-1 can be detected in RA synovium, as well as increased serum concentrations of soluble ICAM-1 in patients with RA (Cush *et al.*, 1993). A mAb against ICAM-1 has shown benefit in acute renal transplant rejection and has been evaluated in an open label pilot study in 31 patients with RA. Twenty-four patients with chronic RA (mean disease duration 18 ± 10 years, failed 4.3 ± 1.4 DMARDs) received four daily infusions of BIRR-1, a murine IgG2a anti-ICAM-1 mAb, following a loading dose on day one of three times the daily dose; 7 others received only one or two doses of mAb. By pharmacokinetic analysis, the target serum level of 10 μg/ml at which (*in vitro*) LFA-1/ICAM-1 interactions are inhibited, was achieved at the mid- and high-dose levels (Kavanaugh *et al.*, 1993, 1994).

A rapid onset of clinical effect was observed on days 8 and 15; maximal on day 29. Of 24 patients who received multiple doses, 13 were improved; benefit continued in 3 for as long as 90 days. Adverse events including fever, headache, and nausea were observed during 74% of the treatments. Several observations made during and immediately following the treatment suggest administration of the mAb led to alterations in lymphocyte recirculation. Peripheral lymphocyte counts increased from a mean of 1.5 cells/mm^3 pretreatment to a maximum of 2.9 on day 5, returning to 1.5 on day 8. Flow cytometric analysis suggested an increase in CD4 cell number, both memory (CD45 RO) and naive (CD45 RA) phenotypes. An increase in activated cells, those expressing MHC class II and CD25, was also noted. Of 16 patients tested for DTH response, 6 were anergic pre- and post treatment, 1 had skin test reactivity pre and post, and 5 (anergic during treatment) regained reactivity afterward. An immune response to the administered mAb was observed, which did not preclude retreatment.

Other agents targeting adhesion molecules are expected to enter clinical trials soon. Oligosaccharide analogues of several cell-bound selectins may offer more selective therapy, without the immunogenicity associated with mAb therapies.

2.5. Antigen-Specific Therapies

Several experimental therapies have been designed to downregulate only those T cells reactive to a specific antigen, believed responsible for initiating and/or perpetuating the autoimmune disease process. By rendering those cells unresponsive or "anergic," "tolerance" to that antigen may be induced. Treatment with peptides based on T-cell receptor (TCR) utilization of the antigen-specific T cells may activate an additional immunoregulatory T-cell subset which downregulates response to the antigen. These peptides may be administered subcutaneously or intradermally on a weekly or monthly basis. Theoretically, this intervention should occur early in the disease process, when an oligoclonal T-cell population is responsible for maintaining the inflammatory process. After an initial course of therapy, readministration, or booster doses, might be required on an intermittent basis. Similarly, peptides may be designed to block antigen binding to MHC class II, subsequent TCR binding, and assembly of the trimolecular complex necessary for T-cell activation. This intervention may be more difficult, as MHC class II molecules are "promiscuous," or capable of binding multiple peptides. Theoretically, treatment with "blocking peptides" would require large doses and regular readministration and the absence of immunogenicity. Alternatively, complexes of MHC class II + peptide could be administered to induce nonresponsiveness in the T-cell population specific to that antigen. Another method for inducing tolerance may occur through oral feeding of antigen. Following digestion in the gut, small amounts of antigen may be taken up by antigen-presenting cells (APCs) in the Peyer's patches and/or gut epithelium, resulting in activation of a regulatory T-cell population.

2.5.1. TCR in MS

Several of these interventions have been studied in a preliminary fashion in patients with MS. MS was chosen because the putative antigen, myelin basic protein (MBP), is characterized while no such knowledge exists in RA; and the animal model, EAE, more closely resembles the human disease. Vandenbark, Offner, and colleagues demonstrated overexpression of Vβ 5.2 and/or Vβ 6.1 genes in the TCR of MBP-reactive T cells in patients with chronic relapsing MS (Kotzin *et al.*, 1991). In a preliminary open label study, synthetic peptides based on these V-region gene sequences were injected intradermally in doses of 100 μg on a weekly to monthly basis (Vandenbark *et al.*, 1993a,b). Peripheral T-cell proliferative responses (T-cell frequencies) to MBP, the administered peptide, a control (noninjected) peptide, and herpes simplex virus (HSV) were assayed. Repeated injection of peptide increased the TCR peptide-specific T-cell frequency, without alteration in the other responses. Over time, there appeared to be a correlation between increased proliferative response to administered peptide, and diminution in MBP reactivity. Treatment was well tolerated. Although further work will be necessary to confirm these preliminary data, this remains an intriguing potential therapy with minimal toxicity.

2.5.2. TCR in RA

In RA, where the putative antigen has yet to be identified, data supporting the overexpression of certain Vβ genes in the TCR of synovial T cells are less clear. In part this may be related to variations in the methods by which Vβ gene utilization has been determined. Some investigators utilize synovial fluid. Others culture synovial tissue T cells after selection (by expression of IL-2R, or stimulation with OKT3); and then allow the outgrowth of synovial infiltrating lymphocytes, sometimes in the presence of a putative antigen: collagen II or *Mycobacterium tuberculosis* (Howell *et al.*, 1991; Paliard *et al.*, 1991; Amento, 1993). Despite the disparate results reported, a clinical trial is under way, administering Vβ 14 and Vβ 17 peptides to patients with RA. In view of the specificity and tolerability of this type of therapy, this study may yield significant results.

2.5.3. Oral Feeding of Antigen

In a Phase I double-blind protocol, Hafler and Weiner studied 30 patients with relapsing remitting MS who swallowed capsules of bovine MBP or control protein daily for 1 year (Hafler *et al.*, 1993; Weiner *et al.*, 1993). Peripheral T-cell reactivity to MBP was decreased in the MBP-treated group, without change in the control group. One or more "flares" or major exacerbations of disease were observed in 12 of 15 patients in the control group, but only 6 of 15 in the treatment group ($p = 0.06$). No toxicity was reported. Although not statistically significant, these data demonstrate a biologic effect and suggest this to be another exceedingly well-tolerated potential therapy for MS. Additional studies are under way in RA, feeding chicken type II collagen; and in uveitis, feeding S antigen.

In a subsequent double-blind study of 60 patients with active RA, 28 received oral doses of chicken collagen type II and 31, placebo. Although there was no washout period following discontinuation of second-line agents, after 3 months, 4 patients in the collagen group experienced remissions in disease activity. However, 4 placebo-treated patients exhibited substantial benefit as well. Again, no toxicity, nor evidence of sensitization to administered collagen was observed (Trentham *et al.*, 1993). Further studies incorporating a washout period and longer treatment duration will be necessary to confirm these initial results.

3. CONCLUSIONS

We have learned much from our recent foray into biologic therapies. Although not the "magic bullets" we hoped for, they have proven to be valuable probes into the underlying pathophysiology of the disease.

In general, administration of biologic agents to patients with autoimmune diseases has resulted in transient benefit. Maximal clinical effects are typically observed within the first weeks of treatment, but are short-lived: of 3 to 6 months' duration. Thus, the long-term benefit (≥ 1 year) we seek in treating chronic diseases may be available only through the use of combination therapies: biologic agent + biologic agent or biologic agent + pharmaceutical product. Thus, we should view the treatment of autoimmune disease much as oncologists view cancer. Certain products could be used as "induction agents," followed by "maintenance therapy."

Experiments in murine systems have underscored the difficulty in accurately predicting, from *in vitro* data, mechanisms of action occurring *in vivo* (Waldor *et al.*, 1987; Alters *et al.*, 1989). This becomes more apparent when reviewing the clinical and biologic effects observed after administration of the various murine anti-CD4 mAbs. The two IgG1 mAbs (MAX 16H5 and BF5; in daily doses of 0.3 mg/kg for 7–10 days) differed in (1) the time course of peripheral CD4 T-cell depletion and reconstitution, (2) the effect on acute-phase reactants, (3) *in vitro* measures of T-cell function, and (4) treatment-associated toxicities. Horneff and colleagues theorize that the effect of the MAX 16H5 mAb is to decrease peripheral monocyte/macrophage counts via repopulation, leading to diminution in serum IL-1, IL-6, and neopterin levels. Further, downmodulation of the CD4 antigen on T cells appears to be monocyte/macrophage dependent (Horneff *et al.*, 1991b, 1993a,b; Burmester and Emmrich, 1993). In comparison, the biologic effects of the BF5 mAb are of shorter duration, yet clinical effects were similar. Racadot and colleagues believe that the dramatic but transient decrease in CD4 as well as CD8 and B cells may have been caused by the activation of CD4 cells leading to the expression of adhesion molecules on endothelial cells, with resultant margination of peripheral mononuclear cells (Racadot *et al.*, 1992).

However, significant and prolonged T-cell depletion has been observed following the administration of chimeric IgG1 anti-CD4 to patients. This was associated with one death in a patient with long-standing cytopenia. A decrease in monocytes to 50% of pretreatment levels was noted in two studies, but not in a third. The xenogeneic antiglobulin response is less than with the murine mAbs and is largely idiotypic. However, it was evident in 70–75% of patients with retreatment. The mechanism for the profound CD4 depletion in humans has not been fully explained. It may occur through mediation of ADCC or CDC, modulation of the CD4 antigen on the T-cell surface, interference with T-cell activation, or induction of apoptosis. There has been no apparent correlation between induced cytopenia and clinical effect. Studies by Wofsy and colleagues in mice demonstrated a dissociation between cell depletion and therapeutic effect (Carteron *et al.*, 1990).

Attempts to explain clinical effects according to changes in the synovium have been equally difficult. Administered mAbs do gain access to the synovial fluid over several days. Burmister and colleagues demonstrated the presence of mAbs within the joints by labeled scans (Reiter *et al.*, 1991). Following a single infusion of chimeric anti-CD4, Choy and colleague observed that 11% of synovial CD4 cells were coated by mAb (versus 90% of peripheral); after five infusions 50% were; but with large variation (Choy and Kingsley, 1993).

Surprisingly, the biologic perturbations following administration of these agents do not correlate with observed clinical response. The significant (and sustained) depletion of peripheral CD4 T cells observed after treatment with the humanized CAMPATH 1H mAb did not predict clinical effect. Administration of the anti-CD5 immunoconjugate resulted in transient depletion of all peripheral T-cell subsets in all but a few patients, yet was associated with sustained ($\geq$ 6 month) benefit in only 25% of patients. Repetitive subcutaneous administration of IL-1Ra appears to be salutory in patients with active disease, but no biologic marker reflecting its effect has been identified. Similarly, treatment with the DAB IL-2 fusion toxin has resulted in transient changes in peripheral IL-2R$^+$ T cells as measured by FACS analysis, but without apparent correlation to clinical effect.

Many of these newer agents appear to have more acute toxicity than therapies currently employed. Systemic symptoms (fever, chills, nausea, malaise, fatigue) can accompany their administration, presumably related to the release of IL-6, IL-1, TNF, either due to cell injury and resultant death, or cell activation. Nonetheless patients appear to tolerate these effects and willingly agree to second and even third courses of treatment.

Almost all biologically based therapeutic agents are immunogenic. Those with a low reported incidence of antibody response may be due to the relatively insensitive techniques used to detect a host immune response (e.g., RIA versus ELISA). Often the clinical effect is not abrogated when such a host response occurs (e.g., IFN-α or insulin) (Lasagna, 1986; Bendtzen *et al.*, 1990; Antonelli *et al.*, 1991). Both the targeted antigen and the isotype determine the immunogenicity of mAbs, limiting the clinical utility of chimeric mAbs as well as murine. Yet repetitive administration of even fully "humanized" mAbs results eventually in an antiidiotype response that may decrease or prevent binding to the target antigen (Choy and Kingsley, 1993b; Watts *et al.*, 1993; Johnston and Spreen, 1994).

A variety of allergic and anaphylactoid reactions have been observed, even with recombinant versions of naturally occurring molecules (Alegre *et al.*, 1991; Abramowicz *et al.*, 1992; Potashnik *et al.*, 1993). Following treatment with IFNs and IL-2, there is a low but recognized incidence of autoimmune manifestations (Atkins *et al.*, 1988;

Conlon *et al.*, 1990; Kung *et al.*, 1990; Mattijssen *et al.*, 1990; Pichert *et al.*, 1991). The occurrence of secondary lymphomas has been reported only after the administration of mitogenic mAbs, such as OKT3, and are believed in part related to the underlying immune status of the host. Recently, several cases of EBV-related lymphomas have been reported in the setting of chronic MTX therapy in patients with RA (Ellman *et al.*, 1991; Shiroky *et al.*, 1991; Kamel *et al.*, 1993). We must view these data with concern, particularly since we have not yet followed patients receiving biologic therapies long enough to exclude the occurrence of secondary lymphomas as an important complication.

Because of their acute and relatively specific effects, biologic agents may help uncover the heterogeneity of the disease population under study. For example, patients at an earlier stage of their disease process may respond differently than those with long-standing disease (Strand and Lee, 1993). Similarly, administration of certain agents, such as chimeric anti-CD4 and CAMPATH 1H mAbs, has not significantly altered acute-phase reactants such as ESR and CRP, yet treatment with one of the murine anti-CD4 mAbs (BF5) and the anti-TNF mAb uniformly decreased these parameters. Effective dosage and dosing regimens may be highly variable, almost patient specific. Thus, it may be difficult to demonstrate a dose–response curve, or a consistent response across a group of patients.

Concomitant polypharmacy, common in diseases such as RA, may impact the efficacy or tolerability profiles of biologic agents, in ways not previously recognized with our current therapies. Decreases in peripheral T-cell counts appear to be more profound in RA patients who have or continue to receive MTX (Moreland *et al.*, 1993b; Strand *et al.*, 1993).

Well-designed clinical trials are critical to the efficient evaluation of biologic products. The importance of blinded, controlled, randomized studies should not be underestimated, even in early Phase I–II studies. This is especially true considering the potentially greater placebo response observed following parenteral treatment. The clinical development of potential AIDS therapies has offered us a paradigm: utilize placebo-controlled trials early in the development phase, and active controls once clinical benefit in humans has been demonstrated. Although the acute effects following administration of biologic agents may pose difficulty for blinded treatment, usually they can be overcome by pretreatment medication (as with oncology therapies) as well as by utilizing different treating and evaluating personnel.

4. FUTURE DIRECTIONS

To date, most clinical trials with biologic agents have been conducted in patients with relatively advanced, if not refractory, disease. Although this may be appropriate when first evaluating a new product in the clinic, it is very possible that the majority of biologic agents will demonstrate superior efficacy in a group of patients with earlier, and therefore more modifiable disease. Signs and symptoms in these patients will more probably demonstrate change within a 3- to 6-month period of time. It may be imperative, then, to gain a safety profile of an agent as soon as possible after its introduction into the clinic, to facilitate its introduction into patients with earlier, more modifiable disease. Biologic interventions in autoimmune diseases are still in their infancy and offer more promise than fulfillment. Given the interests of biotechnology and our rapidly expanding knowledge of etiopathogenesis, biotherapy is certainly here to stay.

ACKNOWLEDGMENTS. These studies were supported by PHS Grant DE09311-03. We sincerely thank Vicki Hurst for her secretarial assistance.

REFERENCES

Abramowicz, D., Crusiaux, A., and Goldman, M., 1992, Anaphylactic shock after retreatment with OKT3 monoclonal antibody, *N. Engl. J. Med.* **327**:736.

Alegre, M., Vandenabeele, P., Depierreux, M., Florquin, S., Flamand, V., Moser, M., Leo, O., Urbain, J., and Fiers, W., 1991, Cytokine release syndrome induced by the 145-2C11 anti-CD3 monoclonal antibody in mice: Prevention by high doses of methylprednisolone, *J. Immunol.* **146**:1184.

Alters, S., Steinman, L., and Oi, V., 1989, Comparison of rat and rat–mouse chimeric anti-murine CD4 antibodies in vitro, *J. Immunol.* **142**:2018.

Amento, E. P., 1993, Is rheumatoid arthritis driven by oligoclonal T cells? *Clin. Exp. Rheum.* **11**:S15.

Antonelli, G., Currenti, M., Turriziani, O., and Dianzani, F., 1991, Neutralizing antibodies to interferon-α: Relative frequency in patients treated with different interferon preparations, *J. Infect. Dis.* **163**:882.

Arend, W., and Dayer, J. M., 1990, Cytokines and cytokine inhibitors or antagonists in rheumatoid arthritis, *Arthritis Rheum.* **33**:305.

Atalla, L., Linker-Israeli, M., Steinman, L., and Rao, N. A., 1990, Inhibition of autoimmune uveitis by anti CD4 antibody, *Invest. Ophthalmol. Visual Sci.* **31**:1264.

Atkins, M. B., Mier, J. W., Parkinson, D. R., Gould, J. A., Berkman, E. M., and Kaplan, M. M., 1988, Hypothyroidism after treatment with interleukin-2 and lymphokine-activated killer cells, *N. Engl. J. Med.* **318**:1557.

Bendtzen, K., Svenson, M., Jonsson, V., and Hippe, E., 1990, Autoantibodies to cytokines—Friends or foes? *Immunol. Today* **11**:167.

Burmester, G., and Emmrich, F., 1993, Anti-CD4 therapy in rheumatoid arthritis, *Clin. Exp. Rheum.* **11**:S139.

Byers, V. S., Henslee, P. J., Kernan, N. A., Blazar, B. R., Gingrich, R., Phillips, G. L., LeMaistre, C. F., Gilliland, G., Antin, J. H., and Martin, P., 1990, Use of an anti-pan T lymphocyte ricin A chain immunotoxin in steroid resistant acute graft vs. host disease, *Blood* **75**:1426.

Carteron, N. L., Wofsy, D., Schimenti, C., and Ermack, T. H., 1990, F(ab′)2 anti CD4 and intact anti CD4 monoclonal antibodies inhibit the accumulation of CD4+ T cells, CD8 T cells, and B cells in the kidneys of lupus prone NZB/W mice, *Clin. Immunol. Immunopathol.* **56**:373.

Chatenoud, L., Ferrari, C., Legendre, C., Franchimont, P., Reuter, A., Kries, H., and Bach, J. F., 1988, Clinical use of OKT3: The role of cytokine release and xenosensitization, *J. Autoimmun.* **1**:631.

Choy, E., and Kingsley, G., 1993a, Anti-CD4 therapy in rheumatoid arthritis, *Clin. Exp. Rheum.* **11**:S147.

Choy, E. H. S., and Kingsley, G. H., 1993b, Immunotherapy, past, present and future, *Br. J. Rheum.* **32**:89.

Choy, E. H. S., Chikanza, I. C., Kingsley, G. H., Corrigall, V., and Panayi, G. S., 1992, Treatment of rheumatoid arthritis with single dose or weekly pulses of chimeric anti-CD4 monoclonal antibody, *Scand. J. Immunol.* **36**:291.

Christadoss, P., and Dauphmee, M. J., 1986, Immunotherapy for myasthenia gravis: A murine model, *J. Immunol.* **136**:2437.

Conlon, K., Urba, W. J., Smith, J. W., Steis, R. G., Longo, D. L., and Clark, J. W., 1990, Exacerbation of symptoms of autoimmune disease in patients receiving α-interferon therapy, *Cancer* **65:**2237.

Cosimi, A. B., Colvin, R. B., Burton, R. C., Goldstein, G., Kung, P. C., Hansen, W. P., Delmonico, F. L., and Russell, P. S., 1981, Use of monoclonal antibodies to T cell subsets for immunologic monitoring and treatment in recipients of renal allografts, *N. Engl. J. Med.* **305:**308.

Cush, J. J., Rothlein, R., Lindsey, H. B., Mainolfi, E. A., and Lipsky, P. E., 1993, Increased levels of circulating intercellular adhesion molecule 1 in the sera of patients with rheumatoid arthritis, *Arthritis Rheum.* **36:**1098.

Dillman, R., 1990, Human antimouse and antiglobulin responses to monoclonal antibodies, *Antibody, Immunoconjugates, Radiopharmaceutics.* **3:**1–15.

Drevlow, B., Capezio, J., Lovis, R., Jacobs, C., Landay, A., and Pope, R. M., 1993, Phase I study of recombinant human interleukin-1 receptor (rHU IL-1R) administered intraarticularly in active rheumatoid arthritis, *Arthritis Rheum.* **36:**S39.

Elliott, M. J., Maini, R., Feldmann, M., *et al.*, 1993, Treatment of rheumatoid arthritis with chimeric monoclonal antibodies to TNFα, *Arth. Rheum.* **36:**1681–1690.

Ellman, M. H., Hurwitz, H., Thomas, C., and Kozloff, M., 1991, Lymphoma developing in a patient with rheumatoid arthritis taking low dose weekly methotrexate, *J. Rheum.* **18:**1741.

Emery, R., and Lake, K., 1991, Post-transplantation lymphoproliferative disorder and OKT3, *N. Engl. J. Med.* **324:**1437.

FDA, 1993, Peripheral and Central Nervous System Drugs Advisory Committee, U.S. Department of Health and Human Services, Washington, DC.

Fishwild, D., and Strand, V., 1994, Treatment with an anti-CD5 immunoconjugate: Effect on peripheral T cells and in vitro assays of immune function in patients with rheumatoid arthritis, *J. Rheum.*, **21:**596–604.

Fox, I., 1991, Interferon gamma in rheumatoid arthritis, in: *Biologic Agents in Autoimmune Diseases II* (V. Strand, E. Amento, and C. Scribner, eds.), Arthritis Foundation, Atlanta, pp. 95–98.

Freundlich, B., Jiminez, S. A., Steen, V. D., Medsger, T. A., Jr., Szkolnicki, M., and Jaffe, H. S., 1992, Treatment of systemic sclerosis with recombinant interferon γ: A phase I/II clinical trial, *Arthritis Rheum.* **35:**1134.

Fung, J. J., Demetris, A. J., Porter, K. A., Iwatsuki, S., Gordon, R. D., Esquivel, C. O., Jaffe, R., Tzakis, A., Shaw, B. W., Jr., and Starzl, T. E., 1987a, Use of OKT3 with cyclosporin and steroids for reversal of acute kidney and liver allograft rejection, *Nephron* **46:**19.

Fung, J. J., Markus, B. H., Gordon, R. D., Esquivel, C. O., Makowka, L., Tzakis, A., and Starzl, T. E., 1987b, Impact of orthoclone OKT3 on liver transplantation, *Transplant. Proc.* **19:**37.

Goldberg, D., Morel, P., Chatenoud, L., Menkes, C. J., Bertoye, P. H., Revillard, J. P., and Bach, J. F., 1991, Immunological effects of high dose administration of anti-CD4 antibody in rheumatoid arthritis patients, *J. Autoimmun.* **4:**617.

Goldstein, G., Fuccello, A. J., Norman, D. J., Shield, C. F., Colvin, R. B., and Cosimi, A. B., 1986, OKT3 monoclonal antibody plasma levels during therapy and the subsequent development of host antibodies to OKT3, *Transplantation* **42:**507.

Hafler, D. A., Zhang, J. W., LaSalle, J., Donnelly, C., Weiner, H. L., and Wucherpfeffnig, K., 1993, The development of antigen specific therapies for autoimmune disease; investigations in multiple, The development of antigen specific therapies for autoimmune disease: in multiple sclerosis as a paradigm for rheumatoid arthritis, *Clin. Exp. Rheum.* **11:**S39.

Hakimi, J., Chizzonite, R., Luke, D. R., Familletti, P. C., Bailon, P., Kondas, J. A., Pilson, R. S., Lin, P., Weber, D. V., and Spence, C., 1991, Reduced immunogenicity and improving pharmacokinetics of humanized anti-Tac in cynomolgus monkeys, *J. Immunol.* **147:**1352.

Hale, G., Clark, M. R., Dyer, M. J., Phillips, J. M., Marcus, R., Riechmann, L., Winter, G., and Waldmann, H., 1988, Remission induction in non-Hodgkins lymphoma with reshaped human monoclonal antibody, CAMPATH-1h, *Lancet* **2:**1394.

Hein, R., Behr, J., Hundgen, M., Hunzelmann, N., Meurer, M., Braun-Falco, O., Urbanski, A., and Krieg, T., 1992, Treatment of systemic sclerosis with γ interferon, *Br. J. Dermatol.* **126:**496.

Herzog, C., Walker, C., Rieber, P., Muller, W., Pichler, W. J., Reiter, C., Riethmuller, G., Wassmer, P., Stockinger, H., and Madic, O., 1987, Monoclonal anti-CD4 in arthritis, *Lancet* **2:**1461.

Herzog, C., Walker, C., Muller, W., Rieber, P., Reiter, C., Riethmuller, G., Wassmer, P., Stockinger, H., Madic, O., and Pichler, W. J., 1989, Anti-CD4 antibody treatment of patients with rheumatoid arthritis: I. Effect on clinical course and circulating T cells, *J. Autoimmun.* **2**:627.

Hirsch, R., Gress, R. E., and Bluestone, J. A., 1989, Anti-CD3 antibody for autoimmune disease: A cautionary note, *Lancet* **1**:1390.

Horneff, G., Burmester, G., Emmrich, F., and Kalden, J. R., 1991a, Treatment of rheumatoid arthritis with an anti-CD4 monoclonal antibody, *Arthritis Rheum.* **34**:129.

Horneff, G., Krause, A., Emmrich, F., Kalden, J. R., and Burmester, G. R., 1991b, Elevated levels of circulating TNFα, IFNγ and IL-2 in systemic reactions induced by anti-CD4 therapy in patients with rheumatoid arthritis, *Cytokine* **3**:266.

Horneff, G., Winkler, T., Kalden, J. R., Emmrich, F., and Burmester, G. R., 1991c, Human anti-mouse antibody response induced by anti-CD4 monoclonal antibody therapy in patients with rheumatoid arthritis, *Clin. Immunol. Immunopathol.* **59**:89.

Horneff, G., Emmrich, F., Reiter, C., Kalden, J. R., and Burmester, G. R., 1992, Persistent depletion of CD4+ T cells and inversion of the CD4/CD8 T cell ratio induced by anti-CD4 therapy, *J. Rheum.* **19**:1845.

Horneff, G., Guse, A., Schulze-Koops, H., Kalden, J. R., Burmester, G. R., and Emmrich, F., 1993a, Human CD4 modulation in vivo induced by antibody treatment, *Clin. Immunol. Immunopathol.* **66**:80.

Horneff, G., Sack, U., Kalden, J. R., Emmrich, F., and Burmester, G. R., 1993b, Reduction of monocyte–macrophage activation markers upon anti-CD4 treatment. Decreased levels of IL-1, IL-6, neopterin and soluble CD14 in patients with rheumatoid arthritis, *Clin. Exp. Immunol.* **91**:207.

Howell, M. D., Diveley, J. P., Lundeen, K. A., Esty, A., Winters, S. T., Carlo, D. J., and Brostoff, S. W., 1991, Limited T cell receptor B chain heterogeneity among IL-2R+ synovial T cells suggests a role for superantigen in rheumatoid arthritis, *Proc. Natl. Acad. Sci. USA* **88**:10921.

Isaacs, J. D., Watts, R. A., Hazleman, B. L., Hale, G., Keogan, M. T., Cobbold, S. P., and Waldmann, H., 1992, Humanized monoclonal antibody therapy for rheumatoid arthritis, *Lancet* **340**:748.

Jacobs, C., 1991, Soluble IL-1 receptor in autoimmune models, in: *Biologic Agents in Autoimmune Diseases II* (V. Strand, E. Amento, and C. Scribner, eds.), Arthritis Foundation, Atlanta, pp. 55–60.

Jacobs, L., Brownschiedle, C. M., and Cookfair, D., 1994, Recombinant beta interferon as treatment for multiple sclerosis, in: *Biologic Agents in Autoimmune Diseases III* (V. Strand, L. Simon, and S. Pillemer, eds.), Arthritis Foundation, Atlanta, pp. 103–112.

Johnston, J., and Spreen, W., 1994, Treatment of rheumatoid arthritis with humanized monoclonal antibody CAMPATH-1H, in: *Biologic Agents in Autoimmune Diseases III* (V. Strand, L. Simon, and S. Pellemer, eds.), Arthritis Foundation, Atlanta, pp. 55–64.

Junghans, R. P., Waldmann, T. A., Landolfi, N. F., Avdalovic, N. M., Schneider, W. P., and Queen, C., 1990, Anti-Tac-H a humanized antibody to the interleukin 2 receptor with new features for immunotherapy in malignant and immune disorders, *Cancer Res.* **50**:1495.

Kahan, A., Amor, B., Menkes, C. J., and Strauch, G., 1989, Recombinant interferon gamma in the treatment of systemic sclerosis, *Am. J. Med.* **87**:273.

Kamel, O. W., van de Rijn, M., Weiss, L. M., Del Zoppo, G. J., Hench, P. K., Robbins, B. A., Montgomery, P. G., Warnke, R. A., and Dorfman, R. F., 1993, Brief report: Reversible lymphomas associated with Epstein Barr virus occurring during methotrexate therapy for rheumatoid arthritis and dermatomyositis, *N. Engl. J. Med.* **328**:1317.

Kavanaugh, A. F., Nichols, L. A., Davis, L. S., Rothlein, R., and Lipsky, P., 1993, Anti-CD54 (ICAM-1) monoclonal antibody therapy in refractory rheumatoid arthritis, *Arthritis Rheum.* **36**:S40.

Kavanaugh, A. F., Davis, L. S., Nichols, L. A., and Lipsky, P. E., 1994, Treatment of rheumatoid arthritis with a monoclonal antibody to intercellular adhesion molecule-1 (ICAM-1; CD54), in: *Biologic Agents in Autoimmune Diseases III* (V. Strand, L. Simon, and S. Pillemer, eds.), Arthritis Foundation, Atlanta, pp. 46–51.

Koike, T., Itoh, Y., Ishii, T., Ito, I., Takabayashi, K., Maruyama, N., Tomioka, H., and Yoshida, S., 1987, Preventive effect of monoclonal anti-L3T4 antibody on development of diabetes in NOD mice, *Diabetes* **36**:359.

Kotzin, B. L., Karuturi, S., Chou, Y. K., Lafferty, J., Forrester, J. M., Better, M., Nedwin, G. E., Offner, H., and Vandenbark, A. A., 1991, Preferential T cell receptor Vb gene usage in myelin basic protein reactive T cell clones from patients with multiple sclerosis, *Proc. Natl. Acad. Sci. USA* **88:**9161.

Kung, A., Jones, B., and Lai, C., 1990, Effects of interferon-γ therapy on thyroid T-lymphocyte subpopulations and induction of autoantibodies, *J. Clin. Endocrinol. Metab.* **71:**1230.

Kyle, V., Roddy, J., Hale, G., Hazleman, B. L, and Waldmann, H., 1991, Humanized monoclonal antibody treatment in rheumatoid arthritis, *J. Rheum.* **18:**1737.

Lasagna, L., 1986, Clinical testing of products prepared by biotechnology, *Reg. Tox. Pharm.* **6:**385.

Lebsack, M. E., Paul, C. C., and Bloedow, F. X., 1991, Subcutaneous IL-1 receptor antagonist in patients with rheumatoid arthritis, *Arthritis Rheum.* **34:**S45.

Lebsack, M. E., Paul, C. C., Martindale, J. J., and Catalano, M. A., 1993, A dose and regimen ranging study of IL-1 receptor antagonist in patients with rheumatoid arthritis, *Arthritis Rheum.* **36:**S39.

Maini, R., Brennan, F., Williams, R., Chu, C. Q., Cope, A. P., Gibbons, D., Elliott, M., and Feldmann, M., 1993, TNF-α in rheumatoid arthritis and prospects of anti-TNF therapy, *Clin. Exp. Rheum.* **11:**S173.

Mathieson, P. W., Cobbold, S. P., Hale, G., Clark, M. R., Oliveira, D. B., Lockwood, C. M., and Waldmann, H., 1990, Monoclonal-antibody therapy in systemic vasculitis, *N. Engl. J. Med.* **323:**250.

Mattijssen, V. J., De Mulder, P. H., Van Liessum, P. A., Corstens, F. H., Franks, C. R., and Wagener, D. J., 1990, Hypothyroidism and goiter in a patient during treatment with interleukin-2, *Cancer* **65:**2686.

Moreland, L., Pratt, P., Mayes, M., Postlethwaite, A., Weisman, M., Schnitzer, T., and Lightfoot, R., 1993a, Minimal efficacy of chimeric anti-CD4 (CM T412) in treatment of patients with rheumatoid arthritis receiving concomitant methotrexate, *Arthritis Rheum.* **36:**S39.

Moreland, L. W., Bucy, R. P., Tilden, A., Pratt, P. W., LoBuglio, A. F., Khazaeli, M., Everson, M. P., Daddona, P., Ghrayeb, J., and Kilgarriff, C., 1993b, Use of a chimeric monoclonal anti-CD4 antibody in patients with refractory rheumatoid arthritis, *Arthritis Rheum.* **36:**307.

Moreland, L. W., Pratt, P. W., Sanders, M. E., and Koopman, W. J., 1993c, Experience with a chimeric monoclonal anti-CD4 antibody in the treatment of refractory rheumatoid arthritis, *Clin. Exp. Rheum.* **11:**S153.

Moreland, L. W., Sewell, K. L., Sullivan, W. F., Shmerling, R. H., Parker, K. C., Swartz, W. G., Woodworth, T. G., and Trentham, D. E., 1993d, Double blind placebo controlled phase II trial of diphtheria interleukin-2 fusion toxin (DAB 486 IL-2) in patients with refractory rheumatoid arthritis, *Arthritis Rheum.* **36:**S39.

Morrison, S. L., and Oi, V. T., 1989, Genetically engineered antibody molecules, *Adv. Immunol.* **44:**65.

Mullarkey, M., Rubin, A., and Roux, E., 1993, Modification of allergic late-phase response by soluble human IL-1 receptor (RHU IL-1R), *J. Cell. Biochem.* **17b:**129.

Nabozny, G. H., Cobbold, S. P., Waldmann, H., and Kong, Y. C., 1991, Suppression in murine experimental autoimmune thyroiditis: In vivo inhibition of CD4+ T cell-mediated resistance by a nondepleting rat CD4 monoclonal antibody, *Cell. Immunol.* **138:**185.

Paliard, X., West, S. G., Lafferty, J. A., Clements, J. R., Kappler, J. W., Marrack, P., and Kotzin, B. L., 1991, Evidence for the effects of a superantigen in rheumatoid arthritis, *Science* **253:**325.

Penn, I., 1990, Cancers complicating organ transplantation, *N. Engl. J. Med.* **323:**1767.

Pichert, G., Jost, L. M., and Fierz, W., 1991, Clinical and immune modulatory effects of alternative weekly IL-2 and IFNγ 2a in patients with advanced renal cell carcinoma and melanoma, *Br. J. Cancer* **63:**287.

Potashnik, G., Lunenfeld, E., Spitz, E., and Glezerman, M., 1993, Anaphylactic reaction to GnRH, *N. Engl. J. Med.* **328:**815.

Racadot, E., Wijdenes, J., and Wendling, D., 1992, Immunological follow-up of 17 patients with rheumatoid arthritis treated in vivo with an anti-T CD4+ monoclonal antibody (B-F5), *Clin. Exp. Rheum.* **10:**365.

Rauges, G. E., Sriram, S., and Cooper, S. M., 1985, Prevention of type II collagen induced arthritis by in vivo treatment with anti L3T4, *J. Exp. Med.* **162:**1105.

Reiter, C., Kakavand, B., Rieber, E. P., Schattenkirchner, M., and Riethmuller, G., and Kruger, K., 1991, Treatment of rheumatoid arthritis with monoclonal CD4 antibody MT-151, *Arthritis Rheum.* **34:**525.

Riechmann, L., Clark, M., Waldmann, H., and Winter, G., 1988, Reshaping human antibodies for therapy, *Nature* **332:**323.

Sanders, M., and Jacobs, C., 1994, Outcome measurements in clinical trials for soluble cytokine receptors in the treatment of inflammatory diseases, in: *Biologic Agents in Autoimmune Diseases III* (V. Strand, L. Simon, and S. Pillemer, eds.), Arthritis Foundation, Atlanta, pp. 98–102.

Schindler, J. D., and Faller, D. V., 1990, Gamma interferon: Mechanism of action and use in rheumatoid arthritis, in: *Immunomodulators in the Rheumatic Diseases* (D. E. Furst and M. E. Weinblatt, eds.), Dekker, New York, 185.

Sewell, K. L., Parker, K. C., Woodworth, T. G., Reuben, J., Swartz, W., and Trentham, D. E., 1993, DAB 486 IL-2 fusion toxin in refractory rheumatoid arthritis, *Arthritis Rheum.* **36:**1223.

Shiroky, J. B., Frost, A., Skelton, J. D., Haegert, D. G., Newkirk, M. M., and Neville, C., 1991, Complications of immunosuppression associated with weekly low dose methotrexate, *J. Rheum.* **18:**1172.

Stafford, F. J., Fleisher, T. A., Brown, M., Lee, G., Austin, H. I., Balow, J. E., and Klippel, J. H., 1993, Clinical and biological effects of anti-CD5 ricin. A chain immunoconjugate in systemic lupus erythematosus, *Arthritis Rheum.* **36:**S227.

Strand, V., and Lee, M. L., 1993, Differential patterns of response in patients with rheumatoid arthritis following administration of an anti-CD5 immunoconjugate, *Clin. Exp. Rheumatol.* **8:**S161.

Strand, V., Lipsky, P. E., Cannon, G. W., Calabrese, L. H., Wiesenhutter, C., Cohen, S. B., Olsen, N. J., Lee, M. L., Lorezn, T. J., and Nelson, B., 1993, Effects of administration of an anti-CD5 immunoconjugate in rheumatoid arthritis, *Arthritis Rheum.* **36:**620.

Swinnen, L. J., Costanzo-Nordin, M. R., Fisher, S. G., O'Sullivan, E. J., Johnson, M. R., Heroux, A. L., Dizikes, G. J., Pifarre, R., and Fisher, R. I., 1990, Increased incidence of lymphoproliferation after bone marrow transplantation, *N. Engl. J. Med.* **323:**1723.

Thistlethwaite, J. R., Jr., Stuart, J. K., Mayes, J. T., Gaber, A. O., Woodle, S., Buckingham, M. R., and Stuart, F. P., 1988, Monitoring and complications of monoclonal therapy, *Am. J. Kidney Dis.* **11:**112.

Thompson, R., 1993, IL-1 receptor antagonist in arthritis and arthritis models, *Clin. Exp. Rheum.* **11:**S169.

Trentham, D. E., Dynesius-Trentham, R. A., Orav, E. J., Combitchi, D., Lorenzo, C., Sewell, K. L., Hafler, D. W., and Weiner, H. L., 1993, Effects of oral administration of type II collagen on rheumatoid arthritis, *Science* **261:**1727.

Vandenbark, A. A., Chou, Y. K., Bourdette, D., Whitham, R., Hashim, G. A., and Offner, H., 1993a, T-cell receptor peptide therapy in EAE and MS, *Clin. Exp. Rheum.* **11:**S51.

Vandenbark, A. A., Hashim, G., and Offner, H., 1993b, TCR peptide therapy in autoimmune disease, *Int. Rev. Immunol.* **9:**251.

van der Lubbe, P., Reiter, C., Breedveld, F. C., Kruger, K., Schattenkirchner, M., Sanders, M., and Riethmuller, G., 1993, Chimeric CD4 monoclonal antibody cM-T412 as a therapeutic approach to rheumatoid arthritis, *Arthritis Rheum.* **36:**1375.

Verwilghen, J., Kingsley, G. H., Ceuppens, J. L., and Panayi, G. S., 1992, Inhibition of synovial fluid T cell proliferation by anti-CD5 monoclonal antibodies. A potential mechanism for their immunotherapeutic action in vivo, *Arthritis Rheum.* **35:**1445.

Wacholtz, M. C., and Lipsky, P., 1992, Treatment of lupus nephritis with CD5 Plus an immunoconjugate of an anti-CD5 monoclonal antibody and ricin A chain, *Arthritis Rheum.* **35:**837.

Waldmann, T., 1991, Monoclonal antibodies in diagnosis and therapy, *Science* **252:**1657.

Waldmann, T. A., Pastan, I. H., Gansow, O. A., and Junghans, R. P., 1992, The multichain interleukin-2 receptor: A target for immunotherapy, *Ann. Intern Med.* **116:**148.

Waldor, M. K., Sriram, S., Hardy, R., Herzenberg, L. A., Lanier, L., Lim, M., and Steinman, L., 1985, Reversal of experimental allergic encephalomyelitis with monoclonal antibody to a T-cell subset marker, *Science* **227:**415.

Waldor, M. K., Mitchell, D., Kipps, T. J., Herzenberg, L. A., and Steinman, L., 1987, Importance of immunoglobulin isotype in therapy of EAE with monoclonal anti-CD4 antibody, *J. Immunol.* **139:**3660.

Walker, C., Herzog, C., Rieber, P., Riethmuller, G., Muller, W., and Pichler, W. J., 1989, Anti-CD4 antibody treatment of patients with rheumatoid arthritis: II. Effect of in vivo treatment on in vitro proliferative response of CD4 cells, *J. Autoimmun.* **2:**643.

Watts, R., Isaacs, J., Hale, G., Hazleman, B., and Waldmann, H., 1993, CAMPATH-1H in inflammatory arthritis, *Clin. Exp. Rheum.* **11:**S165.

Weinblatt, M. E., Maier, A. L., and Emery, P., 1990, Substantial placebo response with parenteral therapy in active rheumatoid arthritis, *Arthritis Rheum.* **33:**S152.

Weiner, H. L., Mackin, G. A., Matsui, M., Orav, E. J., Khoury, S. J., Dawson, D. M., and Hafler, D. A., 1993, Double-blind pilot trial of oral tolerization with myelin antigens in multiple sclerosis, *Science* **259:**1321.

Wendling, D., Wijdenes, J., Racadot, E., and Morel-Fourier, B., 1991, Therapeutic use of monoclonal anti-CD4 antibody in rheumatoid arthritis, *J. Rheumatol.* **18:**325.

Wendling, D., Racadot, E., Morel-Fourier, B., and Wijdenes, J., 1992, Treatment of rheumatoid arthritis with antiCD4 monoclonal antibody. Open study of 25 patients with the B-F5 clone, *Clin. Rheumatol.* **11:**542.

Wilks, D., Byrom, N., Walker, L., Habeshaw, J., and Dalgleish, A., 1990, Characteristic immunophenotyping artefact seen in patients with anti-mouse immunoglobulin antibodies, *Cytometry* **11:**318.

Wofsy, D., 1987, Reversal of advanced murine lupus in NZB/W mice by treatment with monoclonal antibody to L3T4, *J. Immunol.* **138:**3247.

Woodworth, T., 1993, Early clinical studies of IL-2 fusion toxin in patients with severe rheumatoid arthritis and recent onset insulin-dependent diabetes mellitus, *Clin. Exp. Rheum.* **11:**S177.

Zutter, M. M., Martin, P. J., Sale, G. E., Shulman, H. M., Fisher, L., Thomas, D. E., and Durnam, D. M., 1988, Epstein–Barr virus lymphoproliferation after bone marrow transplantation, *Blood* **72:**520.

PART VI

NEUROIMMUNOMODULATION

CHAPTER 10

NEUROENDOCRINE–IMMUNE INTERACTIONS

NICOLA FABRIS

1. INTRODUCTION

A body of experimental evidence now supports the existence of numerous interactions among the nervous, endocrine, and immune systems. Communication between these networks is mediated by humoral mediators, such as hormones, neurotransmitters and immune-derived cytokines, which are to a large extent shared by the different homeostatic systems. Common to nervous, neuroendocrine, and immune cells are also the receptor sites sensitive to such signals. Hormones and neurotransmitters, in addition to regulating various target tissues in the body, also reach lymphoid organs and cells through blood circulation or through direct autonomic nervous system (ANS) connections between the nervous tissue and the organs of the lymphoid system itself (for review see Guillemin *et al.*, 1985; Cotman *et al.*, 1988; Blalock, 1992; Fabris *et al.*, 1992). The neuroendocrine–immune interactions supported by circulating humoral mediators are mainly due to and mediated by the hypothalamus–pituitary axis. This axis may influence the immune system either by releasing various hormones and neuropeptides into the blood with direct modulatory action on the immune effectors or by regulating the hormonal secretion of peripheral endocrine glands which in turn exert an immunomodulating action.

In addition, neuroendocrine–immune interactions are based on direct neuro-immune connections (Bulloch, 1987; Felten and Felten, 1991): anatomical studies have shown that the nerve endings of the sympathetic and parasympathetic systems

NICOLA FABRIS • Immunology Center, Gerontological Research Department, INRCA, 60100 Ancona, and Institute of Haematology, Medical Faculty, University of Pavia, 27100 Pavia, Italy.

Immunopharmacology Reviews, *Volume 2*, edited by John W. Hadden and Andor Szentivanyi. Plenum Press, New York, 1996.

innervate various organs of the immune system such as thymus, spleen, bone marrow, and lymph nodes. Furthermore, ANS-related neurosubstances such as substance P, vasoactive intestinal peptide (VIP), somatostatin, neurotensin, oxytocin, and calcitonin have been immunocytochemically identified in lymphoid organs (Geenen *et al.*, 1986; Bulloch *et al.*, 1991).

The existence of signals generated within the immune system capable of modulating various nervous–neuroendocrine functions has been originally suggested by the alterations that can be induced in the neuroendocrine balance either by removal of relevant lymphoid organs, such as the thymus (for review see Fabris, 1993), or by the functioning of the immune system itself, such as reactions to immunogenic or tolerogenic doses of antigen (for review see Besedovsky and del Rey, 1992). The discovery that the majority of such effects could be mimicked by various immune-derived factors, such as thymic peptides and lymphokines, has given molecular support to those findings (Besedovsky et al., 1991; Milenkovic *et al.*, 1992; McCann *et al.*, 1993).

Besides, it has been found that lymphoid and accessory cells may, in given circumstances and particularly following antigenic stimulation, synthesize and secrete neurohormonal factors, such as adrenocorticotropic hormone (ACTH), growth hormone (GH), thyroid stimulating hormone (TSH), prolactin (PRL), gonadotropins, and endogenous opioids (Blalock, 1988; Hejinen et al., 1991; Panerai, 1993) which are likely to have an autocrine effect, as well as contribute to the neuroendocrine balance. This discovery has further added other humoral signals shared by the immune and the neuroendocrine systems.

In spite of the great understanding reached in recent years on these kinds of interconnections, little effort has been made to confront new notions that we have of the classical neuroendocrinological pathways. Hormones, neurotransmitters, and immune cytokines may both exert developmental actions related to the structural and functional organization of target organ or cell and play roles in the actual performance of mature cells, such as those required to counteract stressful conditions and antigenic insults (for review see Jasmine and Cantin, 1991; Fabris, 1992, 1993). The findings related to neuroendocrine–immune interactions responsible for developmental steps should, therefore, be clearly distinguished from those related to emergency events in fully matured systems (Fig. 1). The stimuli required to activate a given npathway as well as the end effects may be quite different, either quantitatively or qualitatively, according to the functional demands ("morphogenetic" or "of actual performance") of the organism.

These considerations have suggested at least two levels of neuroendocrine–immune interrelationships (Fabris et al., 1988; Fabris, 1992). The first level is based on the interactions between the neuroendocrine system and the thymus (Fig. 1A) an organ devoted to the proliferation and differentiation of stem cells into mature T lymphocytes. Such interactions should take into account the fact that the thymus synthesizes and secretes various hormonelike peptides with differentiation properties on the T-cell lineage (Goldstein, 1984; Hadden, 1993). The second level of interaction is at the periphery (Fig. 1B), between neuroendocrine signals and the humoral

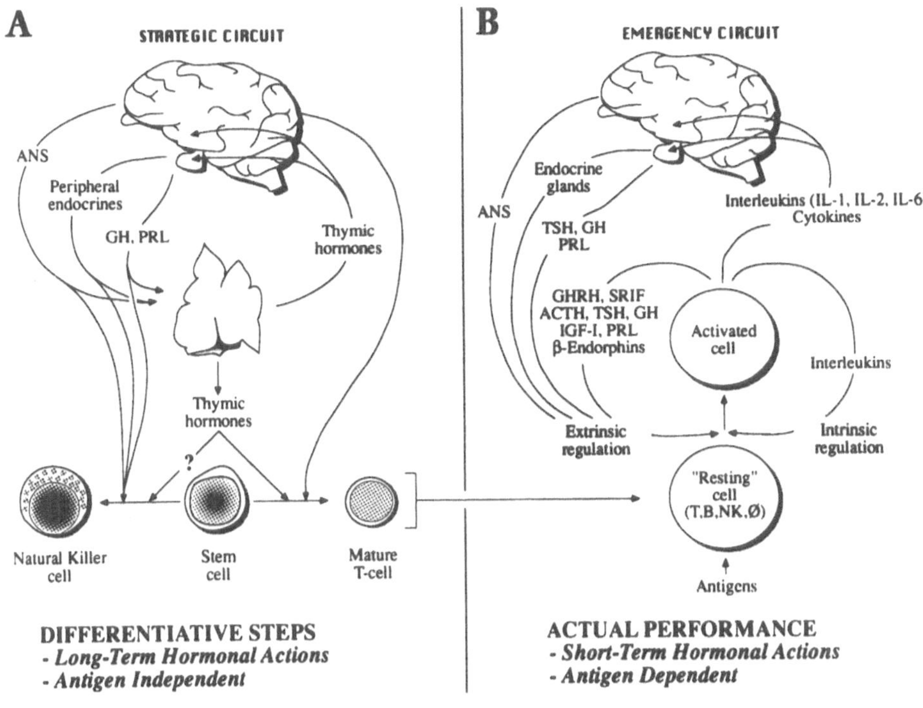

FIGURE 1. Schematic representation of immune–neuroendocrine pathways. (A) The strategic circuit; (B) the emergency circuit. For explanation see text.

products that are secreted by immune cells during specific reactions to various antigens (Blalock, 1992; Besedovsky and del Rey, 1992). The rationale for discriminating between these two levels is based on various considerations. The first level of interaction is primarily involved in maturational steps of both immune and neuroendocrine systems, which occurs independent of the degree of antigenic stimulation: in fact, neuroendocrine–thymus interactions are observable in animals maintained under germfree conditions. This level could be considered "strategic" in nature. The second level of interaction, in contrast, requires the presence of fully differentiated immune cells and the occurrence of a specific antigenic or stress-mediated hormonal stimulus. The main role played by these interactions appears to be that of recovering to normal the neuroendocrine or immune balance when suddenly altered by a stressful cognitive or noncognitive event (Blalock, 1984, 1988), that is, a "tactical" or "emergency" circuit.

Due to the different roles and targets of these two levels of interactions, the kinetics are quite different: "long wave" actions for the first level, supported by long-acting fluctuations of neurohormonal or thymic peptides, and "short wave" actions for the second level, mainly supported by humoral mediators with short-term effects.

This classification does not to assume that the humoral products involved in the two levels of interaction are different. It is a generally accepted notion in neuroendocrinology that the same hormone may exert both long-wave and short-wave actions according to the physiological situation in which the hormone has been recruited (Tata, 1984).

The present chapter aims to summarize the data available on the existence of neuroendocrine–immune interactions, and to analyze the possible integration between neuroendocrine and the immune factors in favoring the development and maintenance of discrete immune and nonimmune functions of the organism.

2. THYMUS–NEUROENDOCRINE INTERACTIONS: THE STRATEGIC CIRCUIT

The thymus is a quite complex organ devoted to proliferation and differentiation of mature T lymphocytes with effector (cytotoxic) and regulatory (helper/suppressor) activities.

The cellular components of the thymus are quite diversified, according to the function accomplished. In addition to T cells at different maturational steps, from stem cells to the mature forms, epithelial cells exist in the thymus capable of producing thymic peptides with differentiation properties on T-cell maturation and, in given circumstances, of synthezing neuropeptides, whose significance is still to be defined.

The steps of thymocyte differentiation in the thymus are now relatively well known and markers have been developed to follow the progressive acquisition of the functional characteristics of mature T lymphocytes. Much less known are the properties of the epithelial components, a subset of which likely plays the major role in neuroendocrine–thymus interactions.

Some of the thymic epithelial cells, particularly in the subcapsular cortex, and in the medullary region, do express major histocompatibility complex (MHC)-encoded antigens. The main function would be that of conferring on developing thymocytes the ability to recognize the self class I and II MHC antigens (Rouse *et al.*, 1974; Salaun *et al.*, 1990; Webb and Sprent, 1990; Bonomo and Matzinger, 1993).

Thymic epithelial cells are thought to synthesize and secrete various thymic peptides (see Chapter 11): some of them have been biochemically characterized such as thymosin α_1 (Goldstein *et al.*, 1977), thymopoietin (Goldstein *et al.*, 1976), thymulin (Bach *et al.*, 1975), and thymic humoral factor (THF) (Trainin *et al.*, 1979) all of which act on maturation and/or differentiation of stem cells into mature T cells (Goldstein, 1984; Hadden, 1993). At an immunohistochemical level, studies using polyclonal and monoclonal antibodies have demonstrated the presence of thymulin, thymosin α_1 and thymopoietin in both murine and human thymic epithelial cells (Savino and Dardenne, 1984). In a few studies, thymic hormone localization has been found to be restricted to $A2B5^+$ cells, i.e., to subcapsular cortical and medullary epithelial cells. This finding has led to the suggestion that these two cell subtypes (epithelial cells and A2B5$^+$ cells) represent the functional (secretory or endocrine) portion of the thymus as opposed to the nonsecreting epithelium of the inner cortical region and of Hassall's corpuscles.

The role of thymic peptides on intrathymic or extrathymic maturation of T cells is still controversial. According to some studies, evidence has shown *in vivo* modulating actions on T cells (Goldstein, 1984), but others were unable to demonstrate effects *in vitro* on surface markers or functional responses of thymocytes (Chen *et al.*, 1983; Hadden *et al.*, 1987). Similar contradictory findings have been obtained by using thymic epithelial cell products (Kruisbeek, 1979; Andrews *et al.*, 1985). This does not exclude a role for thymic factors but they tend to restrict such a role to chemotactic attraction of prothymocytes into the thymus, commitment for the first step of differentiation, i.e. Thy 1.2 marker acquisition in the mouse (Champion *et al.*, 1986), and maintenance of responses to interleukin 1 (IL-1) nad 2 (IL-2) (Hadden, 1992; Coto *et al.*, 1992).

Subsequent steps of intrathymic maturation may depend on other factors and in particular on IL-1 and IL-2. It has in fact been demonstrated that IL-1 and IL-2 are able to act synergistically on the proliferation rate of "double-negative" (Thy 1.2$^+$, Ly2$^-$, L3T4$^-$) cells, which possess IL-2 receptors and immature thymocytes (Ceredig *et al.*, 1985; Raulet, 1985; Hadden, 1992). Interleukins are produced at the intrathymic level (Hadden *et al.*, 1989). IL-1 is secreted by thymic epithelial cells (Ranson *et al.*, 1987; Hadden *et al.*, 1989) and induces thymulin secretion (Coto *et al.*, 1992); IL-2 is produced by thymocytes. The intrathymic production of these interleukins does not exclude the possibility that peripherally produced interleukins may also modulate thymic cell maturation. *In vivo* experimental models have clearly shown that injected interleukins enhance the evolution of T cells by marker and functional criteria (Hadden *et al.*, 1989; Hadden, 1992). This fact has been interpreted as expression of a feedback control on thymic function by signals from the periphery, leading to replenishment of the peripheral pool whenever required.

Recent findings have shown the presence in the human thymus of cells secreting neuropeptides (oxytocin, vasopressin, and neurophysin) which share antigenic properties with the neuropeptides secreted at the hypothalamic–pituitary level (Geenen *et al.*, 1986; Robert and Geenen, 1992). Immunohistochemical studies have revealed that such cells show the same distribution of A2B5$^+$ cells, mainly in the subcapsular cortex and the medulla, suggesting that at least a part of A2B5$^+$ cells can be vasopressin- or oxytocin-secreting cells (Geenen *et al.*, 1988).

The discovery of intrathymic synthesis of these neuropeptides has raised the question as to whether they might exert intrathymic paracrine action on thymocytes. In this context, both vasopressin and oxytocin were shown to replace IL-2 for interferon (IFN)-γ production by mouse splenocytes and by human peripheral blood lymphocytes (Johnson *et al.*, 1985). Thus, thymic vasopressin and oxytocin may have IL-2-like properties, and this could be of relevance with regard to the recent observation of IL-2 receptor expression as a differentiation marker on intrathymic stem cells (Ceredig et al., 1985).

More recently, it has been proposed that the role of such peptides is one of offering a cryptocrine signaling for the induction of immune tolerance to the hypothalamic neurohypophyseal-related peptides (NHP) system (Geenen *et al.*, 1993).

Both thymic peptide- and neuropeptide-secreting epithelial cells play a role in the context of the neuroendocrine–thymus interactions since, at least for thymic peptide-secreting cells, receptors for hormones have been demonstrated (see below). The exact nature of such a role remains, however, to be established (Dardenne and Savino, 1992).

2.1. Neuroendocrine Influence on Thymic Function

Initial evidence of the existence of thymus–neuroendocrine interactions was based on the discovery that congenital mutation affecting pituitary dwarf mice caused concomitant alterations in the thymus and in the thymus-dependent system (Fabris *et al.*, 1972).

Pituitary dwarf mice show a normal development of the lymphoid system during the first 2 weeks of life; however, following weaning, not only is the usual further development not observed but a progressive involution of the entire immune system and mainly of the thymus occurs. The thymus shows a reduction in size and is histologically characterized by a decrease of the cellularity in the cortex and a loss of the corticomedullary distinction (for review see Fabris, 1993).

Such a thymic involution causes underdevelopment of the thymus-dependent system, as indicated by the prolonged allogeneic skin-graft survival, the depressed capability of spleen cells to induce graft-versus-host reaction, to react to T mitogens, or to give rise *in vitro* to T-cell colonies, and the reduced humoral antibody response to thymus-dependent antigens.

The relevance of the pituitary–thymus interactions for the immunodeficiency state of the dwarf mouse is supported by the findings that the underdevelopment of the thymus and the immunologic deficiencies may be completely corrected by daily treatment of dwarf mice with growth hormone and thyroxine for 30 days (Fabris, 1993).

These findings have been recently confirmed in a strain of dwarf dogs (weimaraner dogs) which show retarded growth, small thymus, absence of thymus cortex, and deficiency in lymphocyte mitogen response (Roth *et al.*, 1980). All of these immunological defects can be corrected by growth hormone treatment (Roth *et al.*, 1984).

A number of experimental designs have further supported these findings obtained in experiments of nature. The majority of them have been based on the removal of endocrine glands and on the observation of the consequent modification of thymic functions, as measured by its size or by its histological picture or, indirectly, by the peripheral efficiency of the thymus-dependent lymphoid system (Fabris and Piantanelli, 1982; Fabris, 1992, 1993).

The discovery that some thymic factors are secreted into the bloodstream and that the circulating level of at least one of them, the facteur thymique serique (FTS)

(Bach *et al.*, 1975), now called *thymulin* in its zinc-bound form (Dardenne *et al.*, 1982), strictly reflects the functional activity of the thymus, has offered a new technical approach to evaluate neuroendocrine–thymus interactions both in animals and in humans.

It has been demonstrated that congenital hypopituitarism, experimental diabetes, and thyroidectomy all cause a rapid reduction of plasma level of thymulin, whereas removal of the gonads or of the adrenals does not induce any significant modification. Reconstitution experiments with hormone therapy have demonstrated that the circulating level of thymulin returns to normal just a few days after beginning the hormonal treatment (Fabris and Mocchegiani, 1985).

Also in humans, many endocrinopathies are associated with alterations of circulating thymulin. Thus, hypopituitarism due to congenital defect (Fabris *et al.*, 1983; Mocchegiani *et al.*, 1990a), and hypothyroidism following surgical thyroidectomy (Fabris, *et al.*, 1986a), are associated with consistent reduction of thymulin level. By contrast, hyperthyroidism, due to diffuse nodular goiter, is associated with high plasma levels of thymulin (Fabris *et al.*, 1986a), particularly evident in old individuals, since at this age the physiological plasma concentration of thymulin is usually quite low (Fabris *et al.*, 1984).

Also, functional alterations of thyroid hormone turnover, such as the "low T3" syndrome associated with premature birth (Fabris et al., 1987) or with trauma (Mocchegiani *et al.*, 1995), show reduced thymulin levels; in these studies a positive correlation has been found between thymulin concentrations and T3, but not T4, levels, suggesting that T3 rather than T4 is the hormone exerting its action on the thymus (Mocchegiani *et al.*, 1990b).

With regard to hypopituitarism in human, it has recently been demonstrated that the low thymulin levels present in these conditions are significantly recovered following growth hormone injection (Mocchegiani *et al.*, 1990a, 1991; Fabris and Mocchegiani, 1994); in these latter studies no correlation has been found between plasma GH and thymulin levels, but a significant positive correlation was found between insulinlike growth factor (IGF-1) and thymulin plasma concentrations, suggesting that GH probably acts on the thymus through somatomedins.

In conditions characterized by hypersecretion of GH, such as acromegaly, thymulin plasma levels are increased, but the increment is relatively modest (Travaglini *et al.*, 1990). Patients suffering from prolactin-secreting tumors, on the contrary, show thymulin level either reduced or in the lower range of normal values when compared to age-matched controls (Travaglini *et al.*, 1992).

The role played by prolactin is still controversial: the findings obtained in hyperprolactinemic patients (Travaglini et al., 1990), together with the consideration that thymulin levels are reduced in GH-deficient children, in spite of the normal PRL production, would suggest that PRL is not of particular relevance for thymic function, though data from other laboratories are not in agreement with our findings (Dardenne *et al.*, 1989).

Another hormone relevant for thymic function is insulin, since low thymulin plasma levels have been observed in type 1 juvenile diabetes; this defect, however, does not depend on thymic failure, but on reduced zinc ion availability, with consequent incomplete saturation (and biological activation) of thymulin molecules (Mocchegiani *et al.*, 1989).

More recently, interest has addressed the immunomodulatory role of the pineal gland (Maestroni, 1993). Pinealectomy has been shown to reduce thymic function, including the production of thymulin (Mocchegiani *et al.*, 1994a). These observations have suggested a possible role of pineal peptides, and primarily of melatonin, on the efficiency of the endocrine thymus (Pierpaoli and Regelson, 1994; Mocchegiani *et al.*, 1994a). Further support of this hypothesis has been offered by studies on aged animals (see Section 5.2).

The effect of hormones on thymic cell maturation may be mediated by a direct action on thymocytes or through the action exerted on thymic epithelial cells. Evidence exists for the presence on thymocytes of receptors for hormones, such as growth hormone (Arrenbrecht, 1974), estrogens (Gillette and Gillette, 1979), testosterone (Abraham and Bug, 1976), and adrenergic agonists (Singh *et al.*, 1979). On a functional basis, evidence supports the idea that other pituitary/CNS products may regulate the differentiation of mature T cells (Robert and Geenen, 1992; Fabris, 1993).

The presence of calcitonin gene-related peptide (CGRP) in the thymus and in the peripheral lymphoid tissues is now well documented. In the thymus, CGRP-immunoreactive material has been found in mast cells, in small cells (thymocytes?), and in nerve endings in the corticomedullary region (Bulloch *et al.*, 1991). In the spleen the presence of CGRP is much less evident. The biological meaning for the presence of such peptides has been related to their capacity to inhibit lymphoid cell proliferation following mitogenic, and presumably antigenic stimuli (Bulloch *et al.*, 1991); this action would prevent mature thymocytes from reacting to antigens arriving in the thymus, while letting lymphocytes in the spleen and lymph nodes proliferate according to specific requirements.

With regard to the endocrine component of the thymus, there is no doubt that many hormones and neuropeptides are capable of modulating thymulin secretion by thymic epithelial cells (TEC). Among neuropeptides, Leu-enkephalin and β-endorphin are able to increase thymulin production by TEC, whereas Met-enkephalin α- and γ-endorphin are inactive (Dardenne and Savino, 1992). Among hormones, GH, PRL, adrenal and sex steroids, and thyroid hormones can modulate thymulin production *in vitro*. Such an *in vitro* effect clearly supports the idea that TEC possess specific receptors for these hormones and neuropeptides. At present, experimental demonstration of receptors on TEC has been obtained for glucocorticoids, progesterone, GH, PRL, and T_3 (Dardenne *et al.*, 1986; 1991; Villa Verde *et al.*, 1992; Timsit *et al.*, 1992).

Other factors of pituitary origin may also modulate TEC: a fibroblast growthlike factor, isolated from bovine pituitaries (Hadden *et al.*, 1987), has been proven to induce proliferation of TEC in culture.

From all of the *in vivo* and *in vitro* findings, it can be concluded that the synthesis and secretion of thymic hormones is regulated by a complex neuroendocrine network, which may exert both stimulatory and inhibitory actions (Fig. 2).

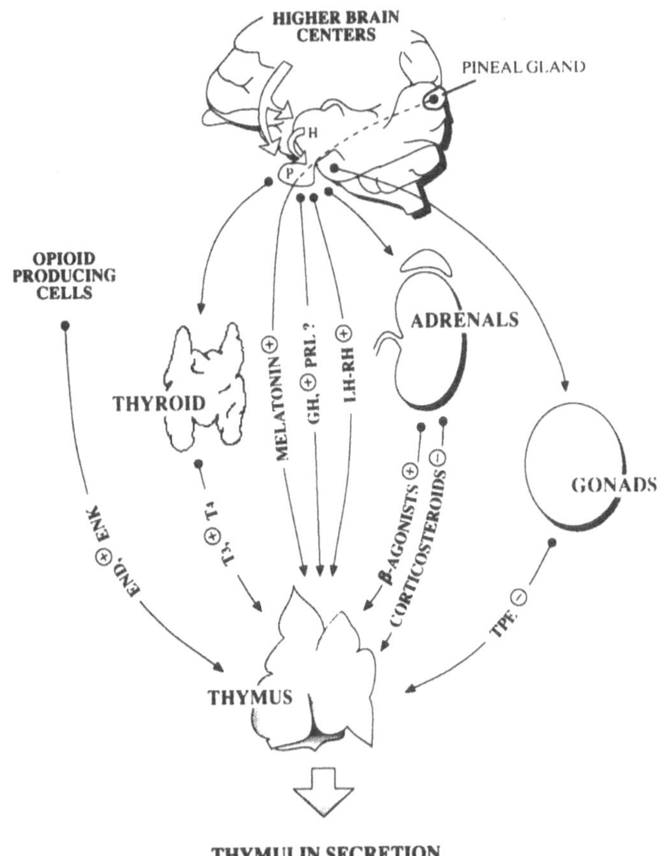

FIGURE 2. Schematic representation of the hormones/neuropeptides capable of modulating the synthesis and/or secretion of thymulin. +, enhancing effect; −, inhibitory action. Data are derived from references reported in Section 2.1.

2.2. Influence of the Thymus on the Neuroendocrine Network

The idea that the thymus may act, particularly during early stages of life, on the physiologic development of nonimmunologic functions has originated from the observation that postthymectomy wasting disease, in addition to the obvious immunologic disturbances, is characterized by pathological signs, which can hardly be linked to the direct effect of immune deficiency itself. Mice thymectomized at birth, show, in fact, a progressive impairment of body growth with reduced length of ears and tail, microsplanchnia, microsomia, thinness of the skin and lack of subcutaneous fat, bone alterations, particularly evident in the vertebrae with consequent hunched posture, and hypotrophy of various tissues including submaxillary gland, hair follicles, and bone marrow. At the pituitary level it was demonstrated that thymectomized mice show a progressive degranulation of pituitary acidophilic GH-producing cells, whereas other cell lineages in the hypophysis are left unmodified (for review see Fabris, 1993).

Degranulation of GH- and PRL-producing cells has also been observed in athymic nude mice. Determination of blood levels of pituitary hormones has demonstrated a reduction of ACTH (transient), GH, PRL plasma level and an increased level of luteotropic hormone (LH) in thymectomized mice. In neonatal thymectomized rats, transitory decrements of ACTH levels and increased blood concentrations of LH were observed.

Both neonatally thymectomized and nude mice have been reported to show an abnormal histological picture of adrenals accompanied by a transient increase of plasma levels of corticosterone. According to other authors, neonatal thymectomy in rats induces a reduction of corticosterone plasma levels, which, in the presence of the concomitant low levels of ACTH, would suggest an action of the thymus on the adrenals via the hypophysis.

Gonadal function in thymus-deprived animals has been investigated extensively, since it was demonstrated that neonatal thymectomy in hamsters had quite different effects according to sex (males undergo wasting diseases, females do not). In mice, thymectomy causes sterility in females, but not in males (Nishizuka and Sakakura, 1969; Besedovsky and Sorkin, 1974). Further investigations in thymectomized and athymic nude mice have shown that both thymus-deprived conditions are characterized by an altered profile of sex hormones (Michael *et al.*, 1980).

With regard to the endocrine pancreas very little is known. Preliminary experiments in nude mice have shown that while there are no differences in the basal levels of plasma insulin between nude and normal littermates, the insulin-dependent hexokinase pattern in the liver is strongly altered in nude animals (Fabris, 1993).

Finally, some physiological reactions induced by the stimulation of β-adrenergic receptors, such as the increased rate of DNA synthesis in submandibular glands or the increment of total water intake shortly after the injection of isoproterenol (IPR), are found deeply reduced in thymectomized and nude mice, and are restored to normal values by a syngeneic neonatal thymus transplant (Piantanelli *et al.*, 1978). Additional data from our laboratory have furthermore demonstrated that the β-adrenoceptor density in different tissues (submandibular glands, brain) is reduced in mice lacking a thymus and recovers with syngeneic thymus transplant (Piantanelli *et al.*, 1985; Rossolini *et al.*, 1992).

With regard to the thymic mechanism of action on the neuroendocrine network, both thymic humoral factors and the cellular products of the thymus, i.e., the mature T lymphocytes, might be involved: the former because of their hormonelike nature, and the latter because, in given circumstances, they may produce lymphokines, capable of influencing some pituitary functions (Besedovsky and del Rey, 1992; McCann *et al.*, 1993), or even pituitary-hormonelike substances, such as ACTH, TSH, PRL, GH, and gonadotropins (Blalock, 1984; Hejinen *et al.*, 1991; Smith, 1992; Panerai, 1993).

The relevance of these pituitary hormonelike products of mature T cells can be questioned; first, because such products are secreted on stimulation with antigens and therefore might exert only a temporary action, and second, because thymus–neuroendocrine interactions also operate in germfree conditions, where even the background antigenic stimulation is supposed to be nearly absent.

Furthermore, at least with respect to some altered neuroendocrine pattern in thymus-deprived animals, such as IPR response and reduced T_3 and T_4 plasma levels, no recovery has been achieved when mature lymphocytes have been used instead of neonatal thymus grafts (Piantanelli, personal communication).

A possible role played by thymic factors may, to the contrary, be supported by the following considerations: (1) they do not require any specific antigenic stimulation; (2) some neuroendocrine abnormalities, such as the degranulation of GH-producing cells in the pituitary of thymus-deprived mice, can be prevented by injection of thymic extracts (Deschaux *et al.*, 1979); (3) evidence has recently been gathered of a direct effect of some thymosins at pituitary and hypothalamic levels. In particular, it has been shown that thymosins may modulate at the hypothalamic level the secretion of corticotropin-releasing factor (CRF) and luteotropin-releasing factor (LRF), thus modulating both the pituitary–adrenal and pituitary–gonadal axis (Rebar, 1984; Spangelo *et al.*, 1987; Milenkovic *et al.*, 1992). By using single peptides it has also been shown that thymosin α_1 acts preferentially on the pituitary–adrenal axis whereas thymosin β_4 acts on the pituitary–gonadal axis, thus suggesting a specific effect of these compounds (Rebar *et al.*, 1981; Hall et al., 1989).

3. IMMUNE–NEUROENDOCRINE INTERACTIONS: THE EMERGENCY CIRCUIT

3.1. Neurohormonal Modulation of Immune Functions

A large and growing number of hormones and neurotransmitters have been identified as exerting a critical action on discrete immune functions. This identification is supported by functional studies based on deprivation designs (such as endocrine gland ablation; or brain or peripheral neural lesions), on exogenous administration of specific substances to otherwise normal animals, or on *in vitro* studies.

Because of the multiple functions of various hormones and neuropeptides and the wide distribution of the secretory cells within the organism, all of these experimental designs have yielded relevant information which is difficult to interpret. More decisive, though functionally limited, is the identification of receptors for different hormones, neuropeptides, and autacoids on lymphoid cells (Fabris and Provinciali, 1989; Carr, 1992) (Table I).

Evidence has been gathered on the existence of receptors for corticosteroids (Cake and Litwack, 1975; Werb *et al.*, 1978), insulin (Hollenberg and Cuatrecasas, 1974; Helderman and Strom, 1978), prolactin (Russell *et al.*, 1984; Hienstand *et al.*,

TABLE I
Evidence of Cellular Receptors for Neurohormonal Substances on Lymphocytes (L) or Natural Killer Cells[a]

	Functional study		Binding study		Competitive antagonism	
	L	NK	L	NK	L	NK
Autacoids						
Histamine	•	•	•		•	
5-HT	•		•			
PG	•	•	•			
Leukotrienes	•	•				
Neuropeptides						
Endorphins	•	•	•		•	•
Enkephalins	•	•	•			
Somatostatin	•		•			
VIP	•	•	•			
Substance P	•		•			
CRH	•	•	•			
Protein hormones						
GH	•	•	•			
PRL	•	•		•		
ACTH	•	•	•			
TSH	•	•				
LH		•				
Insulin	•		•			
Calcitonin	•	•	•			
PTH	•					
Nonprotein hormones						
Thyroxine	•	•	•			
Glucocorticoids	•	•		•		
Androgens	•					
Estrogens	•	•				
Progesteroids	•					
ACh			•			
Catecholamine	•	•	•		•	•
Melatonin	•	•	•			

[a]As demonstrated by functional or binding studies or by competitive antagonism. Data from references cited in Section 3.1.

1986), α and β-adrenergic agents (Hadden *et al.*, 1970; Bourne *et al.*, 1974; Landmann *et al.*, 1981, 1989; Hadden, 1983), acetylcholine (Strom *et al.*, 1974; Richman and Arnason, 1979; Sibinga and Goldstein, 1988), endorphins (Hazum *et al.*, 1979), enkephalins (Wybran *et al.*, 1979), substance P, vasoactive intestinal peptide (VIP) (Payan *et al.*, 1984; Stanisz *et al.*, 1987), and more recently melatonin (Lopez-Gonzales *et al.*, 1992).

In general, glucocorticoids, estrogens, progesterone, and testosterone depress the immune response, whereas growth hormone, prolactin, thyroxine, insulin, and melatonin increase the response (Billingham *et al.*, 1951; Dougherty *et al.*, 1964; Wolstenholme and Knight, 1970; Claman, 1975; Fabris, 1977; Fabris *et al.*, 1983; Cooper, 1984; Guillemin *et al.*, 1985; Locke *et al.*, 1985; Hadden *et al.*, 1989; O'Dorisio and Panerai, 1990; for review see Berczi and Kovacs, 1987).

Because of the concurrent presence of both agonist and antagonist hormones, and the periodicity of most hormonal secretions (Reiter, 1990), the efficiency of an immune response at any one time will be affected by the current balance of neurohormonal influences.

The impact, however, of such a balance in the economy of the immune system may vary according to the relevance of the target function of the neuroendocrine signals. Thus, hormones acting on developmental stages of the immune system induce more relevant modifications, sometimes irreversible, than hormonal substances acting on the functional performance of mature cells. The positive action exerted by developmental hormones, such as growth hormone, thyroxine, and insulin, on the proliferation of stem cells toward more mature stages , as well as the suppressive effect due to corticosteroids, gonadotropins, progesteroids, and testosterone, may have a long-lasting effect on the development of the major branches of the immune system (Fabris, 1977, 1981a; Fabris and Piantanelli, 1982; Fabris and Provinciali, 1989).

Many of the neuroendocrine signals are effective only on activated immune cells since, on stimulation, these cells are induced to express various hormonal receptors, such as those for insulin (Hollenberg and Cuatrecasas, 1974; Helderman and Strom, 1978) and for muscarinic and β-adrenoceptors (Strom *et al.*, 1981; Daily *et al.*, 1988; Carlson *et al.*, 1991), which are not present in resting cells.

Of the nonprotein hormones and autacoids, β-adrenergic amines, histamines, and prostaglandin E, in addition to their known effect on the inflammatory processes, act on both B and T cells. In particular, they inhibit both cytolytic functions and the production of lymphokines by effector T cells and suppressor T cells. They can also (except for histamine) inhibit the production and the release of antibody by B cells. On the other hand, cholinergic drugs, particularly of the muscarinic type, increase T-cell proliferation after mitogen stimulation and T-cell-mediated cytolysis (Hadden *et al.*, 1977; Hadden, 1983). These findings have been interpreted in the light of the role played by cyclic nucleotides, cAMP and cGMP, in the physiological control of proliferation and differentiation of lymphocytes (Hadden, 1983; Carlson *et al.*, 1991).

Also, opioids have been shown to modulate many immune functions, both *in vivo* and *in vitro*. *In vivo*, classical opioids, such as morphine, reduce antibody production (Weber *et al.*, 1987; Dinari *et al.*, 1989), cellular immune response (Bryant et al., 1990; Molitar *et al.*, 1992), graft-versus-host and delayed-type hypersensitivity reactions (Bryant and Roudebush, 1990), and natural killer cell activity (Weber and Pert, 1989; Bayer *et al.*, 1990; Provinciali *et al.*, 1991a). Consequences of such an immunosuppressive effect are increased susceptibility to bacterial and viral infections (Tubaro *et al.*, 1983; Watson and Nguyen, 1990) and decreased resistance to tumor growth in experimental animals (Lewis *et al.*, 1983, 1985). According to recent findings, the action of opioids on the immune system may be mediated either by the activation of the HPA axis (Gibson *et al.*, 1979; Bryant *et al.*, 1988), particularly when the administration is chronic (Gonzalves *et al.*, 1991), or through the involvement of the central nervous system and in particular of the periaqueductal gray matter (Weber and Pert, 1989; Band *et al.*, 1992).

The experimental designs used to evaluate the effect of hormones and neuropeptides on NK-mediated cytotoxicity and/or resistance to tumor growth have been quite similar to those chosen for studies on specific immunity: *in vivo* models based primarily on deprivation of relevant endocrine glands or of nervous centres or on administration of hormones or neuropeptides; and *in vitro* designs aimed at demonstrating direct effects of these substances on the capacity of NK cells to bind and/or to lyse target cells.

Both types of designs have limitations. First, any *in vivo* manipulation may reveal a role for some hormone or neuropeptide in NK activity, without indicating whether the effect is direct or mediated by other hormonal substances or hormone-dependent metabolic events. Second, NK cells have a life span of at least 2 weeks and the generation of functional elements from undifferentiated precursors requires several weeks (Hochman *et al.*, 1978). Studies *in vitro* are, therefore, unlikely to reveal effects at the level of generation or survival of NK cells, which, in contrast, may be suggested by studies *in vivo*.

NK activity is physiologically regulated by macrophages with suppressor activity (Brunda *et al.*, 1979) as well as by different lymphokines, such as interferon (Herberman *et al.*, 1979) and IL-2 (Henney *et al.*, 1981). Since all of these functions may be sensitive to the action of various hormones and neuropeptides, and the experiments often use mixed cell populations, the interpretation of data on neurohormonal modulation of NK activity should seek to discriminate direct effects on NK cells or their precursors from actions mediated through the activation of macrophages or lymphokine-secreting cells.

In addition, the sensitivity of NK cells to the boosting effect of IL-2 and IFN appears at different stages during ontogenetic development; it has been suggested that basal activity, IL-2 sensitivity, and IFN sensitivity may represent three consecutive stages in the maturation of the NK lineage (Yoshiki *et al.*, 1985; Provinciali *et al.*, 1989). Most of the studies on neurohormonal modulation of NK activity have taken this into account and have tried to define the stage at which a neurohormonal influence is exerted.

With regard to the demonstration of receptors for hormones and neuropeptides on NK cells, the available data mainly concern glucocorticoids, β-endorphins, and prolactin (Fig. 3).

Binding techniques have demonstrated receptors for glucocorticoids (Katz *et al.*, 1985), whereas receptors for β-endorphin and enkephalin have been demonstrated only by competitive antagonism with naloxone (Mathews *et al.*, 1983). This last assumption is, however, quite controversial, since a variety of different receptors for endogenous opioids have been identified and nonopiate receptors have also been found in lymphoid cells (Hazum *et al.*, 1979).

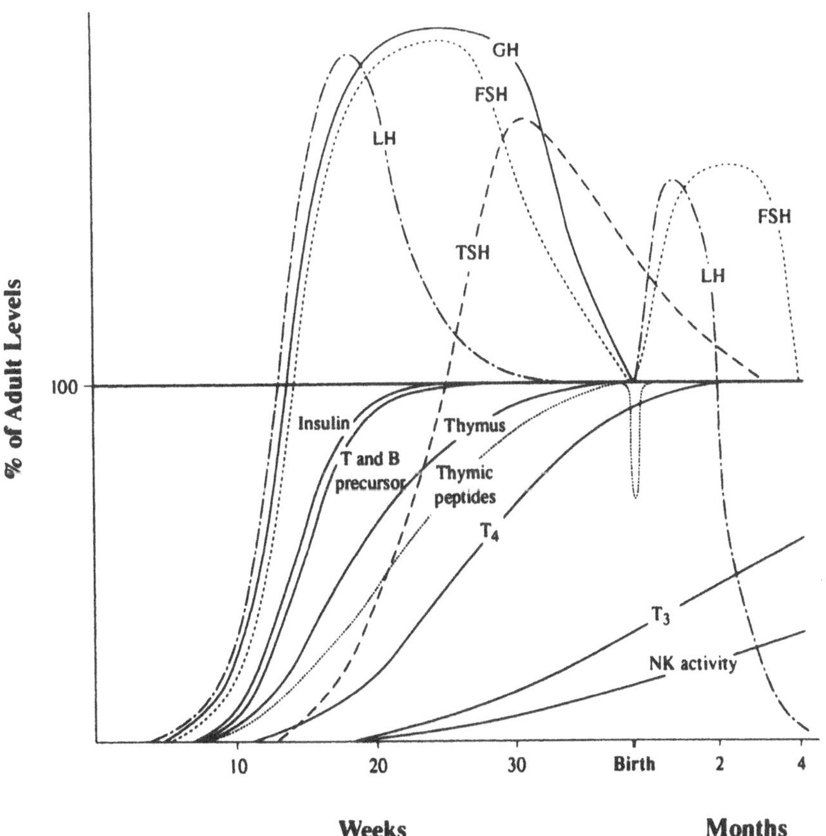

Figure 3. Schematic representation of timing of ontogenetic development of various endocrine and immune functions, compatible with the existence of neuroendocrine–immune interactions.

The existence of PRL receptors on NK cells has been reported. The number of PRL receptors on NK cells is comparable to that previously found on T and B cells (Matera et al., 1988).

The effect of GH and PRL on peripheral immune function in humans is unclear. In general, no major modifications in the lymphocyte subsets as well as in NK activity have been detected in patients suffering from chronic elevation of GH or PRL (Matera *et al.*, 1988; Sobharwal *et al.*, 1992), although defective NK activity in hyperprolactinemic subjects (Gerli *et al.*, 1986; Nicollete et al., 1989) has also been reported. In contrast, positive effect of exogenous GH was observed on NK activity in women with impaired endogenous GH secretion (Crist *et al.*, 1987).

3.2. Immune Effects on the Neuroendocrine System

Antigenic stimulation may affect the neuroendocrine system and particularly the pituitary-adrenal axis. Increased ACTH and corticosterone blood levels have been observed after injection with various antigens (Besedovsky *et al.*, 1975), viruses (Besedovsky *et al.*, 1986; Dunn *et al.*, 1987), and tumor cells (Besedovsky *et al.*, 1985; Normann *et al.*, 1988). Other endocrine mechanisms affected by antigenic challenges with innocuous material or tumor cells are thyroid hormones (Besedovsky *et al.*, 1975), PRL, insulin, and testosterone (Besedovsky *et al.*, 1985). Also, the ANS is influenced by the immune response (Saphier *et al.*, 1987; Carlson *et al.*, 1987).

From the immune side, the mediation of all of these effects is due to lymphokines and monokines secreted by immune cells on stimulation (for review see Besedovsky *et al.*, 1991; Milenkovic *et al.*, 1992; McCann *et al.*, 1993). In particular, IL-1 causes pituitary ACTH release, through the mediation of CRF (Besedovsky *et al.*, 1986; Sapolsky *et al.*, 1987). IL-6, tumor necrosis factor (TNF), and IFN-γ also stimulate the pituitary–adrenal axis (Holsboer *et al.*, 1988; Naitoh *et al.*, 1988; Sharp *et al.*, 1989).

IL-1, IL-6, TNF, and IFN-γ are able to influence the pituitary–thyroid axis (Dubuis *et al.*, 1988; Zakarija *et al.*, 1988; Krog-Rasmussen *et al.*, 1988; Milenkovic *et al.*, 1989; Fujii *et al.*, 1989; Yamasjita *et al.*, 1989; Pang *et al.*, 1989; Sato *et al.*, 1990), pituitary–gonadal axis (Roby and Terranova, 1988; Darbon *et al.*, 1989; Gottschall *et al.*, 1989; Gaillard et al., 1990; Mealy *et al.*, 1990; Rivier and Vale, 1990; Schettini *et al.*, 1990), and GH secretion (Rettori *et al.*, 1989; Walton and Cronin, 1989; Spangelo and MacLeod, 1990; Vankezecom *et al.*, 1990).

Cytokines may also affect metabolism: it has been demonstrated that IL-1, TNF, and IL-6 can affect intermediate metabolism (Beutler *et al.*, 1985; Tracey *et al.*, 1986; del Rey and Besedovsky,1987; Besedovsky and del Rey, 1992). IL-1 causes decreased glucose level (del Rey and Besedovsky, 1987); the mechanism seems to be independent of insulin turnover since it is observed also in insulin-resistant diabetic animals (del Rey and Besedovsky, 1989). Lipid metabolism results were also modified following IL-1 injection (Besedovsky and del Rey, 1990).

The relevance of cytokines for the neuroendocrine pathways should take into account the fact that humoral factors can be synthesized and secreted also by cells other than immune cells. In particular, IL-1 has been found in nerve and in glial cells and astrocytes on stimulation with pyrogenic material (Fontana *et al.*, 1984; Giulian *et al.*, 1986; Lechan *et al.*, 1990) and receptors have been identified in discrete brain areas (Cunningham *et al.*, 1992; Ban *et al.*, 1992; for review see Rothwell and Dantzer, 1992). Other cytokines, such as IL-2, IL-3, IL-6, and TNF, have been detected in discrete brain areas and in pituitary cells (Araujo *et al.*, 1989; Kamegai *et al.*, 1990; Spangelo *et al.*, 1990). The role for such a production is still not completely defined. While IL-1 production may be required for mediating pyrogen stimuli (Fontana *et al.*, 1984; Schettini *et al.*, 1990) and for modulating the HPA and gonadal axis (Berkenbosch *et al.*, 1987; Sapolsky *et al.*, 1987; Yamaguchi et al., 1990), all of the cytokines reported above may exert growth as well as neuromodulatory actions on nerve cells (Giulian and Lachman, 1985; Bindoni *et al.*, 1988; Kamegai *et al.*, 1990; Blatteis, 1990).

The production of these cytokines within the CNS may be justified by their difficulty crossing the blood–brain barrier (Coceani *et al.*, 1988; Stitt, 1990; Banks and Kastin, 1993). The connection between the production of cytokines by the peripheral tissues and by the CNS remains to be explained; the link may be represented by prostaglandins (Stitt, 1986; Morimoto *et al.*, 1986) or prostaglandinlike molecules (Morimoto *et al.*, 1986; Katsura *et al.*, 1988; Cornell, 1989).

4. MECHANISMS OF NEUROENDOCRINE–IMMUNE INTERACTIONS

In order to understand the mechanisms of neuroendocrine–immune interactions, at least two main levels of action must be taken into consideration: (1) a direct action on target cells and (2) the involvement of other humoral and/or cellular events, which may in turn affect target cells. The direct action implies either a change in membrane permeability, resulting in enhanced influx of ions (Ca^{2+}, Na^{+}), amino acids, sugars, nucleosides or the activation of relevant metabolic intermediates (cAMP, cGMP), or the induction of enzymatic activities, or, finally, changes at the level of transcriptional and translational processes (Tata, 1984). The direct action is ensured by the presence on target cells (lymphocytes or endocrine cells) of specific receptors for hormones or cytokines (Fabris and Provinciali, 1989).

The second level of action of endocrine/immune factors may be mediated by the induction of other cell/humoral factors. Neuroendocrine agents may modulate the production of several lymphokines and monokines. Thus, glucocorticoids affect IL-1, 2, and 4, TNF, colony-stimulating factor, and IFN-γ (Wahl *et al.*, 1975; Gillis *et al.*, 1979; Snyder and Unanue, 1982; Kelso and Munck, 1984; Beutler *et al.*, 1986; Daynes and Araneo, 1989). Somatostatin and VIP decrease IFN-γ; substance P and substance K increase IL-1, TNF, and IL-6 release from peripheral blood white cells (Lotz *et al.*, 1988; Muscettola and Grasso, 1990).

Norepinephrine decreases IL-1 production (Koff *et al.*, 1986), α-adrenergic agonists increase TNF release by stimulated macrophages (Spengler *et al.*, 1990).

Relatively little data exist on the modulation by hormones and neurotransmitters of receptor expression for lymphokines. Glucocorticoids induce IL-1 receptor on B cells (Akahoshi *et al.*, 1988) and decrease IL-6 receptor on monocytes (Bauer *et al.*, 1989); insulin decreases TNF receptors on monocytes (Bermudez et al., 1990); PRL (Mukherjee *et al.*, 1990) and TSH (Provinciali and Fabris, 1990) induce IL-2 receptors on monocytes.

Epinephrine and somatostatin reduce receptor for TNF on monocytes (Bermudez *et al.*, 1990); β-agonists reduce IL-2 receptors on lymphocytes (Feldman *et al.*, 1987) and substance P enhances IL-2 receptors in gut-associated lymphocytes (Hart et al., 1988).

Hormones and neuropeptides can also directly or indirectly influence the expression of class I and class II MHC antigens in both immune cells and their targets. Thus, glucocorticoids affect cytokine-mediated induction of class II antigens on macrophages (Snyder and Unanue, 1982; Rhodes *et al.*, 1986; Shen *et al.*, 1986) and norepinephrine and VIP inhibit class II antigen expression on astrocytes (Frohman *et al.*, 1988).

Conversely, leukocytes, either spontaneously or after induction, may produce and secrete immunoreactive and endocrine-active hormones such as TSH, GH, ACTH, gonadotropins, and endorphins (Smith *et al.*, 1983, 1986; Ebaugh and Smith, 1987; Weigent et al., 1988). Also, neurotensins, considered modulators of dopaminergic system activity in the CNS (Nemeroff, 1986; Brouard *et al.*, 1992), have been shown, by indirect evidence, to be produced by peripheral blood lymphocytes (Schimpff *et al.*, 1992).

The existence of so many neurohormonal substances capable of modulating discrete immune functions by such different mechanisms of action raises the question as to what regulates all of these interactions. The answer to such a question should take into account that (1) the immune system has developed quite efficient mechanisms of self-regulation, (2) the effects of neurohormonal inputs into the immune system are, in physiological conditions, small though biologically relevant, and (3) the same bidirectional interaction studied *in vivo* or *in vitro* may give even opposite results.

With regard to the last point, for instance, PRL shows an immunopotentianting effect *in vivo* but is ineffective on the same immune response *in vitro* (Bernton, 1989). On the contrary, endorphins show an immunopotentiating effect *in vitro* but an immunosuppressive effect *in vivo* (Shavit *et al.*, 1984; Wybran, 1985). The high frequency of such discrepancies cannot be considered as merely coincidental, but suggests another frequent phenomenon, i.e., that many hormones/neurotransmitters have an opposite effect based on whether they are administered before or after antigenic or target challenge. This is true for adrenalin, VIP, and prostaglandins (Fabris and Provinciali, 1989).

An interesting approach to the first two points of the question has been proposed on the basis of the role of second messengers of lymphocyte activation (Coffey and Hadden, 1985; Carlson *et al.*, 1991). The hypotheses rely on a two-signal model based on the concept that both the neural stimulus (neurotransmitter, neurohormone, neuropeptide) and the immune stimulus (antigen, lymphokine, cell contact) act on their specific receptors and that the stimulation of these receptors results in the induction of different sets of second messengers. The more or less synergistic action of these sets on the cAMP or cGMP intracellular level offers the basis of a cross talk between the two signals. Such a two-signal model represents a nice approach to support neuro-immune interactions, but it does not offer a solution for the complex inputs that an immune cell receives from the neuroendocrine system, since the model is limited by the low number of sets of second messengers. Additional mechanisms should be recruited in the network in order to accommodate the variety of inputs that a cell can accept.

According to classical neuroendocrinology, every response of a cell to hormones or neuropeptides is the result of a number of coordinated events which follow the interaction of the factor(s) with the target cell.

An example of a sequential interaction of many hormones is found in the growth and maturation of the mammary gland (Topper, 1970; Turkington, 1972). In fact, ductal development is dependent on the interactions between estrogen, GH, and glucocorticoids; alveolar development may be regulated by estrogen–glucocorticoid–GH or estrogen–progesterone–prolactin interactions. On the basis of these preparatory events, coordinated interactions among prolactin, glucocorticoids, estrogen, and progesterone lead to lactogenesis, whereas insulin, glucocorticoids, and prolactin act synergistically to control the synthesis of milk proteins (Lockwood *et al.*, 1966). Another example of a multihormone-dependent physiological process is the synthesis of α-2m globulin by mammalian liver which is regulated by thyroid hormones, estrogens, androgens, and GH (Kurtz and Feigelson, 1978).

One of the main mechanisms involved in these sequential activation systems is the heterologous regulation of receptors. In fact, the activities of some receptors may be modulated not only by the homologous hormone, but also by other factors. For example, the hormones that interact with prolactin in the control of lactation, such as thyroid hormones, sex steroids, and glucocorticoids, influence prolactin receptor expression in a variety of target cells (Tata, 1984).

As observed for the endocrine system, multifactor coordinated events intrinsic to the immune network exist which are indispensable for the differentiation of immune cells and the amplification of immune responses. It is well known that the activation of many various immune functions requires the sequential actions of many lymphokines.

With regard to NK activity, which has represented an interesting model for investigating hormone/lymphokine interplay, the requirement for a sequential action of two different lymphokines has been demonstrated: IL-2 acts initially on the growth and differentiation of NK cells from nonlytic precursors, and IFN exerts its action later on NK cell differentiation for lytic activity (Koo and Manyac, 1986; Kalland, 1986).

The sequence IL-2/IFN also has been observed in the course of ontogenetic development of NK activity, both in humans (Yoshiki *et al.*, 1985) and in rodents (Provinciali *et al.*, 1989).

Does sequentiality represent a kind of communication between the neuroendocrine and immune systems? Studies performed on the interactions between thyrotropic/

thyroid hormones and IL-2/IFN on the activation of NK cells have produced some interesting results.

In mice early in life, NK lytic activity is very low and progressively increases; the sensitivity to IL-2 precedes that to IFN. Only IL-2 can boost NK cell activity in 25 day-old animals and both IL-2 and IFN act on the cytotoxicity of spleen cells in mice over 50 days old (Provinciali *et al.*, 1989).

By using, as a model, the sequentiality IL-2/IFN observed in the ontogenetic development of NK cells, it has been shown that the *in vitro* administration of physiological concentrations of thyroxine (T_4) induces an earlier development of IFN responsiveness of NK cells determining the appearance of IFN-sensitivity in spleen cells from 25-day-old mice, but not in spleen cells from 15 day-old mice. On the other hand, the preincubation of spleen cells with thyrotropic hormone (TSH) determines an earlier development of IL-2 responsiveness of NK cells whereas IFN sensitivity is not affected.

These findings clearly suggest that NK development requires a multisignal sequence represented by TSH/IL-2/T_4-T_3/IFN (Provinciali *et al.*, 1991b). The sequence TSH/IL-2 is based on the capacity of TSH to induce synthesis and/or expression of IL-2 receptors, while the mechanism of the sequence T_3/IFN is yet unknown. The capacity of hormones/neurotransmitters to modulate various lymphokine receptors, as reported above, suggests that this mechanism may operate in immune functions other than NK activity.

As a working hypothesis, it may also be suggested that hormone/lymphokine and neurotransmitters/lymphokines in multisignal sequential mechanism of cell activation apply to target cells other than immune cells. Models suitable for such an investigation may be represented by: neurons devoted to body temperature control and sensitive to IL-1 and MSH (Hiltz *et al.*, 1992; Watanabe *et al.*, 1993); pituitary endocrine cells sensitive to hormones and various lymphokines (Bertnon *et al.*, 1987; McCann *et al.*, 1993); ovarian cells sensitive to gonadotropins and interleukins (Kasson and Gorospe, 1989) and many other tissue cells (osteoclasts, hepatocytes, adipocytes), which can be stimulated by both hormone/neurotransmitters and lymphokines.

Taken together, these observations and concepts deal with a hormone–lymphokine interplay which cannot be based only on the two-signal model suggested by Carlson *et al.* (1991). A multisignal coded sequence, based on heterologous receptor regulation, in addition to the mechanism represented by the activation of different sets of second messengers, may better explain the variety of neuroendocrine–immune interactions.

5. IMPLICATIONS FOR DEVELOPMENT AND AGING

5.1. Neuroendocrine–Immune Interactions during Ontogeny

The idea that neuroendocrine–immune interplay is relevant for ontogenetic steps should satisfy at least one major criterion: that humoral factors from both homeostatic systems have to appear in the course of embryonic or fetal life in the orderly sequence required by the suspected neuroendocrine–immune interaction.

This assumption implies that phenomena of refractoriness to a given stimulus should be detectable in both homeostatic systems, if timing of neuroendocrine and immune development is not respected.

The available data cannot, at present, give a definite and comprehensive picture of these interconnections during ontogeny, but some suggestions can certainly be put forward. Figure 3 is a simple impression of neuroendocrine and immune development during ontogeny in humans. The orderly sequence of events in the neuroendocrine and immune development seems to be quite compatible with the existence of bidirectional interactions between the two systems. In fact, the precocious appearance of some pituitary hormones (GH, FSH, LH, TSH) and insulin in the fetal blood is closely related to the growth of the thymus and the increase in lymphoid cells bearing T and B markers. It is interesting to note that the later development of thyroid function is strictly coupled to the acquisition of NK cell cytotoxicity, thereby suggesting an important role of the pituitary–thyroid axis on the development of NK cells.

While these kinds of thoughts may support the existence of neuroendocrine–immune interactions during ontogenetic development, they do not define the orderly sequence of events which may condition the development of a given function. At present, little information is available, but it may certainly indicate the validity of such an approach.

In fact, congenital alterations of neuroendocrine development, as they occur in mice or dogs, or experimentally induced endocrinopathies early in life (for review see Fabris, 1993), cause desynchronization of the physiological development of the immune system, affecting the thymus and the thymus-dependent functions more than other immune functions, such as pure B-dependent antibody response or macrophage activity. It is interesting to note that the timing of an experimental "ectomy" may have quite different end effects.

Thus, neonatal adrenalectomy causes a retarded development of thymus-dependent humoral antibody responses when performed during the first days of life. The same adrenalectomy performed at 20 days of age has no effects and, later, induces an increment of immune responses (Fabris, 1981b).

Neonatal thyroidectomy causes a profound underdevelopment of the thymus and of thymus-dependent functions, whereas adult thyroidectomy has minor effects and more time is required after the operation in order to detect them (Fabris, 1973).

The experimentally induced hypothyroidism produced by treatment of mice from birth with propylthiouracil (PTU) prevents the appearance of responsiveness of NK cells to interferon, the defect being reversed by the cessation of PTU treatment (Provinciali *et al.*, 1991b).

In supplementation studies, it was demonstrated that the neonatal administration of GH to normal mice accelerates the development of immune reactions when compared to untreated animals (Pierpaoli *et al.*, 1970, 1976).

On the contrary, the administration of testosterone to chicken embryos causes underdevelopment of the bursa of Fabricius with consequent defect in B-cell responses, which cannot be resumed by the physiological development of sexual hormones (Glick, 1964). Perinatal treatment of female mice with the nonsteroidal estrogen diethylstilbestrol (DES) gives rise to persistent alterations in immunological functions, mainly through its interference with T-cell differentiation (Kalland *et al.*, 1979).

Another example of the influence of sex steroids on immune development is offered by New Zealand mice. Female New Zealand mice frequently develop a lethal glomerulonephritis between 8 and 14 months of age. Castration or testosterone treatment of females prolongs survival whereas castration or estradiol treatment of males has opposite effects (Roubinian et al., 1978; Steinberg *et al.*, 1979). It is important to note that castration of males results in accelerated mortality for autoimmune disease only if performed at 2–3 weeks of age with minor effects at 5 weeks of age. The effects disappear when castration is performed at 14–15 weeks of age (Steinberg *et al.*, 1979).

This strict relationship between modifications of immune responses and age of operation shows that the physiological functions progressively acquired by endocrine glands during their ontogenetic maturation may have a different and even opposite effect on the development of immunological response.

This observation would suggest that differentiation steps may be reached by an orderly sequence of events, receptor development included, but that the further maturation of the system requires other factor(s) which are defective, or have been removed, in these experimental models.

The immune system, besides being subjected to neuroendocrine influences for its development, is also involved in the ontogenetic maturation of the neuroendocrine network.

The main models to study the influence of the immune system on the neuroendocrine system have utilized animals deprived of important immune organs such as the thymus or the bursa of Fabricius. Athymic nude mice and neonatally thymectomized mice display a profoundly disturbed neuroendocrine system revealed by altered hypophyseal synthesis and/or release of GH and prolactin or luteotropic hormone, hypofunctioning of thyroid and sexual glands, and hyperproduction of corticosteroids (Pierpaoli *et al.*, 1971; Pierpaoli and Besedovsky, 1975). These defects could be largely corrected by thymus implantation (Besedovsky and Sorkin, 1974). The timing of thymus removal is very important for the development of endocrine imbalances. This is demonstrated by the fact that neonatal thymectomy in mice consistently results in developmental arrest of the ovary when performed at 3 days of age. Ovarian dysgenesia is not observed when the mice are thymectomized at 7 days or later (Nishizuka and Sakakura, 1969; Michael *et al.*, 1980).

Bursectomy in chick embryos after 68 hr of embryonic life causes the appearance, at 17 days of development and at hatching, of reduced levels of corticosteroid and increased production of testosterone. Bursal grafting is able to prevent these endocrine alterations (Pedernera *et al.*, 1980).

Animals maintained in germfree conditions, and, therefore, deprived of normal antigenic stimulation during early life, show insufficiency of thyroid, adrenal, and testicular function (Miyakawa and Ukai, 1970; Nomura *et al.*, 1973). Similarly, the prolongation of the stage of immunologic immaturity through sequential inoculation of mice with different allogeneic cells during the neonatal and perinatal period can induce alteration and retardation in the maturation of the endocrine system (Pierpaoli *et al.*, 1977).

Taken together, the findings reported to date on the reciprocal influence of the neuroendocrine and immune systems clearly indicate that such interactions do exist and may condition in positive or negative ways the maturation of the two systems.

5.2. Neuroendocrine–Immune Interactions during Aging

Since it has been demonstrated that modifications induced by experimental manipulation of the thymus (and of the immune system) alter the neuroendocrine system and vice versa, it may also be expected that the physiological decline with advancing age of either the immune or the neuroendocrine system may be in part responsible for the alterations observed in the other partner.

As a matter of fact, regrowth of an old thymus with recovery of its endocrine activity was observed when the thymus was implanted into young syngeneic recipients, thus confirming that the "old" microenvironment cannot support thymic function (Bach and Beaurain, 1979). Following this observation, experiments have obtained similar results by various endocrine manipulations. Thus, it has been demonstrated that regrowth of the thymus, with recovery of the plasma level of zinc–thymulin, may be achieved in old animals by treatment with thyroid hormones (Fabris *et al.*, 1982), with GH (Davila *et al.*, 1987; Goff *et al.*, 1987), with analogues of LH-RH (Greenstein *et al.*, 1987; Marchetti *et al.*, 1991), and, more recently, with either melatonin or intrathymic graft of young pineal (Mocchegiani *et al.*, 1994b).

Interestingly, similar thymic "rejuvenation" was obtained in mice by treatment with arginine (Fabris *et al.*, 1986b) which has a secretagogue activity on pituitary GH, and with zinc salts (Fabris *et al.*, 1991) which certainly may have a direct action on the thymus, but are also capable of acting on the pituitary–thyroid axis (Licastro *et al.*, 1992).

In humans, very few trials have been done, but, at least, with regard to thymic endocrine activity, both arginine (Fabris et al., 1986b; Mocchegiani *et al.*, 1990c) and zinc (Travaglini et al., 1989) are effective in old age. On the other hand, the capacity of thyroid hormones and of GH to restore thymic function in old age is further supported by the clinical observation that hyperthyroidism in old humans is associated with thymic enlargement (Simpson *et al.*, 1975) and that both hyperthyroidism and acromegaly in old subjects are associated with high circulating plasma levels of thymic hormones, comparable to those recorded in young normal individuals (Fabris *et al.*, 1986a; Travaglini *et al.*, 1990, 1992).

The major deductions from these findings are that age-related thymic involution is not an irreversible process, and that functional recovery can be achieved even in old age.

Further, reconstitution of thymic efficiency in old mice greatly influences neuroendocrine functions.

In mice, with advancing age, there are modifications of the plasma level of some hormones, such as increased insulin and decreased T_3 level and reduction of the adaptive reaction to β-adrenergic stimuli (Piantanelli et al., 1978). This latter change is probably due to a decreased density of β-adrenoceptors on cell membranes of various tissues, including the submandibular gland and some parts of the brain (Piantanelli *et al.*, 1985; Rossolini *et al.*, 1992). All of these deficits are fully restored in old animals by neonatal thymus grafts. Furthermore, a neonatal thymus graft can also correct the increased polyploidy present in aged liver cells (Pieri *et al.*, 1980).

The majority of the neuroendocrine changes demonstrated in these studies are strictly age-dependent, i.e., they display a linear progression starting early in life. Their interconnection with the thymus, which shows a quite similar age-dependent progressive deterioration, does not seem, therefore, to be merely coincidental.

Focusing on the "strategic" circuit reported in Fig. 1A, there does not seem to be any single intrinsic and critical event with advancing age to account for the progressive deterioration of the neuroendocrine-thymus functions in old age.

Quite similar considerations apply to the emergency circuit. In the case of neurohormonal modulation of peripheral immune functions, some, although not exhaustive, data suggest that the age-related deterioration of T-cell and NK-cell functions do not represent irreversible processes, but rather defects that can be corrected *in vivo* and in some cases even *in vitro* by appropriate hormonal treatments (Table II).

Thus, it has been demonstrated that lymphocyte proliferation may be enhanced by treatments with GH (Davila *et al.*, 1987), TSH (Provinciali *et al.* 1992), thyroid hormones (Fabris *et al.*, 1982), enkephalins (Jankovic and Maric, 1991), melatonin (Pierpaoli and Regelson, 1994; Mocchegiani *et al.*, 1994b), arginine (Fabris *et al.*, 1986b; Mocchegiani *et al.*, 1990a), and zinc salts (Fabris *et al.*, 1991). With regard to NK activity, GH (Davila *et al.*, 1987; Crist *et al.*, 1987), endorphins (Solomon *et al.*, 1988) and melatonin (Bulian *et al.*, 1994) are able to increase basal NK activity, whereas treatments with TSH increase only IL-2-induced NK cytotoxicity and with T_3 IFN-boosted NK activity (Provinciali and Fabris, 1990, 1991).

Do leukocyte-derived immunotransmitters play a role in the age-related deterioration of some neuroendocrine functions? This might be deduced from the known effects of some interleukins on hypothalamic and pituitary functions (Besedovsky and del Rey, 1992; McCann *et al.*, 1993), but to our knowledge, no investigations have been carried out to answer this question.

The findings discussed above clearly demonstrate that at least some age-related alterations of the neuroendocrine and immune networks are not intrinsic "per se" and irreversible, and that the seat of age-related deterioration cannot easily be assigned to one or another homeostatic apparatus.

TABLE II
Recovery of Immune Effectiveness by Neurohormonal or Nutritional Treatments in Old Age

Treatment	Species	Target	References
GH	Rat	Lymphocyte proliferation	Davila *et al.* (1987)
	Rat	Basal NK activity	Davila *et al.* (1987)
	Human	Basal NK activity	Crist *et al.* (1987)
Analogues of LH-RH	Rat	Thymocyte proliferation	Marchetti *et al.* (1991)
TSH	Mouse	Lymphocyte proliferation	Provinciali *et al.* (1992)
	Human, mouse	IL-2-induced NK activity	Provinciali *et al.* (1990)
T_3/T_4	Human, mouse	IFN-induced NK activity	Provinciali *et al.* (1991)
T_4	Mouse	Lymphocyte proliferation	Fabris *et al.* (1982)
β-Endorphin	Human	Basal NK activity	Solomon *et al.* (1988)
Enkephalins	Mouse	Lymphocyte proliferation	Jankovic and Maric (1991)
Melatonin	Mouse	Delayed hypersensitivity	Pierpaoli and Regelson (1994)
	Mouse	Lymphocyte proliferation	Mocchegiani *et al.* (1994)
	Mouse	Basal NK activity	Bulian *et al.* (1993)
Arginine	Human, mouse	Lymphocyte proliferation	Mocchegiani *et al.* (1990)
Zinc salts	Mouse	Lymphocyte proliferation	Fabris *et al.* (1991)

These considerations suggest that we need to revise, at a theoretical level, both the "nervous–neuroendocrine" (Everitt and Burgess, 1976; Frolkis, 1982; Meites *et al.*, 1986) and the "immune" hypotheses of aging (Walford, 1969; Burnet, 1970), especially the assumption that there is a genetically determined hierarchy among the three homeostatic systems of the body and that the deterioration of one of them, according to each single theory, is a primary, intrinsic, and irreversible event. If this were true, the age-associated alterations of the other systems would necessarily follow. As an alternative to both the "neuroendocrine" and the "immune" theories of aging, we hypothesize that, due to the continuous interactions existing among the nervous, neuroendocrine, and immune systems during the entire life of the organism, it is the disruption of such interactions in old age which is responsible for most of the age-associated dysfunctions (Fabris, 1991).

The deterioration of neuroendocrine-immune interactions with aging, in addition to depending on age-related alterations at the level of one of the homeostatic systems involved, might also depend on modifications of some basic mechanisms capable of influencing all of the homeostatic systems. A putative factor in this context is zinc metabolism (Fabris *et al.*, 1991), since it has been demonstrated that zinc is required for the functional efficiency of the nervous, neuroendocrine, and immune systems (Fabris *et al.*, 1991; Licastro *et al.*, 1992; Fabris, 1994). These findings, together with the observations that (1) zinc turnover is altered with advancing age both in humans and in other animals and (2) that zinc supplementation in old age is able to restore thymic function, restore various immune deficiencies, and also can correct some age-related hormonal defects (Fabris *et al.*, 1991), suggest a crucial role for zinc in neuroendocrine–immune interactions during aging.

ACKNOWLEDGMENTS. I thank my colleagues Eugenio Mocchegiani and Mauro Provinciali for fruitful discussions and suggestions. Thanks are given to Isabella Cappanera, Clara Chesi and Marzio Marcellini for technical assistance.

REFERENCES

Abraham, A. D., and Bug, G., 1976, ^{3}H-testosterone distribution and binding in rat thymus cells in vivo, *Mol. Cell. Biochem.* **13:**157.

Akahoshi, T., Oppenheim, J. J., and Matsushima, K. J., 1988, Induction of high-affinity interleukin 1 receptors on human peripheral blood lymphocytes by glucocorticoid hormone, *J. Exp. Med.* **167:**924.

Andrews, P., Shortman, K., Scollay, R., Potworowski, E. F., Kruisbeek, A. M., Goldstein, G., Trainin, N., and Bach, J. F., 1985, Thymus hormones do not induce proliferative ability or cytolytic function in PNA + cortical thymocytes, *Cell. Immunol.* **91:**455.

Araujo, D. M., Lapchak, P. A., Collier, B., and Quiron, R. M., 1989, Localization of interleukin-2 receptors in the rat brain: interaction with the cholinergic system, *Brain Res.* **498:**257.

Arrenbrecht, S., 1974, Specific binding of growth hormone to thymocytes, *Nature* **252:**255.

Bach, J. F., Dardenne, M., Pleau, J. M., and Bach, A. M., 1975, Isolation, biochemical characteristic and biological activity of a circulating thymic hormone in the mouse and in the human, *Ann. N.Y. Acad. Sci.* **249:**186.

Bach, M. A., and Beaurain, G., 1979, Respective influence of extrinsic and intrinsic factors on the age-related decrease of thymic secretion, *J. Immunol.* **122:**2505.

Ban, E., Haour, F., and Lenstra, R., 1992, Brain interleukin-1 gene expression induced by peripheral lipopolysaccharides administration, *Cytokines* **4(10):**48.

Band, L. C., Pert, A., and Williams, W., 1992, Central μ-opioid receptors mediate suppression of natural killer activity in vivo, *Prog. NeuroEndocrine Immunol.* **5(2):**95.

Banks, W. A., and Kastin, A. J., 1993, Measurement of transport of cytokines across the blood–brain barrier, in: *Neurobiology of Cytokines—A Volume of Methods in Neurosciences* (E. B. De Souza, ed.), Academic Press, London, in press.

Bauer, J., Lengyel, G., Bauer, T. M., Acs, G., and Gerok, W., 1989, Regulation of interleukin-6 receptor expression in human monocytes and hepatocytes, *FEBS Lett.* **249:**27.

Bayer, B. M., Daussin, S., Hernandez, M., and Irvin, L., 1990, Morphine inhibition of lymphocyte activity is mediated by an opioid dependent mechanism, *Neuropharmacology* **29:**369.

Berczi, I., and Kovacs, K., eds., 1987, *Hormones and Immunity*, MTP Press, Lancaster.

Berkenbosch, F., van Oers, J., del Rey, A., Tilders, F., and Besedovsky, H., 1987, Corticotropin-releasing factor producing neurons in the rat activated by interleukin-1, *Science* **238:**524.

Bermudez, L. E., Wu, M., and Young, L. S., 1990, Effect of stress-related hormones on macrophage receptors and response to tumor necrosis factor, *Lymphokine Res.* **9:**137.

Bernton, E. W., 1989, Prolactin and immune host defenses, *Prog. NeuroEndocrine Immunol.* **2(1):**21.

Bernton, E. W., Beach, J. E., Holaday, J. W., Smallridge, R., and Fein, H. G., 1987, Release of multiple hormones by a direct action of interleukin 1 on pituitary cells, *Science* **238:**519.

Besedovsky, H. O., and del Rey, A., 1990, Metabolic and endocrine actions of interleukin-1. Effects on insuln-resistant animals, *Ann. N.Y. Acad. Sci.* **594:**214.

Besedovsky, H. O., and del Rey, A., 1992, Immune-neuroendocrine circuits: Integrative role of cytokines, in: *Frontiers in Neuro-endocrinology*, Volume 13(1), Raven Press, New York, pp. 61–94.

Besedovsky, H. O., and Sorkin, E., 1974, Thymus involvement in female sexual maturation, *Nature* **249:**356.

Besedovsky, H. O., Sorkin, E., and Keller, M., 1975, Changes in blood hormone levels during the immune response, *Proc. Soc. Exp. Biol. Med.* **150:**466.

Besedovsky, H. O., del Rey, A., and Sorkin, E., 1985, Changes in plasma hormone profile after tumor transplantation into syngeneic and allogeneic rats, *Int. J. Cancer* **36:**209.

Besedovsky, H. O., del Rey, A., Sorkin, E., and Dinarello, C. A., 1986, Immunoregulatory feedback between interleukin-1 and glucocorticoid hormones, *Science* **233:**652.

Besedovsky, H., del Rey, A., Klusman, I., Furukawa, H., Monge-Arditi, G., and Kabiersch, A., 1991, Cytokines as modulators of hypothalamo-pituitary-adrenal axis, *J. Steroid Biochem. Mol. Biol.* **40(4–6):**613.

Beutler, B., Milsark, I.W., and Cerami, A. C., 1985, Cachectin tumor necrosis factor: Production, distribution and metabolic fate in vivo, *J. Immunol.* **135:**3972.

Beutler, B., Krochin, N., Milsark, I. W., Luedke, C., and Cerami, A., 1986, Control of cachectin (tumor necrosis factor) synthesis: Mechanisms of endotoxin resistance, *Science* **232:**977.

Billingham, R. E., Krohn, P. L., and Medawar, P. B., 1951, The effect of cortisone on the survival of skin homografts in the rabbit, *Br. Med. J.* **2:**1049.

Blalock, J. E., 1984, The immune system as a sensory organ, *J. Immunol.* **132:**1067.

Blalock, J. E., 1988, Production of neuroendocrine peptide hormones by the immune system, in: Progress in Allergy, Volume 43 (J. E. Blalock and K. L. Bost, eds.), Karger, Basel, pp. 1–13.

Blalock, J. E., ed., 1992, Neuroimmunoendocrinology, Volume 52, Karger, Basel.

Blatteis, C. M., 1990, Neuromodulative actions of cytokines, *Yale J. Biol. Med.* **63:**133.

Bonomo, A., and Matzinger, P., 1993, Thymus epithelium induces tissue-specific tolerance, *J. Exp. Med.* **177:**1153.

Bourne, H. R., Lichtenstein, L. M., Melmon, K. L., Henney, C. S., Weinstein, Y., and Shearer, G. M., 1974, Modulation of inflammation regulates many leukocyte functions, *Science* **184:**19.

Brouard, A., Pelaprat, D., Dana, C., Vial, M., Lhiaubet, A.M., and Rostene, W., 1992, Mesencephalic dopaminergic neurons in primary cultures express functional neurotensin receptors, *J. Neurosci.* **12:**1409.

Brunda, J. M., Taranelli, D., Holden, H. T., and Varesio, L., 1979, Suppression of in vitro maintenance and interferon-mediated augmentation of natural killer cell activity by adherent peritoneal cells from normal mice, *J. Immunol.* **130:**1974.

Bryant, H. U., and Roudebush, R. E., 1990, Suppressive effects of morphine pellet implants on in vivo parameters of immune function, *J. Pharmacol. Exp. Ther.* **255:**410.

Bryant, H. U., Bernton, E. W., and Holaday, J. W., 1988, Morphine pellet-induced immunomodulation in mice: Temporal relationships, *J. Pharmacol. Exp. Ther.* **245:**913.

Bryant, H. U., Bernton, E. W., and Holaday, J. W., 1990, Immunomodulatory effects of chronic morphine treatment: Pharmacologic and mechanistic studies, *Res. Monogr.* **96:**131.

Bulian, D., Provinciali, M., Di Stefano, G., Tibaldi, A., Pierpaoli, W., and Fabris, N., 1993, Recovery of NK cell activity by melatonin treatment in old mice, *II° Int. Congress ISNIM*. Paestum, Italy Sept. 1993, p. 203 (abstract).

Bulloch, K., 1987, The innervation of immune system tissues and organs, in: *The Neuro-immune-endocrine Connection* (C.W. Cotman, R. E. Brinton, A. Galaburda, B. McEwen, and D. M. Schneider, eds.), Raven Press, New York, pp. 33–47.

Bulloch, K., Hausman, J., Radojcic, T., and Short, S., 1991, Calcitonin gene related peptide in the developing and aging thymus: an immunocytochemical study, *Ann. N.Y. Acad. Sci.* **621:**218.

Burnet, F. M., 1970, Immunological Surveillance, Pergamon Press, Elmsford, NY.

Cake, M. H., and Litwack, G., 1975, The glucocorticoid receptors, in: *Biochemical Actions of Hormones*, Volume 3 (G. Litwack, ed.), Academic Press, New York, pp. 317–390.

Carlson, S. L., Felten, D. L., Livnat, S., and Felten, S. Y., 1987, Alterations of monoamines in specific central autonomic nuclei following immunization in mice, *Brain Behav. Immun.* **1:**52.

Carlson, S. L., Brooks, W. H., Roszman, T. L., 1991, Neurotransmitter–lymphocyte interaction: Dual receptor modulation of lymphocyte proliferation and cAMP production, *J. Neuroimmunol.* **24**:155.

Carr, D. J. J., 1992, Neuroendocrine peptide receptors on cells of the immune system, in: *Neuroimmuno-endocrinology*, Volume 52 (E. Blalock, ed.) Karger, Basel, pp. 84–96.

Ceredig, R., Lowenthal, J. W., Nahholz, M., and MacDonald, H. R., 1985, Expression of interleukin-2 receptors as a differentiation marker on intrathymic stem cells, *Nature* **314:**98.

Champion, S., Imhof, B. A., Savagner, P., and Thiery, J. P., 1986, The embryonic thymus produces chemotactic peptides involved in the homing of hemopoietic precursors, *Cell* **44:**781.

Chen, S. S., Tung, J. S., Gillis, S., Good, R. A., and Hadden, J. W., 1983, Changes in surface antigens of immature thymocytes under the influence of interleukin 2 and thymic factors, *Proc. Natl. Acad. Sci. USA* **80:**5980.

Claman, H. N., 1975, How corticosteroids work, *J. Allergy Clin. Immunol.* **55:**145.

Coceani, F., Lees, J., and Dinarello, C. A., 1988, Occurrence of interleukin-1 in cerebrospinal fluid of the conscious cat, *Brain Res.* **446:**245.

Coffey, R. G., and Hadden, J. W., 1985, Neurotransmitters, hormones, and cyclic nucleotides in lymphocyte regulation, FASEB **263:**9063.

Cooper, E. L., ed., 1984, *Stress, Immunity and Aging*, Dekker, New York.

Cornell, R. P., 1989, Central interleukin 1-elicited hyperinsulinemia is mediated by prostaglandins but not autonomics, *Am. J. Physiol.* **257:**R839.

Cotman, C. W., Brinton, R. E., Galaburda, A. B., McEwen, B., and Schneider, D. M., eds., 1988, *The Neuro-immune Endocrine Connection*, Raven Press, New York.

Coto, J. A., Hadden, E. M., Sauro, M., Zorn, N., and Hadden, J. W., 1992, Interleukin 1 regulates secretion of zinc-thymulin by human thymic epithelial cells and its action on T lymphocyte proliferation and nuclear protein kinase C, *Proc. Natl. Acad. Sci. USA* **89:**7752.

Crist, D. M., Peale, G. T., Mackinnon, L. T., Sibbitt, W. L., and Kraner, J. C., 1987, Exogenous growth hormone treatment alters body composition and increases natural killer cell activity in women with impaired endogenous growth hormone secretion, *Metabolism* **36:**115.

Cunningham, E. T., Wada, E., Carter, D. B., Tracey, D. E., Battey, J. F., and De Souza, E. B., 1992, In situ histochemical localization of type I interleukin-1 receptor messenger RNA in the central nervous system, pituitary and adrenal gland of the mouse, *J. Neurosci.* **12(3):**11001.

Daily, M. O., Shreurs, J., and Schulman, H., 1988, Hormone receptors on cloned T lymphocytes. Increased responsiveness to histamine, prostaglandins and beta-adrenergic agents as a late stage in T cell activation, *J. Immunol.* **140:**2931.

Darbon, J. M., Oury, F., Laredo, J., and Bayard, F., 1989, Tumor necrosis factor-alpha inhibits follicle stimulating hormone-induced differentiation in cultured rat granulosa cells, *Biochem. Biophys. Res. Commun.* **163:**1038.

Dardenne, M., and Savino, W., 1992, Neuroendocrine circuits controlling the physiology of the thymic epithelium, *Ann. N.Y. Acad. Sci.* **650:**85.

Dardenne, M., Pleau, J. M., Nabama, B., Lefancier, P., Denien, M., Choay, J., and Bach, J. F., 1982, Contribution of zinc and other metals to the biological activity of the serum thymic factor, *Proc. Natl. Acad. Sci. USA* **79:**5370.

Dardenne, M., Itoh, T., and Homo-Delaroche, F., 1986, Presence of glucocorticoid receptors in cultured thymic epithelial cells, *Cell Immunol.* **100:**112.

Dardenne, M., Savino, W., Gagnerault, M. C., Itoh, T., and Bach, J. F., 1989, Neuroendocrine control of thymic hormonal production. I. Prolactin stimulates in vivo and in vitro the production of thymulin by human and murine thymic epithelial cells, *Endocrinol.* **125:**3.

Dardenne, M., Kelly, P. A., Bach, J. F., and Savino, W., 1991, Identification and functional activity of prolactin receptors in thymic epithelial cells, *Proc. Natl. Acad. Sci. USA* **88:**9700.

Davila, D. R, Brief, S., Simon, J., Hammer, R. E., Brinster, R. L., and Kelly, K. W., 1987, Role of growth hormone in regulating T-dependent immune events in aged, nude and transgenic rodents, *J. Neurosci. Res.* **18:**108.

Daynes, R. A., and Araneo, B. A., 1989, Contrasting effects of glucocorticoids on the capacity of T cells to produce the growth factors interleukin 2 and interleukin 4, *Eur. J. Immunol.* **19:**2319.

del Rey, A., and Besedovsky, H. O., 1987, Interleukin-1 affects glucose homeostasis, *Am. J. Physiol.* **253**:R794.

del Rey, A., and Besedovsky, H. O., 1989, Antidiabetic effects of interleukin-1, *Proc. Natl. Acad. Sci. USA* **86**:5943.

Deschaux, P., Massengo, B., and Fontanges, R., 1979, Endocrine interaction of the thymus with the hypophysis, adrenals and testes: Effect of two thymic extracts, *Thymus* **1**:95.

Dinari, G., Ashkenazi, S., Marcus, H., Rosenbach, Y., and Zahavi, I., 1989, The effect of opiates on the intestinal immune response to cholera toxin in mice, *Digestion* **44**:14.

Dougherty, T. F., Berliner, M. L., Schneebeli, G. L., and Berliner, D. L., 1964, Hormonal control of lymphatic structure and function, *Ann N.Y. Acad. Sci.* **113**:825.

Dubuis, J. M., Dayer, J. M., Siegrist-Kaiser, C. A., and Burger, A. G., 1988, Human recombinant interleukin-1 beta decreases thyroid hormone and thyroid stimulating hormone levels in rats, *Endocrinology* **123**:2175.

Dunn, A. J., Powell, M. L., Moreshead, W. V., Gaskin, J. M., and Hall, N. R., 1987, Effect of Newcastle disease virus administration to mice on the metabolism of cerebral monoamines, plasma corticosterone and lymphocyte proliferation, *Brain Behav. Immun.* **1**:216.

Ebaugh, M. J., and Smith, E. M., 1987, Human lymphocyte production of immunoreactive luteinizing hormone, *Fed. Proc.,* **46**:7811.

Everitt, A. V., and Burgess, J. A., eds., 1976, *Hypothalamus Pituitary and Aging*, Thomas, Springfield, IL.

Fabris, N., 1973, Immunodepression in thyroid-deprived animals, *Clin. Exp. Immunol.* **15**:601.

Fabris, N., 1977, Hormones and aging, in: *Immunology and Aging* (T. Makinodan and E. Yunis, eds.), Plenum Medical, New York, pp. 73–89.

Fabris, N., 1981a, Body homeostatic mechanism and aging of the immune system, in: *Immunology and Aging* (M. M. B. Kay and T. Makinodan, eds.), CRC Press, Boca Raton, FL, pp. 61–78.

Fabris, N., 1981b, Ontogenetic and phylogenetic aspects of neuroendocrine–immune network, *Dev. Comp. Immunol.* **5**:49.

Fabris, N., 1991, Neuroendocrine–immune interactions: A theoretical approach to aging, *Arch. Gerontol. Geriatr.* **12**:219.

Fabris, N., 1992, Biomarkers of aging in the neuroendocrine–immune domain. Time for a new theory of aging? *Ann. N.Y. Acad. Sci.* **663**:335.

Fabris, N., 1993, Neuroendocrine/thymus interactions during development and aging, in: *Hormones and Immunity. Bilateral Communication between the Endocrine and Immune Systems* (C. Grossman, ed.), Springer-Verlag, Berlin, pp. 265–299.

Fabris, N., 1994, Neuroendocrine–immune aging: The role of zinc and an integrative view, *Ann. N.Y. Acad. Sci.*, **719**:353–368.

Fabris, N., and Mocchegiani, E., 1985, Endocrine control of thymic serum factor production in young-adult and old mice, *Cell. Immunol.* **91**:325.

Fabris, N., and Mocchegiani, E., 1994, Immunomodulating role of growth hormone, in: *Growth Hormone II: Basic and Clinical Aspects* (B. B. Bercu and R. R. Walker, eds.), Springer-Verlag, Berlin, pp. 116–130.

Fabris, N., and Piantanelli, L., 1982, Thymus–neuroendocrine interactions during development and aging, in: *Endocrine and Neuroendocrine Mechanism of Aging* (R. C. Adelman and G. S. Roth, eds.), CRC Press, Boca Raton, FL, pp. 186–195.

Fabris, N., and Provinciali M., 1989, Hormones, in: *Natural Immunity* (D. Nelson, ed.), Academic Press, New York, pp. 306–347.

Fabris, N., Pierpaoli W., and Sorkin, E., 1972, Lymphocytes, hormones and ageing, *Nature* **240**:557.

Fabris, N., Muzzioli, M., and Mocchegiani, E., 1982, Recovery of age-dependent immunological deterioration in BALB/c mice by short term treatment with L-thyroxine, *Mech. Age. Dev.* **18**:327.

Fabris, N., Mocchegiani, E., Muzzioli, M., and Imberti, R., 1983, Thymus-neuroendocrine network, in: *Immunoregulation* (N. Fabris, E. Garaci, J. Hadden, and N. A Mitchison, eds.), Plenum Press, New York, pp. 341–362.

Fabris, N., Mocchegiani, E., Amadio, L., Zannotti, M., Licastro, F., and Franceschi, C., 1984, Thymic hormone deficiency in normal aging and Down's syndrome: Is there a primary failure of the thymus? *Lancet* **1**:983.

Fabris, N., Mocchegiani, E., Mariotti, S., Pacini, F., and Pinchera, A., 1986a, Thyroid function modulates thymus endocrine activity, *J. Clin. Endocrinol. Metab.* **62**:474.

Fabris, N., Mocchegiani, E., Muzzioli, M., and Piloni, S., 1986b, Recovery of yage related decline of thymic endocrine activity and PHA response by lysine-arginine combination, *Int. J. Immunopharmacol.* **8**:677.

Fabris, N., Mocchegiani, E., Mariotti, S., Caramia, G., Bracilli, T., Pacini, F., and Pinchera, A., 1987, Thymulin deficiency and low 3, 5, 3′-triiodothyronine syndrome in infants with low birth weight syndromes, *J. Clin. Endocrinol. Metab.* **65**:247.

Fabris, N., Mocchegiani, E., Muzzioli, M., and Provinciali, M., 1988, Neuroendocrine-thymus interactions: Perspectives for intervention in aging, *Ann. N.Y. Acad. Sci.* **521**:72.

Fabris, N., Mocchegiani, E., Muzzioli, M., and Provinciali, M., 1991, Role of zinc in neuroendocrine-immune interactions during aging, *Ann. N.Y. Acad. Sci.* **621**:314.

Fabris, N., Jankovic, B. D., Markovic, B., and Spector, N. H., eds., 1992, *Ontogenetic and Phylogenetic Mechanisms of Neuroimmunomodulation from Molecular Biology to Psychosocial Sciences*, Ann. N.Y. Acad. Sci. **650**.

Feldman, R. D., Hunninghake, G. W., and McArdle, W. L., 1987, Beta-adrenergic-receptor-mediated suppression of interleukin 2 receptors in human lymphocytes, *J. Immunol.* **139**:3355

Felten, S. Y., and Felten, D. L., 1991, Innervation of lymphoid tissue, in: *Psychoneuroimmunology* (R. Ader, D.L. Felten, and N. Cohen, eds.), Academic Press, New York, p. 27.

Fontana, A., Weber, E., and Dayer, J. M., 1984, Synthesis of interleukin l/endogenous pyrogen in the brain of endotoxin-treated mice: A step in fever induction, *J. Immunol.* **133**:1696.

Frohman, E., Frohman, T., Vayuvegula, B., Gupta, S., and van den Noort, S., 1988, Vasoactive intestinal polypeptide inhibits the expression of the MHC class II antigens on astrocytres, *J. Neurol. Sci.* **88**:339.

Frolkis, V. V., 1982, *Aging and Life Prolonging Process*, Springer-Verlag, Berlin.

Fujii, T., Sato, K., and Ozawa, M., 1989, Effect of interleukin-1 (IL-1) on thyroid hormone metabolism in mice: Stimulation by IL-1 of iodothyronine 5′-deiodinating activity (type 1) in the liver, *Endocrinology* **124**:167.

Gaillard, R. C., Turnill, D., Sappino, P., and Muller, A. F., 1990, Tumor necrosis factor alpha inhibits the hormonal response of the pituitary gland to hypothalamic releasing factors, *Endocrinology* **127**:101.

Geenen, V., Legros, J. J., Franchimont, P., Baudrihaye, M., Defrense, M. P., and Boniver, J., 1986, The neuroendocrine thymus: Coexistence of oxytocin and neurophysin in the human thymus, *Science* **232**:508.

Geenen, V., Defrense, M. P., Robert, F., Legros, J. J., Franchimont, P., and Boniver, J., 1988, Immunocytochemical evidence that thymic nurse cells are neuroendocrine cells, *Neuroendocrinology* **47**:365.

Geenen, V., Cormann-Goffin, N., Martens, H., Vandersmissen, E., Robert, F., Benhida, A., Legros, J. J., Martial, J., and Franchimont, P., 1993, Thymic neurohypophysial-related peptides and T cell selection, *Regul. Peptides* **45**:273.

Gerli, R., Rambotti, P., Nicoletti, I., Orlandi, S., Migliorati, G., and Riccardi, C., 1986, Reduced number of natural killer cells in patients with pathological hyperprolactinenia, *Clin. Exp. Immunol.* **64**:399.

Gibson, A., Ginsberg, M., Hall, M., and Hart, S. L., 1979, The effects of opiate receptor agonist and antagonist on the stress-induced secretion of corticosterone in mice, *Br. J. Pharmacol.* **65**:139.

Gillette, S., and Gillette, R., 1979, Changes in thymic estrogen receptor expression following orchidectomy, *Cell. Immunol.* **42**:194.

Gillis, S., Crabtree, G. R., and Smith, K. A., 1979, Glucocorticoid-induced inhibition of T-cell growth factor production. I. The effect on mitogen induced lymphocyte proliferation, *J. Immunol.* **123**:1624.

Giulian, D., and Lachman, L. B., 1985, Interleukin-1 stimulates astroglial proliferation after brain injury, *Science* **228**:497.

Giulian, D., Baker, T. J., Shih, L. N., and Lachman, L. B., 1986, Interleukin 1 of the central nervous system is produced by ameboid microglia, *J. Exp. Med.* **164**:594.

Glick, B., 1964, The bursa of Fabricius and the development of immunologic competence, in: *The Thymus in Immunobiology* (R. A. Good and A. E. Gabrielson, eds.), Harper & Row (Hoeber), New York, pp. 343–360.

Goff, B. L., Roth, J. A., Arp, L. H., and Incefy, G. S., 1987, Growth hormone treatment stimulates thymulin production in aged dogs, *Clin. Exp. Immunol.* **65:**580.

Goldstein, A. L., ed., 1984, *Thymic Hormones and Lymphokines*, Plenum Press, New York.

Goldstein, A. L., Low, T. L. K., McAdoo, M., McClure, J., Thurman, G. B., Lay, C. Y., Chang, D., Wang, S. S., Harvey, C., Ramel, A. N., and Meinhofer, J., 1977, Thymosin. I. Isolation and sequence analysis of an immunologically active thymic polypeptide, *Proc. Natl. Acad. Sci. USA* **74:**711.

Goldstein, G., Scheid, M., Hammertring, U., Bose, E. A., Schlesinger, D. H., and Niall, H. D., 1976, Isolation of a polypeptide that has lymphocyte-differentiating properties and is probably represented universally in living cells, *Proc. Natl. Acad. Sci. USA* **72:**11.

Gonzalves, M. L., Milanes, M. V., and Vargas, M. L., 1991, Effects of acute and chronic administration of μ- and δ-opioid agonists on the hypothalamic–pituitary–adrenocortical (HPA) axis in the rat, *Eur. J. Pharmacol* **200:**155.

Gottschall, P. E., Katsuura, G., and Arimura, A., 1989, Interleukin-1 beta is more potent than interleukin-1 alpha in suppressing follicle-stimulating hormone-induced differentiation of ovarian granulosa cells, *Biochem. Biophys. Res. Commun.* **163:**764.

Greenstein, B. D., Fitzpatrick, F. T., Kendall, M. D., and Wheeler, M. J., 1987, Regeneration of the thymus in old male rats treated with a stable analogue of LHRH, *J. Endocrinol.* **112:**345.

Guillemin, R., Cohn, M., and Melnechuk, T., eds., 1985, *Neural Modulation of Immunity*, Raven Press, New York.

Hadden, J. W., 1983, Cyclic nucleotides and related mechanism in immune regulation: a mini review, in: *Immunoregulation* (N. Fabris, E. Garaci, J. Hadden, and N.A. Mitchison, eds.), Plenum Press, New York, pp. 201–230.

Hadden, J. W., 1992, Thymic endocrinology, *Int. J. Immunopharmacol.* **14:**345–352.

Hadden, J. W., 1993, Immunostimulants, *Immunol. Today* **14(6):**275.

Hadden, J. W., Hadden, E. M., and Middleton, E., Jr., 1970, Lymphocyte blast transformation. I. Demonstration of adrenergic receptors in human peripheral lymphocytes, *J. Cell. Immunol.* **1:**583–595.

Hadden, J. W., Coffey, R. G., and Spreafico, F., 1977, *Immunopharmacology*, Volume 3, Plenum Press, New York.

Hadden, J. W., Specter, S., Galy, A., Touraine, J. L., and Hadden, E. M., 1987, Thymic hormones, interleukins, endotoxin and thymomimetic drugs, in: *Immunopharmacology III* (L. Chedid, J. Hadden, F. Spreafico, P. Dukor, and D. Willoughby, eds.), Pergamon Press, Elmsford, NY, pp. 487–492.

Hadden, J. W., Galy, A., Chen, H., Wang, Y., and Hadden, E. M., 1989, The hormonal regulation of thymus and T lymphocyte development and function, in: *Interactions among CNS, Neuroendocrine and Immune Systems* (J. W. Hadden, K. Masek, and G. Nisticò, eds.), Pythagora Press, Rome, pp. 126–135.

Hall, N. R. S., O'Grady, M. P., and Farah, J. M., Jr., 1989, Activation of the hypothalamic-pituitary-adrenal axis by thymic peptides, in: *Interactions among CNS, Neuroendocrine and Immune Systems* (J. W. Hadden, K. Masek, and G. Nisticò, eds.), Pythagora Press, Rome, pp. 114–125.

Hart, R., Dancygier, H., Wagner, F., Niedrmeyer, H., and Classen, M., 1988, Substance P. modulates lymphokine activities in supernatants of cultured human duodenal biopsies, *Immunol. Lett.* **119**:133–136

Hazum, E., Chang, K. J., and Cuatrecasas, P., 1979, Specific nonopiate receptors for betaendorphins, *Science* **205:**1303.

Hejinen, C. J., Kavelaars, A., and Ballieux, R. E., 1991, Beta-endorphin: Cytokine and neuropeptide, *Immunol. Rev.* **119:**41.

Helderman, J. H., and Strom, T., 1978, Specific insulin binding site on T and B lymphocytes as a marker of cell activation, *Nature* **274:**62.

Henney, C. S., Kuribayashi, K., Kern, D. E., and Gillis, S., 1981, Interleukin-2 augments natural killer cell activity, *Nature* **291:**335.

Herberman, R. B., Ortaldo, J. R., and Bonnard, G. D., 1979, Augmentation by interferon of human natural and antibody-dependent cell-mediated cytotoxicity, *Nature* **227**:221.

Hienstand, P. C., Mekler, P., Nordmann, R., Grieder, A., and Permmongkol, C., 1986, Prolactin as a modulator of lymphocyte responsiveness provides a possible mechanism of action for cyclosporine, *Proc. Natl. Acad. Sci. USA* **83**:335.

Hiltz, M. E., Catania, A., and Lipton, J. M., 1992, α-MSH peptides inhibit acute inflammation induced in mice by rIL-1, rIL-6, rTNF-α and endogenous pyrogen but not that caused by LTB4, PAF and rIL-8, *Cytokine* **4**:320.

Hochman, P. S., Cudkowicz, G., and Dausset, J., 1978, Decline of natural killer cell activity in sublethally irradiated mice, *J. Natl. Cancer Inst.* **61**:265.

Hollenberg, M. D., and Cuatrecasas, P., 1974, Hormone receptors and membrane glycoproteins during in vitro transformation of lymphocytes, in: *Control of Proliferation of Animal Cells* (B. Clarkson and R. Baserga, eds.), Cold Spring Harbor Press, Cold Spring Harbor, NY, pp. 423–434.

Holsboer, F., Stalla, G. K., von Bardeleben, U., Hamman, K., Muller, H., and Muller, O. A., 1988, Acute adrenocortical stimulation by recombinant gamma interferon in human controls, *Life Sci.* **42**:1.

Jankovic, B. D., and Maric, D., 1991, Enkephalin-induced stimulation of humoral and cellular immune reactions in aged rats, *Ann. N.Y. Acad. Sci.* **621**:135.

Jasmine, G., and Cantin, M., eds., 1991, *Stress Revised, Methods Exp. Pathol.*, Volume 14, Karger, Basel.

Johnson, H. M., Farrar, W. L., and Torres, B. A., 1985, Regulation of lymphokine production by arginine vasopressin and cytokines: Modulation of lymphocyte function by neurohypophyseal hormones, *J. Immunol.* **129**:983.

Kalland, T., 1986, Generation of natural killer cells from bone marrow precursors in vitro, *Immunology* **57**:493.

Kalland, T., Strand, O., and Forsberg, J. G., 1979, Long-term effects of neonatal estrogen treatment on mitogen responsiveness of mouse spleen lymphocytes, *J. Natl. Cancer Inst.* **63**:413.

Kamegai, M., Niijima, K., Kunishita, T., Nishizawa, M., Ogawa, M., Araki, M., Ueki, A., Konishi, Y., and Tabira, T., 1990, Interleukin 3 as a trophic factor for central cholinergic neurons in vitro and in vivo, *Neuron* **2**:429.

Kasson, B., and Gorospe, W., 1989, Effects of interleukins 1, 2 and 3 on follicle-stimulating hormone-induced differentiation of rat granulosa cells, *Mol. Cell. Endocrinol.* **62**:103.

Katsura, G., Gottschall, P. E., Dahl, R. R., and Arimura, A., 1988, Adrenocorticotropin release induced by intracerebroventricular injection of recombinant human interleukin-1 in rats: Possible involvement of prostaglandin, *Endocrinology* **122**:1773.

Katz, P., Zaytovn, A. M., and Lee, J. H., Jr., 1985, Characterisation of corticosteroid receptors in natural killer cells: Comparison with circulating lymphoid cells, *Cell. Immunol.* **94**:347.

Kelso, A., and Munck, A., 1984, Glucocorticoid inhibition of lymphokine secretion by alloreactive T lymphocyte clones, *J. Immunol.* **133**:784.

Koff, W. C., Fann, A. V., Dunegan, M. A., and Lachman, L. B., 1986, Catecholamine-induced suppression of interleukin-1 production, *Lymphokine Res.* **5**:239.

Koo, G. B., and Manyak, C. L., 1986, Generation of cytotoxic cells from murine bone marrow by human recombinant IL-2, *J. Immunol.* **137**:1751.

Krog-Rasmussen, A., Bech, K., and Feldt-Rasmussen, U., 1988, Interleukin-1 affects the function of cultured human thyroid cells, *Allergy* **43**:435.

Kruisbeek, A. M., 1979, Thymic factors and T cell maturation in vitro: A comparison of the effects of thymic cultures with thymic extracts and thymus dependent serum factors, *Thymus* **1**:163.

Kurtz, D. T., and Feigelson, P., 1978, Multihormonal control of the messengers RNA for the hepatic protein alpha-2-macroglobulin, in: *Biochemical Actions of Hormones*, Volume 5 (G. Litwack, ed.), Academic Press, New York, pp. 433–455.

Landmann, R. M. A., Bittinger, H., and Buhler, F. R., 1981, High affinity beta-2-adrenergic receptors in mononuclear leucocytes: Similar density in young and old normal subjects, *Life Sci.* **29**:1761.

Landmann, R. M. A., Wesp, M., Box, R., Keller, U., and Buhler, F. R., 1989, Distribution and function of beta-adrenergic receptors in human blood lymphocytes, in: *Interactions among CNS, Neuroendocrine and Immune Systems* (J. W. Hadden, K. Masek, and G. Nisticò, eds.), Pythagora Press, Rome, pp. 251–264.

Lechan, R. M., Toni, R., Clark, B. D., Cannon, J. G., Shaw, A. R., and Dinarello, C. A., 1990, Immunoreactive interleukin-1-beta localization in the rat forebrain, *Brain Res.* **514:**135.

Lewis, J. W., Shavit, Y., Terman, G. W., Nelson, L. R., Martin, F. C., Gale, R. P., and Liebeskind, J. C., 1983, Stress and morphine affect survival of rats challenged with a mammary ascites tumor (MAT 13762B), *Nat. Immun. Cell Growth Regul.* **3:**43.

Lewis, J. W., Shavit, Y., Terman, G. W., Nelson, L. R., Martin, F. C., Gale, R. P., and Liebeskind, J. C., 1985, Involvement of opioid peptides in the analgesic, immunosuppressive and tumor-enhancing effects of stress, *Psychopharmacol. Bull.* **21:**479.

Licastro, F., Mocchegiani, E., Zannotti, M., and Fabris, N., 1992, Zinc affects the metabolism of thyroid hormones in children with Down's syndrome: Normalization of thyroid stimulating hormone and reversal of triiodothyronine plasmic levels by dietary zinc supplementation. Evaluation of clinical impact, *Int. J. Neurosci.* **65:**259.

Locke, S., Ader, R., Besedovsky, H., Hall, N., Solomon, G., and Strom, T., eds., 1985, *Foundations of Psychoneuroimmunology*, Aldine, New York.

Lockwood, D. H., Turkington, R. W., and Topper, Y. J., 1966, Hormone-dependent development of milk protein synthesis in mammary gland in vitro, *Biochim. Biophys. Acta* **130:**493.

Lopez-Gonzales, M. A., Calvo, J. R., Osuna, C., and Guerrero, J. M., 1992, Interaction of melatonin with human lymphocytes: Evidences for binding sites coupled to potentiation of cyclic AMP stimulated by vasoactive intestinal peptide and activation of cyclic GMP production, *J. Pineal Res.* **12:**97.

Lotz, M., Vaughan, J. H., Carson, D. A., and Effect, D. A., 1988, Effect of neuropeptides on the production of inflammatory cytokines by human monocytes, *Science* **241:**1218.

McCann, S. M., Milenkovic, L., Gonzales, M. C., Lyson, K., Karanth, S., and Rettori, V., 1993, Endocrine aspects of neuroimmunomodulation: Methods and overview, in: *Neurobiology of Cytokines—A Volume of Methods in Neurosciences* (E. B. De Souza, ed.), Academic Press, London, pp. 187.

Maestroni, G. J., 1993, The immunoneuroendocrine role of melatonin, *J. Pineal Res.* **14:**1.

Marchetti, B., Morale, M. C., Batticane, N., Gallo, F., Farinelli, Z., and Cioni, M., 1991, Aging of the reproductive–neuroimmune axis, *Ann. N.Y. Acad. Sci.* **621:**159.

Matera, L., Muccioli, G., Casano, A., Bellussi, G., and Genazzani, E., 1988, Prolactin receptors on large granular lymphocytes: Dual regulation by cyclosporin A, *Brain Behav. Immun.* **2:**1.

Mathews, P. M., Froelich, C. J., Sibbitt, W. R., Jr., and Bankhurst, A.D., 1983, Enhancement of natural cytotoxicity by beta-endorphin, *J. Immunol.* **130:**1658.

Mealy, K., Robinson, B., Millette, C.F., Majazoub, J., and Wilmore, D.W., 1990, The testicular effects of tumor necrosis factor, *Ann. Surg.* **211:**470.

Meites, J., Goya, R., and Takahashi, S., 1986, Why the neuroendocrine system is important in aging processes. A review, *Exp. Gerontol.* **22:**1.

Michael, S. D., Taguchi, O., and Nishizuka, Y., 1980, Effect of neonatal thymectomy on ovarian development and plasma LH, FSH, GH and PRL in the mouse, *Biol. Reprod.* **22:**343.

Milenkovic, L., Rettori, V., Snyder, G.D., Beutler, B., and McCann, S.M., 1989, Cachectin alters anterior pituitary hormone release by a direct action in vitro, *Proc. Natl. Acad. Sci. USA* **86:**2418.

Milenkovic, L., Lyson, K., Aguila, M. C., and McCann, S. M., 1992, Effect of thymosin alpha-1 on hypothalamic hormone release, *Neuroendocrinology* **56:**674.

Miyakawa, M., and Ukai, M., 1970, Adrenal gland functions in germfree animals, *Jpn. J. Clin. Med.* **28:**2178.

Mocchegiani, E., Boemi, M., Fumelli, P., and Fabris, N., 1989, Zinc-dependent low thymic hormone level in type I diabetes, *Diabetes* **38(7):**932.

Mocchegiani, E., Paolucci, P., Balsamo, A., Cacciari, E., and Fabris, N., 1990a, Influence of growth hormone on thymic endocrine activity in humans, *Horm. Res.* **33:**248.

Mocchegiani, E., Amadio, L., and Fabris, N., 1990b, Neuroendocrine–thymus interactions. I. In vitro modulation of thymic factor secretion by thyroid hormones, *J. Endocrinol. Invest.* **13:**139.

Mocchegiani, E., Cacciatore, L., Talarico, M., Lingetti, M., and Fabris, N., 1990c, Recovery of low thymic hormone levels in cancer patients by lysine–arginine combination, *Int. J. Immunopharmacol.* **12(4):**365.

Mocchegiani, E., Fabris, N., Travaglini, P., Sartorio, A., and De Min, C., 1991, Thymic endocrine activity in children with idiopathic growth-hormone deficiency, *Inter. J. Neurosci.* **59:**151.

Mocchegiani, E., Bulian, D., Santarelli, L., Tibaldi, A., Pierpaoli, W., and Fabris, N., 1994a, Zinc–melatonin interrelationship: A work hypothesis, *Ann. N.Y. Acad. Sci.*, **719**:298–307.

Mocchegiani, E., Bulian, D., Santarelli, L., Muzzioli, M., Tibaldi, A., Pierpaoli, W., and Fabris, N., 1994b, Immuno-enhancing effect of melatonin in old mice may be mediated by zinc turnover, *J. Neuroimmunol.*, **53**:189–201.

Mocchegiani, E., Imberti, R., Testasecca, D., Zandri, M., Santarelli, L., and Fabris, N., 1995, Thyroid and thymic endocrine function and survival in severely traumatised patients with or without head injury, *Intensive Care Med.*, **21**:334–341.

Molitar, T. W., Morilla, A., Risdal, J. M., Murtaugh, M. P., Chao, C. C., and Peterson, P. K., 1992, Chronic morphine administration impairs cell-mediated immune responses in swine, *J. Pharmacol. Exp. Ther.* **260:**581.

Morimoto, A., Murakami, N., Nakamori, T., Sukata, Y., and Watanabe, T., 1986, Possible involvement of PGE in development of ACTH response induced by human recombinant interleukin-1, *J. Physiol. (London)* **411:**245.

Mukherjee, P., Mastro, A. M., and Hymer, W. C., 1990, Prolactin induction of interleukin-2 receptors on rat splenic lymphocytes, *Endocrinology* **126:**88.

Muscettola, M., and Grasso, G., 1990, Somatostatin and vasoactive intestinal peptide reduce interferon gamma production by human peripheral blood mononuclear cells, *Immunobiology* **180:**419.

Naitoh, Y., Fukata, J., and Tominaga, T., 1988, Interleukin-6 stimulates the secretion of adrenocorticotropic hormone in conscious, freely-moving rats, *Biochem. Biophys. Res. Commun.* **155:**1459–1463.

Nemeroff, C. B., 1986, The interaction of neurotensin with dopaminergic pathways in the central nervous system: Basic neurobiology and implications for the pathogenesis and treatment of schizophrenia, *Psychoneuroendocrinology* **11:**15.

Nicollete, L., Gerli, R., Orlandi, S., Migliorati, G., Rambotti, P., and Riccardi, C., 1989, Defective natural killer cell activity in puerperal hyperprolactinemia, *J. Reprod Immunol.* **15:**113.

Nishizuka, Y., and Sakakura, T., 1969, Thymus and reproduction: Sex-linked dysgenesis of the gonad after neonatal thymectomy in mice, *Science* **166:**753.

Nomura, T., Ohsawa, N., Kageyama, K., Saito, M., and Tajima, Y., 1973, Testicular functions of germfree mice, in: *Germfree Research* (J. B. Heneghan, ed.), Academic Press, New York, pp. 515–528.

Normann, S., Besedovsky, H. O., Schardt, M., and del Rey, A., 1988, Hormonal changes following tumor transplantation and the relationship of corticosterone to tumor induced anti-inflammation, *Int. J. Cancer* **41:**850.

O'Dorisio, M. S., and Panerai, A., eds., 1990, Neuropeptides and immunopeptides: Messengers in a neuroimmune axis, *Ann N.Y. Acad Sci.* **594**.

Panerai, A., 1993, Lymphocytes as a source of hormones and peptides, *J. Endocrinol. Invest.* **16:**549.

Pang, X. P., Hershman, J. M., Mirell, C. J., and Pekary, A. E., 1989, Impairment of hypothalamic–pituitary–thyroid function in rats treated with human recombinant tumor necrosis factor-alpha (cachectin), Endocrinology **125:**76.

Payan, D., Brewster, D., Missirian-Bastian, A., and Goetzl, E., 1984, Substance P: Recognition by a subset of human T lymphocytes, *J. Clin Invest.* **74:**1532.

Pedernera, E. A., Romano, M., Besedovsky, H. O., and Aguilar, M., 1980, The bursa of Fabricius is required for normal endocrine development in chicken, *Gen. Comp. Endocrinol.* **42:**413.

Piantanelli, L., Basso, A., Muzzioli, M., and Fabris, N., 1978, Thymus-dependent reversibility of physiological and isoproterenol-evoked age-related parameters in athymic nude and old normal mice, *Mech. Ageing Dev.* **7:**171.

Piantanelli, L., Gentile, S., Fattoretti, P., and Viticchi, C., 1985, Thymic regulation of brain cortex beta-adrenoceptors during development and aging, *Arch. Gerontol. Geriatr.* **4:**179.

Pieri, C., Giuli, C., Del Moro, M., and Piantanelli, L., 1980, Electron microscopic morphometric analysis of mouse liver II. Effect of aging and thymus transplantation in old animals, *Mech. Ageing Dev.* **13**:275.

Pierpaoli, W., and Besedovsky, H. O., 1975, Role of the thymus in programming of neuroendocrine function, *Clin. Exp. Immunol.* **20**:325.

Pierpaoli, W., and Regelson, W., 1994, Pineal control of aging: Effect of melatonin and pineal grafting on aging mice, *Proc. Natl. Acad. Sci. USA*, **91**:787–791.

Pierpaoli, W., Fabris, N., and Sorkin, E., 1970, Developmental hormones and immunological maturation, in: *Hormones and the Immune Response* (G. E. W. Wolstenholme and J. Knight, eds.), Churchill Ciba Study Group No. 36, London, pp. 126–143.

Pierpaoli, W., Bianchi, E., and Sorkin, E., 1971, Modification of the growth-hormone producing cells in the hypophysis of neonatally thymectomized mice, *Clin. Exp. Immunol.* **9**:889.

Pierpaoli, W., Kopp, H. G., and Bianchi, E., 1976, Interdependence of thymic and neuroendocrine functions in ontogeny, *Clin. Exp. Immunol.* **24**:501.

Pierpaoli, W., Kopp, H. G., Muller, J., and Keller, M., 1977, Interdependence between neuroendocrine programming and the generation of immune recognition in ontogeny, *Cell. Immunol.* **29**:16.

Provinciali, M., and Fabris, N., 1990, Role of pituitary–thyroid–axis on basal and lymphokine induced NK cell activity in aging, *Int. J. Neurosci.* **51**:273.

Provinciali, M., and Fabris, N., 1991, Models and mechanisms of neuroendocrine–immune interactions during ontogeny, *Adv. Neuroimmunol.* **1**:124.

Provinciali, M., Muzzioli, M., and Fabris, N., 1989, Timing of appearance/ disappearance of IFN and IL-2 induced natural cytotoxicity during ontogenetic development and aging, *Exp. Gerontol.* **24**:227.

Provinciali, M., Di Stefano, G., Raffaeli, W., Pari, G., Desiderio, F., and Fabris, N., 1991a, Evaluation of NK and LAK cell activities in neoplastic patients during treatment with morphine, *Int. J. Neurosci.* **59**:127.

Provinciali, M., Di Stefano, G., Bressani, N., and Fabris, N., 1991b, Sequential activation of hormone/ cytokines in the differentiation of NK cells, *J. Chemother.* **3**:81.

Provinciali, M., Di Stefano, G., and Fabris, N., 1992, Improvement of proliferative capacity of murine spleen lymphocytes by thyrotropin, *Int. J. Immunopharmacol.* **14**:865.

Ranson, J., Fischer, M., Mercer, L., and Zlotnik, A., 1987, Lymphokine-mediated induction of antigen-presenting ability in thymic stromal cell, *J. Immunol.* **139**:2620.

Raulet, D. H., 1985, Expression and function of interleukin-2 receptors on immature thymocytes, *Nature* **314**:101.

Rebar, R. W., 1984, Effects of thymic peptides on hypothalamic–pituitary function, in: *Thymic Hormones and Lymphokines* (A. L. Goldstein, ed.), Plenum Press, New York, pp. 325–334.

Rebar, R. W., Miyake, A., Low, T. L. K., and Goldstein, A. L., 1981, Thymosin stimulates secretion of luteinising hormone releasing factor, *Science* **214**:669.

Reiter, R. J., ed., 1990, *Advances in Pineal Research*, John Libbey, London.

Rettori, V., Milenkovic, L., Beutler, B. A., and McCann, S. M., 1989, Hypothalamic action of cachectin to alter pituitary hormone release, *Brain Res. Bull.* **23**:471.

Rhodes, J., Ivanyi, J., and Cozens, P., 1986, Antigen presentation by human monocytes: Effects of modifying major histocompatibility complex class II antigen expression and interleukin 1 production by using recombinant interferons and corticoids, *Eur. J. Immunol.* **16**:370.

Richman, D. P., and Arnason, B. G., 1979, Nicotinic acetylcholine receptor: Evidence for a functionally distinct receptor on human lymphocytes, *Proc. Natl. Acad. Sci. USA* **76**:4632.

Rivier, C., and Vale, W., 1990, Cytokines act within the brain to inhibit luteinizing hormone secretion and ovulation in the rat, *Endocrinology* **127**:849.

Robert, F., and Geenen, V., 1992, Thymic neuropeptides and T-lymphocyte development, *Ann. N.Y. Acad. Sci.* **650**:99.

Roby, K. F., and Terranova, P. F., 1988, Tumor necrosis factor alters follicular steroidogenesis in vitro, *Endocrinology* **123**:2952.

Rossolini, G., Basso, A., Piantanelli, L., Tacconi, R., Amici, D., and Gianfranceschi, G. L., 1992,

Neuroendocrine thymus and beta-adrenergic responsiveness in aging mice, *Arch. Gerontol. Geriatr.* **3**:311.

Roth, J. A., Roth, J. A., Lamax, L. G., Alszuler, N., Hampshire, J., Laeberle, M. L., Shelton, M., Draper, D. D., and Ledet, A. A. E., 1980, Thymic abnormalities and growth hormone deficiency in dogs, *Am. J. Vet. Res.* **41**:1256.

Roth, J. A., Roth, J. A., Laeberle, M. L., Grier, D. L., Hopper, J. G., Spiegel, H. E., and Macallister, H.A., 1984, Improvement in clinical condition and thymus morphological features associated with growth treatment of immuno-deficient dwarf-dogs, *Am. J. Vet. Res.* **45**:1151.

Rothwell, N. J., and Dantzer, R. S., eds., 1992, *Interleukin in the Brain*, Pergamon Press, Elmsford, NY.

Roubinian, J. R., Tala, N., Greenspan, J. S., Goodman, J. R., and Siiteri, P. K., 1978, Effect of castration and sex hormone treatment on survival, antinucleic acid antibodies, and glomerulonephritis in NZB/NZW F1 mice, *J. Exp. Med.* **147**:1568.

Rouse, R. V., Ewijk, W., Van-Joes, P. P., and Weissman, I. L., 1974, Expression of MHC antigens by mouse dendritic cells, *J. Immunol.* **122**:2508.

Russell, D. H., Matrision, L., Kibler, R., Larson, D., Poulps, B., and Magun, B., 1984, Prolactin receptors on human lymphocytes and their modulation by cyclosporin, *Biochem. Biophys. Res. Commun.* **121**:899.

Salaun, J. C., Bandeira, A., Khazaai, I., Calman, F., Caltey, M., Coutinho, A., and Le Douarin, N. M., 1990, Thymic epithelium tolerizes for histocompatibility antigens, *Science* **247**:1471.

Saphier, D., Abramsky, O., Mor, G., and Ovadia, H., 1987, Multiunit electrical activity in conscious rats during an immune response, *Brain Behav. Immun.* **1**:40.

Sapolsky, R. M., Rivier, C., Yamamoto, G., Plotsky, P. M., and Vale, W., 1987, Interleukin-1 stimulates the secretion of hypothalamic corticotropin-releasing factor, *Science* **238**:522.

Sato, K., Satoh, T., and Shizume, K., 1990, Inhibition of ^{125}I organification and thyroid hormone release by interleukin-1, tumor necrosis factor-alpha, and interferon-gamma in human thyrocytes in suspension culture, *J. Clin. Endocrinol. Metab.* **70**:1735.

Savino, W., and Dardenne, M., 1984, Thymic hormone-containig cells. IV. Immunohistologic evidence for the simultaneous presence of thymulin, thymopentin and thymosin a-1 in normal and pathological human thymuses, *Eur. J. Immunol.* **14**:987.

Schettini, G., Florio, T., and Meucci, O., 1990, Interleukin-1-beta modulation of prolactin secretion from rat anterior pituitary cells: Involvement of adenylate cyclase activity and calcium mobilization, *Endocrinology* **126**:1435.

Schimpff, R. M., Lhiaubet, A. M., Vial, M., and Rostene, W., 1992, Blood peripheral human leukocytes; a possible source for plasma levels of neurotensin, *Progr. NeuroEndocrine Immunol.* **5(2)**:126.

Sharp, B. M., Matta, S. G., Peterson, P. K., Newton, R., Chao, C., and McAllen, K., 1989, Tumor necrosis factor-alpha is a potent ACTH secretagogue: Comparison to interleukin-1 beta, *Endocrinology* **124**:3131.

Shavit, Y., Lewis, J. W., Terman, G. W., Gale, R. P., and Liebeskind, J.C., 1984, Opioid peptides mediate the suppressive effect of stress on natural killer cell cytotoxicity, *Science* **223**:188.

Shen, L., Guyre, P., Ball, E., and Fanger, M., 1986, Glucocorticoid enhances gamma interferon effects on human monocyte antigen expression and ADCC, *Clin Exp. Immunol.* **65**:387.

Sibinga, N. E. S., and Goldstein, A., 1988, Opioid peptides and opioid receptors in cells of the immune system, *Annu. Rev. Immunol.* **6**:219.

Simpson, J. C., Gray, E. S., Michie, W., and Beck, J. S., 1975, The influence of preoperative drug treatment on the extent of hyperplasia of the thymus in primary thyrotoxicosis, *Clin. Exp. Immunol.* **22**:249.

Singh, U., Millson, D. S., Smith, P. A., and Owen, J. J. T., 1979, Identification of beta-adrenoceptors during thymocyte ontogeny in mice, *Eur. J. Immunol.* **9**:31.

Smith, E. M., 1992, Hormonal activities of cytokines, in: *Neuroimmunoendocrinology* (J. E. Blalock, ed.), Volume 52, Karger, Basel, pp.154–169.

Smith, E. M., Mai Phan, Kruger, T. E., Coppenhaver, D. H., and Blalock, E., 1983, Human lymphocyte production of immunoreactive thyrotropin, *Proc. Natl. Acad. Sci. USA* **80**:6010.

Smith, E. M., Morrill, A. C., Meyer, W. J., III, and Blalock, E., 1986, Corticotropin releasing factor induction of leukocyte-derived immunoreactive ACTH and endorphins, *Nature* **321:**881.

Snyder, D. S., and Unanue, E. R., 1982, Corticosteroids inhibit murine macrophage Ia expression and interleukin-1 production, *J. Immunol.* **129:**1803.

Sobharwal, P., Zwilling, B., Glaser, R., and Malarkey, W. B., 1992, Cellular immunity in patients with acromegaly and prolactinomas, *Prog NeuroEndocrine Immunol.* **5(2):**120.

Solomon, G. F., Fiatarone, M. A., Benton, D., Morley, J. E., Bloom, E., and Makinodan, T., 1988, Psychoimmunologic and endorphin function in the aged, *Ann N.Y. Acad. Sci.* **521:**43.

Spangelo, B. L., and MacLeod, R. M., 1990, Regulation of the acute phase response and neuroendocrine function by interleukine 6, *Prog. NeuroEndocrine Immunol.* **3:**167.

Spangelo, B. L., Judd, A. M., Ross, P. C., Login, I. S., Jarvis, W. D., Badamchian, M. Goldstein, A. L., and MacLeod, R. M., 1987, Thymosin fraction 5 stimulates prolactin and growth hormone release from anterior pituitary cells in vitro, *Endocrinology* **121:**2035.

Spangelo, B. L., Judd, A. M., MacLeod, R. M., Goodman, D. W., and Isakson, P. C., 1990, Endotoxin-induced release of interleukin-6 from rat medial basal hypothalamus, *Endocrinology* **127:**1779.

Spengler, R. N., Allen, R. M., Remick, D. G., Strieter, R. M., and Kunkel, S. L., 1990, Stimulation of alpha-adrenergic receptor augments the production of macrophage-derived tumor necrosis factor, *J. Immunol.* **145:**1430.

Stanisz, A., Scicchitano, R., Payan, D., and Bienenstock, J., 1987, In vitro studies of immunoregulation by substance P and somatostatin, *Ann. N.Y. Acad. Sci.* **496:**217.

Steinberg, A. D., Melez, K. A., Raveche, E. S., Reeves, J. P., Boegel, W. A., Smathers, P. A., Taurog, J. D., Weinlein, L., and Duvic, M., 1979, Approach to the study of the role of sex hormones in autoimmunity, *Arthritis Rheum.* **22:**1170.

Stitt, J. T., 1986, Prostaglandin E as a neural mediator of the febrile response, *Yale J. Biol. Med.* **59:**137.

Stitt, J.T., 1990, Passage of immunomodulators across the blood–brain barrier, *Yale J. Biol. Med.* **63:**121.

Strom, T. B., Sytkowski, A. J., Carpenter, C. B., and Merrill, J. P., 1974, Cholinergic augmentation of lymphocyte-mediated cytotoxicity. A study of the cholinergic receptor of cytotoxic T lymphocytes, *Proc. Natl. Acad. Sci. USA* **71:**1330.

Strom, T. B., Lane, M. A., and George, K., 1981, The parallel, time-dependent, bimodal change in lymphocyte cholinergic binding activity and cholinergic influence upon lymphocyte-mediated cytotoxicity after lymphocyte activation, *J. Immunol.* **127:**705.

Tata, J. R., 1984, The action of growth and developmental hormones, in: *Biological Regulation and Development*, Volume 3B (R. F. Goldberg and K. R. Yamamoto, eds.), Plenum Press, New York, pp. 1–58.

Timsit, J., Savino, W., Safieh, B., Chanson, P., Gagnerault, M. C., Bach, J. F., and Dardenne, M., 1992, Growth hormone and insulin-like growth factor-I stimulate hormonal function and proliferation of thymic epithelial cells, *J. Clin. Endocrinol. Metab.* **75:**183.

Topper, Y. J., 1970, Multiple hormone interactions in the development of mammary gland in vitro, *Recent Prog. Horm. Res.* **26:**287.

Tracey, K. J., Beutler, B., and Lowry, S. F., 1986, Shock and tissue injury induced by recombinant human cachectin, *Science* **234:**470.

Trainin, N., Rotter, V., Yakir, Y., and Leve, R., 1979, Biochemical and biological properties of THF in animal and human models, *Ann. N.Y. Acad. Sci.* **332:**9.

Travaglini, P., Moriondo, P., Togni, E., Venegoni, P., Bochicchio, D., Conti, A., Faglia, G., Ambroso, G., Ponticelli, C., Mocchegiani, E., and Fabris, N., 1989, Effect of oral zinc administration on prolactin and thymulin circulating levels in patients with chronic renal failure, *J. Clin. Endocrinol. Metab.* **68:**186.

Travaglini, P., Mocchegiani E., Togni, E., Muratori, M., Re, T., Bassani, N., and Fabris, N., 1990, Thymulin and zinc circulating level in patient with GH and PRL secreting pituitary adenomas, *Int. J. Neurosci.* **51:**269.

Travaglini, P., Mocchegiani, E., De Min, C., Re, T., and Fabris, N., 1992, Modifications of thymulin titers in patients affected with prolonged low or high zinc circulating levels are independent of patients'age, *Arch. Gerontol. Geriatr.* Suppl 3:349.

Tubaro, E., Borelli, G., Croce, C., Cavallo, G., and Santiangeli, C., 1983, Effect of morphine on resistance to infection, *J. Infect. Dis.* **148:**656.

Turkington, R. W., 1972, Multiple hormonal interactions. The mammary gland, in: *Biochemical Action of Hormones*, Volume 2 (G. Litwack, ed.), Academic Press, New York, pp. 55–80.

Vankezecom, H., Carmeliet, P., and Heremans, H., 1990, Interferon-gamma inhibits stimulated adrenocorticotropin, prolactin, and growth hormone secretion in normal rat anterior pituitary cell cultures, *Endocrinology* **126:**2919.

Villa Verde, D. M. S., Defrense, M. P., Vannier dos Santos, M. A., Dussault, J. H., Boniver, J., and Savino, W., 1992, Identification of nuclear triiodothyronine receptors in the thymic epithelium, *Endocrinology* **131:**1313.

Wahl, S. M., Altman, L. C., and Rosenstreich D. L., 1975, Inhibition of in vitro lymphokine synthesis by glucocorticoids, *J. Immunol.* **115:**476.

Walford, R. L., 1969, *The Immunological Theory of Aging*, Munksgaard, Copenhagen.

Walton, P. E., and Cronin, M. J., 1989, Tumor necrosis factor-alpha inhibits growth hormone secretion from cultured anterior pituitary cells, *Endocrinology* **125:**925.

Watanabe, T., Hiltz, M. E., Catania, A., and Lipton, J. M., 1993, Inhibition of IL-1 induced peripheral inflammation by peripheral and central administration of analogs of the neuropeptide α-MSH, *Brain Res. Bull.* **32:**311.

Watson, R. R., and Nguyen, T. H., 1990, Suppression by morphine and ethanol of tumor cell cytotoxic activity released by macrophages from retrovirally infected mice upon in vitro stimulation by beta carotene, *Prog. Clin. Biol. Res.* **325:**79.

Webb, S., and Sprent, J., 1990, Tolerogenicity of thymic epithelium, *Eur. J. Immunol.* **20:**2525.

Weber, R. J., and Pert, A., 1989, The periaqueductal gray matter mediates opiate-induced immunosuppression, *Science* **245:**188.

Weber, R. J., Ikejiri, B., Rice, K. C., Pert, A., and Hagan, A., 1987, Opiate receptor mediated regulation of the immune response in vivo, *NIDA Res. Monogr.* **76:**341.

Weigent, D. A., Baxter, J. B., Wear, W. E., Smith, L. R., Bost, K. L., and Blalock, E., 1988, Production of immunoreactive growth hormone by mononuclear leukocytes, *FASEB J.* **2:**2812.

Werb, Z., Foley, R., and Munck, A., 1978, Interaction of glucocorticoids with macrophages. Identification of glucocorticoid receptors in monocytes and macrophages, *J. Exp. Med.* **147:**1684.

Wolstenholme, G. E. W., and Knight, J., eds., 1970, *Hormones and the Immune Response*, Churchill Ciba Foundation Study Group No. 36, London.

Wybran, J., 1985, Enkephalins and endorphins: Activation molecules for the immune system and natural killer activity? *Neuropeptides* **5:**371.

Wybran, J., Appelboom, T., Famey, J. P., and Govaerts, A., 1979, Suggestive evidence for morphine and methionine-enkephalin receptor-like structures on normal blood T lymphocytes, *J. Immunol.* **123:**1068.

Yamaguchi, M., Yoshimoto, Y., Komura, H., Koile, K., Matsuzaki, N., Hirota, K., Miyake, A., and Tanizawa, O., 1990, Interleukin 1 beta and tumor necrosis factor alpha stimulate the release of gonadotropin-releasing hormone and interleukin 6 by primary cultured rat hypothalamic cells, *Acta Endocrinol.* **123:**476.

Yamasjita, S., Kimura, H., and Ashizawa, K., 1989, Interleukin-1 inhibits thyrotropin-induced human thyroglobulin gene expression, *J. Endocrinol.* **122:**177.

Yoshiki, U., Miyawaki, T., and Seki, H., 1985, Differential effects of recombinant human interferon-gamma and interleukin-2 on natural killer cell activity of peripheral blood in early human development, *J. Immunol.* **135:**180.

Zakarija, M., Hornicek, F. J., Levis, S., and McKenzie, J. M., 1988, Effects of gamma-interferon and tumor necrosis factor alpha on thyroid cells: Induction of class II antigen and inhibition of growth stimulation, *Mol. Cell Endocrinol.* **58:**129.

CHAPTER 11

THYMIC ENDOCRINOLOGY AND PROSPECTS FOR TREATING THYMIC INVOLUTION

JOHN W. HADDEN

1. INTRODUCTION

In the early 1960s, the central role of the thymus in cellular immunity was simultaneously and independently discovered by R. A. Good and co-workers and J. F. A. P. Miller and co-workers (Good, 1991; Miller, 1991). The thymus has only recently been analyzed in a manner that allows an understanding, on the one hand, of the complicated and stepwise manner by which T cells mature and acquire the many surface receptors necessary for identifying antigen and the molecular and cellular world around them and, on the other hand, of the autocrine, paracrine, and endocrine influences that regulate their differentiation, proliferation, secretion, and cytotoxicity. It is the purpose of this review to focus on the endocrine thymus and to elaborate on those factors and mechanisms that contribute to thymic development and involution. The possibilities for therapeutic intervention to reverse thymic involution and induce new T-cell development for the treatment of secondary cellular immune deficiencies associated with diseases such as cancer, infection, and autoimmunity will be discussed.

While it is not possible at the present time to offer a completely integrated view of the thymus within the context of its neurological and endocrine framework, an attempt will be made to emphasize these aspects of thymic function. The reader is

JOHN W. HADDEN • Department of Internal Medicine, Division of Immunopharmacology, University of South Florida College of Medicine, Tampa, Florida 33612.

Immunopharmacology Reviews, Volume 2, edited by John W. Hadden and Andor Szentivanyi. Plenum Press, New York, 1996.

referred to the chapters by Szentivanyi *et al.* and Fabris in this volume for complementary views of the neuroendocrine immunology involved.

1.1. Normal Thymic Development

The thymus evolves in the mouse embryo from day 10 after gestation and just before and after birth there are three cycles of seeding of γd T cells to various sites including the skin, gut, and endocrine organs (Scollay *et al.*, 1986; Lobach and Haynes, 1987; Rothenberg, 1992). At birth, there is an ample thymus with αβ T cells but no αβ T cells are distributed to the periphery. Following the first week of life there is a distribution of αβ T cells to the various other lymphoid organs of the body, including spleen, gut, and other tissue-associated lymphoid systems. Eighty percent of circulating lymphocytes in the peripheral blood are T lymphocytes. These circulate out of the blood, into the tissues, to lymph nodes via the lymphatics and then reenter blood. T lymphocytes mediate a variety of functions related to the expression of immunity. Regulatory helper and suppressor activities are central to B-lymphocyte responses and antibody production. Clonal expansion is critical to mounting a cellular immune response (CMI). Cytokine production expands the process and incurs the involvement of a variety of other effector cell populations, particularly the monocyte-derived macrophage in delayed-type hypersensitivity (DTH). Finally, direct cytotoxicity is an important mechanism for eradicating pathogen-infected cells and tumor cells.

The thymus grows in proportion to body weight until puberty is reached. During this period of time, the organism is challenged by multiple environmental pathogens and develops long-lasting immunity. Thus, the peripheral lymphoid tissues become replete with memory cells capable of resisting a broad variety of pathogen challenges. At puberty, thymic involution occurs which is probably a result of increase in androgen and estrogen production as both can act to involute the thymus (Grossman, 1984, 1985). This involution is progressive and marked by midlife; however, it is not irreversible.

Following challenge as a result of depletion of lymphocytes through irradiation (e.g., Chernobyl) or as a result of intensive chemotherapy as occurs in the treatment of leukemia with bone marrow transplantation, the organ can revitalize and process new T cells. Similarly, experimental manipulations in the mouse with pituitary hormones as with GH3 transplants (Kelley *et al.*, 1986) demonstrate that normal thymic weight and morphology can be restored in involution caused by aging.

Presumably throughout life when new T lymphocytes are needed on a selective basis, the partially involuted thymus is capable of delivering them and when massive replacement is needed the organ can recover full function. Throughout adult life the thymus is thought to contribute an endocrine function mediated by one or more circulating hormones (Bach, 1983). These substances have been detected in the circulation by bioassay and decline in the fourth decade of life (Bach *et al.*, 1975;

Twomey *et al.*, 1977; Lewis *et al.*, 1978). These hormones are thought to regulate T-lymphocyte production and sensitivity to cytokines, particularly interleukin 2 (IL-2) (Hadden, 1992). Throughout the life of normal individuals, blood T-lymphocyte levels remain remarkably stable (approximately 1600/mm^3) so that these and other mechanisms yet to be defined are operant to maintain a stable and functional pool of T lymphocytes in the body.

1.2. Thymocyte Development

Normally, marker-negative precursor populations in bone marrow become sensitized, presumably through the action of circulating thymic hormones, to a program of development that involves initially traffic to the thymus. Such traffic to the thymus may involve chemotactic factors; at least one such factor has been isolated (Champion *et al.*, 1986). On arrival to the thymus, subcapsular intrathymic precursors are directly associated with thymic epithelial cells of neural crest origin containing a number of secretory peptides. Various growth-promoting factors act on these precursors including IL-2, IL-7, and stem cell growth factor (Ceredig *et al.*, 1985; Scollay, 1985; Mizutani *et al.*, 1987; Godfrey *et al.*, 1992). The resupply of immature T cells in the recovery from thymic involution proceeds from the subcapsular population of precursors and the forward flow of cells must be critically regulated by endocrine and/or neuronal means.

When early T cells enter the subcapsular area, they develop the pan T marker CD2 but are negative for CD4 and CD8 and are thus referred to as the double-negative population. This population then evolves into the large double-positive immature cortical population (85% of thymocytes). Subsets of this population can be delineated. In general, this is a cycling population and the vast majority of cells are destined for programmed cell death (apoptosis). In this phase, the genes for the T-cell antigen receptor (Tcr) and related proteins (CD3) are expressed, rearranged, and displayed on the surface of these cells as part of the maturation process. During this period both negative and positive selection are thought to occur. This population is highly sensitive to depletion caused by glucocorticoids and sex hormones and is the major population depleted as a result of either stress-induced or age-related involution. Presumably, in a way that is related to antigenic stimulation, positive selection of responsive populations leads to maturation which is associated with the conversion of double-positive cells to either single-positive CD4 or single-positive CD8 cell populations. These single-positive cells distribute either to the periphery directly or to the medulla and then to the periphery. The corticomedullary junction has been emphasized as the transitional point and the thymic stromal cells there regulate these events (Papiernik *et al.*, 1987; Papiernik, 1990). Supportive information derived from studies of growth hormone and prolactin focus on this as a restriction point of development sensitive to growth hormone/prolactin action (Russell, 1989; Murphy *et al.*, 1992). Although this may be a hormonally regulated step, it would appear that antigen is also crucial to this developmental process. Following antigen administration, newly mature T lymphocytes from thymus travel to nodes regional to the antigenic stimulation (Mojcik *et al.*, 1991; Hosseinzadeh and Goldschneider, 1993). These cells show thymocyte markers which disappear within a week. These thymic émigrés are thought to reflect antigen-activated T cells and thus indicate that the thymus is exposed to and processes antigen. Thus, antigen seems to be the critical issue in the positive selection of T lymphocytes at the cortical–medullary junction. It would seem important to know the impact of involution on the production of thymic émigrés.

The molecules that are extrinsic to the thymus and act to induce T-cell development are not well understood. In addition to antigen, it is likely that interleukins which derive from activation of leukocytes in the periphery play a role. A number of interleukins have been detected in the circulation under such circumstances. Many interleukins contribute to T-cell development. Central to the issue is the synergy observed between IL-1 and IL-2. IL-1 at low levels (i.e., noninflammatory levels of about 1 ng/ml) induces high-affinity IL-2 receptor expression (via induction of the α chain which with the β chain forms the high-affinity receptor) and contributes to the production of IL-2. IL-2 acting via these receptors induces T-cell cloning in the absence of antigen. We have emphasized this genetic program as key in the development of T lymphocytes (Hadden *et al.*, 1989b,d; Hadden, 1992) and presented evidence that cytokines, particularly IL-1 and IL-2, constitute signals from the periphery for T-cell renewal. Thymic peptides like thymosin α_1 and zinc thymulin influence this pathway (Serrate and Sztein, 1989; Coto *et al.*, 1992); other endocrine factors must also contribute (see Section 4 for further discussion).

2. THYMIC ENDOCRINOLOGY

The development of the thymus is dependent on the pituitary and thyroid glands but not on the gonads or adrenals (see Fabris, this volume). Steroids from both gonads and adrenals at sufficient levels can induce thymic involution through mass apoptosis of the double-positive population of immature cortical thymocytes. The upregulation by growth hormone/prolactin of thymic hormone would appear to be via the subcortical/medullary thymic epithelial cells (TEC).

The thymic stroma contains a variety of cell populations besides lymphocytes, the major of which are TEC. In addition, there are macrophages, dendritic cells, nurse cells, and Hassall's corpuscles. These latter populations are thought to be critical for antigen processing, negative and positive selection, and cleanup after apoptosis of immature cells. The TEC and particularly the subcortical/medullary population of TEC are the focus of the endocrine thymus since they produce in a regulated manner a number of cytokines and several thymic peptides (thymosin α_1 and zinc thymulin). Interestingly, these cells appear to be of neural crest origin and bind A2B5, an antibody that recognizes neural cells and other peptide-secreting endocrine cells (Haynes and Eisenbarth, 1983). The CNS influences discussed by Szentivanyi *et al.*

and Fabris in their chapters may well be reflected in significant part via these neural crest-derived cells (Bockman and Kirby, 1984).

2.1. Thymic Epithelial Cells

Studies of TEC in culture began in the late 1970s (Hensen *et al.*, 1978). Kruisbeek and Astaldi (1979) showed that thymic epithelial supernatants (TES) enhance the proliferation of immature PNA^+ (double positive) thymocytes in response to phytohemagglutinin (PHA). A number of investigators confirmed the observation of one or more mitogenic factors present in TES (Nieburgs *et al.*, 1984, 1987; Koninky *et al.*, 1984; Pfeifer *et al.*, 1986; Ogata *et al.*, 1987; Hadden *et al.*, 1989d; Kasai and Hirokawa, 1991; Schreiber *et al.*, 1991). Others implicated TES in thymocyte differentiation (Hadden *et al.*, 1989b; Kurtzberg *et al.*, 1989; Dalloul *et al.*, 1991) but the nature of the factors remained obscure.

TEC identification was advanced by the development of monoclonal antibodies to surface markers on TEC (Kampinga *et al.*, 1989). Such TEC identification showed different subtypes of TEC; subcapsular/medullary and cortical TEC form the two major classifications. It was known from histological observations that these cells differ in their morphology and their secretory products. The pattern that emerged from these studies showed that the medullary phenotype was similar to the subcapsular phenotype. Both of these populations secrete IL-1, IL-6, IL-8, G-, M-, and GM-CSF, and TGF-β, and contain and constitutively secrete thymosin α_1 and zinc thymulin. Cells of the cortical region produce IL-7 and IL-1 (Haynes and Eisenbarth, 1983; Kampinga *et al.*, 1989; Farr *et al.*, 1989; Gutierrez and Palacios, 1991; Ropke and Elbroend, 1992). Galy *et al.* (1993) described SV40-transformed clones (presumably cortical TEC) which produce IL-7, IL-6, GM-CSF, and TGF-β_1. In these cells, IL-1 induced GM-CSF and, to a lesser extent, IL-6. Most of the subsequent studies likely employed the subcapsular/medullary population of TEC.

TEC were found to bind to T lymphocytes to form rosettes (Singer *et al.*, 1986; Munoz-Blay *et al.*, 1987; Palmer *et al.*, 1991). It was found that $CD2^+$ thymocytes bind to LFA-3 on the TEC (Vollger *et al.*, 1987; Denning *et al.*, 1987a). Subsequently, it was shown that TEC bind activated thymocytes through LFA-1 on the T cell and ICAM-1 on the TEC (Singer *et al.*, 1990). Makgoba *et al.* (1989) have reviewed the significance of interactions of CD2:LFA-3 and ICAM-1:LFA-1 in other aspects of T-lymphocyte biology. Other novel adhesion ligands between TEC and thymocytes have been identified (Couture *et al.*, 1990; Giunta *et al.*, 1991; Utsumi *et al.*, 1991; Sawada *et al.*, 1992).

It was shown that when both mature and immature T cells bind TEC, they change their responsiveness. Denning *et al.* (1987b) observed enhanced PHA proliferative responses of mature thymocytes. Wiranowska *et al.* (1987) showed enhanced proliferation of prothymocytes with synergy on the further addition of IL-2. This observation was confirmed by Papiernik *et al.* (1987) and Denning *et al.* (1988). Further, coculture of TEC with prothymocytes resulted in the increased expression of the pan-

T marker Thy-1 (Wiranowska *et al.*, 1987; Brightman *et al.*, 1989) and other characteristics of maturation including TCR/CD3 complex expression (Palacios *et al.*, 1989; Savino *et al.*, 1989; Nagamine *et al.*, 1991; Muller and Kyewski, 1993; Tjonnfjord *et al.*, 1993; Takahama *et al.*, 1994).

The role of TEC–thymocyte interaction in positive and negative selection has been an issue of study and controversy (Sprent *et al.*, 1988; Nakashima *et al.*, 1990; Salaun *et al.*, 1990; Gutierrez and Palacios, 1991; MacDonald, 1992; Burkly *et al.*, 1993; Aguilar *et al.*, 1994; Degermann *et al.*, 1994; Hugo *et al.*, 1994). Review of these studies indicates that TEC are thought to play a role in positive selection while bone marrow-derived cells, macrophages, dendritic cells, and nurse cells are generally thought to mediate negative selection.

With the identification of growth factors for TEC in the late 1980s, a period of in-depth characterization of the endocrinology of TEC *in vitro* began (Nieburgs *et al.*, 1987; Galy *et al.*, 1989, 1990a,b; Eshel *et al.*, 1990; Schreiber *et al.*, 1991). Epidermal growth factor (EGF), IL-1, and β fibroblast growth factor (β-FGF) were found to be growth factors for these cells. Galy *et al.* (1989) showed that tumor necrosis factor α (TNF-α) and interferon γ (IFN-γ) potentiated the effect of IL-1 on TEC growth. TEC were found to produce PGE_2 and thromboxane (Nieburgs *et al.*, 1987; Sun *et al.*, 1990; Liu *et al.*, 1992). PGE_2 and IL-1 are also produced by reticular cells and nurse cells (Papiernik *et al.*, 1984; Lafontaine *et al.*, 1991; McCormack *et al.*, 1991). Several groups showed that TEC produce IL-1 and colony-stimulating factors (CSFs) (Le *et al.*, 1987; Ransom *et al.*, 1987). Some studies failed to show constitutive production of IL-1 (Eshel *et al.*, 1990; Galy *et al.*, 1990a).

Subsequently, GM-CSF, G-CSF, M-CSF, fibronectin, collagen type IV, laminin, thymosin α_1, and zinc–thymulin were added to the list of TEC products (Hashimura *et al.*, 1987; Galy *et al.*, 1991; Meilin *et al.*, 1992; Coto *et al.*, 1992; Shu *et al.*, 1996). Subcortical/medullary TEC presumably secrete three separate classes of peptides: interleukins, ground substance, and thymic hormone peptides. Savino *et al.* (1993) have recently suggested that the ground substance constitutes a matrix for the presentation of cytokine paracrine influences as a major component of the thymic microenvironment.

Studies on the regulation of secretion of these TEC have been useful. IL-1 induces IL-6, IL-8, GM-CSF, LIF, and zinc–thymulin but not IL-1, fibronectin, or thymosin α_1 (Galy *et al.*, 1990a, 1991; Cohen-Kaminsky *et al.*, 1991; Coto *et al.*, 1992; Shu *et al.*, 1996). The effects of IL-1 can be distinguished at least in part from its effects on proliferation (Coto *et al.*, 1992; Shu *et al.*, 1996). Endotoxin (LPS) and IL-4 enhance IL-1 induction of IL-6 (Galy *et al.*, 1991). EGF and its analogue TGF induce IL-1 and IL-6 (Le *et al.*, 1991). IFN-γ increases IL-1-induced secretion of IL-6 and class II expression and, at low doses (< 1 unit/ml), induces proliferation and laminin, collagen, and fibronectin secretion (Berrih *et al.*, 1985; Lannes-Vieira *et al.*, 1991; Colic *et al.*, 1992; Galy *et al.*, 1993). At higher doses, IFN-γ inhibits secretion of fibronectin, collagen, laminin, and proliferation and IL-1 induction of GM-CSF (Lannes-Vieira *et al.*, 1991; Galy and Spits, 1991). Activation of LFA-3 by anti-LFA-3 and ICAM-1 with anti-ICAM-1 both induce IL-1, IL-6, GM-CSF but not IL-8, LIF, fibronectin, or thymosin α_1 (Le *et al.*, 1991; Shu *et al.*, 1996). Hydrocortisone, which promotes the growth of TEC (Eshel *et al.*, 1990), inhibits the production of IL-8 and GM-CSF but not IL-6 and GM-CSF induced by IL-1, anti-ICAM-1, and anti-LFA-3 (Shu *et al.*, 1996). While not yet complete, these studies show important differential regulation of TEC secretion.

TEC secretion is unusual in that the cells contain large electron-dense vacuoles which vary in size, presumably related to secretory activity (Nabarra and Andrianarison, 1987a). The appearance in media of cytokines, ground substance, and thymic peptides is slow, occurring over days, unlike other secretory glands. Also, the regulation of secretion is unique (Nabarra and Andrianarison, 1987b). How differential secretion occurs is not clear, but cytokine secretion likely does not involve vacuole release.

In addition, it has been reported that various neuropeptides can be localized in the thymus to TEC and that TEC make oxytocin and vasopressin and possibly other neuropeptides (Gepetti *et al.*, 1987; Savino *et al.*, 1990; Lorton *et al.*, 1990; Bellinger *et al.*, 1990; Gomariz *et al.*, 1990; Robert *et al.*, 1991, 1992; Martin-Fontecha *et al.*, 1993). The role of these neuropeptides in thymic endocrine function and/or T-cell development and function remains to be determined. Nerve growth factor has been implicated in TEC secretion of IL-6 (Screpanti *et al.*, 1992; Galy and Spits, 1992; Table I).

Table I presents a summary of our recent data on the effects of various agents to induce secretion of IL-6 and GM-CSF from human fetal TEC in culture. IL-1, monoclonal antibodies against the two T-cell ligands (ICAM-1 and LFA-3), insulinlike growth factor-1 (IGF-1), growth hormone (GH), prolactin, and nerve growth factor (NGF) all significantly augmented the constitutive secretion of IL-6. IL-1, GH, prolactin, and NGF significantly induced GM-CSF but the other agents did not. In

TABLE I
Effects of Various Agents on Secretion of Human Thymic Epithelial Cells[a]

	Secretion	
Agent	IL-6	GM-CSF
Control	38 ± 14	ND[b]
IL-1 (20 ng/ml)	>300	267 ± 16
Anti-ICAM-1	165 ± 16	ND
Anti-LFA-3	104 ± 20	ND
IGF-1 (10 ng/ml)	>300	ND
GH (10 ng/ml)	165 ± 5	42 ± 3
Prolactin (2 ng/ml)	201 ± 9	38 ± 2
NGF (750 ng/ml)	137 ± 11	44 ± 3

[a]Secretion is pg/ml measured by ELISA (R&D Systems, Minneapolis, MN), ± *SEM* 9 samples). TEC were incubated for 48 hours with the agents in serum-free media as described (Shu *et al.*, 1996).
[b]Not detectable.

addition to emphasizing the differential regulation of cytokine secretion by TEC, these data are particularly notable in the pronounced effects of the various CNS-related growth factors (GH, prolactin, and NGF).

In addition to TEC-derived cytokines, activated thymocytes secrete the spectrum of cytokines also produced by mature T cells. These cytokines may function in autocrine and paracrine ways. IFN-γ and perhaps other T-cell cytokines may further act on TEC. TEC-produced cytokines act to promote thymocyte proliferation and also differentiation; thus, a complicated interaction between TEC and T cells exists involving cytokine signals in both directions (see Fig. 1) leading to T-cell development. Further cytokines rather than thymic hormones appear to be the driving forces for T-cell development (Hadden *et al.*, 1989b,d; Cardin *et al.*, 1991; Hadden, 1992).

In summary, then, the best studied are the medullary/subcapsular TEC which produce IL-1, IL-6, IL-8, GM-, G-, and M-CSF, LIF, fibronectin, collagen, laminin, thymosin α_1, and zinc–thymulin. Secretion from these cells seems to be regulated differentially by the three major ligands, IL-1 and the two T-cell-binding ligands (ICAM-1 and LFA-3). It is not known whether this differential regulation results from different cell populations or the same cell population. Importantly, no coordinant regulation exists between cytokine secretion and the large constitutive production of ground substance and thymosin α_1.

2.2. Thymic Hormone Exocrine Secretion

The thymic hormone story, as related to TEC, is less clear. Thymosin α_1, thymopoietin, and thymulin have been localized in TEC and are thought to be vacuole located (Auger *et al.*, 1987; Fabien *et al.*, 1988; Talle *et al.*, 1991). Of these three thymic peptides, only thymulin has been shown to be regulated in its secretion by prolactin, hydrocortisone, sex steroids, and thyroid hormone (Savino *et al.*, 1984, 1988; Dardenne *et al.*, 1986, 1989; Coto *et al.*, 1992) and is thymus-dependent, i.e., thymectomy removes the presence in serum of zinc–thymulin complex (Safieh *et al.*, 1990).

Thymulin is a zinc-binding nonapeptide found in the circulation (Dardenne *et al.*, 1984) but has a modified structure in the thymus involving a folate molecule (Ernstrom *et al.*, 1988, 1990; Sandberg and Ernstrom, 1991; Ernstrom, 1991).

The zinc–thymulin complex potentiates the action of low doses of mitogen on the proliferation of IL-2 receptor-positive mature T cells with further effects of IL-6 and GM-CSF in its presence (Coto *et al.*, 1992; J. W. and E. M. Hadden, unpublished observations). The zinc–thymulin complex acts in growth-promotion as a cytokine-sensitizer for IL-2 and perhaps other cytokines.

The promotion of T-cell responses to mitogen and to IL-2 and other cytokines seems a logical action for a thymic hormone circulating in the periphery. Such actions could enhance T-cell proliferation and secretory responses to antigen and generally promote the responsiveness of the cellular immune system.

With the interpretation that zinc–thymulin is the only thymus-dependent hor-

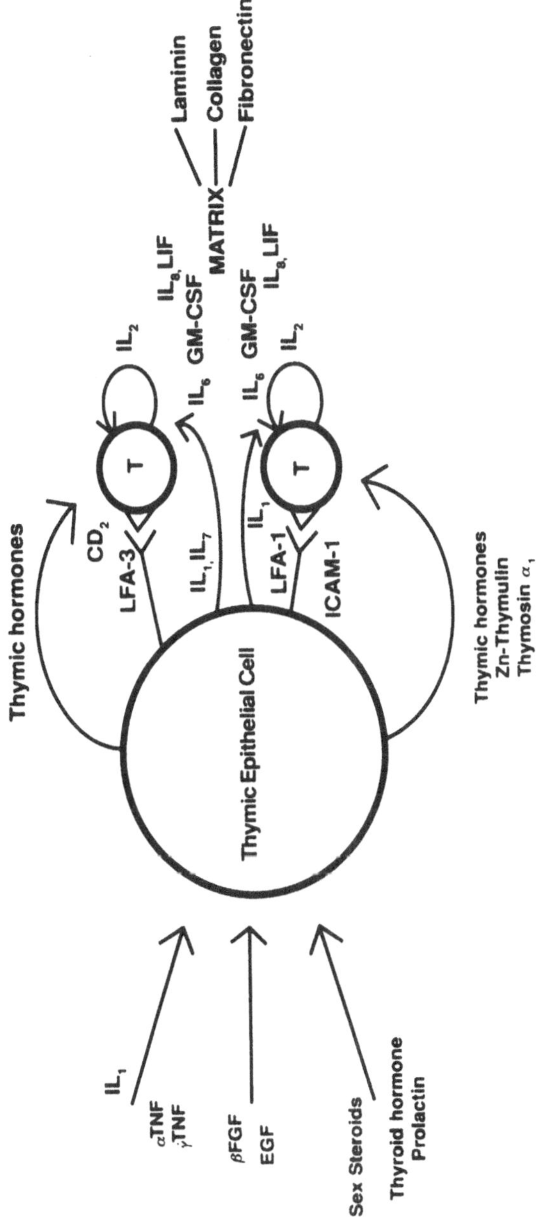

FIGURE 1. Thymocyte–thymic epithelial cell interactions.

mone regulated in its secretion and exported to the periphery, it is important to elaborate on its endocrinology, particularly as relates to the discussion of Fabris's chapter. Zinc is taken up by TEC in the thymus to make zinc–thymulin complex for secretion. Thymulin binds zinc and delivers it in the circulation at picogram per milliliter levels to T lymphocytes. Thymulin may circulate but needs zinc to act. Circulating levels of zinc are in the 1 μg/ml range, thus the T lymphocyte is unaffected by free zinc at > 10,000-fold excess levels. With zinc deficiency, thymic involution and a secondary cellular immune deficiency like AIDS develop.

In vitro, IL-1, prolactin, and zinc promote zinc–thymulin secretion by TEC (Dardenne *et al.*, 1989; Coto *et al.*, 1992; Hadden, unpublished). Also, IL-1 induces prolactin secretion from pituitary cells (Bernton *et al.*, 1987). *In vivo* IL-1 induces zinc uptake into thymus (and liver and bone marrow) with induction of metallothionein (Cousins and Leinert, 1988). Zinc–thymulin secretion is augmented *in vivo* by zinc loading and by prolactin (Dardenne *et al.*, 1989; Mocchegiani *et al.*, 1992). IL-1, zinc–thymulin, and prolactin all act in concert to promote IL-2 production and IL-2 receptor expression in T lymphocytes (Russell, 1989; Mukherjee *et al.*, 1990; Coto *et al.*, 1992). Further, high concentrations of zinc induce T-cell proliferation, promote IL-1 action, increase protein kinase C (PKC) activity and binding, and promote IL-2R expression (Winchurch, 1988; Csermely *et al.*, 1988; Malave *et al.*, 1990). It is reasonable to suggest that a critical issue of thymic function is the packaging and delivery of zinc to the T-cell system and that this process is under exquisite neuroendocrine control and may, as Fabris suggests, be central in the process of immune senescence following thymic involution.

While it is outside of the scope of this review to discuss the biochemical mechanisms involved in the action of these various cytokines and peptide hormones (see Hadden *et al.*, 1991), it is important to note that IL-1 and zinc–thymulin in the presence of IL-1 activate PKC in the nuclei of T cells (Coto *et al.*, 1992). The effect of zinc–thymulin is not reproduced by zinc or thymulin alone. This action on nuclear PKC is shared by thymosin α_1 (Sauro, Zorn, and Hadden, unpublished) and prolactin (Russell *et al.*, 1990). Notably, prolactin and growth hormone binding to their receptors is zinc-dependent (Cunningham *et al.*, 1990). PKC contains two zinc fingers and zinc is required for PKC action (Forbes *et al.*, 1991). This symmetry of PKC regulation by this collection of zinc-related factors all of which have similar actions to promote IL-2-dependent T-cell proliferation suggests a neuroendocrine theme of some significance (Fig. 2).

3. NEUROENDOCRINE REGULATION OF THE THYMUS

The picture of the thymus established so far emphasizes regulation by products of the immune system itself, both interleukins and thymic hormones. In addition, there are several critical areas of endocrine and neuronal regulation of thymus development and function (Fabris and Szentivanyi *et al.*, this volume; Fabris *et al.*,

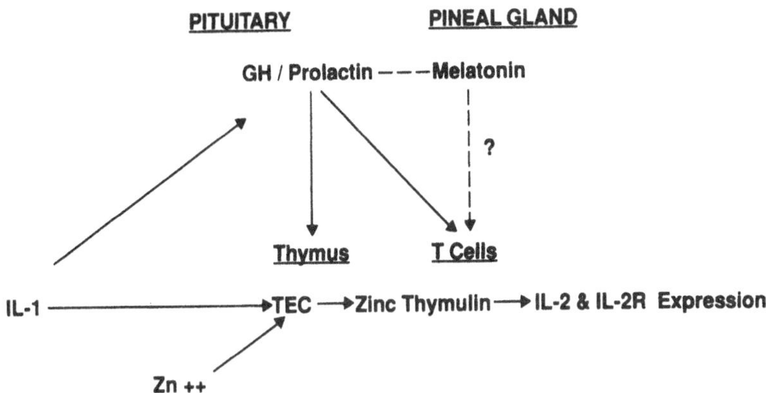

FIGURE 2. Regulation of zinc–thymulin production and action.

1989; Hadden *et al.*, 1991; Batanero *et al.*, 1992; de Leeuw *et al.*, 1992; Saha *et al.*, 1993). Anterior hypothalamic lesions are associated with thymic atrophy (Phelps, Chen, and Menzies, personal communication). The pituitary gland is a source of growth hormone and prolactin which play a role in the development and function of the thymus (see Fabris, this volume; Russell, 1989; Gala, 1991).

The maternal pituitary in genetically dwarf mice is adequate for initial development of the thymus in the embryo and breast-feeding provides endocrine support for its continuance (Duquesnoy and Good, 1970). At weaning, the thymus involutes and pituitary factors will restore it. Hypophysectomy results in only partial involution (Smith, 1930) and once the cellular immune system is already established, CMI persists (Saha *et al.*, 1993). If hypophysectomized animals are given hydrocortisone to induce more profound involution, they recover pretreatment thymus weights more slowly (3 weeks versus 1 week; Saha *et al.*, 1993). Finally, the involuted thymuses of aged animals can be substantially restored with treatment with pituitary peptides (Kelley *et al.*, 1986, 1987). Targets of growth hormone action include TEC (zinc–thymulin production), T lymphocytes, and macrophages (IL-1 production) (for review see Kelley *et al.*, 1987; Gala, 1991). Other pituitary hormones like TSH via the thyroid may be active, as well. A thymotropic hormone has been postulated (Duquesnoy and Good, 1970) but while pituitary extracts were found to promote TEC proliferation (Hadden *et al.*, 1989c), only a βFGF-like factor purified therefrom was active (Galy *et al.*, 1990b). A more comprehensive study of pituitary hormones on TEC secretion of cytokines (± IL-1) is needed to complete the picture.

The pineal gland has been related to thymic function (Maestroni, 1993; Mocchegiani *et al.*, 1994). Pinealectomy induces thymic involution and defects in CMI correctable by melatonin administration. Pineal grafts and melatonin reverse age- and stress-related thymic involution. Melatonin levels decline with age and correlate with age-related zinc and zinc–thymulin deficiency. In aged mice melatonin treatment restores zinc balance, zinc–thymulin serum levels, and CMI as measured by mitogen responses. The target of melatonin action in thymus has not been shown and whether lymphocytes have receptors for melatonin is disputed. Mocchegiani *et al.* (1996) have postulated that melatonin acts to increase zinc uptake and turnover including incorporation by the thymus into zinc–thymulin.

The maintenance of an appropriate endocrine environment is important to normal thymic function (see Fabris, this volume). The gonads have been linked to negative regulation of the thymus (see Fabris, this volume; Grossman, 1984, 1985); however, sex steroids may be important to subset differentiation within the thymus with estrogens favoring CD4 thymocyte development and function and androgens favoring CD8 thymocyte development and function (Nagel *et al.*, 1981; Olsen *et al.*, 1991). Androgen and estrogen receptors in lymphocytes and TEC would appear to be present. Unclear is any differential impact of menopause on thymus in the female. In any case, sex steroids may not be critical for maintenance of thymic integrity and function.

The thymus is innervated by sympathetic fibers by way of the superior cervical ganglion (Bulloch and Moore, 1981; Bulloch and Pomerantz, 1984; Felten *et al.*, 1985, 1987; Nance *et al.*, 1987; Felten and Felten, 1989). Cholinergic innervation is controversial and is generally thought to be absent. In addition, the pineal is sympathetically innervated. We have presented evidence showing that 6-hydroxy dopamine treatment induces thymic involution and retards thymic recovery following hydrocortisone administration, indicating an important role of the sympathetic nervous system in supporting thymic function (Saha *et al.*, 1993). The sympathetic nervous innervation may very possibly be functionally related to diurnal variations in thymic function directly or indirectly via melatonin.

In addition, neuropeptides secreted by peptidergic fibers may play important roles in thymic function (Savino *et al.*, 1990; Lorton *et al.*, 1990; Bellinger *et al.*, 1990) and a nerve growth factor with a link to zinc function is suspected (Hadden and Levi, unpublished). The translation of such influences from the central nervous system into immunologic responses as are seen in the conditioning and stress experiments (Ader and Cohen, 1991) probably occurs through these pathways involving neuropeptides and neurohormones.

Our data in hypothysectomized and sympathectomized adult mice (Saha *et al.*, 1993) indicate that the pituitary and sympathetic nervous system are both important in maintaining a normal thymus but their absence is associated with only partial involution and the ability of the thymus in the absence of a pituitary to respond to antigenic stimulation or to respond to correct lymphocytopenia has yet to be determined.

All in all, the thymic neuroendocrine environment is mediated by the capacity of antigen-sensitive T cells to interact with that environment including TEC and peptidoglycan intercellular matrix, to receive hormonal and cytokine signals of several types, and to secrete cytokines all leading to a stepwise development of T cells toward maturity. As thymocytes mature in the thymus, TEC ligands through adhesion molecules and adherence to matrix would appear to be important components of this system that induce autocrine and paracrine hormonal signals. All of these processes can be envisioned to be regulated by the neuroendocrine environment. The mature cells then exit to the periphery and are influenced by both thymic and nonthymic hormone action.

4. THYMIC INVOLUTION AND IMMUNE SENESCENCE

As discussed earlier, thymic involution occurs normally following puberty, yet the T-cell system is replete with T cells capable of mediating normal CMI and DTH (Clark and Maclennan, 1986). In this case, thymic involution seems incidental since recovery can take place when T-cell depletion occurs. It is important to note that throughout life mature T lymphocytes are destroyed or naturally die. These cells are replaced. Their replacements come from the expansion of the peripheral pool or from the thymus. In order for the organism to detect T lymphocytopenia and to correct it, a sensing device must exist akin to the Barrow receptors for blood pressure or the renal sensors for oxygen content and thus erythrocyte levels (via erythropoietin). Such a sensing device must then instruct the thymus via endocrine and/or neuronal means to supply new T cells. Such a sensing device should be sought. The large impact of neck irradiation on T-lymphocyte counts in x-ray-treated head and neck cancer patients (Wolf *et al.*, 1985) suggests that it may be located in the neck region. The response for self-renewal involves both subsets of T lymphocytes equally (CD4 and CD8) and, therefore, the sensing mechanism does not discriminate between subsets (Rocha *et al.*, 1989). More information is needed on this topic.

It is difficult to say when exactly thymic involution becomes pathological or irreversible. Much as been written about stress-induced thymic involution. In the mouse, endogenous glucocorticoid production can reach levels in stress capable of inducing an almost complete lysis and removal of the cortex with its double-positive population. This process recovers spontaneously within a week (Rothenberg, 1980). The mechanisms involved in the apoptotic process have been studied intensively yet the signals and mechanisms involved in the recovery are not known. In humans the sensitivity of T lymphocytes to the lytic effects of glucocorticoids is 1/10–1/100 that of mouse (Mishell *et al.*, 1977) and it is not clear whether a similar glucocorticoid-induced thymic involution occurs in humans. Certainly, thymic involution has been observed in postmortem studies of young humans with chronic infections and cancer; thus, disease induces thymic involution. Perhaps the best studied area is cancer (author's experience). The murine tumor models show progressive CMI defects with T-lymphocyte depletion and thymic involution. Similarly in humans, anergy, CMI defects, and lymphocytopenia occur with cancer, are more severe as the disease progresses, and are prognostically significant.

In aging, thymic involution may be normal, yet in mice a stage is reached where thymic involution is present, lymphocytopenia and CMI defects occur, and no recovery takes place (see Machinodan and Kay, 1980; Fabris *et al.*, 1992). At this point, thymic involution appears to be pathological and irreversible. In humans, a similar state has been assumed yet has not been clearly demonstrated.

Analyses of immune function of aged humans show relatively normal lymphocyte levels but impaired function. Defects of antigen responses occur with decreased protective responses to influenza immunization and increased autoimmune phenomena (without disease) suggesting dysfunction of regulatory mechanisms. Several studies on lymphocyte counts in midlife indicate a tendency of lymphocyte levels to decline progressively in the fourth, fifth, and sixth decades (Augener *et al.*, 1974; Alexopoulos and Babitis, 1976). The data predicted that the aged (70–90) would be lymphocytopenic yet they have generally normal lymphocyte levels (Falcoa *et al.*, 1987; Reibnegger *et al.*, 1988; Dworsky *et al.*, 1989; E. M. and J. W. Hadden, unpublished). An analysis of these data suggested to me that declining lymphocyte levels might be a harbinger of death and I was delighted to see this confirmed (Bender *et al.*, 1986). This interpretation implies that thymic involution is pathological when irreversible and contributes to premature mortality.

Transfer experiments from old to young mice *in vivo* and *in vitro* generally indicate that when transferred to young animals, thymic precursors can contribute to normal T-cell development (Greiner *et al.*, 1984; Scollay *et al.*, 1986; Goldschneider *et al.*, 1986; Donskoy and Goldschneider, 1992). The aged thymic environment can induce involution of young thymus (Hirokawa *et al.*, 1982). Development of normal T cells occurs in the aged somewhat more slowly (Scollay *et al.*, 1980). The reconstitution experiments of Kelley *et al.* (1986, 1987) indicate that the basic machinery is intact. Thus, deficiency of intra- and extrathymic endocrine influences which operate to keep the thymus capable of a self-renewal response seems implicated as the central mechanism.

It is clear that antigen drives T-cell development either directly or indirectly via interleukins. It is also clear that hormones and neuropeptides and transmitters play a role. The thymus at the level of the T cells and TEC are producers of various neuropeptides and hormones. How these substances act in relation to antigen is not known. It is known that the system develops to a certain level without antigen since gnotobiotic animals show normal thymic development and only slowed seeding of T cells into the periphery (Y. B. Kim, personal communication). The development of T cells in the absence of antigen must result from endocrine influences extrinsic to thymus operating in conjunction with intrathymic influences. In the aged, antigen stimulation of self-renewal of T cells is probably limited by the deficiencies of these latter influences. The endocrine and antigen influences can thus be viewed as complementary in promoting T-cell development.

The notion that thymic involution may be bypassed by extrathymic routes deserves discussion as an alternative pathway (Rocha *et al.*, 1992). A significant percentage, perhaps 20%, of T lymphocytes may be educated outside the thymus and be unrestricted by MHC. Data indicate that intraepithelial Tcr^+, $CD4^-$, and $CD8^-$ T cells evolve in gut apparently early in life and are maintained as a separate linage. It is not known whether this population is affected by thymic involution. In the nude mouse, T cells evolve in varying numbers and with varying degrees of function as the animals age. These cells have been characterized (Chen *et al.*, 1984) but it is not clear whether these cells evolve through the residual cords of the thymus of this animal (Ikehara *et al.*, 1987) or through skin or other sites (Rocha *et al.*, 1992). Our own efforts to boost the development of these populations in the nude mouse using a variety of stimuli such as interleukins and thymic hormones which have been used successfully to enhance reconstitution following hydrocortisone-induced thymic involution were completely unsuccessful (Hadden *et al.*, 1989a). It seems likely that these extrathymic routes evolve for the purposes of regional defense or regional regulation and unlikely that they represent alternative sources to meet body needs in the case of severe thymic involution.

5. PROSPECTS FOR CORRECTION

The issue of the treatment of thymic involution focuses not only on the thymus itself but also on the peripheral pool of T cells and their function (Hadden *et al.*, 1992a,b). In this regard, one finds a variety of treatment possibilities but few that analyze the latter (Table II). Fetal or neonatal thymus transplantation corrects thymic involution yet such treatment is impractical from a clinical standpoint. The activities of pituitary-derived hormones or related substances [growth hormone, prolactin, growth hormone releasing factor (GHRF), insulin-like growth factor-1 (IGF-1)] are also important in demonstrating activity yet injection of such materials in humans may yield unacceptable endocrine and other abnormalities (e.g., acromegaly).

The work of Mocchegiani *et al.* (1992, 1995, 1996) indicating that oral zinc repletion in the aged will produce a normal thymus, increase thymulin-containing

TABLE II
Agents Used to Treat Thymic Involution

Agent[a]	Thymic weight or cellularity	Zinc–thymulin levels	Peripheral T cells or CMI
Pituitary implants and extracts (GH)[1]	+	?	+
Growth hormones[1,2]	+	+	+
GHRF analogue[3]	+	+	?
LHRH analogue[4]	+	?	?
Arginine[5]	+	+	?
GH and IGF-1[6]	+	?	?
Melatonin[7]	+	+	?
Zinc salts[8]	+	+	+

[a]References: 1, Kelley *et al.*, (1986, 1987); 2, Goff *et al.* (1987); 3, Walker *et al.* (1994); 4, Greenstein *et al.* (1987); 5, Fabris *et al.* (1986); 6, Beschorner *et al.* (1991); 7, Mocchegiani *et al.* (1995); 8, Mocchegiani *et al.* (1992).

cells, increase serum zinc–thymulin levels, and induce recovery of T-cell function in the periphery is very strong in suggesting a practical clinical approach.

Our own studies have focused on mixed interleukins and thymic peptides to reverse hydrocortisone-induced thymic involution in middle-aged mice (9–12 months) (Hadden *et al.*, 1992a,b; 1995). Mixed natural interleukins (NI) but not individual recombinant interleukins 1 and 2 or their mixture increase immature and mature thymocytes and splenic T cells. The treatment with NI enhances thymocyte and splenocyte responses to *in vitro* stimulation with interleukins (IL-1, IL-2, NI) and T-cell mitogens (PHA and Con A). Thymosin fraction V is inactive alone; however, with NI it potentiates the responses of thymocytes to ILs and mitogens and splenocytes to ILs. Thymosin α_1 is active in a manner similar to NI and the effect of NI and thymosin α_1 was additive (Hadden *et al.*, 1995). The impact of the combination is striking in its magnitude. The combination needs to be studied in aged humans. Another alternative is the use of other thymic products. Our own work indicates that thymic epithelial supernatants, when injected in this model, will enhance recovery (unpublished results), suggesting that TEC-derived thymic peptides may be therapeutically useful.

Another major aspect of thymic involution refers to the "thymic menopause," i.e., the endocrine failure of the thymus. The biological activity attributable to thymic hormone falls off in circulation in the fourth decade paralleling the gonadal menopause of the female (Bach *et al.*, 1975; Twomey *et al.*, 1977). Although adult thymectomy does not have an acute impact on the T-cell system, a variety of evidence would indicate that loss of endocrine function of the thymus is accountable for progressive hyporesponsiveness of cells in the periphery.

A variety of thymic hormone materials have been described (for reviews see Goldstein, 1984; Byrom and Hobbs, 1984). Crude preparations include thymosin fraction V and thymomodulin (TP-1). Pure, synthetic preparations include thymosin α_1 and zinc–thymulin complex. The two thymic hormone factors serve to synergize with IL-1 in the activation of T lymphocytes by mitogens like PHA, leading to enhanced display of IL-2 receptors, production of IL-2, and expansion of T-cell population (Serrate and Sztein, 1989; Coto *et al.*, 1992; E. M. and J. W. Hadden, unpublished). Thus, hyporesponsiveness of T lymphocytes associated with aging may be attributable to thymic hormone deficiency. This may be manifest in the defective responsiveness of aged individuals to stimulation by new antigens, e.g., the failure of influenza immunization in the aged to promote antibody levels and adequate protection. In these circumstances, one can envision that zinc replacement, thymic factors, the products of TEC, and mixed interleukins may all act to reverse these defects in responsiveness.

There are two groups of drugs that may be useful in enhancing thymic involution-related function of T lymphocytes (Hadden, 1985). The drugs are referred to as "thymomimetic" drugs and are exemplified by levamisole and isoprinosine. Both of these types of agents have been shown to augment immune responses in aged animals (Tsang *et al.*, 1984; Bruley-Rousset *et al.*, 1986). Methyl inosine monophosphate (MIMP), a relative of isoprinosine, also reverses the effects of aging on PHA responses of lymphocytes (E. M. and J. W. Hadden, unpublished). It is important to note that oral treatments (zinc and these thymomietic drugs) are more practical than injections on the bases of physician acceptance and patient compliance.

6. CONCLUSIONS

From an immunologic standpoint, T-lymphocyte development is a genetically predetermined process beginning in precursor cells and evolving within the thymus as a result of interaction of T-cell receptors with TEC, cytokines, and other intrathymic factors and resulting in antigen-responsive cells capable of mediating CMI through proliferation, cytokine production, and cytotoxicity. The process is antigen-driven in all aspects. Thymic involution is a pathological event leading to immune senescence and defective antigen responses.

From a neuroendocrine standpoint, T-lymphocyte development is a genetically determined process regulated at every step by endocrine, paracrine, and autocrine hormonal signals and by neuropeptides and neurotransmitters. While antigen is important, the neuroendocrine axis provides critical maintaining and perhaps determining influences necessary for normal antigen response. Thymic involution is viewed as a failure of the axis to provide necessary neuroendocrine input to sustain T-cell responses to antigen.

The integrated view accepts the importance of both and recognizes the many unknowns contributing to the interaction. Effective reversal of thymic involution has been achieved with interleukin products of immune cells and thymic peptides of various types, on the one hand, and with endocrine products, particularly pituitary and pineal hormones, on the other. Apparent is a central role for zinc in thymus and T-cell function and in the treatment of thymic involution. Emerging is an integrated view of IL-1, zinc–thymulin, prolactin, and melatonin in the turnover of zinc and actions of zinc–thymulin to promote T-lymphocyte proliferation in response to mitogen and interleukin signals.

The clinical application of agents to reverse thymic involution is predicated on the assumption that it is closely linked to T-lymphocyte dysfunction. Defective T-lymphocyte responses may be treated with zinc replacement, thymic peptides, or thymomimetic drugs like levamisole and isoprinosine (see Hadden, 1994). Where T-cell depletion and dysfunction occur in association with thymic involution, corrective attempts to produce new T lymphocytes are warranted and may be achieved with interleukin mixtures with or without thymic peptides, with pituitary hormones and other endocrine factors, or with combinations with or without appropriate antigenic stimulation.

REFERENCES

Ader, R., and Cohen, N., 1991, The influence of conditioning in immune responses, in: *Psychoneuroimmunology*, 2nd ed. (R. Ader, D. L. Felten, and N. Cohen, eds.), Academic Press, New York, pp. 611–646.

Aguilar, L. K., Aguilar-Cordova, E., Cartwright, J., Jr., and Belmont, J. W., 1994, Thymic nurse cells are sites of thymocyte apoptosis, *J. Immunol.* **152:**2645.

Alexopoulos, C., and Babitis, P., 1976, Age dependence of T lymphocytes, *Lancet* **1:**426.

Augener, W., Cohnen, G., Reuter, A., and Brittinger, G., 1974, Decrease of T lymphocytes during ageing, *Lancet* **1:**1164.

Auger, C., Stahli, C., Fabien, N., and Monier, J.-C., 1987, Intracellular localization of thymosin alpha 1 by immunoelectron microscopy using a monoclonal antibody, *J. Histochem. Cytochem.* **35:**181.

Bach, J.-F., 1983, Physiology of the endocrine function of the thymic epithelium, in: *Progress in Immunology* (Y. Yamamura and T. Tada, eds.), Academic Press, New York, pp. 1563–1579.

Bach, J.-F., Dardenne, M., Pleau, J. M., and Bach, A. M., 1975, Isolation, biochemical characterization and biological activity of a circulating thymic hormone in the mouse and in the human, *Ann. N.Y. Acad. Sci.* **249:**186.

Batanero, E., de Leeuw, F.-E., Jansen, G. H., van Wichen, D. F., Huber, J., and Schuurman, H.-F., 1992, The neural and neuroendocrine component of the human thymus II. Hormone immunoreactivity, *Brain Behav. Immun.* **6:**249.

Bellinger, D. L., Lorton, D., Romano, T. D., Olschowka, J. A., Felten, S. Y., and Felten, D. L., 1990, Neuropeptide innervations of lymphoid organs, *Ann. N.Y. Acad. Sci.* **594:**17.

Bender, B. S., Nagel, J. E., Adler, W. H., and Andres, R., 1986, Absolute peripheral blood lymphocyte count and subsequent mortality of elderly men. The Baltimore longitudinal study of aging, *J. Am. Geriatr. Soc.* **34:**649.

Bernton, E. W., Beach, J. E., Holaday, J. W., Smallridge, R. C., and Fein, H. G., 1987, Release of multiple hormones by a direct action of interleukin-1 on pituitary cells, *Science* **238:**519.

Berrih, S. F., Arenzana-Seisdedos, F., Cohen, S., Devos, R., Charron, D., and Virelizier, J. L., 1985, Interferon-γ modulates HLA class II antigen expression on cultured human thymic epithelial cells, *J. Immunol.* **135:**1165.

Beschorner, W. E., Divic, J., Pulido, H., Yao, X., Kenworth, P., and Bruce, G., 1991, Enhancement of thymic recovery after cyclosporine by recombinant human growth hormone and insulin-like growth factor 1, *Transplantation* **52:**879.

Bockman, D. E., and Kirby, M. L., 1984, Dependence of thymus development on derivatives of the neural crest, *Science* **223:**498.

Brightman, B. K., Chandy, K. G., Spencer, R. H., and Fan, H., 1989, A T lymphoid cell line responds to a thymic stromal cell line by expression of Thy-1 and CD4, *J. Immunol.* **143:**2775.

Bruley-Rousset, M., Vergnon, I., and Renoux, G., 1986, Influences of sodium diethyldithiocarbamate, DTC (Imuthiol®) on T cell defective responses of aged BALB/c mice, *Int. J. Immunopharmacol.* **8:**287.

Bulloch, K., and Moore, R. Y., 1981, Innervation of the thymus gland by brain stem and spinal cord in mouse and rat, *Am. J. Anat.* **162:**157.

Bulloch, K., and Pomerantz, W., 1984, Autonomic nervous system innervation of thymic-related lymphoid tissue in wildtype and nude mice, *J. Comp. Neurol.* **228:**57.

Burkly, L. C., Degermann, S., Longley, J., Hagman, J., Brinster, R. L., Lo, D., and Flavell, R. A., 1993, Clonal deletion of $V\beta5^+$ T cells by transgenic I-E restricted to thymic medullary epithelium, *J. Immunol.* **151:**3954.

Byrom, N. A., and Hobbs, J. R., eds., 1984, *Thymic Factor Therapy*, Volume 16, Serono Symposia Publications, Raven Press, New York.

Cardin, S. R., Hayday, A. C., and Bottomly, K., 1991, Cytokines in T-cell development, *Immunol. Today* **12:**239.

Ceredig, R., Lowenthal, J. W., Nanholz, M., and MacDonald, H. R., 1985, Expression of interleukin-2 receptor as a differentiation marker on intrathymic stem cells, *Nature* **314:**98.

Champion, S., Imhof, B. A., Savagner, P., and Thiery, J. P., 1986, The embryonic thymus produces chemotactic peptides involved in the homing of hemopoietic precursors, *Cell* **44:**781

Chen, W.-F., Scollay, R., Shortman, K., Skinner, M., and Marbrook, J., 1984, T-cell development in the absence of a thymus: The number, the phenotype, and the functional capacity of T lymphocytes in nude mice, *Am. J. Anat.* **170:**339.

Clark, A. G., and Maclennan, K. A., 1986, The many facets of thymic involution, *Immunol. Today* **7:**204.

Cohen-Kaminsky, S., Delattre, R.-M., Devergne, O., Rouet, P., Gimond, D., Berrih-Akhin, S., and Galanaud, P., 1991, Synergistic induction of interleukin-6 production and gene expression in human thymic epithelial cells by LPS and cytokines, *Cell. Immunol.* **138:**79.

Colic, M., Pejnovic, N., Kataranovski, M., Popovic, L., Gasic, S., and Dujic, A., 1992, Interferon gamma alters the phenotype of rat thymic epithelial cells in culture and increases interleukin-6 production, *Dev. Immunol.* **2:**151.

Coto, J. A., Hadden, E. M., Sauro, M., Zorn, N., and Hadden, J. W., 1992, Interleukin 1 regulates secretion of zinc-thymulin by human thymic epithelial cells and its action on T-lymphocyte proliferation and nuclear protein kinase C, *Proc. Natl. Acad. Sci. USA* **89:**7752.

Cousins, R. J., and Leinart, A. S., 1988, Tissue-specific regulation of zinc metabolism and metallothionein genes by interleukin-1, *FASEB J.* **2:**2884.

Couture, C., Patel, P. C., and Potworowski, E. F., 1990, A novel thymic epithelial adhesion molecule, *Eur. J. Immunol.* **20:**2769.

Csermely, P., Szamel, M., Resch, K., and Somogyi, J., 1988, Zinc can increase the activity of protein kinase C and contributes to its binding to plasma membranes in T lymphocytes, *J. Biol. Chem.* **263:**6487.

Cunningham, B. C., Bass, S., Fuh, G., and Wells, J. A., 1990, Zinc mediation of the binding of human growth hormone to the human prolactin receptor, *Science* **250:**1709.

Dalloul, A. H., Fourcade, C., Debre, P., and Mossalayi, M. D., 1991, Thymic epithelial cell-derived supernatants sustain the maturation of human prothymocytes: Involvement of interleukin 1 and CD23, *Eur. J. Immunol.* **21:**2633.

Dardenne, M., Savino, W., Gastinel, L., and Bach, J.-F., 1984, Thymulin: New biochemical aspects, in: *Thymic Hormones and Lymphokines* (A. L. Goldstein, ed.), Plenum Press, New York, pp. 37–42.

Dardenne, M., Savino, W., Duval, D., Kaiserlian, D., Hassid, J., and Bach, J.-F., 1986, Thymic hormone containing cells. VII. Adrenals and gonads control the in vivo secretion of thymulin and its plasmatic inhibitor, *J. Immunol.* **136:**1303.

Dardenne, M., Savino, W., Gagnerault, M.-C., Itoh, T., and Bach, J.-F., 1989, Neuroendocrine control of thymic hormonal production. I. Prolactin stimulates in vivo and in vitro the production of thymulin by human and murine thymic epithelial cells, *Endocrinology* **125:**3.

Degermann, S., Surh, C. D., Glimcher, L. H., Sprent, J., and Lo, D., 1994, B7 expression on thymic medullary epithelium correlates with epithelium-mediated deletion of $V\beta5^+$ thymocytes, *J. Immunol.* **152:**3254.

DeJouanen, E., Strickland, R. G., and Williams, R. C., 1975, Studies of human lymphocytes in the newborn and the aged, *Am. J. Med.* **58:**620.

de Leeuw, F. E., Jansen, G. H., Batanero, E., Whichen, D. F. V., Huber, J., and Schuurman, H. J., 1992, The neural and neuro-endocrine component of the human thymus, *Brain Behav. Immun.* **6:**234.

Denning, S. M., Tuck, D. T., Vollger, L. W., Springer, T. A., Singer, K. H., and Haynes, B. F., 1987a, Monoclonal antibodies to CD2 and lymphocyte function-associated antigen 3 inhibit human thymic epithelial cell-dependent mature thymocyte activation, *J. Immunol.* **139:**2573.

Denning, S. M., Tuck, D. T., Singer, K. H., and Haynes, B. F., 1987b, Human thymic epithelial cells function as accessory cells for autologous mature thymocyte activation, *J. Immunol.* **138:**680.

Denning, S. M., Kurtzberg, J., Le, P. T., Tuck, D. T., Singer, K. H., and Haynes, B. F., 1988, Human thymic epithelial cells directly induce activation of autologous immature thymocytes, *Proc. Natl. Acad. Sci. USA* **85:**3125.

Donskoy, E., and Goldschneider, I., 1992, Thymocytopoiesis is maintained by blood-borne precursors throughout postnatal life. A study in parabiotic mice, *J. Immunol.* **148:**1604.

Duquesnoy, R. J., and Good, R. A., 1970, Prevention of immunologic deficiency in pituitary dwarf mice by prolonged nursing, *J. Immunol.* **104:**1553.

Dworsky, R., Paganini-Hill, A., Ducey, B., Hechinger, M., and Parker, J. W., 1989, Lymphocyte immunophenotyping in an elderly population: Age, sex, and medication effects—a flow cytometry study, *Mech. Ageing Dev.* **48:**255.

Ernstrom, U., 1991, Identification of a mammalian growth factor as a ribofolate peptide, *Biosci. Rep.* **11:**119.

Ernstrom, U., Karlsson, P., and Soder, O., 1988, Isolation of a thymocyte growth peptide from human thymus, *Int. Arch. Allergy Appl. Immunol.* **85:**434.

Ernstrom, U., Gafvelin, G., and Rudja, J.-M., 1990, Purification of thymocyte growth peptide (TGP) from sheep thymus. Relationship to FTS/thymulin, *Biosci. Rep.* **10:**403.

Eshel, I., Savion, N., and Shoham, J., 1990, Analysis of thymic stromal cell subpopulations grown in vitro on extracellular matrix in defined medium. II. Cytokine activities in murine thymic epithelial and mesenchymal cell culture supernatants, *J. Immunol.* **144:**1563.

Fabien, N., Auger, C., and Monier, J.-C., 1988, Immunolocalization of thymosin alpha 1, thymopoietin and thymulin in mouse thymic epithelial cells at different stages of culture: A light and electron microscopic study, *Immunology* **63:**721.

Fabris, N., Mocchegiani, E., Mariotti, S., Pacini, F., and Pinchera, A., 1986, Thyroid function modulates thymus endocrine activity, *J. Clin. Endocrinol. Metab.* **62:**474.

Fabris, N., Mocchegiani, E., Muzzioni, M., and Provinciali, M., 1989, Neuroendocrine–thymus interactions, in: *Interactions Among Central Nervous System, Neuroendocrine System, Neuroendocrine and Immune System* (J. W. Hadden, K. Masek, and G. Nistico, eds.), Pythagora Press, Rome, pp. 177–189.

Fabris, N. Harman, D., Knook, D. L., Steinhafen-Thiessen, E., and Zs.-Nagy, I., eds., 1992, *Physiopathological Processes of Aging Towards a Multicausal Interpretation, Ann. N.Y. Acad. Sci.* Volume 673.

Falcao, R. P., Ismael, S. J., and Donadi, E. A., 1987, Age-associated changes of T lymphocyte subsets, *Diagn. Clin. Immunol.* **5:**205.

Farr, A. G., Hosier, S., Braddy, S. C., Anderson, S. K., Eisenhardt, D. J., Yan, Z. J., and Robles, C. P., 1989, Medullary epithelial cell lines from murine thymus constitutively secrete IL- 1 and hematopoietic growth factors and express class II antigens in response to recombinant interferon-γ, *Cell. Immunol.* **119:**427.

Felten, D. L., and Felten, S. Y., 1989, Innervation of the thymus, *Thymus* **2:**73.

Felten, D. L., Felten, S. Y., Carlson, S. L., Olschowka, J. A., and Livnat, S., 1985, Noradrenergic and peptidergic innervation of lymphoid tissue, *J. Immunol.* **135:**755.

Felten, D. L., Felten, S. Y., Bellinger, D. L., Carlson, S. L., Ackerman, K. D., Madden, K. S., Olschowka, J. A., and Livnat, S., 1987, Noradrenergic sympathetic neural interaction with the immune system: Structure and function, *Immunol. Rev.* **100:**225.

Forbes, I. J., Zalewski, P. D., and Giannakis, C., 1991, Role for zinc in a cellular response mediated by protein kinase C in human B lymphocytes, *Exp. Cell Res.* **195:**224.

Gala, R. R., 1991, Prolactin and growth hormone in the regulation of the immune system, *Proc. Soc. Exp. Biol. Med.* **198:**513.

Galy, A. H. M., and Spits, H., 1991, IL-1, IL-4, and IFN-γ differentially regulate cytokine production and cell surface molecule expression in cultured human thymic epithelial cells, *J. Immunol.* **147:**3823.

Galy, A. H. M., and Spits, H., 1992, CD40 is functionally expressed on human thymic epithelial cells, *J. Immunol.* **149:**775.

Galy, A. H. M., Hadden, E. M., Touraine, J.-L., and Hadden, J. W., 1989, Effects of cytokines on thymic epithelial cells in culture: IL-1 induces thymic epithelial proliferation and change in morphology, *Cell. Immunol.* **124:**13.

Galy, A. H. M., Dinarello, C. A., Kupper, T. S., and Hadden, J. W., 1990a, Effects of cytokines on human thymic epithelial cells in culture: Recombinant IL_1 stimulates thymic epithelial cells to produce IL_6 and GM-CSF, *Cell. Immunol.* **129:**161.

Galy, A. H. M., Jolivet, M., Jolivet, C., and Hadden, J. W., 1990b, Fibroblast growth factor (FGF) and an FGF-like molecule in pituitary extracts stimulate thymic epithelial cells proliferation, *Thymus* **15:**199.

Galy, A. H. M., Malefyt, R. D. W., Barcena, A., Peterson, M. S., and Spits, H., 1993, Untransfected and SV40-transfected fetal and postnatal human thymic stromal cells, *Thymus* **22**:13.

Geppetti, P., Maggi, C. A., Zecchia-Orlandi, S., Santicioli, P., Meli, A., Frilli, S., Spillantimi, M. G., and Amenta, F., 1987, Substance P-like immunoreactivity in capsaicin-sensitive structures of the rat thymus, *Regul. Peptides* **18**:321.

Giunta, M., Favre, A., Ramarli, D., Grossi, C. E., and Corte, G., 1991, A novel integrin involved in thymocyte–thymic epithelial cell interactions, *J. Exp. Med.* **173**:1537.

Godfrey, D. I., Zlotnik, A., and Suda, T., 1992, Phenotypic and functional characterization of c-kit expression during intrathymic T cell development, *J. Immunol.* **149**:2281.

Goff, B. L., Roth, J. A., Arp, L. H., and Incefy, G. S., 1987, Growth hormone treatment stimulates thymulin production in aged dogs, *Clin. Exp. Immunol.* **65**:580.

Goldschneider, I., Komschlies, K. L., and Greiner, D. L., 1986, Studies of thymocytopoiesis in rats and mice. I. Kinetics of appearance of thymocytes using a direct intrathymic adoptive transfer assay for thymocyte precursors, *J. Exp. Med.* **163**:1.

Goldstein, A. L., ed., 1984, *Thymic Hormones and Lymphokines: Basic Chemistry and Clinical Applications*, Plenum Press, New York.

Gomariz, R. P., Lorenzo, M. L., Cacicedo, L., Vicente, A., and Zapata, A. G., 1990, Demonstration of immunoreactive vasoactive intestinal peptide (IR-VIP) and somatostatin (IR-SOM) in rat thymus, *Brain Behav. Immun.* **4**:151.

Good, R. A., 1991, Experiments of nature in the development of modern immunology, *Immunol. Today* **12**:283.

Greenstein, B. D., Fitzpatrick, F. T., Kendall, M. D., and Wheeler, M. J., 1987, Regeneration of the thymus in old male rats treated with a stable analog of LHRH, *J. Endocrinol.* **112**:345.

Greiner, D. L., Goldschneider, I., and Lubaroff, D. M., 1984, Identification of thymocyte progenitors in hemopoietic tissues of the rat. I. A quantitative assay system for thymocyte regeneration, *Thymus* **6**:181.

Grossman, C. J., 1984, Regulations of the immune system by sex steroids, *Endocrine Rev.* **5**:435.

Grossman, C. J., 1985, Interactions between gonadal steroids and the immune system, *Science* **227**:257.

Gutierrez, J. C., and Palacios, R., 1991, Heterogenicity of thymic epithelial cells in promoting T-lymphocyte differentiation in vivo, *Proc. Natl. Acad. Sci. USA* **88**:642.

Hadden, J. W., 1985, Thymomimetic drugs, in: *Serono Symposium on Immunopharmacology*, Volume 23 (P. A. Miescher, L. Bolis, and M. Ghione, eds.), Raven Press, New York, pp. 183–192.

Hadden, J. W., 1992, Thymic endocrinology, *Int. J. Immunopharmacol.* **14**:345.

Hadden, J. W., 1994, T cell adjuvancy, *Int. J. Immunopharmacol.* **16**:703.

Hadden, J. W., Caspritz, G., Zheng, Q. Y., Chen, H., Wolstencroft, R., and Hadden, E. M., 1989a, Thymosin, interleukins, isoprinosine and imuthiol do not reconstitute T cells in athymic nude mice, *Int. J. Immunopharmacol.* **11**:13.

Hadden, J. W., Galy, A., Chen, H., Wang, Y., and Hadden, E. M., 1989b, The hormonal regulation of thymus and T lymphocyte development and function, in: *Interactions Among Central Nervous System, Neuroendocrine and Immune Systems* (J. W. Hadden, K. Masek, and G. Nistico, eds.), Pythagora Press, Rome, pp. 147–164.

Hadden, J. W., Galy, A., Chen, H., and Hadden, E. M., 1989c, A pituitary factor induces thymic epithelial cell proliferation in vitro, *Brain Behav. Immun.* **3**:149.

Hadden, J. W., Chen, H., Wang, Y., and Hadden, E. M., 1989d, Strategies of immune reconstitution: Effects of lymphokines on murine T cell development in vitro and in vivo, *Life Sci. AIDS Comm.* **44**:5.

Hadden, J. W., Hadden, E. M., and Coffey, R. G., 1991, First and second messengers in the development and function of thymus-dependent lymphocytes, in: *Psychonueroimmunology*, 2nd ed. (R. Ader, D. L. Felten, and N. Cohen, eds.), Academic Press, New York, pp. 529–560.

Hadden, J. W., Malec, P., Coto, J., and Hadden, E. M., 1992a, Thymic involution in aging. Prospects for correction, in: *Physiopathological Processes of Aging Towards a Multicausal Interpretation*, Volume 673 (N. Nistico, D. Harman, D. L. Knook, E. Steinhagen-Thiessen, and I. Zs-Nagy, eds.), New York Academy of Sciences, New York, pp. 231–239.

Hadden, J. W., Malec, P., Saha, A., and Hadden, E. M., 1992b, Cytokine synergy in immunotherapy, in: *Combination Therapies 2* (A. Goldstein and E. Garaci, eds.), Plenum Press, New York, pp. 1–10.

Hadden, J. W., Saha, A., Sosa, M., and Hadden, E. M., 1995, Immunotherapy with natural interleukins and/or thymosin γ, potently augments T-lymphocyte responses of hydrocortisone-treated aged mice, *Int. J. Immunopharmacol.* **17**:821.

Hashimura, H., Toyokawa, T., Hato, F., Oshitani, N., Kimura, S., and Kinoshita, Y., 1987, Separation of biologically active polypeptides from rat thymus-epithelial-cell-culture-supernatant by high-performance liquid chromatography, *Cell. Mol. Biol.* **33**:375.

Haynes, B. F., and Eisenbarth, G. S., 1983, Use of monoclonal antibodies to identify cell-surface antigens of human neuroendocrine thymic epithelium, *Monoclonal Antibodies* **3**:47.

Hensen, E. J., Hoefsmit, C. M., and Van Den Tweel, J. G., 1978, Augmentation of mitogen responsiveness in human lymphocytes by a humoral factor obtained from thymic epithelial cultures, *Clin. Exp. Immunol.* **32**:309.

Hirokawa, K., Sato, K., and Makinodan, T., 1982, Influence of age of thymic grafts on the differentiation of T cells in nude mice, *Clin. Immunol. Immunopathol.* **24**:251.

Hosseinzadeh, H., and Goldschneider, I., 1993, Demonstration of large scale migration of cortical thymocytes to the peripheral lymphoid tissues of cyclosporine-treated rats, *J. Exp. Med.* **178**:285.

Hugo, P., Kappler, J. W., Godfrey, D. I., and Marrack, P. C., 1993, Thymic epithelial cell lines that mediate positive selection can also induce thymocyte clonal deletion, *J. Immunol.* **152**:1022.

Ikehara, S., Shimizu, J., Yasumizu, R., Hakamura, T., Inaba, M., Inoue, S., Oyaizu, N., Sugiura, K., Oo, M. M., Hamashima, Y., and Good, R. A., 1987, Thymic rudiments are responsible for induction of functional T cells in nu/nu mice, *Thymus* **10**:93.

Kampinga, J., Berges, S., Boyd, R. L., Brekelmans, P., Colic, M., Van Ewijk, W., Kendall, M. D., Ladyman, H., Nieuwenhuis, P., Ritter, M. A., Schuurman, H.-J., and Tournefier, A., 1989, Thymic epithelial antibodies: Immunohistological analysis and introduction of nomenclature, *Thymus* **13**:165.

Kasai, M., and Hirokawa, K., 1991, A novel cofactor produced by a thymic epithelial cell line: Promotion of proliferation of immature thymic lymphocytes by the presence of interleukin-1 and various mitogens, *Cell. Immunol.* **132**:377.

Kelley, K. W., Brief, S., Westly, H. J., Novakfski, J., Bechtel, P. J., Simon, J., and Walker, E. B., 1986, GH3 pituitary adenoma cells can reverse thymic aging in rats, *Proc. Natl. Acad. Sci. USA* **83**:5663.

Kelley, K. W., Brief, S., Westly, H. J., Novakfski, J., Bechtel, P. J., Simon, J., and Walker, E. B., 1987, Hormonal regulations of the age-associated decline in immune function, in: *Neuroimmune Interactions: Proceedings of the 2nd International Workshop on Neuroimmune Modulations* (B. D. Jankovic, B. M. Markovic, and N. H. Spector, eds.), New York Academy of Sciences, New York, p. 469.

Koninky, J. F. J. G., Schreurs, J. M., Penninks, A. H., and Seinen, W., 1984, Induction of postthymic T-cell maturation by thymic humoral factor(s) derived from a tumor cell of thymic epithelial origin, *Thymus* **6**:395.

Kruisbeek, A. M., and Astaldi, G. C. B., 1979, Distinct effects of thymic epithelial culture supernatants on T cell properties of mouse thymocytes separated by the use of peanut agglutinin, *J. Immunol.* **123**:984.

Kurtzberg, J., Denning, S. M., Nycum, L. M., Singer, K. H., and Haynes, B. F., 1989, Immature human thymocytes can be driven to differentiate into nonlymphoid lineages by cytokines from thymic epithelial cells, *Proc. Natl. Acad. Sci. USA* **86**:7575.

Lafontaine, M., Landry, D., Blanc-Brunat, N., Pelletier, M., and Montplaisir, S., 1991, IL-1 production by human thymic dendritic cells: Studies on the interrelation with DC accessory function, *Cell. Immunol.* **135**:431.

Lannes-Vieira, J., van der Meide, P. H., and Savino, W., 1991, Extracellular matrix components of the mouse thymic microenvironment. II. In vitro modulation of basement membrane proteins by interferon-γ: Relationship with thymic epithelial cell proliferation, *Cell. Immunol.* **137**:329.

Le, P. T., Tuck, D. T., Dinarello, C. A., Haynes, B. F., and Singer, K. H., 1987, Human thymic epithelial cells produce interleukin 1, *J. Immunol.* **138**:2520.

Le, P. T., Kurtzberg, J., Brandt, J., Niedel, J. E., Haynes, B. F., and Singer, K. H., 1988a, Human thymic epithelial cells produce granulocyte and macrophage colony-stimulating factors, *J. Immunol.* **141**:1211.

Le, P. T., Fredrickson, G., Ries, L. F. L., Diamanstein, T., Hirano, T., Kishimoto, T., and Vilcek, J., 1988b, Interleukin-2-dependent and interleukin 2-independent pathways of regulation of thymocyte function by interleukin 6, *Proc. Natl. Acad. Sci. USA* **85**:8643.

Le, P. T., Lazorick, S., Whichard, L. P., Yang, Y.-C., Clark, S. C., Haynes, B. F., and Singer, K. H., 1990a, Human thymic epithelial cells produce IL-6, granulocyte-monocyte-CSF, and leukemia inhibitory factor, *J. Immunol.* **145**:3310.

Le, P. T., Vollger, L. W., Haynes, B. F., and Singer, K. H., 1990b, Ligand binding to the LFA-3 cell adhesion molecule induces IL-1 production by human thymic epithelial cells, *J. Immunol.* **144**:4541.

Le, P. T., Lazorick, S., Whichard, L. P., Haynes, B. F., and Singer, K. H., 1991, Regulation of cytokine production in the human thymus: Epidermal growth factor and transforming growth factor α regulate mRNA levels of interleukin 1α (IL-1α), IL-1β, and IL-6 in human thymic epithelial cells at a posttranscriptional level, *J. Exp. Med.* **174**:1147.

Lewis, V. M., Twomey, J. J., Bealmear, P., Goldstein, G., and Good, R. A., 1978, Age, thymic involution, and circulating thymic hormone activity, *J. Clin. Endocrinol. Metab.* **47**:145.

Liu, P.-S., Sun, L., Wen, M., and Hayashi, J., 1992, Stimulation of prostaglandin production in rat thymic epithelial cells by protein kinase C mediated activation of phospholipase A2, *Biochem. Int.* **27**:931.

Lobach, D. F., and Haynes, B. F., 1987, Ontogeny of the human thymus during fetal development, *J. Clin. Immunol.* **7**:81.

Lorton, D., Bellinger, D. L., Felten, S. Y., and Felten, D. L., 1990, Substance P innervation of the rat thymus, *Peptides* **11**:1269.

McCormack, J. E., Kappler, J., Marrack, P., and Westcott, J. Y., 1991, Production of prostaglandin E_2 and prostacyclin by thymic nurse cells in culture, *J. Immunol.* **146**:239.

MacDonald, H. R., 1992, Enigma variations, *Curr. Biol.* **2**:653.

Machinodan, T., and Kay, M. M., 1980, Age influence on the immune system, *Adv. Immunol.* **29**:287.

Maestroni, G. J. M., 1993, The immunoneuroendocrine role of melatonin, *J. Pineal Res.* **14**:1.

Makgoba, M. W., Sanders, M. E., and Shaw, S., 1989, The CD2-LFA-3 and LFA-1 -ICAM pathways: Relevance to T-cell recognition, *Immunol. Today* **10**:417.

Malave, I., Rodriguez, J., Araujo, Z., and Rojas, I., 1990, Effect of zinc on the proliferative response of human lymphocytes: Mechanism of its mitogenic action, *Immunopharmacology* **20**:1.

Martin-Fontecha, A., Broekhuizen, R., de Heer, C., Zapata, A., and Schuurman, H.-J., 1993, The neuroendocrine component of the rat thymus: Studies on cultured thymic fragments before or after transplantation in congenitally athymic and euthymic rats, *Brain Behav. Immun.* **7**:1.

Meilin, A., Shoham, J., and Sharabi, Y., 1992, Analysis of thymic stromal cell subpopulations grown in vitro on extracellular matrix defined medium. IV. Cytokines secreted by human thymic epithelial cells in culture and their activities on murine thymocytes and bone marrow cells, *Immunology* **77**:208.

Miller, J. F. A. P., 1991, Analysis of the thymus influence in leukemogenesis, *Immunol. Today* **191**:248.

Mishell, R. I., Lucas, A., and Mishell, B. B., 1977, The role of activated accessory cells in preventing immune suppression by hydrocortisone, *J. Immunol.* **119**:118.

Mizutani, S., Watt, S. M., Robertson, D., Hussein, S., Healy, L. E., Furley, A. J. W., and Greaves, M. F., 1987, Cloning of human thymic subcapsular cortex epithelial cells with T-lymphocyte binding sites and hemopoietic growth factor activity, *Proc. Natl. Acad. Sci. USA* **84**:4999.

Mocchegiani, E., Muzzioli, M., Santarelli, L., and Fabris, N., 1992, Restoring effect of oral supplementation of zinc and arginine on thymic endocrine activity and peripheral immune functions in aged mice, *Arch. Gerontol. Geriat.* **3**:267.

Mocchegiani, E., Muzzioli, M., Santarelli, L., and Fabris, N., 1994, Zinc and immune system: "In vivo" effect of zinc on thymic endocrine activity and on peripheral immune functions in old mice, *Int. J. Immunopharmacol.* **17**:703.

Mocchegiani, E., Bulian, D., Santarelli, L., Tibaldi, A., Muzzioli, M., Pierpaoli, W., and Fabris, N., 1996,

The immuno-reconstituting effect of melatonin or pineal grafting and its relation to zinc pool in aging mice, *J. Pharm. Exp. Therapeutics*, in press.

Mojcik, C., Greiner, D. L., and Goldschneider, I., 1991, Characterization of RT6 bearing rat lymphocytes II. Developmental relationships of $RT6^-$ and $RT6^+$ T cells, *Dev. Immunol.* **1**:191.

Mukherjee, P., Mastro, A. M., and Hymer, W. C., 1990, Prolactin induction of interleukin-2 receptors on rat splenic lymphocytes, *Endocrinology* **126**:88.

Muller, K.-P., and Kyewski, B. A., 1993, T cell receptor targeting to thymic cortical epithelial cells in vivo induces survival, activation and differentiation of immature thymocytes, *Eur. J. Immunol.* **23**:1661–1670.

Munoz-Blay, T., Nieburgs, A. C., and Cohen, S., 1987, Thymic epithelium in vitro. V. Binding of thymocytes to cultured thymic epithelial cells, *Cell. Immunol.* **109**:371.

Murphy, W. J., Durham, S. K., and Longo, D. L., 1992, Role of neuroendocrine hormones in murine T cell development. Growth hormone exerts thymopoietic effects in vivo, *J. Immunol.* **149**:3851.

Nabarra, B., and Andrianarison, I., 1987a, Ultrastructural studies of thymic reticulum. I. Epithelial component, *Thymus* **9**:95.

Nabarra, B., and Andrianarison, I., 1987b, Pattern of secretion in thymic epithelial cells: Ultrastructural studies of the effect of blockage at various levels, *Cell Tissue Res.* **249**:171.

Nagamine, J., Takeda, K., Tatsumi, Y., Ogata, M., Miyake, K., Hamaoka, T., and Fujiwara, H., 1991, Role of a thymic stromal cell clone in inducing the stage-specific differentiation of various subpopulations of double-negative thymocytes, *J. Immunol.* **147**:1147.

Nagel, J. E., Chrest, F. J., and Adler, W. H., 1981, Enumeration of T lymphocyte subsets by monoclonal antibodies in young and aged humans, *J. Immunol.* **127**:2086.

Nakashima, M., Mori, K., Maeda, K., Kishi, H., Hirata, K., Kawabuchi, M., and Watanabe, T., 1990, Selective elimination of double-positive immature thymocytes by a thymic epithelial cell line, *Eur. J. Immunol.* **20**:47.

Nance, D. M., Hopkins, D. A., and Bieger, D., 1987, Re-investigation of the innervation of the thymus gland in mice and rats, *Brain Behav. Immun.* **1**:134.

Nieburgs, A. C., Korn, J. H., Picciano, P., and Cohen, S., 1984, The production of regulatory cytokines for thymocyte proliferation by murine thymic epithelium in vitro, *J. Immunol.* **124**:1287.

Nieburgs, A. C., Korn, J. H., Picciano, P. T., and Cohen, S., 1987, Thymic epithelium in vitro. IV. Regulation of growth and mediator production by epidermal growth factor, *Cell. Immunol.* **108**:396.

Ogata, M., Sato, S., Sano, H., Hamaoka, T., Doi, H., Nakanishi, K., Asano, Y., Itoh, T., and Fujiwara, H., 1987, Thymic stroma-derived T cell growth factor (TSTGF). Functional distinction of TSTGF from interleukin 2 and 4 and its preferential growth-promoting effect on helper T cell clones, *J. Immunol.* **139**:2675.

Olsen, N. J., Watson, M. B., Henderson, G. S., and Kovacs, W. J., 1991, Androgen deprivation induces phenotypic and functional changes in the thymus of adult male mice, *Endocrinology* **129**:2471.

Palacios, R., Studer, S., Samaridis, J., and Pelkonen, J., 1989, Thymic epithelial cells induce in vitro differentiation of PRO-T lymphocyte clones into TCRα, $\beta/T3^+$ and TCR, $/T3^+$ cells, *EMBO J.* **8**:4053.

Palmer, D. K. Brown, K. M., and Basch, R. S., 1991, Thymic stromal cells in culture. 2. Binding of normal thymocytes to a cloned thymic stromal cell line, *Cell. Immunol.* **138**:473.

Papiernik, M., 1990, Thymic accessory cells, cytokines and thymocyte activation, *Res. Immunol.* **141**:275.

Papiernik, M., Homo-Delarche, F., and Duval, D., 1984, Prostaglandins and interleukin 1 produced by phagocytic cells of the thymic reticulum in culture are able to regulate thymocyte proliferation, in: *Icosanoids and Cancer* (H. Thaler-Dao, ed.), Raven Press, New York, pp. 267–270.

Papiernik, M., Penit, C., and El Rouby, S., 1987, Control of prothymocyte proliferation by thymic accessory cells, *Eur. J. Immunol.* **17**:1303.

Pfeifer, J. D., Wetzel, G. D., and Dutton, R. W., 1986, Partial purification and characterization of a factor from a cloned thymic epithelial cell line, *J. Immunol.* **136**:555.

Ransom, J., Fischer, M., Mercer, L., and Zlotnik, A., 1987, Lymphokine-mediated induction of antigen-presenting ability in thymic stromal cells, *J. Immunol.* **139**:2620.

Reibnegger, G., Huber, L. A., Jurgens, G., Schonitzer, D., Werner, E. R., Wachter, H., Wick, G., and Traill, K. N., 1988, Approach to define normal aging in man. Immune function, serum lipids, lipoproteins and neopterin levels, *Mech. Ageing Dev.* **46**:67.

Robert, F., Geenen, V., Schoenen, J., Burgeon, E., De Groote, D., Defresne, M. P., Legros, J. J., and Franchimont, P., 1991, Colocalization of immunoreactive oxytocin, vasopressin and interleukin-1 in human thymic epithelial neuroendocrine cells, *Brain Behav. Immun.***5**:102.

Robert, F. R., Martens, H., Cormann, N., Benhida, A., Schoenen, J., and Geenen, V., 1992, The recognition of hypothalamo-neurohypophysial functions by developing T cells, *Dev. Immunol.* **2**:131.

Rocha, B., Dautigny, P., and Pereira, R., 1989, Peripheral T lymphocytes: Expansion potential and homeostatic regulation of pool sizes and CD4/CD8 ratios in vivo, *J. Immunol.* **19**:905.

Rocha, B., Vassalli, P., and Guy-Grand, D., 1992, The extrathymic T-cell development pathway, *Immunol. Today* **13**:449.

Ropke, C., and Elbroend, J., 1992, Human thymic epithelial cells in serum-free culture: Nature and effects on thymocyte cell lines, *Dev. Immunol.* **2**:111.

Rothenberg, E. V., 1980, Expression of differentiation antigens in subpopulations of mouse thymocytes: Regulation at the level of de novo synthesis, *Cell* **20**:1.

Rothenberg, E. V., 1992, The development of functionally responsive T cells, *Adv. Immunol.* **51**:85.

Russell, D. H., 1989, New aspects of prolactin and immunity: A lymphocyte-derived prolactin-like product and nuclear protein kinase C activation, *Trends Pharmacol. Sci.* **10**:40.

Russell, D. H., Zorn, N. E., Buckley, A. R., Crowe, P. D., Sauro, M. D., Hadden, E. M., Farese, R. V., and Laird, H. E., 1990, Prolactin and known modulators of rat splenotypes activate nuclear protein kinase C, *Eur. J. Pharmacol.* **188**:139.

Safieh, B., Kendall, M. D., Norman, J. C., Metreau, E., Dardenne, M., Bach, J.-F., and Pleau, J. M., 1990, A new radioassay for the thymic peptide thymulin, and its application for measuring thymulin in blood samples, *J. Immunol. Methods* **127**:255.

Saha, A. R., Hadden, E. M., Sosa, M., and Hadden, J. W., 1993, Thymus in neuroendocrine perspective, in *Nitric Oxide: Brain and Immune System* (S. Moncada, G. Nistico, and E. A. Higgs, eds.), Portland Press, London, pp. 43–54.

Salaun, J., Bandeira, A., Khazaal, I., Calman, F., Cotley, M., Coutinho, A., and le Douarin, N. M., 1990, Thymic epithelium tolerizes for histocompatibility antigens, *Science* **247**:1471.

Sandberg, G., and Ernstrom, U., 1991, In vivo stimulation of thymocyte proliferation by thymocyte growth peptide (TGP), *Int. J. Immunopharmacol.* **13**:649.

Savino, W., Wolf, B., Aratan-Spire, S., and Dardenne, M., 1984, Thymic hormone containing cells. IV. Fluctuation in the thyroid hormone levels in vivo can modulate the secretion of thymulin by the epithelial cells of young mouse thymus, *Clin. Exp. Immunol.* **55**:629.

Savino, W., Bartoccioni, E., Homo-Delarche, F., Gagnerault, M. C., Itoh, T., and Dardenne, M., 1988, Thymic hormone containing cells—IX. Steroids in vitro modulate thymulin secretion by human and murine thymic epithelial cells, *J. Steroid Biochem.* **30**:479.

Savino, W., Itoh, T., Hertogs, H., and Shoham, J., 1989, Contact-mediated maturational effects of thymic stromal cells on murine thymocytes in culture, *Immunology* **67**:496.

Savino, W., Ban, E., Ville-Verde, D. M., and Dardenne, M., 1990, Modulation of thymic endocrine function, cytokeratin expression and cell proliferation, by hormones and neuropeptides, *Int. J. Neurosci.* **51**:201.

Savino, W., Ville-Verde, D. M. S., and Lannes-Viera, J., 1993, Extracellular matrix proteins in intrathymic T-cell migration and differentiation? *Immunol. Today* **14**:158.

Sawada, M., Nagamine, J., Takeda, K., Utsumi, K., Kosugi, A., Tatsumi, Y., Hamaoka, T., Miyame, K., Nakajima, K., Watanabe, T., Sadakibara, S., and Fujiwara, H., 1992, Expression of VLA-4 on thymocytes. Maturation stage-associated transition and its correlation with their capacity to adhere to thymic stromal cells, *J. Immunol.* **149**:3517.

Schreiber, L., Eshel, I., Meilin, A., Sharabi, Y., and Shoham, J., 1991, Analysis of thymic stromal cell subpopulations grown in vitro on extracellular matrix in defined medium. III. Growth conditions of human thymic epithelial cells and immunomodulatory activities in their culture supernatant, *Immunology* **74**:621.

Scollay, R., 1985, Control of T-cell development, *Nature* **314:**97.

Scollay, R. G., Butcher, E. C., and Weissman, I. L., 1980, Thymus cell migration quantitative aspects of cellular traffic from the thymus to the periphery in mice, *Eur. J. Immunol.* **10:**210.

Scollay, R. G., Smith, J., and Stauffer, V., 1986, Dynamics of early T cells: Prothymocyte migration and proliferation in the adult mouse thymus, *Immunol. Rev.* **91:**129.

Screpanti, I., Meco, D., Scarpa, S., Morrone, S., Frati, L., Gulino, A., and Modesti, A., 1992, Neuromodulatory loop mediated by a nerve growth factor and interleukin 6 in thymic stromal cell cultures, *Proc. Natl. Acad. Sci. USA* **89:**3209.

Serrate, S. A., and Sztein, M. B., 1989, Characterization of the immunoregulatory properties of thymosin α_1 on interleukin-2 production and interleukin-2 receptor expression in normal human lymphocytes, *Int. J. Immunopharmacol.* **11:**789.

Shu, S., Naylor, P., Touraine, J.-L., and Hadden, J. W., 1996, IL-1, ICAM-1, LFA-3 and hydrocortisone differentially regulate cytokine secretion by human fetal thymic epithelial cells, *Thymus*, **24**:89.

Singer, K. H., Wolf, L. S., Lobach, D. F., Denning, S. M., Tuck, D. T., Robertson, A. L., and Haynes, B. F., 1986, Human thymocytes bind to autologous and allogeneic thymic epithelial cells in vitro, *Proc. Natl. Acad. Sci. USA* **83:**6588.

Singer, K. H., Denning, S. M., Whichard, L. P., and Haynes, B. F., 1990, Thymocyte LFA-1 and thymic epithelial cell ICAM-1 molecules mediate binding of activated human thymocytes to thymic epithelial cells, *J. Immunol.* **144:**2931.

Smith, P. E., 1930, Effect of hypophysectomy upon the involution of the thymus in the rat, *Anat. Rec.* **47:**119.

Sprent, J., Lo, D., Gao, E. K., and Ron, Y., 1988, T cell selection in the thymus, *Immuol. Rev.* **101:**173.

Sun, L., Riltch, A. S., Liu, P.-S., Johnson, L. A., and Hayashi, J., 1990, Thymocytes stimulate metabolism of arachidonic acid in rat thymic epithelial cells, *Cell. Immunol.* **131:**86.

Takahama, Y., Letterio, J. J., Suzuki, H., Farr, A. G., and Singer, A., 1994, Early progression of thymocytes along the CD4/CD8 developmental pathway is regulated by a subset of thymic epithelial cells expressing transforming growth factor β, *J. Exp. Med.* **179:**1495.

Talle, M. A., Brown, M. J., Blynn, C. M., Audhya, T. K., and Goldstein, G., 1991, Use of monoclonal antibodies to identify thymopoietin in cultured human thymic epithelial cells, *Thymus* **18:**169.

Tjonnfjord, G. E., Veiby, O. P., Steen, R., and Egeland, T., 1993, T lymphocyte differentiation in vitro from adult human prethymic CD34$^+$ bone marrow cells, *J. Exp. Med.* **177:**1531.

Tsang, K. Y., Fudenberg, H. H., Hoehler, F. K., and Hadden, J. W., 1984, Immunostimulating compounds: Isoprinosine and NPT 15392, in: *Immune Modulation Agents and Their Mechanisms* (R. L. Fenichel and M. A. Chirigos, eds.), Dekker, New York, pp. 79–95.

Twomey, J. J., Goldstein, G., Lewis, V. M., Bealmear, P. M., and Good, R. A., 1977, Bioassay determination of thymopoietin and thymic hormone levels in human plasma, *Proc. Natl. Acad. Sci. USA* **74:**2541.

Utsumi, K., Sawada, M., Narumiya, S., Nagamine, J., Sakata, T., Iwagami, S., Kita, Y., Teraoka, H., Hirano, H., Ogata, M., Hamaoka, T., and Fujiwara, H., 1991, Adhesion of immature thymocytes to thymic stromal cells through fibronectin molecules and its significance for the induction of thymocyte differentiation, *Proc. Natl. Acad. Sci. USA* **88:**5685.

Vollger, L. W., Tuck, D. T., Springer, A., Hayners, B. F., and Singer, K. H., 1987, Thymocyte binding to human thymic epithelial cells is inhibited by monoclonal antibodies to CD2 and LFA-3 antigens, *J. Immunol.* **138:**358.

Walker, R., Engelman, R., Pross, S., and Bercu, B., 1994, Effects of growth hormone secretagogues on age-related changes in the rat immune system, *Endocrine* **2:**857.

Winchurch, R. A., 1988, Activation of thymocyte responses to interleukin-1 by zinc, *Clin. Immunol. Immunopathol.* **47:**174.

Wiranowska, M., Kaido, T., Caspritz, G., Cook, J., and Hadden, J. W., 1987, Interleukin-2 and coculture with thymic epithelial cells synergistically induce prothymocyte differentiation and proliferation, *Thymus* **10:**231.

Wolf, G. T., Amendola, B. E., Diaz, R., Lovett, E. J., III, Hammerschmidt, R. M., and Peterson, K. A., 1985, Definitive vs. adjuvant radiotherapy. Comparative effects of lymphocyte subpopulations in patients with head and neck squamous carcinoma, *Arch. Otolaryngol. Head Neck Surg.* **111:**716.

CHAPTER 12

SOME EVOLUTIONARY, MORPHOREGULATORY, AND FUNCTIONAL ASPECTS OF THE IMMUNE–NEUROENDOCRINE CIRCUITRY

ANDOR SZENTIVANYI, CHRISTINE M. ABARCA, STUART M. BROOKS, RICHARD F. LOCKEY, and LEON D. PROCKOP

1. INTRODUCTION

David Wilson Talmage, one of the most important pioneers of the molecular biology of immunoregulation, in discussing recently (1988) what is beyond molecular immunology, poses the following questions:

> What will we study after we understand all the genes and their products that impact on the immune system? Surely, in a few years we will understand how lymphocytes differentiate and are activated, how they synthesize, secrete, kill, migrate. What will we study then? My prediction is that immunology will then have its greatest challenge. How can we put it all together for the benefit of mankind? How will we prevent allergies, autoimmunity, trans-

---

ANDOR SZENTIVANYI and RICHARD F. LOCKEY • Departments of Internal Medicine, Neurology, Pharmacology, and Environmental and Occupational Health, University of South Florida Colleges of Medicine and Public Health, Tampa, Florida 33612. CHRISTINE M. ABARCA • Department of Internal Medicine, University of South Florida Colleges of Medicine and Public Health, Tampa, Florida 33612. STUART M. BROOKS • Department of Environmental and Occupational Health, University of South Florida Colleges of Medicine and Public Health, Tampa, Florida 33612. LEON D. PROCKOP • Department of Neurology, University of South Florida Colleges of Medicine and Public Health, Tampa, Florida 33612.

Immunopharmacology Reviews, Volume 2, edited by John W. Hadden and Andor Szentivanyi. Plenum Press, New York, 1996.

> plant rejection, and how will we cure cancer? The coming era of immunology will be a stage of synthesis—a return to Stage 1 and the immunology of the whole animal. [Talmage, 1988]

This return to stage one, the immunology of the whole animal, has already begun as reflected by this chapter.

Indeed, of the various evolving views on immunologic inflammation, immunity, and hypersensitivity, this paper discusses the irrevocable shift and turnabout in our concepts of immunoregulation as connected with our growing understanding of the immune–neuroendocrine circuitry. This network, powerful enough both conceptually and in de facto functioning to bring about a radical change in our perceptions of the human immune, endocrine, and nervous systems, has already enlisted the minds, hearts, and resources of a large number of our leading laboratories in many areas of life sciences on an international scale.

The immune–neuroendocrine circuitry represents an immensely complex, powerful, and wide-ranging charter of human physiological and pathologic possibilities that, among others, is working its way to the creation of a new immunology based on a vastly enlarged vision of immunologic potential in health and disease.

2. THE DISCOVERY OF THE IMMUNE–NEUROENDOCRINE CIRCUITRY AND THE CONCEPTS OF PREVAILING IMMUNOLOGIC THOUGHT THAT IMPEDED THE TIMELY RECOGNITION OF ITS ROLE IN IMMUNE HOMEOSTASIS

The role of hypothalamic influences in the induction and expression of immunologic inflammation, immunity, and hypersensitivity was first discovered in the fall of 1951 at the University of Debrecen School of Medicine in Hungary. The rationale behind the decision for a systematic exploration of the hypothalamus was as follows. Historically, the interpretation of the symptomatology and the underlying reaction sequence of human asthma was patterned after those of the anaphylactic guinea pig. However, the range of atopic responsiveness in asthma includes a variety of stimuli that are nonimmunologic in nature. Foremost among these is a broad range of pharmacologically active mediators that today could be considered as the chemical organizers of central and peripheral autonomic regulation. Therefore, it was believed that anaphylaxis could not be used as a model for the investigation of the constitutional basis of atopy in asthma. It was postulated that such a model, if it were to be meaningful, must be able to imitate both the immunologic and autonomic abnormalities of the disease. Since at that early time (1951) none of the currently existing neuroactive agents (e.g., agonists, antagonists) that one could conceivably use as an experimental tool to induce an autonomic imbalance were in existence, it was concluded that the best chance to develop such a condition could be through various manipulations at the neuroendocrine regulatory level of the hypothalamus. Consequently, hypothalamically imbalanced anaphylactic animals were used. These were produced by the electrolytic lesion, and conversely, the electrical stimulation of various nuclear groupings in the hypothalamus through permanently implanted depth electrodes placed stereotaxically into the hypothalamus. The resulting cumulative findings obtained on such a model indicated that the hypothalamus has a modulatory influence on all cellular and humoral immune reactivities and that both neural as well as endocrine pathways are required for hypothalamic modulation of immune responses (Filipp *et al.*, 1952; Szentivanyi *et al.*, 1952, 1978, 1980, 1987b, 1988a,c,d,e, 1989a, 1990; Filipp and Szentivanyi, 1953, 1956, 1957, 1958, 1985; Szentivanyi, 1953, 1961, 1988a,b, 1989; Szentivanyi and Filipp, 1956, 1958; Szentivanyi and Szekely, 1956, 1957a, 1958; Szentivanyi and Fishel, 1965, 1966; Szentivanyi and Fitzpatrick, 1980; Szentivanyi and Szentivanyi, 1982a,b, 1987, 1988; J. Szentivanyi *et al.*, 1988, 1989a–c; Schwartz *et al.*, 1988).

Concurrently with these developments, however, an unparalleled expansion of information on the basic aspects of immunology, in general, and on the nature of antibody diversity, in particular, started to occupy the center stage of immunologic interest. Most importantly, the new perceptions surrounding the nature of antibody diversity began to surface in the late 1950s with the first conclusive genetic studies having been completed and a new set of concepts defined. These circumstances led to a total transformation of prevailing immunologic thought ultimately leading to the replacement of instructionist theories by the selective theories as advanced by Talmage (spring, 1957) and Burnet (fall, 1957).

Three major postulates were implicit in these theories of heritable cellular commitment: (1) the antigen receptor site and the antibody combining site whose synthesis that cell controls are identical and are derived at least partially from the same structural gene; (2) the condition guaranteeing the correspondence of the immunoglobulin synthesized with the antigen is that they are limited to the same cell that is the cell specialized for the synthesis of a single antibody; (3) the cell specialization stipulated in item 2 is inherited and, therefore, clonal (the clonal selection theory of acquired immunity). Subsequently, it became established that virtually all antibody diversity and specificity encoded in the immune system can be accounted for in genetic terms and thus the controls for the antibody response must reside largely within the major histocompatibility complex where different genes appear to code for immune response, suppression, and cell interaction. Another impediment in the timely recognition of the significance of the immune–neuroendocrine circuitry in immune homeostasis was the ability to have immune reactivities proceed *in vitro*. This further supported the concept that the immune system is a totally autonomous and self-regulating unit (this view has overlooked the rich neurohormonal milieu in which most *in vivo* immune responses occur). Sporadic refutations of these postulates have occurred and continue to surface in the literature, but the great bulk of the evidence is supportive of the clonal selection theory. The theory's sheer eloquence, however, has probably been most responsible for its dominant role in immunologic thought and its acceptance as dogma since the early 1960s. In any case, these concepts and the large body of supportive evidence have so permeated the field that it became difficult, if not impossible, to think of immunology outside of this framework (Szentivanyi, 1989).

In the late 1950s and throughout the 1960s the two conceptual centers of these ideas were under the leadership of D. W. Talmage at the University of Chicago and later at Colorado, and the group at Walter and Eliza Hall Institute in Australia under M. Burnet. Because of the close association with Talmage, extending over a period of 10 years, I was very much under the influence of these views and developed reservations against the significance of the above-mentioned hypothalamic findings in immunoregulation. Nevertheless, by 1966 in a chapter of a German text (Szentivanyi and Fishel, 1966) through an extensive analysis of these findings and the dominant immunologic concepts, the following conclusions were articulated: (1) the significance of the immunopharmacologic mediators of immune manifestations in normal mammalian physiology is that they are the chemical organizers of central and peripheral autonomic action; (2) the preceding suggests the inseparability of the immune response system from the neuroendocrine system; (3) such inseparability indicates the de facto existence of immune–neuroendocrine circuits and the necessity for a bidirectional flow of information between the two systems; (4) one must distinguish between the concepts of autoregulation as one that primarily revolves around one effector molecule of immunity, the antibody, and satisfies the requirements of antibody diversity and specificity in contrast to the more complex requirements of immune homeostasis; (5) in contrast to autoregulation that is always self-contained, homeostatic control is always beyond the constraints of one single cell or tissue system; and (6) thus, immune homeostasis must represent a far more sophisticated level of control than autoregulation, and is based on immune–neuroendocrine circuits. Indeed, as Gail Schechter (1989) points out, no bodily system is as simple, sacred, or singular as once thought. Instead, as in any good relationship, the separate components strive for sensitivity, synchrony, and synergy. Recognition and communication among the immune, endocrine, and nervous systems exemplify the formula for harmony and homeostasis.

While the manifold similarities between the immune and nervous systems are fully realized (see below), the immune system has a major additional level of complexity over that of the nervous system. Although the nervous system with its spectacular masses of much-revealing and well-defined projection patterns is well-moored in the body in a static web of axons, dendrites, and synapses, the elements of the immune system are in a continuously mobile phase incessantly scouring over and percolating through the body tissues, returning via an intricate system of lymphatic channels and then blending again in the blood. This dynamism is relieved only by scattered concentrations called *lymphoid organs*. These circumstances would appear to indicate that the functional plasticity of the immune system is far greater than that of the nervous system, and consequently, its regulation must require a more complex and sophisticated level of control. For these reasons, we have raised the frivolous question in the above-mentioned text in 1966 whether the immune system is more "intelligent" than the brain.

When these conclusions were reached (in the 1960s), our understandings of cellular immunology were in an early phase. The 1970s saw the discovery of the lymphokines, monokines, and a broad range of other effector molecules of immunologic inflammation, immunity, and hypersensitivity. But it was only in the 1980s that we began to recognize that the cells of the immune system synthesize, store, and release neurotransmitters, hypothalamo-hypophyseal hormones, etc., and by all criteria serve as neuroendocrine cells "par excellence" (Szentivanyi and Fishel, 1965, 1966; Szentivanyi *et al.*, 1978, 1980, 1989a; Hadden and Szentivanyi, 1985).

3. DEVELOPMENTAL INTERRELATIONSHIPS AMONG THE CELLULAR AND HUMORAL COMPONENTS OF THE IMMUNE–NEUROENDOCRINE CIRCUITRY

These interrelationships may be briefly stated through a discussion of (1) the cells involved in the synthesis, storage, secretion, and/or release of the effector molecules of immunologic reactivities; (2) neural crest interactions in the development of the immune system; (3) cerebral dominance or lateralization and immune disorders; (4) the ancient superfamily of immune recognition molecules and the neural cell adhesion molecule; (5) neuroactive immunoregulatory cytokines and growth factors; (6) coevolution of cytokine receptor families in the immune and nervous systems; (7) shared molecular mechanisms in the development of immune and neuronal memories; and (8) the unique recognition and communication powers of the immune and nervous systems as shared characteristics.

3.1. The Cells Involved in the Synthesis, Storage, Secretion, and/or Release of the Effector Molecules of Immunologic Reactivities

The functions of the immune system are the properties of cells distributed throughout the body. They include (1) free or circulating cells of the blood, lymph, and intravascular spaces; (2) similar cells collected into units that allow for close interaction with lymph or circulating blood—lymph nodes, spleen, liver, and bone marrow; and (3) two major control organs for the system, the thymus gland and the hypothalamic–pituitary–adrenal complex. The cells involved in the synthesis, storage, secretion, and/or release of the effector molecules of immunologic inflammation, immunity, and immunologically based hypersensitivity (allergy) represent a continuous spectrum of related cell types specialized in the production and storage of various physiopharmacologically active effector substances in variable proportions, i.e., of cells that have a common developmental origin with differentiation being determined by the specific requirements of the local neurohumoral regulation. Accounting only for those effector molecules for which the cell type has been identified, this incomplete spectrum of cells and effector substances includes macrophages and lymphocytes (interleukins 1–17, interferons, tumor necrosis factors, lysosome and complement components, prostaglandins, leukotrienes, acid hydrolases, neutral proteinases, arginase, nucleotide metabolites, various neuroactive immunoregulatory peptides including ACTH, CRF-like activity, bombesin, endorphins, enkephalins,

TSH, growth hormone, prolactin, neurotensin, chorionic gonadotropin, VIP, tachykinin neuropeptides including substance P, substance K, neuromedin K, somatostatins, mast cell growth factor, catecholamines, etc.), neutrophil leukocytes (SRS-A, ECF-A, enzymes, PAF and other vascular permeability factors, kinin-generating substances, a complement-activating factor, histamine releasers, a neutrophil inhibitory factor, VIP, 5-HETE, etc.), basophilic leukocytes (histamine, SRS-A, ECF-A, NCF, PAF, SP, SOMs, etc.), murine basophilic leukocytes (the same as in humans plus serotonin), eosinophilic leukocytes (PAF, 8, 15-diHETE, SRS-1, eosinophil peroxidase, major basic protein, etc.), serosal, connective tissue or TC mast cells (histamine, SRS-A, ECF-A, NCF, PAF, VIP, SP, SOMs, etc.), mucosal or T mast cells (histamine, SRS-A, ECF-A, NCF, PAF, VIP, SP, SOMs, etc.), "chromaffin-positive" mast cells (dopamine in ruminants; in other species possibly norepinephrine and neuropeptide Y), the so-called P cells (histamine, serotonin), enterochromaffin cells (serotonin), chromaffin cells (epinephrine, norepinephrine, dopamine, neuropeptide Y, IL-1α, etc.), platelets (depending on species, histamine, serotonin, catecholamines, prostaglandins, 12-HETE), neurosecretory cells (histamine, serotonin, catecholamines, acetylcholine, prostaglandins, and other eicosanoids, kinins, the various hypothalamic substances that release or inhibit the release of the anterior pituitary hormones, and the group of neuroactive immunoregulatory peptides including ACTH, bombesin, neurotensin, endorphins, enkephalins, TSH, growth hormone, prolactin, chorionic gonadotropin, VIP, the tachykinin neuropeptides, somatostatins, neuropeptide Y, IL-1α, IL-1β, IL-6, etc.), medullary thymic epithelial cells and the Hassall's corpuscles (thymosins and other thymic factors), SIF cells (dopamine), and other nerve cells including essentially all of the effector molecules listed under the neurosecretory cells. For more detailed information on the foregoing cell types and effector molecules, see Szentivanyi *et al.* (1990).

Many of these cell types possess different morphologic, physicochemical, and general biologic characteristics. Nevertheless, in passing from one member of this cell spectrum to another, obvious transitions are seen in all of these characteristics. Furthermore, when one surveys their properties and their probable physiologic function in the higher organism, significant cohesive features become apparent that set them apart from other body constituents as a distinct single class of cells that must be included in current concepts of neurosecretion.

There are some workers who postulated that the cellular components of the immune–neuroendocrine circuitry and their effector molecules could be viewed as two different divisions of this network. The two major divisions according to these workers may be defined as involved in neurovascular immunology and neuroendocrine immunology. Neurovascular immunology is concerned with immune response-related actions of vasoactive neurotransmitter substances that function as potent, short-lived local "hormones" first identified and studied as mediators of immunologic inflammation and hypersensitivity. They also play important roles in blood flow, vascular permeability, and pain transmission. These soluble effector molecules are simple compounds (i.e., amine mediators), short-chain peptides (i.e., kinins, substance P, etc.), and short-chain lipids (i.e., prostaglandins, leukotrienes) and have a long evolutionary history in biological defense. They use paracrine and synaptic signaling on their effector cells. The second major division, defined above as involved in neuroendocrine immunology, represents all of the immune response-related hypothalamic, pituitary, and other hormones that use endocrine signaling and are primarily immunomodulatory in character. This perhaps convenient but arbitrary functional separation of these two divisions is intrinsically incorrect as discussed in Szentivanyi (1993b).

3.2. Neural Crest Interactions in the Development of the Immune System

In discussing neural crest interactions in the development of the immune system at first we must briefly characterize the developmental biology of this structure. The neural crest is produced from ectodermal cells which are released from the apical portions of the neural folds at about the time fusion occurs to form the neural tube and a separate overlying ectodermal layer. The basement membrane underlying the neural crest cells breaks down, the cellular characteristics change, and they become separated from the other components of the neural fold. There is a change in relative spatial relationship, or migration, of the neural crest cells to varied associations and destinies (Goodman and Pearson, 1982).

We have known for some time that neural development is conducted in several distinct, consecutive steps but it is only recently that we have begun to understand the nature of the molecular mechanisms underlying these steps. The first step is primarily controlled by inductive mechanisms, i.e., by established diffusible factors of vertebrate embryonic induction. This is followed by intracellular regulation of a set of transcriptional factors containing, for instance, Hox and Pou domains (He and Rosenfeld, 1991; Willkinson and Krumlauf, 1990). When the neural tube is formed, neural crest cells, i.e., multipotent stem cells, start to differentiate into the various cell types that comprise the nervous system. This is the stage at which neuronal immunoglobulin gene superfamilies (IgSFs) and cytokine receptors play important roles. Three processes take place at this stage to form the nervous system: cell migration, pathway finding, and determination of cell lineage. Recent studies suggest that the molecules involved in these three processes may have originated from the same protein molecule that has also evolved to generate major molecules in the immune system (see discussion of coevolution of cytokine receptors in the immune and nervous systems below).

The portion of the neural crest pertinent to this discussion is that which is closely associated with the developing brain, specifically, the hindbrain. Crest cells in this cranial portion (anterior to the fifth somite) differentiate into mesenchyme, in addition to other connective tissue, muscular and nervous components. Neural crest cells migrate ventrolaterally through the bronchial arches and contribute mesenchymal cells to a number of structures. It is this mesenchyme that forms the layers around the epithelial primordia of the thymus (LeDouarin, 1982).

The full significance of the foregoing will be even more appreciated when viewed in the context of three additional considerations: (1) the thymus is formed by contributions from different sources which must interact in a precisely timed sequence for proper development; (2) ablation of small portions of neural crest prevents or alters the development of the thymus; and (3) formation of the thymus precedes that of the more secondary, peripheral lymphoid tissues reflecting a critical thymic role already in the early development of the immune system. Taken together, development of the immune system is inherently linked to the neural crest and any aberration in this link results in defective immune development such as that seen for instance in the DiGeorge syndrome.

3.3. The Ancient Superfamily of Immune Recognition Molecules and the Neural Cell Adhesion Molecule (N-CAM)

The ancient superfamily of immune recognition molecules and the N-CAM represent another aspect of the interrelationships among the cellular and molecular components of the immune–neuroendocrine circuitry. Most of the glycoproteins that mediate cell–cell recognition or antigen recognition in the immune system contain related structural elements, suggesting that the genes that encode them have a common evolutionary history. Included in this Ig superfamily are antibodies, T-cell receptors, MHC glycoproteins, the CD2, CD4, and CD8 cell–cell adhesion proteins, some of the polypeptide chains of the CD3 complex associated with T-cell receptors and the various Fc receptors on lymphocytes and other white blood cells—all of which contain one or more Ig-like domains (Ig homology units). Each Ig homology unit is usually encoded by a separate exon, and it seems likely that the entire supergene family evolved from a gene coding for a single Ig homology unit similar to that encoding Thy-1 or β_2-microglobulin which may have been involved in mediating cell–cell interactions. Since a Thy-1-like molecule has been isolated from the brain of squids, it is probable that such a primordial gene arose before vertebrates diverged from their invertebrate ancestors some 400 million years ago. New family members presumably arose by exon and gene duplications, and similar duplication events probably gave rise to the multiple gene segments that encode antibodies and T-cell receptors (Cunningham *et al.*, 1987).

An increasing number of cell-surface glycoproteins that mediate Ca^{2+}-independent cell–cell adhesion in vertebrates are being discovered to belong to the Ig superfamily. One of these is the so-called N-CAM, which is a large, single-pass transmembrane glycoprotein (about 1000 amino acid residues long). N-CAM is expressed on the surface of nerve cells and glial cells and causes them to stick together by Ca^{2+}-independent mechanisms. When these membrane proteins are purified and inserted into synthetic phospholipid vesicles, the vesicles bind to one another, as well as to cells that have N-CAM on their surface; the binding is blocked if the cells are pretreated with monovalent anti-N-CAM antibodies. Thus, N-CAM binds cells together by a homophilic interaction that directly joins two N-CAM molecules (Milner *et al.*, 1989).

Anti-N-CAM antibodies disrupt the orderly pattern of retinal development in tissue culture and when injected into the developing chick eye, disturb the normal growth pattern of retinal nerve cell axons. These observations suggest that N-CAM plays an important part in the development of the central nervous system by promoting cell–cell adhesion. In addition, the neural crest cells that form the peripheral nervous system have large amounts of N-CAM on their surface when they are associated with the neural tube, lose it while they are migrating, and then reexpress it when they aggregate to form a ganglion suggesting that N-CAM plays a part in the assembly of the ganglion.

There are several forms of N-CAM, each encoded by a distinct mRNA. The different mRNAs are generated by alternative splicing of an RNA transcript produced from a single large gene. The large extracellular part of the polypeptide chain (~ 680 amino acid residues) is identical in most forms of N-CAM and is folded into five domains characteristic of antibody molecules. Thus, N-CAM belongs to the same ancient superfamily of recognition proteins to which antibodies belong (Williams and Barclay, 1988; Brümmendorf and Rathjen, 1994).

I have mentioned earlier the guidance provided by the neural crest in the development of the thymus, that is, a central regulatory organ for the immune system. The converse also appears to be true: the immune system has a special role in the development of the nervous system. In this context, the most critical feature of the immune system is its tremendous polymorphism so that lymphocytes that are produced can recognize enormous numbers of different antigens. For this reason, the immune system is ideally suited to provide markers or "anchoring sites" that enable developing structures to be built up in precisely the correct form. In no organ system is this type of detailed anchorage mechanism as important as in the developing nervous system in which many millions of nerve fibers traverse great distances and establish connections with particular groups of target cells. Marking by means of histocompatibility antigens provides exactly such a system, as indeed the original function of the MHC antigens was defined in the 1970s as the general plasma membrane anchorage site of organogenesis-directing proteins (Edelman, 1987).

3.4. Extracellular Matrix Proteins with Neurite-Promoting Activity and Their Relation to the Immunoglobulin Superfamily

Nerve cells, i.e., neurons, have two special properties that distinguish them from all other cells in the body. First, they conduct bioelectric signals for long distances without any loss of signal strength. Second, they possess specific intercellular connections with other nerve cells and with innervated tissues such as muscles and glands. These connections determine the types of information a neuron can receive and the range of responses it can yield in return (Szentivanyi and Fishel, 1966). The functionally most revealing structural feature of the neuron is the characteristic specialized contact zone that has been presumptively identified as the site of interneuronal communication, i.e., the synapse.

This specialized contact zone is composed of presumed proteinaceous material lining the intracellular portions of the pre- and postsynaptic membranes and filling the synaptic cleft between the apposed cell surfaces. Such types of specialized contacts are a general form of the specialized cell contacts seen between many types of cells derived from the embryonic ectoderm, of which the nerve cell is but one. However, the specialized contact between neurons is polarized; that is, the presynaptic terminal intracellular material is composed of interrupted presynaptic dense projections measuring about 500–700 Å in diameter and separated from each other by 300–400 Å. This material may be present only to bind specific presynaptic nerve endings permanently to specific postsynaptic cell sites. Alternatively, the specialized contact zone could assist in the efficiency of transmission of the nerve impulse and could constitute a method for modulating synaptic transmission in terms of discharge frequency (Szentivanyi *et al.*, 1980; Szentivanyi and Fitzpatrick, 1980). For these reasons, this specialized contact zone must be regarded as a unique association of two cells, and therefore, the synapse represents a special *sui generis* neuronal feature (see below).

Neurite promotion from the neurons is one of the most important events in the process of synapse formation. Therefore, this section focuses on extracellular matrix (ECM) proteins with neurite-promoting activity including their receptors, cell adhesion molecules in addition to the above-described NCAM, and their relation to members of the immunoglobulin superfamily.

Although many ECM proteins have been isolated recently, the ECM proteins that exhibit the neurite-promoting activity are type IV collagen, fibronectin, laminin, and a newly discovered protein, the so-called *neurite outgrowth factor* (NOF) which promotes neurite outgrowth from various neurons (Kato *et al.*, 1983, 1992; Taniura *et al.*, 1991; Taira *et al.*, 1993) such as sympathetic, parasympathetic, sensory, motor, and central neurons. Laminin, and its family proteins, exhibit the highest activity for promoting neurite outgrowth.

Laminin is a glycoprotein of about 900 kDa, a main component of the basement membrane, and possesses a variety of cellular functions such as neurite outgrowth-promoting (Evercooren *et al.*, 1982), cell adhesive (Graf *et al.*, 1987), growth factor-like (Panayotou *et al.*, 1989), calcium-binding, and metastatic activities. Compared with other ECM proteins, the neurite outgrowth-promoting activity is the strongest. Structurally, laminin is composed of three subunits of A chain (440 kDa), B_1 chain (230 kDa), and B_2 chain (220 kDa) that are assembled by disulfide bonds to form a cruciform structure.

NOF, a glycoprotein of about 720 kDa, has been shown to be present in the extracellular matrix of muscle fibers and the ciliary ganglion. A partial primary structure of NOF is homologous (80%) with laminin B_1 chain, indicating NOF belongs to the laminin family. The neurite outgrowth by NOF is strictly dependent on the developmental stage. Thus, ciliary neurons until embryonic 10 day can fully extend the neurites in the presence of NOF, but thereafter the neurons rapidly lose this ability.

Study of the receptors for ECM proteins started in 1984 with the work of Tamkun *et al.* who isolated a fibronectin receptor cDNA and named it *integrin*. Thereafter, integrin has been used as a general term for ECM protein receptors. The cDNA cloning of the NOF receptor indicates that there are at least two mRNAs that encode NOF receptor which may be produced by alternative splicing occurring in the region that codes a cytoplasmic domain, because C-terminal length differs in obtained cDNA clones. Since no homology could be found with any known nucleic acid sequences, it is suggested that NOF receptor is a novel protein. The receptor is composed of 583 amino acids including a signal sequence. The deduced amino acid sequence revealed that the NOF receptor has five repeats of immunoglobulin (Ig)-like domain in its extracellular region, indicating that the NOF receptor belongs to the Ig superfamily. Weak homology (20–30%) is observed with other Ig superfamily molecules such as SCI, NCAM, and VCAM in amino acid sequence.

In the nervous system, many Ig superfamily proteins are found to participate in the cell attachment (Salzer and Colman, 1989). In the vertebrate brain, NCAM (Edelman, 1988), SCI (Tanaka *et al.*, 1991), LI (Rathjen and Schachner, 1984), MAG (Arquint *et al.*, 1987), and PO (Sakamoto *et al.*, 1987) are the major Ig superfamily proteins (Brümmendorf and Rathjen, 1994).

4. NEUROPOIETIC IMMUNOMODULATORY CYTOKINES AND GROWTH FACTORS

Many immunomodulatory cytokines and growth factors, when studied for neuroactivity, were found to possess such capacity. At the time of this writing, however, there are only a few agents whose neuropoietic characterization progressed to a point that their separate and individual discussion is both indicated and possible. They include the ciliary neurotropic factor, the leukemia inhibitory factor, oncostatin M, and beta-nerve growth factor.

4.1. Ciliary Neurotropic Factor (CNTF)

Human CNTF is a 200-amino-acid-residue, single-chain polypeptide of 22.7 kDa. It is highly conserved across species lines as amino acid sequence comparisons of human with rat and rabbit CNTF show 83 and 87% identity, respectively (Lam *et al.*, 1991; Lin *et al.*, 1989; Stockli *et al.*, 1989). To date, CNTF has been localized to Schwann cells and type 1 astrocytes (Stockil *et al.*, 1991; Rende *et al.*, 1992; Rudge *et al.*, 1994). It has demonstrated activity as a survival and differentiation factor for cells of the nervous system.

Originally identified as a tropic factor for 8-day chick embryo ciliary (parasympathetic) ganglion neurons (Barbin *et al.*, 1984), that is, cells that normally died without tropic supplement(s), CNTF has subsequently been shown to exhibit *in vitro* survival-promoting activity on sensory (dorsal root) ganglion neurons, nonautonomic motor neurons, and sympathetic motor neurons (Barbin *et al.*, 1984; Manthorpe *et al.*, 1986; Martinou *et al.*, 1992; Magal *et al.*, 1991a,b; Forger *et al.*, 1993; Kotzbauer *et al.*,

1994). This enhanced neuronal survival activity was also confirmed in *in vivo* studies. CNTF has been proposed to be a rescue factor for damaged or axotomized neurons which is supported by the observations that (1) motor neuron death that follows axotomy of the rat facial nerve may be reversed by applying rat CNTF to the proximal axonal segment (Sendtner *et al.*, 1992) and (2) recombinant human CNTF injected into rat lateral ventricles prevents the death of axotomized medial septal neurons (axons of cholinergic and GABAergic neurons) projecting to the hippocampus (Lams and Isacson, 1988; Hagg *et al.*, 1992).

CNTF also serves as a neuronal differentiation factor capable of influencing the phenotype of a neuron. Thus, this cytokine can dictate the type of neurotransmitter used, neuropeptide produced, and the type of synapses made between two neurons (Landis, 1990; Patterson and Nawa, 1993). Indeed, CNTF has been shown *in vitro* to induce cholinergic properties in otherwise adrenergic motor neurons including the expression of acetylcholine (ACh) as neurotrasmitter and substance P (SP) and vasoactive intestinal peptide (VIP) as ACh-associated neuropeptides (Saadat *et al.*, 1989; Rao *et al.*, 1992). Although usually associated with the cholinergic phenotype, CNTF has also been shown to promote the adrenergic phenotype in rat fetal locus coeruleus cell cultures (Louis *et al.*, 1993), and adrenal chromaffin cells (Tokiwa *et al.*, 1994). Another function of CNTF is in glial differentiation. In cultures of oligodendroglia type 2 astrocyte progenitors, if applied in the presence of the extracellular matrix, CNTF promotes the development of either oligodendroglia or type astrocytes (Mayer *et al.*, 1994) which is in functional agreement that type 1 astrocytes are known to synthesize CNTF (Stockli *et al.*, 1991; Hughes *et al.*, 1988). Finally, like IL-6 CNTF induces fever following intravenous injection (Shapiro *et al.*, 1993).

4.2. Leukemia Inhibitory Factor (LIF)

This cytokine was originally identified as a factor that inhibited proliferation and induced macrophage differentiation of the murine myeloid leukemic cell line MI. Subsequent to its purification and molecular cloning, LIF was recognized to be a pleiotropic factor that is identical to a number of other proteins previously purified as based on numerous other biological activities. These circumstances led to the development of a variety of synonyms* for LIF. LIF expression has been detected in a number of cell lines. Of these we list here only those that are clearly important for the objectives of this chapter such as stimulated T lymphocytes and monocytes (Anegon and Grolleau, 1991; Gillett *et al.*, 1993), mast cells (Lorenzo *et al.*, 1994), Schwann cells (Marshall *et al.*, 1993), astrocytes (Aloisi *et al.*, 1994), bone marrow stromal cells, and thymic epithelial cells (Metcalf, 1992; Bhatt *et al.*, 1991). In some of these

*Synonyms for LIF include differentiating stimulating factor (D factor) or differentiation inducing factor (DIF); differentiation-inhibition activity (DIA) or differentiation retarding factor (DRF); hepatocyte-stimulating factor III (HSFIII); cholinergic neuronal differentiation factor (CNF/CDF/CNDF); human interleukin for DA cells (HILDA); osteoclast-activating factor (OAF); and melanoma-derived lipoprotein lipase inhibitor (MLPLI).

cell types, synthesis of LIF has been induced by LPS, phorbol ester, calcium ionophore, retinoic acid, and TNF-α (Metcalf, 1992; Kurzrock *et al.*, 1991; Gough, 1992; Van Vlasselaer, 1992; Aggarwal and Gutterman, 1992).

Human LIF cDNA encodes a 202-amino-acid-residue polypeptide that is cleaved to yield a 180-amino-acid-residue mature human LIF. Native human and murine LIFs are highly glycosylated single-chain molecules varying in molecular mass from 38 to 67 kDa.

LIF has multiple effects on both hematopoietic and nerve cell populations. Its activities overlap those of IL-6, IL-11, CNTF, and oncostatin M (shared gp130 signal-transducing subunit in their receptor complexes). LIF also shows synergistic activity with IL-3 to increase the production of primitive hematopoietic progenitor (Leary *et al.*, 1990) and megakaryocyte colonies (Metcalf *et al.*, 1991). In the nervous system, LIF regulates the levels of both muscarinic and substance P receptor mRNAs in sympathetic neurons and can induce neurotransmitter switching of sympathetic neurons from noradrenergic to cholinergic *in vitro* and *in vivo* (Bamber *et al.*, 1994; Ludlam *et al.*, 1994). It selectively increases CNS cholinergic differentiation in neurons whose projections are peripheral targets (Mayer *et al.*, 1994) and probably plays a role in early neural crest-derived sensory neuron development (Qui *et al.*, 1994; Murphy *et al.*, 1993). Moreover, LIF has the potential to rescue sensory and motor neurons from axotomized death through retrograde axonal LIF transport (Cheema *et al.*, 1994a,b). In cultures of O-2A progenitors, LIF induces oligodendroglia formation and in the presence of endothelial cell-derived extracellular matrix it promotes the differentiation of O-2A progenitors into type 2 astrocytes (Mayer *et al.*, 1994).

4.3. ONCOSTATIN M (OSM)

This substance was originally isolated as a growth inhibitor of A375 melanoma cells from the conditioned medium of phorbol-ester-treated U937 human histiocytic lymphoma cells (Zarling *et al.*, 1986). In subsequent studies, OSM became recognized as a member of a family of cytokines that includes LIF, IL-6, IL-11, and CNTF. These cytokines have similar protein tertiary structures and gene organization, have overlapping biological activities, and share gp130 as a signal transducer (Rose and Bruce, 1991; Bazan, 1991; Nishimoto *et al.*, 1994; Zhang *et al.*, 1994; Hirano *et al.*, 1994; Gearing, 1993; Bruce *et al.*, 1992a,b). OSM is produced by activated monocytes/macrophages and T lymphocytes (Rose and Bruce, 1991), expressed in AIDS-related Kaposi's sarcoma (KS)-derived spindle cells, and is an autocrine growth factor for KS (Cai *et al.*, 1994). With a molecular mass of approximately 28 kDa, OSM is a single-chain glycoprotein the DNA of which has been cloned (Malik *et al.*, 1989). The gene for OSM has been mapped to chromosome 22 at q12 (Jeffery *et al.*, 1993; Giovannini *et al.*, 1993) within 19-kb of the LIF gene. The two genes are arranged in a head- to-head orientation, suggesting that common regulatory elements may lie within the 19-kb region between the two genes (Kallestad *et al.*, 1991).

Additional OSM activities beyond those shared with LIF, IL-6, IL-11, or CNTF include the induction of differentiation of MI murine myeloid leukemia cells (Bruce *et al.*, 1992a,b), the stimulation of G-CSF and GM-CSF production by human endothelial cells, and the blockade of IL-6 in those cell lines that express gp130 but lack functional OSM receptors (Sporeno *et al.*, 1994).

4.4. Nerve Growth Factor (NGF or β-NGF)

Nerve growth factor is a 26-kDa, nonglycosylated, homodimeric polypeptide originally identified as a neurotropic factor for embryonic sympathetic neurons (Levi-Montalcini and Hamburger, 1951; Ullrich *et al.*, 1983; Iwane *et al.*, 1990). In addition to NGF, three other NGF-related molecules have been identified: brain-derived neurotropic factor (BDNF), neurotropin-3 (NT-3), and neurotropins 4/5 (NT-4/5) (Berkemeier *et al.*, 1991; Jones and Reichardt, 1990; Rosenthal *et al.*, 1990; Ip *et al.*, 1992a). Cells known to synthesize either NGF or NGF mRNA include submandibular duct epithelium, neurons, Schwann cells, fibroblasts, smooth muscle cells, astrocytes, $CD4^+$ T cells, macrophages, mast cells, and embryonic keratinocytes (Bradshaw *et al.*, 1993; Missale *et al.*, 1994; Meakin and Shooter, 1992; Korsching, 1993; Ebendal, 1992; Chao, 1992; Szeberenyi and Erhardt, 1994; Kakihana *et al.*, 1993; Ehrhard *et al.*, 1993a; Leon *et al.*, 1994). Factors known to regulate NGF secretion in astrocytes include IL-1, IL-4, and IL-5 (Carman-Krzan *et al.*, 1991; Awatsuji *et al.*, 1993).

Within the nervous system, NGF has a remarkably broad spectrum of documented activities. It includes the blocking of natural cell death in developing sensory and sympathetic neurons, the rescue of basal forebrain cholinergic neurons following axotomy, the induction of proliferation and differentiation of adult adrenal chromaffin cells, and support provided to cerebellar granule neurons during ontogenesis (Tischler *et al.*, 1993; Morimoto *et al.*, 1994; Muller *et al.*, 1994). NGF plays a significant role in hematopoiesis and the immune system. In early hematopoiesis, NGF is as effective as IL-1 in synergizing with M-CSF (CSF-1) to generate early hematopoietic progenitors with or without pluripotent stem cells and GM-CSF colonies (Chevalier *et al.*, 1994). NGF is chemotactic for neutrophils, enhances threefold the *in vitro* survival of neutrophils, increases by twofold neutrophil phagocytic activity, induces superoxide production (DeSimone *et al.*, 1990), and has a significant role in monocyte maturation (Ehrhard *et al.*, 1993).

In humoral immunity, NGF induces B-cell differentiation and promotes IgM, IgA, and, most significantly, IgG4 synthesis in mononuclear cells (Kimata *et al.*, 1991; Otten *et al.*, 1989). Both B cells and $CD3^+$ T cells proliferate in response to NGF. In the field of allergy, NGF has established effects on cells of the mast cell/basophil lineage. Thus, NGF enhances the activity of T-cell-derived GM-CSF in the promotion of basophil differentiation from basophil progenitors and prepares basophils for histamine release in response to anti-IgE exposure (Tsuda *et al.*, 1991; Bischoff and Dahinden, 1992). NGF has been demonstrated to induce mast cell degranulation in a calcium-independent manner with a substantial increase in histamine release in response to antigen stimulation (DeSimone *et al.*, 1990; Bischoff and Dahinden, 1992). Also, there is a strong correlation between serum NGF levels and systemic lupus erythematosus, an autoimmune disease (Bracci-Laudiero *et al.*, 1993). Finally, NGF protection of cholinergic neurons arrests and/or improves memory decline and it was shown to reverse age-related cognitive dysfunction in aged rats (Barinaga, 1994; Markowska *et al.*, 1994).

5. COEVOLUTION OF CYTOKINE RECEPTOR FAMILIES IN THE IMMUNE AND NERVOUS SYSTEMS

Established members of neurotropic factors (NTFs) and neuronal differentiation factors (NDFs) belong to two major groups: cytokines and growth factors. The family of cytokines may be divided into three subclasses based on structural homology of their receptors (Bazan, 1990, 1991): (1) class I receptors: IL-1R, -3R, -4R, -5R, -6R, and -7R, granulocyte–macrophage colony-stimulating factor receptor (GMCSFR), erythropoietin receptor (EPR), cholinergic differentiation factor receptor (CDFR), leukemia inhibitory factor receptor (LIFR), ciliary neutropic factor receptor (CNTFR); (2) class II receptors: interferon-α receptor (INF-αR), interferon-γ receptor (INF-γR), and tissue factor receptor (TFR); and (3) class III receptors, i.e., those receptors whose primary structures belong to immunoglobulin gene superfamilies (IgSFs) such as IL-1. Growth factors can be classified into gene families based on the homology of their structures: nerve growth factor (NGF) family, fibroblast growth factor (FGF) family, epidermal growth factor (EGF) family, insulin growth factor (IGF) family, etc.

Class I cytokine receptors can be further divided into at least two subtypes, class Ia and class Ib, based on structural differences (Yamamori and Sarai, 1992). Class Ia includes IL-2R, -3R, and -5R, and GM-CSFR (Miyajima *et al.*, 1992) and consists of the common cytokine domain with four conserved cysteines and a Trp-Ser-X(variable residues)-Trp-Ser motif near the transmembrane domains. Class Ib contains IL-6R, CNTFR, LIFR, and G (granulocyte)-CSFR, and has additional elements, i.e., three fibronectinlike domains near the transmembrane domain and an Ig-like domain at the N-terminus in the extracellular sites. It is the group of cytokines in class Ib that is of special interest to us in the context of this discussion. As briefly mentioned above, a number of NTFs and NDFs have been identified recently together with their receptors at molecular levels. It was shown that NTFs enhance survival of certain types of neurons whereas NDFs affect neuronal phenotype without having any influence on neuronal survival. Cholinergic differentiation factor (CDF) that has a potent NDF activity on sympathetic neurons is identical to leukemia inhibitory factor (LIF) that plays an important role in the immune system (Yamamori *et al.*, 1989). Ciliary neutropic factor (CNTF) with an NTF activity on ciliary ganglion neurons also possesses NDF activity as that of CDF/LIF by inducing cholinergic differentiation of sympathetic neurons in culture (Saadat *et al.*, 1989). Another member of this group (class Ib), IL-6, an established immunoregulatory molecule, improves the survival of messencephalic catecholaminergic and septal cholinergic neurons from postnatal rats (2 weeks old) in cultures (Hama *et al.*, 1991), and triggers the association of its receptor (IL-6R) with the signal transducer gp130 (Taga *et al.*, 1989). Generation of sensory neurons is stimulated by LIF (Murphy *et al.*, 1991) and LIFR is structurally related to the IL-6 signal transducer gp130 (Gearing *et al.*, 1991). Furthermore, there is evidence that not only LIF but also CNTF act on neuronal cells via a shared signal pathway that involves the IL-6 signal transducing receptor component (Ip *et al.*, 1992b).

In view of the very similar NTF and NDF activities of all cytokine members of class Ib, Yamamori (1992) proposed that their receptors are likely to have a closely similar structure. This suggestion was considerably strengthened by findings in a number of laboratories showing that their receptors belong to a subclass of receptors for cytokines with both neuronal and immunoregulatory activities (Davis *et al.*, 1991; Gearing and Cosman, 1991; Hall and Rao, 1992; Jessell and Melton, 1992; Patterson, 1992). This close structural relationship between the nervous and immune systems at the molecular level may be explained by evolutionary mechanisms in agreement with the proposal of Edelman (1989) that the structural resemblance of immunoglobulin and neural cell surface molecules may have resulted from a common evolutionary origin, and with the analysis of Bazan (1990) of the structural design and molecular evolution of the cytokine receptor superfamily. Finally, Yamamori and Sarai (1992), in an attempt to trace the evolutionary origin of the cytokine receptors, constructed a higher subdomain structure of the receptor for CDF/LIF based on its known primary structure. In their study, the receptor appears to contain immunoglobulin and fibronectin-like domains in addition to common domains of the cytokine receptor, similar to those cell surface molecules of the neural IgSFs. Taken together, these and other above-mentioned findings indicate that the class Ib cytokine receptor evolved as a consequence of fusion of the genes for a more primitive cytokine receptor in class Ia and for the IgSF, and similarly that a large number of molecules regulating neural development and vertebrate immunoregulation have a common evolutionary background. Thus, the origin of cytokine receptors represents a classical example of molecular coevolution in the immune and nervous systems (Yamamori and Sarai, 1992).

6. CEREBRAL DOMINANCE OR LATERALIZATION AND IMMUNE DISORDERS

The recognition of cerebral lateralization grew out of the discovery in the last century of cerebral dominance, that is, the superior capacity of each side of the brain to acquire particular skills. Over the past 120 years, it was believed that hemispheric dominance was based on functional asymmetry—on the differences in function of the two sides of the brain and of specific regions within them. In the face of the prevalent belief that cerebral dominance lacked an anatomic correlate, work over the past three decades has conclusively established that cerebral dominance is based on asymmetries of structure. An example of this is the early detectable asymmetry in the human brain that involves the upper surface of the posterior portion of the left temporal lobe, the *planum temporale*. The larger size of the left *planum temporale* reflects the greater extent of a particular temporoparietal cytoarchitectonic area on the left. There are other asymmetries in the human brain and the same applies to the findings throughout the animal kingdom. In addition to genetics, several other factors in the course of development, both prenatal and postnatal, influence the direction and extent of these structural differences (Geschwind and Galaburda, 1985).

Associations of anomalous cerebral dominance include not only developmental disorders such as dyslexia, autism, stuttering, mental retardation, and learning disorders, as well as some extraordinary musical, mathematic, athletic, and other talents,* but also alterations in many bodily systems including the immune system. In these situations, the same influences that modify structural asymmetry in the brain also modify other systems such as the immune system. The suspected molecular mechanisms involved in the influence of structural asymmetry on the development of immune reactivities are discussed in more detail in two larger reviews (Szentivanyi, 1991, 1993b). Here I shall only mention that animal experiments in the past 10 years provided some insight into the nature of the association between anomalous hemispheric dominance and immune reactivities.

Thus, beginning in 1980 and continuing throughout the decade, Renoux and coworkers showed that immunomodulation of the T-cell lineage in rodents can be a phenomenon of hemispheric lateralization. In 1980, the initial observation yielded data indicating that lesioning the left cerebral neocortex depresses T-cell-mediated responses in mice without affecting B-cell responses. These observations were extended in experiments where animals with a right cortical lesion served as controls for animals with a left cortical ablation. The findings demonstrated a balanced brain asymmetry in which the right hemisphere controls the inductive influence on T cells of signals emitted by the left hemisphere. In addition, most recent studies found that ditiocarb sodium (Imuthiol), an immunostimulant specifically active on the T-cell lineage, can replace the signals emitted by the left neocortex, since mice without a left neocortex were stimulated to increase T-cell-dependent responses by treatment with ditiocarb sodium, whereas the agent did not modify the responses already increased in right decorticates. B-cell-dependent and some macrophage-dependent responses are not affected by either neocortical ablation or ditiocarb sodium. This lateralization of cortical influences on immune function in rodents is likely to be predictive of an even greater influence in humans with more profound and complex cortical functions (Renoux *et al.*, 1987).

*It is difficult to speak in some of these cases of extraordinary talents as the "pathology of superiority" but that is what the evidence dictates.

7. IMMUNE AND NEURONAL MEMORY

The immune system and the nervous system possess short- or long-term memory, or both. The latter may be defined as the recording of experiences that can modify behavior. This general definition encompasses a broad spectrum of phenomena from the bacterial capacity of sensing chemical gradients to cognitive learning in humans.

The clonal selection theory of acquired immunity provides a useful conceptual framework for understanding the cellular basis of immunologic memory. According to this scheme, immunologic memory is generated during the primary immune response because (1) the proliferation of antigen-triggered virgin cells creates a large number of memory cells—a process known as clonal expansion; (2) the memory cells have a much longer life span than do virgin cells and recirculate between the blood and secondary lymphoid organs; and (3) each memory cell is able to respond more readily to antigen than does a virgin cell.

One reason, if not the most important reason, for the increased responsiveness of memory B cells is the higher affinity (avidity) of their antibody receptors for the homologous antigen. Thus, with the passage of time after immunization there is a progressive increase in the affinity of antibodies produced against the immunizing antigen. This phenomenon is known as affinity maturation and is the result of the accumulation of somatic mutations in variable (V)-region coding sequences after antigenic stimulation of B lymphocytes. The rate of somatic mutation in these sequences is estimated to be 10^{-3} per nucleotide pair per cell generation which is about a million times greater than the spontaneous mutation rate in other genes. This process is called somatic hypermutation. Since B cells are stimulated to proliferate by the binding of antigen, any mutation occurring during the course of an immune response that increases the affinity of a cell surface antibody molecule will cause the preferential proliferation of the B cell making the antibody, especially when antigen concentration decreases with increasing time after immunization. Thus, affinity maturation is the consequence of repeated cycles of somatic hypermutation followed by antigen-driven selection in the course of an antibody response.

Research in the field of neuronal memory is still in an early phase primarily because of methodologic difficulties and the validity of approaches currently used. The human brain is extraordinarily complex (10^{12} neurons) and intricate (an average neuron may have 10,000 dendrites interacting with other neurons), dictating the use of reductionist approaches which always require a correlation with the whole organism to verify the conclusions reached at the molecular level. Such relationship emphasizes the importance relating the biochemical events in single cells to the more complex organisms such as *Aplysia*, *Drosophila*, rodents, cats, and humans. The fact, however, that adjacent neurons are almost never identical means that the quantity of material needed to perform biochemical analyses necessitates a cell line approach. Both bacteria and neural cell lines provide a homogeneous population of cells that can be studied biochemically. Bacteria detect chemical gradients using a memory obtained by the combination of a fast excitation process and a slow adaptation process. This model system, which has the advantages of extensive genetic and biochemical information, shows no features of long-term memory.

To study long-term memory, other biologic systems that exhibit two phenomena associated with learning and memory, habituation and potentiation, must be used. Habituation is defined as the decreased responsiveness to a stimulus when it is presented repetitively over time. Potentiation, on the other hand, is defined as the increased responsiveness to a stimulus when that stimulus is presented repetitively over time. In the mammalian brain, the hippocampus plays a special role in learning: when it is destroyed on both sides of the brain, the ability to form new memories is largely lost although previous long-established memories remain. The evidence obtained on hippocampal slices indicates that the biochemical changes in the synapse represent the molecular bases for long-term memory (Malinow and Tsien, 1990; Bekkers and Stevens, 1990). Despite the wealth of information provided by investigations in mammalian brain slices, it became increasingly clear that the study of cultured neural cells is more desirable because only in such a system could one be certain that the complete biochemical pathway, that is, the complete signal transduction pathway from stimulatory input to a behavioral output, could be analyzed. To study memory, however, some modifiable behavior needs to be observed. Because neurons communicate with each other chemically through the release of a neurotransmitter, the secretion of neurotransmitters (the output) evoked by various chemical stimuli (input) could be used to monitor the responsiveness of the cell. This experimental system was used to study the input–output properties of a particular neuron. Both habituation and potentiation could be demonstrated in neuronal cell lines indicating that they can serve as good model systems for the memory process, except that they do not possess synaptic connections. In the early phase of these studies the absence of synaptic connections posed a substantial problem for two major reasons: (1) as stated before, current evidence favors (in more organized neural tissue such as brain slices) the idea that the biochemical changes in the synapse are the molecular basis of long-term memory and (2) the synapse is a unique anatomic association of two cells that occurs only in the nervous system and therefore represents a special *sui generis* neuronal feature.

Whether memories, however, are generally recorded in presynaptic changes or in postsynaptic changes, in synaptic chemistry or in synaptic structure, or indeed in synapses at all, are still open questions. Regardless of the validity of any of these questions, it appears that the biochemical features of all memory-forming processes (i.e., habituation, potentiation, and associative learning in invertebrates, mammalian brain slices, and cultured clonal neural cell lines) are highly similar [the PC 12 cells (McFadden and Koshland, 1990a,b) and HT4 cells (Morimoto and Koshland, 1990a,b)]. They can be characterized as follows: (1) a monoamine (primarily serotonin) and a glutamate receptor (known as NMDA receptor because it is selectively activated by the artificial glutamate analogue *N*-methyl-D-aspartate) are involved; (2) binding of the neurotransmitter (serotonin, glutamate) by these receptors initiates a cascade of enzymatic reactions; (3) the first step in this cascade is the activation of a

G-protein which may either interact directly with ion channels or control the production of cyclic adenosine monophosphate (AMP) or Ca^{2+}; (4) the two second messengers in turn regulate ion channels directly or activate kinases that phosphorylate various proteins including ion channels; (5) at many synapses both channel-linked and non-channel-linked receptors are present, responding either to the same or to different neurotransmitters; (6) responses mediated by non-channel-linked receptors (serotonin) have a slow onset and long duration and modulate the efficacy of subsequent synaptic transmission providing the basis for memory formation; (7) channel-linked receptors that allow Ca^{2+} to enter the cell (NMDA receptor) also mediate long-term memory effects; and (8) either too much or too little cyclic AMP can interfere with memory formation (Dudai, 1988).

In all of these processes, the interaction between serotonin and glutamate and their respective receptor systems can be illustrated by the studies carried out on the HT4 neural cell line (Jessell and Melton, 1992). The HT4 cells do not habituate to repetitive membrane depolarization but after exposure of these cells to various neurotransmitters, serotonin has the capacity to potentiate cellular responsiveness. Depending on the strength of the serotonin stimulus, both short- and long-term potentiation can be induced. For instance, a 2-min exposure to serotonin results in a transient increase in cellular responsiveness, where a 5-min presentation gives rise to a more permanent potentiation, the difference between the two involving the activation of NMDA receptors. Thus, the stronger (5 min) serotonin stimulus results in the endogenous release of excitatory amino acids with activation of NMDA receptors. Consistent with this mechanism, long-term secretory potentiation can also be produced with a 2-min stimulus of serotonin only if glutamate or NMDA is given simultaneously.

Comparison of Immunologic versus Neuronal Memory Mechanisms

As we now begin a comparison of immunologic versus neuronal memory, we have to return to an earlier statement that immunologic memory is related to clonal selection and lymphocyte maturation. Although this is correct in cellular terms, in molecular terms the problem of clonal selection and expansion reduces to the issue of affinity maturation of the antibody on the surface of the lymphocyte. In other words, the entire antigen-driven selection of antibody-producing lymphocytes is based on the strength of the antibody–antigen interaction, which depends on both the affinity and the number of binding sites. The affinity of an antibody reflects the strength of binding of an antigenic determinant to a single antigen-binding site and it is independent of the number of sites. However, the total avidity of an antibody for a multivalent antigen, such as a polymer with repeating subunits, is defined as the total binding strength of all of its binding sites together. When a multivalent antigen combines with more than one antigen-binding site on an antibody, the binding strength is greatly increased because all of the antigen–antibody bonds must be broken simultaneously before the antigen and antibody can dissociate. Thus, a typical IgG molecule will bind at least 1000 times more strongly to a multivalent antigen if both antigen-binding sites are engaged than if only one site is involved. For the same reason, if the affinity of the antigen-binding sites in an IgG and an IgM molecule are the same, the IgM molecule (with ten binding sites) will have a much greater avidity for a multivalent antigen than an IgG molecule (with two sites). This difference in avidity, often 10^4-fold or more, is important because antibodies produced early in an immune response usually have much lower affinities than those produced later. Because of its high total avidity, IgM—the major Ig class produced early in immune responses—can function effectively even when each of its binding sites has only a low affinity (Szentivanyi *et al.*, 1987a).

In the late 1950s and early 1960s an excellent correlation was shown between the body temperature of rabbits and the affinity and avidity of the antibody produced against the radiolabeled antigen as tested in equilibrium dialysis experiments (Szentivanyi and Filipp, 1962). The higher the body temperature was, the greater the affinity and avidity were. In the beginning of these studies, commercially available *E. coli* endotoxin was used, but later the rise in temperature was reproduced by electrical stimulation of the posterior hypothalamus or hippocampus through stereotaxically implanted permanent depth electrodes in studies without endotoxin administration (Szentivanyi *et al.*, 1986). Discovery of the peptidoglycan and its derivatives as powerful immunologic adjuvants opened up a new window for the consideration of the relationship between immunologic and neuronal memory. The peptidoglycan, which is the basal layer of the bacterial cell wall, is a rigid macromolecule surrounding the cytoplasmic membrane. It is formed by the polymerization of a disaccharide tetrapeptide subunit; in the intact peptidoglycan, disaccharides form linear chains whereas peptides are linked by interpeptide linkages (Hadden and Szentivanyi, 1985). The recognition of the immunomodulating properties of peptidoglycans and peptidoglycan fragments is the result of the work aimed at identifying the structure responsible for the adjuvant activity of the mycobacterial cells in Freund's adjuvant (Friedman *et al.*, 1981). Simple active molecules were soon produced by organic synthesis followed by a vast array of analogues and derivatives that can be classified into several categories. The one that is most pertinent to this discussion is the group of "simple muramyl peptides." Of these the smallest immunoactive synthetic muramyl peptide is *N*-acetylmuramyl-L-alanyl-D-isoglutamine (MDP) (Szentivanyi *et al.*, 1983; Klein *et al.*, 1983). This substance has a pyrogenic effect that originally was attributed to its ability to induce the release of endogenous pyrogen from mononuclear phagocytes. However, a direct central nervous system action could not be excluded since MDP was found to be active by the intracerebroventricular route [MDP was shown to cross the blood–brain barrier (Krueger *et al.*, 1988)], and in rabbits made leukopenic by nitrogen mustard treatment (Hadden and Szentivanyi, 1985). In addition, it was subsequently shown that MDP can also induce sleep, and the somnogenic effect can be separated from its pyrogenic activity. MDP's pyrogenic activity does not affect brain temperature changes that are tightly coupled to sleep states (Krueger *et al.*, 1989). More importantly with respect to the direct central nervous system neuronal effects of MDP, this substance is capable of specific binding to serotonin receptors of synaptosomal membranes of brain tissue and competes with serotonin for these binding sites, and the kinetics of serotonin binding to brain homogenates is altered after sleep deprivation (Fillion *et al.*, 1989). Additional findings on the capacity of MDP to act directly and specifically on central neurons include the following: MDP alters neuronal firing rates in different regions of the brain (Dougherty and Dafny, 1987), humoral antibody responses are enhanced by lowering serotonin levels in the brain (Eremina and Devoino, 1973), administration of *para*-chlorophenylalanine which markedly decreases the level of brain serotonin completely abolishes the MDP-induced rise in body temperature and the somnogenic effect (Masek *et al.*, 1989). Finally, it has been established that immunization decreases the concentration of serotonin in the hypothalamus and the hippocampus (Vekshina and Magaeva, 1974).

Although the foregoing evidence is fragmentary, it does establish a set of future reference points to begin to undertake a more informed comparison of the molecular mechanisms involved in immune and neuronal memory. One of the reference points involves a novel proto-oncogene, bcl-2, that by all available information plays a significant role in both immune and neuronal memory. The other possible reference point may be represented by an IL-1α that so far has been found to be present only in a subset of T-memory cells and hippocampal neurons.

The bcl-2 Gene

The bcl-2 Gene and Immune Memory. The germinal center forms a specialized microenvironment that plays a key role in the induction of antibody synthesis, affinity maturation of B cells, isotype switching, and memory B-cell formation. Furthermore, it is believed that the germinal center is also involved in the maintenance of T-cell memory. The bcl-2 protein, originally discovered as a proto-oncogene, has proved to be unique in being localized to the mitochondria and in blocking programmed cell death rather than affecting proliferation. It was identified at the chromosomal breakpoint of t(14;18)-bearing B-cell lymphomas. In adults, bcl-2 is topographically restricted to progenitor cells and long-lived cells in tissues characterized by apoptotic cell death and it is confined to the zones of surviving B cells in germinal centers (Korsmeyer, 1992a; Hockenbery, 1992). Within the thymus, bcl-2 is present in the surviving mature thymocytes of the medulla but absent from the majority of immature cortical thymocytes, most of which die by apoptosis. Transgenic mice that overexpress bcl-2 in the B-cell lineage demonstrate extended cell survival and prolonged immune responses, and conclusively support a role for bcl-2 in B-cell memory. Transgenic models that overexpress bcl-2 in the thymus have expanded the involvement of bcl-2 to multiple apoptopic pathways and indicate its critical role in thymocyte maturation (Graninger, 1992).

Another source of information on the role and functioning of bcl-2 is provided by some recent observations on B chronic lymphocytic leukemia (B-CLL). In the natural history of CLL, at least three categories of genes are believed to be involved: (1) genes that are responsible for the transforming event(s) in the target cells, (2) genes that help the progressive accumulation of malignant cells, and (3) genes that cause the progression toward a more aggressive lymphoma. The possibility that the clonal expansion of B-CLL is related to a prolonged life span of monoclonal B cells rather than to an acceleration of their proliferative activity is now suggested by recent findings on the expression of the bcl-2 gene in B-CLL cells (Schena *et al.*, 1993). As discussed earlier, the bcl-2 gene product regulates programmed cell death and recent studies indicate that blc-2 is involved in the selection and maintenance of long-lived memory B cells rescuing them from apoptotic death and leading to their accumulation in the G0 phase of the cell cycle. Variant chromosomal translocations have been detected in a small fraction (5–10%) of B-CLL involving blc-2 and the Ig light chain gene. Despite the low percentage of bcl-2 rearrangements, the expression of mRNA and protein is appreciable in most samples of fresh B-CLL cells in an amount comparable to that observed in Karpas 422 cells which contain a t(14;18).

The bcl-2 gene is translocated into the Ig loci in about 80% of human follicular lymphomas and in 10% of B-type chronic lymphocytic leukemias (B-CLL), resulting in a high level of expression of bcl-2 transcripts and protein in B-CLL cells in their normal equivalent $CD5^+$ B cells and in normal B-cell populations representative of different *in vivo* and *in vitro* stages of activation and proliferation. bcl-2 was found to be expressed in all of 11 cases of $CD5^+$ B-CLL clones, contrasting with the absent expression in normal $CD5^+$ B cells. Activation of B-CLL cells by phorbol esters to IgM secretion without concomitant DNA synthesis resulted in a rapid but transient downregulation of bcl-2 expression. In contrast, the reduction of bcl-2 at both the mRNA and protein levels was sustained after mitogenic stimulation, suggesting that bcl-2 expression and proliferation are inversely related in these cells. Furthermore, the pattern of bcl-2 expression in B-CLL resembled that of normal tonsillar follicular B cells in which a high level of expression was found in resting mantle zone B cells but not in the proliferating germinal center B cells. Based on these findings, and the role of bcl-2 in maintaining B-cell memory, Schena *et al.* (1992) proposed that the phenotype of B-CLL cells corresponds to a mantle zone memory-type B cell. Studying bcl-2 protein expression in high-grade B-cell lymphomas derived from lymph node or mucosa-associated lymphoid tissue (MALT), a significant difference has been found in bcl-2 expression between nodal (39/48) and MALT high-grade B-cell lymphoma (1/15). bcl-2 was usually expressed by memory or resting B cells, most activated B cells being bcl-2 negative, except in lymph node-originated, high-grade B-cell lymphomas, which appear to be mainly bcl-2-positive. Presence of bcl-2 protein in nodal large-cell lymphomas seems to be independent of a t(14;18) translocation, only being found in 19 to 28% of these lymphomas, although it constitutes a definitive difference between both tumors, suggesting the existence of different molecular genetic characteristics and pathogenesis (Villuendas *et al.*, 1991).

Another dimension of the significance of bcl-2 in B-cell memory has to do with the maintenance of the remarkably constant number of lymphocytes in an animal in the face of antigen-driven proliferation and a high rate of B-cell lymphopoiesis. This reflects the relatively brief life span of many newly generated B cells and argues for a well-regulated death mechanism. Even so, a secondary immune response can be generated years after a primary exposure to antigen. Antigen that might restimulate B cells persists for extended periods on follicular dendritic cells in the light zone of germinal centers. Antigen-binding B cells have also been found months after the end of manifest cell division. It is increasingly apparent that the precise signal that enables certain B cells to emerge as long-term surviving memory cells is bcl-2. Consequently, this agent must have a critical role in the maintenance of immune responsiveness. Indeed, transgenic mice overproducing bcl-2 have a long-term persistence of immunoglobulin-secreting cells and an extended lifetime for memory B cells (Nunez *et al.*, 1991). Systemic lupus erythematosus (SLE) provides another example reflecting the same. In SLE, spontaneous hyperreactivity of the cells of the immune system leads to the production of pathogenic autoantibodies. A hyperproliferative state of lymphocytes is indicated by the increased expression of bcl-2. In 19 of 24 patients with SLE, an increased concentration of bcl-2 mRNA was found in unstimulated circulating blood lymphocytes. The overexpression of the bcl-2 gene was more pronounced in patients with active SLE suggesting a pathogenic role of increased bcl-2 expression and prolonged survival of autoimmune memory cells in this disease (Graninger, 1992).

The foregoing discussion was focused on B-cell memory and its relation to the bcl-2 gene. One of the central questions in T-cell immunity is how the generation of T-cell memory may proceed simultaneously with the maintenance of T-cell homeostasis. Akbar *et al.* (1993b) in their recent article present the role of bcl-2 in regulating T-cell memory as a balancing act between cell death and survival. More specifically, these authors have investigated the bcl-2 protein expression by resting and activated mature T-cell populations. Freshly isolated $CD45RO^+$ T cells within $CD4^+$ and $CD8^+$ subsets expressed significantly less bcl-2 than $CD45RO^-$ ($CD45RA^+$) T cells. When $CD45RA^+$ T cells within both $CD4^+$ and $CD8^+$ subsets were activated *in vitro*, the transition to CD45RO phenotype was associated with a decrease in bcl-2 expression. In these studies, a significant correlation was seen between low bcl-2 expression by activated T cells and their apoptosis in culture. These findings suggest that the primary activation of T cells leads to the expansion of a population that is destined to perish unless rescued by some extrinsic event. Thus, the suicide of $CD45RO^+$ T cells could be prevented by the addition of IL-2 to the culture medium which resulted in a concomitant increase in the bcl-2 expression of these cells. The paradox that the $CD45RO^+$ population contains the primed/memory T-cell pool yet expresses low bcl-2 and is susceptible to apoptosis can be reconciled by the observations that maintenance of T-cell memory may be dependent on the continuous restimulation of T cells which increases their bcl-2 expression (Akbar *et al.*, 1993a).

The bcl-2 Gene and Neuronal Memory. To assess the role of bcl-2 in neuronal apoptosis, Allsopp *et al.* (1993) microinjected a bcl-2 expression vector into neurotropic factor-deprived embryonic neurons. Sensory neurons that depend for survival on one or more members of the nerve growth factor family of neurotropic factors (nerve growth factor, brain-derived neurotropic factor, and neurotropin-3) were rescued by bcl-2, whereas ciliary neurotropic factor (CNTF)-dependent ciliary neurons were not. Sensory neurons, however, became refractory to bcl-2 after exposure to CNTF. These findings indicate that at least two memory (death) pathways operate in neurons that are distinguished by their susceptibility to bcl-2.

Abe-Dohmae *et al.* (1993) have developed an analytical method for quantification of the RNA transcripts of the murine bcl-2 gene. The PCR products from bcl-2 alpha and bcl-2 beta mRNA were fluorometrically analyzed and their specific contents calculated by the internal standard method. Both bcl-2 mRNAs in adult mice were transcribed at the highest level in the thymus and at a comparable level in the spleen. Aside from the immune system, the brain gave the most abundant levels of the bcl-2 mRNAs. During development of the brain, the bcl-2 alpha and bcl-2 beta mRNA levels were highest on embryonic day 15 and about two and three times higher than those of adults, respectively. The results suggest that the bcl-2 gene is highly expressed during neurogenesis and functions to regulate development, memory, and survival of neurons in the central nervous system.

There are at least three additional examples of the effects of bcl-2 in neuronal systems. The first example involves glutamate toxicity. At high concentrations (5–10 mM), this substance has been shown to kill cells of the phenochromocytoma cell line PC12. Zhong *et al.* (1993) have recently reported that similar concentrations of glutamate also kill immortalized central neural cell lines and that the expression of bcl-2 in these cell lines blocks glutamate neurotoxicity.

The experiences obtained in Sindbis virus (SV) encephalitis could serve as a second example of neuronal activity by bcl-2. As known, encephalitis in mice provides a model for studying age-dependent susceptibility to acute viral encephalitis. The AR 339 strain of SV causes fatal encephalitis in newborn mice but weanling mice recover uneventfully. Weanling mice with normal immune systems clear the virus from neurons through an antibody-mediated mechanism. This does not happen in newborn mice because the infected neurons die soon after they are infected. Death in immature neurons infected with SV occurs by induction of apoptosis. This can be prevented by cellular expression of bcl-2, an inhibitor of apoptosis, which is expressed by mature neurons in culture (Griffin *et al.*, 1994).

A third example of the neural or neurally related involvement of bcl-2 is provided by the recent study of Novack and Korsmeyer (1994). These workers have assessed bcl-2's pattern of expression during murine embryogenesis. Immunohistochemical analysis demonstrated that bcl-2 is widely expressed early in mouse fetal development and that this expression becomes restricted with maturation. For this discussion it is important to note that retinal neuroepithelial cells uniformly express bcl-2 until cells begin to differentiate and then display the topographic distribution maintained into adulthood. The wide distribution of bcl-2 in the developing mouse suggests that many immature cells require a death repressor molecule or that bcl-2 may have roles beyond regulating developmental cell death.

bcl-X, a bcl-2-Related Gene. Boise *et al.* (1993) reported the isolation of a bcl-2-related gene that can function as a bcl-2-independent regulator of programmed cell death. Alternative splicing results in two distinct bcl-X mRNAs. The protein product of the larger mRNA, bcl-XL, is similar in size and predicted structured to bcl-2. When stably transfected into an IL-3-dependent cell line, bcl-XL inhibits cell death on growth factor withdrawal at least as well as bcl-2. The second mRNA species, bcl-XS, encodes a protein that inhibits the ability of bcl-2 to enhance the survival of growth factor-deprived cells. *In vivo*, bcl-XS mRNA is expressed at high levels in cells that undergo a high rate of turnover, such as developing lymphocytes. In contrast, bcl-XL is found in tissues containing long-lived, postmitotic cells such as adult brain. Together, these data suggest that bcl-X plays an important role in both positive and negative regulation of programmed cell death as well as cell memory, respectively.

8. ADRENERGICALLY ACTIVE LYMPHOCYTE SUBSTANCES

Three macromolecular fractions with adrenergic activity can be identified in lymphocyte conditioned medium by diethylaminoethanol (DEAE) ion-exchange high-performance liquid chromatography (HPLC), immunoneutralization, molecular mass, sequence analysis, and biologic characterizations. One of these fractions contains a secretory variant of β-arrestin and an IL-1α antagonist, both of which downregulate β_2-adrenergic receptors in A549 human lung epithelial cells. The two other fractions represent protein components that upregulate β_2-adrenergic receptors. One of these contains a mixture of IL-1α and IL-1β, whereas the adrenergically active components(s) of the remaining fraction is currently being characterized. The first question that may be asked in the context of this chapter is whether the adrenergically highly active IL-1α obtained from the corresponding macromolecular fraction of lymphocyte conditioned medium has a specific receptor on airway cells. Recent studies designed to explore this question used human bronchial epithelial cells isolated and cultured from the normal bronchi of patients undergoing surgery (for standard clinical reasons) essentially as described by Mattoli *et al.* (1990). Using this method, 99% of the final cell population contains epithelial cells. The latter were then incubated with IL-1α radiolabeled by a modified chloramine-T method. In addition to binding of specific, single-class IL-1α receptors, the latter were also identified by internalization of the receptor, affinity cross-linking, and sodium dodecyl sulfate–polyacrylamide gel electrophoresis (SDS–PAGE). Using unlabeled IL-1α and [^{3}H]dihydroalprenolol (DHA) for measuring β-adrenergic mRNA with the guanidium thiocyanate method, the IL-1α-induced accumulation of β_2-adrenoceptor mRNA is demonstrable within 2 hr and an increase in β-adrenoceptor concentration within 4 hr. In other words, concentrated IL-1α derived from human T lymphocytes binds to a specific, single-class surface receptor on human bronchial epithelial cells and induces production of β_2-adrenoceptor mRNA via an associated or separate receptor-linked signaling pathway leading to an increase in epithelial β_2-adrenoceptor concentration (Robicsek *et al.*, 1992).

Subsequently, it was shown that lymphocytic IL-1α is a cell- and species-specific factor in increasing β-adrenoceptor concentration and induction of its gene. In this study, we used A549 human lung epithelial cells, A431 human epidermoid cells, DDT_1MF_2 hamster smooth muscle cells, cultured human bronchial epithelial cells and smooth muscle cells, cultured canine tracheal epithelial and tracheal smooth muscle cells. Concentrated human lymphocytic IL-1α was then cocultured with these various cell populations for 24 hr and β_2-adrenoceptors measured radioactively. The originally shown synergistic β-adrenoceptor upregulation between IL-1α and cortisol (Szentendrei *et al.*, 1991) was present in the A549 and A431 cells, as well as the human bronchial epithelial cells. Northern blot hybridization showed that levels of β_2-adrenoceptors and β_2-adrenoceptor mRNAs increased significantly by both IL-1α and cortisol, whereas Gs-α, Gi-2α, Gi-3α mRNA levels remained unchanged (see below). In all of these situations, the increase in β_2-adrenoceptor mRNAs always preceded the enhanced expression of the receptor. When DDT_1MF_2 cells, human and canine tracheal smooth muscle cells were used, IL-1α had no effect on either β_2-adrenoceptors or β_2-adrenoceptor mRNAs whereas cortisol remained active (Szentivanyi *et al.*, 1992). This extraordinary degree of cell and species specificity of the β_2-adrenoceptor upregulating effect of lymphocytic IL-1α makes these observations highly important both for normal airway physiology as well as for the possible nature of the β-adrenergic dysregulation in asthma by adding an entirely new dimension to the β-adrenergic theory of the atopic abnormality in bronchial asthma as postulated 26 years ago by Szentivanyi (1968).

9. THE UNIQUE RECOGNITION AND COMMUNICATION POWERS OF THE IMMUNE AND NEUROENDOCRINE SYSTEMS AS SHARED CHARACTERISTICS

Earlier we cited Schechter, pointing out that a good relationship between two biologic systems must be sensitive, synchronized, and synergistic (Schechter, 1989). There are no two biologic systems where such characterization of an ideal relationship would be more valid than in the case of the immune and neuroendocrine systems as reflected by their unique recognition and communication powers as shared characteristics. Indeed, if intelligence is the capacity to adapt to changing circumstances, then the central nervous system and the immune system manifest this ability beyond all others. As pointed out by Geschwind (1983), it would be remarkable if each of these supreme examples of rapid and subtle adaptation did not tap the other's almost limitless potential for variation. While at one time the concept existed that stress might alter immune reactivity through some relatively diffuse activation of the endocrine system of the hypothalamus (Selye, 1936, 1943, 1946, 1949; Karady *et al.*, 1938), we now find that there are specific interactions at every level, as discussed below. The latter are based on four critical features shared by both systems: (1) they are composed of extraordinarily large numbers of phenotypically distinct cells organized into intricate networks. Moreover, the size of this extensive cellular arsenal continuously increases as new sequence information becomes available and enormous numbers of new members of the IgSF surface each year (see Brümmendorf and Rathjen, 1994). Within these cell networks, the individual cells can interact either positively or negatively and the response of one cell reverberates through the system by affecting many other cells. (2) Cells of both systems synthesize, secrete, and/or release the same effector molecules. (3) Recognition of these effector molecules is realized by the same cellular receptors and second messenger mechanisms of both cell systems. (4) These cellular and molecular determinants make a continuous, bilateral flow of information, the sine qua non of the unique interactions within the immune–neuroendocrine circuitry, possible.

A more amplified view on the basic biochemistry and molecular biology of receptor–effector coupling by G-proteins (i.e., the fundamental mechanism used by hormones, neurotransmitters, and the immunomodulatory cytokines for signal transmission by G-proteins) is presented by Szentivanyi (1993a), Lochrie and Simon (1988), and Birnbaumer and Brown (1990). Here we shall only mention that about 80% of all known neurohormones, neurotransmitters, immunomodulatory lymphokines, and other autocrine and paracrine factors that regulate cellular interactions in the immune–neuroendocrine circuitry, called "primary" messengers, elicit cellular responses by combining with specific receptors that are coupled to effector functions by G-proteins. Although the primary messengers are many, the number of physicochemically and biologically distinct receptors that mediate their action is even larger. So far about 80 distinct receptors that recognize 40 hormones, neurotransmitters, and so on, can be identified. It is reasonable to assume that the total number of distinct receptors coupled by G-proteins will be 100 to 150. In contrast to receptors, the number of final effector functions regulated by these receptors and the number of G-proteins that provide for receptor–effector coupling are much lower, probably not much more than 15 each.

In mammals, a total of 8 G-proteins have been purified essentially free from each other (Gt, Gs, Gi1, Gi2, Gi3, G01, G02, and Gz/x) and the cDNAs derived from a total of 9 genes encoding G-alpha subunits have been cloned and designated alpha$_s$, alpha$_{i1}$, alpha$_{i2}$, alpha$_{i3}$, alpha$_0$, alpha$_{tr}$, alpha$_{tc}$, alpha$_{01f}$, and alpha$_{z/x}$, giving rise to 12 mRNAs because of the fourfold variation in the splicing of the alpha$_s$ precursor mRNA. In addition, there is evidence for the existence of at least 7 additional G-alpha genes. Homology cloning has also revealed that there are at least 4 G-beta genes and 3 G-gamma genes.

The G-proteins are heterotrimeric membrane proteins (alpha, beta, gamma; 1:1:1), distinguished by unique alpha subunits, but sharing common beta subunits. Stated in a different way, G-proteins may be viewed as being composed of a unique, but homologous alpha subunit in reversible association with a complex comprised of a beta and a gamma subunit commonly shared by several different G-protein alpha subunits. Thus, the alpha subunit of Gs (the G-protein that stimulates adenylate cyclase) may share beta–gamma complex in common with the alpha subunits of the family of G-proteins that mediate inhibition of adenylate cyclase (G1), or other

G-proteins like G0, Gz, and Gt. The alpha subunits bind and hydrolyze GTP, and are often the substrates for NAD^+-dependent ADP ribosylation by bacterial toxins (i.e., pertussis, cholera). Activated β-adrenoceptors catalyze the exchange of GTP for bound guanosine diphosphate (GDP) by the alpha subunit of the holoprotein, promoting the dissociation of the GTP-bound alpha subunit from the beta–gamma complex. It is the "free" GTP ligand alpha subunit of a G-protein that regulates the activity of the membrane-bound effector units such as adenylate cyclase.

The primary sequences of several G-protein-linked effectors, including adenylate cyclase and phospholipase C, have been determined and molecular cloning of phospholipase A2 and Ca^{2+} and K^+ channels are in an advanced stage in several laboratories. As mentioned earlier, G-alpha$_s$ mediates the stimulation of adenylate cyclase and has been shown to regulate Ca^{2+} channel activity. The G-proteins that mediate the inhibition of adenylate cyclase, termed Gi, constitute a family with at least three members, G-alpha$_{i1}$, G-alpha$_{i2}$, and G-alpha$_{i3}$, each the product of a separate gene. Of these, it is G-alpha$_{i2}$ that mediates the inhibition of adenylate cyclase (Szentivanyi, 1993a).

At the time of writing, receptors for simple substances, such as the amine mediators and short-chain peptides as well as lipids, and for more than 20 different hypothalamopituitary peptides have been identified in the cells of the immune system, essentially in lymphocytes. In addition to the hypothalamopituitary hormones, lymphocytes also express receptors for peptides secreted from neurons together with other neurotransmitters. These neuropeptides take on added significance as immunomodulators, since it is now known that lymphoid organs are directly innervated with nerves secreting these agents. From the standpoint of the integration of information in the immune–neuroendocrine circuitry, future studies will have to examine these parallel signaling pathways in isolation. In other words, it will be necessary to determine how an individual cell completely processes and integrates information from these individual pathways. This is all the more remarkable because the cell is faced with the task of balancing the need to communicate with other cells with the need for growth and maintenance of the differentiated state while preserving adequate flexibility to support regulation, sensitivity, and gain. One early result of such inquiries is the demonstration of cross-regulation (crosstalk) between the various G-protein-mediated signaling pathways. Thus, it was shown that in the cross-regulation between α_1- and β_2-adrenergic receptor-mediated pathways, activation of β_2-adrenergic receptors increased α_1-adrenergic receptor mRNA levels (Morris *et al.*, 1991). Conversely, activation of the $G_{1\alpha}$-mediated inhibitory pathway of adenylate cyclase cross-regulates the stimulatory ($G_{s\alpha}$-mediated) β-adrenergic-sensitive adenylate cyclase system by (1) upregulating β_2-adrenergic receptors and enhancing the activation of the stimulatory ($G_{s\alpha}$-mediated) adenylate cyclase pathway and (2) downregulating elements of the inhibitory adenylate cyclase pathway, $G_{1\alpha2}$ and A_1-adenosine receptor binding, respectively (Hadcock *et al.*, 1991). It may be added that cross-regulation is also observed between signaling pathways that do not share the same effectors. Although much more work remains to be done to unravel the complexities of the coordinated regulation of information processing and integration by the cell, it is already possible to state that there is cross-regulation between neurally derived substances and lymphokines.

The foregoing leads us to a general consideration of the "endocrine" hypothalamus and its regulation by cytokines.

10. THE ENDOCRINE HYPOTHALAMUS AND CYTOKINES

As indicated earlier, the existence of an immune–neuroendocrine circuitry was discovered in Szentivanyi's laboratory in the fall of 1951 together with the demonstration that the integrative center of this circuitry is the hypothalamus. The cumulative findings in these studies showed that the hypothalamus has a modulatory influence on all cellular and humoral immune reactivities and that either or both neural as well as endocrine pathways are required for hypothalamic modulation of immune responses (Filipp *et al.*, 1952; Szentivanyi *et al.*, 1952, 1978, 1980, 1987b, 1988a–d, 1989a, 1990; Filipp and Szentivanyi, 1953, 1956, 1957, 1958, 1985; Szentivanyi, 1953, 1961, 1988a,b, 1989; Szentivanyi and Filipp, 1956, 1958; Szentivanyi and Szekely, 1956, 1957a,b, 1958; Szentivanyi and Fishel, 1965, 1966; Szentivanyi and Fitzpatrick, 1980; Szentivanyi and Szentivanyi, 1982a,b, 1987, 1988; J. Szentivanyi *et al.*, 1988, 1989a–c; Schwartz *et al.*, 1988).

The hypothalamus is a small anatomically complex region of the diencephalon which in a variety of ways contributes to a number of regulatory systems. The functional and anatomic complexity of the hypothalamus is the consequence of its role as a nodal region for (1) convergence of input from the limbic system which contributes to a coordination between visceral and behavioral functions, (2) bidirectional bundles of neurons with their perikarya in the telencephalon or brain stem, and (3) local neurons coordinating and integrating distant organ system activities through the effector functions of the endocrine and autonomic nervous systems. It is the last role that is the subject of our discussion below and the reason for referring to this structure as the "endocrine" hypothalamus. The control of anterior pituitary hormone secretion is dependent primarily on the release of putative neurotransmitters and other messenger substances, mostly peptides, produced by hypophysiotropic neurons in the hypothalamus. These peptidergic neurons act as "neuroendocrine transducers" that transform neural input into neurochemical commands (hypophysiotropic hormones or factors, HPT). Nearly 40 of these, mostly peptides, are present in the median eminence (ME) of the hypothalamus (the ME constitutes the final common hypothalamic pathway for signals from the brain to the pituitary). The majority of these agents are produced in perikarya located in different hypothalamic nuclei: (1) corticotropin-releasing factor (CRF) in the paraventricular nucleus (PVN), (2) growth hormone-releasing hormone (GHRH) in the arcuate nucleus, (3) somatostatin (SRIF) in the anterior periventricular area, (4) thyrotropin-releasing hormone (TRH) in the PVN, and (5) dopamine (DA) in the A12 region of the hypothalamus and the A2 and A4 regions of the brain stem. In contrast to these restricted locations, the neurons containing luteinizing hormone-releasing hormone (LHRH) are scattered in the diagonal band of Broca, the medial septum, the medial preoptic and suprachiasmatic areas, and the lateral basal hypothalamus.

Except for SRIF, the classic hypophysiotropic hormones are colocalized with other transmitters. For example, in the PVN, CRF is colocalized with arginine VP (AVP), oxytocin (OT), neurotensin (NT), enkephalin (ENK), cholecystokinin (CCK), galanin (GAL), angiotensin II (ANGII), vasoactive intestinal peptide (VIP), peptide histidine isoleucine (PHI), and γ-aminobutyric acid (GABA). Thyrotropin-releasing hormone (TRH) in the PVN is colocalized with GAL and δ-sleep-inducing peptide (DSIP). In the anterior nucleus (AN), GHRH is colocalized with dopamine (DA), GAL, NT, neuropeptide Y (NPY), and glutamic acid decarboxylase (GAD). Fibers from the PEV and PVN form a curved fan of fibers above the optic chiasm and enter the medial basal hypothalamus through the lateral basal retrochiasmatic area. Then they run toward the ME. Fibers from the LHRH-containing neurons follow other pathways. For a more comprehensive discussion of the endocrine hypothalamus, see Szentivanyi and Fishel (1966), Szentivanyi *et al.* (1978, 1980), Szentivanyi and Fitzpatrick (1980).

In the foregoing sections, discussions of the reciprocal, regulatory interplay between the immune and neuroendocrine systems have mainly covered the peripheral pathways by which the neuroendocrine influences are able to affect immune functions. However, as stated earlier, the flow of information in the immune–neuroendocrine circuitry is bidirectional, and there is conclusive evidence that products of the immune system are capable of modulating neuroendocrine, i.e., hypothalamic, processes. There are two lines of evidence indicating that the products of the immune system can influence the hypothalamus or the pituitary gland, or both. The first is provided by correlational studies showing that changes occur in the hypothalamus during the course of an immune response. Along this line, Korneva and Klimenko (1976) recorded single-unit activity in the hypothalamus showing significant changes in the neuronal firing patterns in the posterior, ventromedial, and supramaxillary nuclei during the course of an immune response. These observations were independently confirmed by Besedovsky *et al.* (1977) who found a considerable increase in the firing rate of neurons in the ventromedial hypothalamus 1 to 5 days following sensitization to trinitrophenol (TNP)-hemocyanin. Srebro *et al.* (1974) found a significant increase in the nuclear volume of neurosecretory cells in the supraoptic nucleus during skin allograft rejection. Changes in the serotonin levels occur in the hypothalamus and hippocampus following immunization with typhoid antigen (Vekshina and Magaeva, 1974), whereas increases in dopamine-stimulated adenylate cyclase activity in caudate homogenates are found following bacille Calmette–Guérin (BCG) antigen administration (Cotzias and Tang, 1977). In recent years, these observations have been expanded by the findings on the effects of Newcastle disease virus on the metabolism of cerebral biogenic amines (Dunn *et al.*, 1987), and similar changes have also been observed with influenza virus.

The second line of evidence implicating the immune system in regulating physiologic processes at the level of the hypothalamus or the pituitary gland, or both, is derived from studies in which products of the cells of the immune system were administered to experimental animals or added to cultured neuronal or pituitary cells. Thus, several cytokines including IL-1α, IL- 1β, IL-2, IL-6, TNF-α, and IFN-γ are now known to affect the release of pituitary hormones by an action on the hypothalamus and/or the pituitary gland. Their predominant effects are to stimulate the hypothalamic–pituitary–adrenal axis and to suppress the hypothalamic–pituitary–thyroid and gonadal axes. It is not clear whether cytokines, which are relatively large molecules, cross the blood–brain barrier (BBB) to exert their effects. Three possible hypotheses have been suggested: (1) they do cross the BBB at the level of the organum vasculosum of the lamina terminalis in the anterior hypothalamus where the integrity of the barrier is at its weakest (Katsuura, 1990); (2) the cytokines stimulate the production of an intermediary substance(s) which then transmits the signal to the hypothalamus; to support this hypothesis there is some evidence suggesting that prostaglandins are involved (see below) in the stimulation of ACTH release by systemically administered IL-1 (Katsuura, 1988; Morimoto *et al.*, 1989); and (3) that in some way they stimulate the release of cytokines locally within the hypothalamus and the pituitary (Jones and Kennedy, 1993).

10.1. Adrenocorticotropin (ACTH)

Without knowing the exact nature of the mechanism(s) involved, it is possible to summarize the factual information that is currently available. Thus, IL-1 is known to release ACTH and glucocorticoids which is mediated by CRF. Indeed, the stimulatory effect of IL-1 can be inhibited by immunoneutralization of endogenous CRF (Uehara *et al.*, 1987). IL-1 added directly to the cerebral ventricles results in an immediate release of CRF (Breder *et al.*, 1988; Berkenbosch *et al.*, 1987), causes depletion of secretory vesicles from CRF neurosecretory axons (Whitnall *et al.*, 1992), enhances CRF and mRNA expression (Suda *et al.*, 1989), and directly stimulates CRF release from rat hypothalami (Allaerts *et al.*, 1990) which is mediated by an eicosanoid cyclooxygenase pathway (Navarra *et al.*, 1991). Specific, high-affinity receptors for IL-1 have also been described in the hypothalamus (Farrar *et al.*, 1987) and their immunoneutralization inhibits IL-1-stimulated ACTH release (Rivier *et al.*, 1989). Vasopressin and CRF are cosecreted from some hypothalamic neurosecretory cells. Vasopressin increases the ACTH stimulatory response to CRF and it has been shown that IL-1 stimulates vasopressin release by acting directly on CRF neurosecretory cells (Whitnall *et al.*, 1992).

IL-6 stimulates ACTH release in rats when given intravenously (Naito *et al.*, 1988) or intracerebroventricularly (Lyson and McCann, 1991). Coadministration of an anti-CRF antibody with IL-6 blocks the effect of this cytokine on ACTH secretion (Naito *et al.*, 1991) suggesting that as in the case of IL-1 above, the IL-6 effect is also mediated by CRF. This is further supported by *in vitro* work demonstrating that IL-6 stimulates CRF secretion from medial basal hypothalamic fragments in the rat (Lyson *et al.*, 1991). IL-2 can also stimulate the release of CRF from superfused rat hypothalami (Cambronero *et al.*, 1992). In contrast to IL-1 and IL-6, the IL-2 effect on ACTH release has a much slower rate of onset (Naito *et al.*, 1989; Loze *et al.*, 1985). TNF stimulates ACTH release in rats when given intravenously (Bernandini *et al.*, 1990; Loze *et al.*, 1985) through a mechanism similar to IL-1 (Vankele-Com *et al.*, 1990).

Based on the currently available evidence, it appears, therefore, that IL-1, IL-2, IL-6, and TNF have stimulatory effects on the hypothalamic–pituitary–adrenal axis with only IFN-α having inhibitory properties. The main effect of cytokines is to stimulate the release of hypothalamic CRF. This effect is then augmented by direct pituitary actions of IL-1 and IL-6 from hypothalamic and/or pituitary sources (possibly from both) on basal and CRF-stimulated ACTH secretion. Conversely, glucocorticoids have been known for some time to have a negative feedback on interleukin synthesis in cells of the immune system (Snyder and Unanne, 1982) by inhibiting gene expression (Lee *et al.*, 1988) as well as by inhibiting the hypothalamic–pituitary axis.

10.2. Gonadotropin

The predominant effect of IL-1 on the hypothalamic–pituitary–gonadal axis is inhibitory via a central action on gonadotropin-releasing hormone (GnRH) secretion (Rivier and Vale, 1989; Kalra *et al.*, 1990a). The inhibitory effect of IL-1 on GnRH is mediated through endogenous opioids as the opiate antagonist naloxone blocks this action (Kalra *et al.*, 1990b). Rivier and Vale (1990) also found that IL-1 induced inhibition of the proestrus LH surge and ovulation was dependent on an opioid-mediated mechanism. CRF has also been shown to inhibit GnRH and LH release (Nikolarakis *et al.*, 1986; Petraglia *et al.*, 1987), and opioids are involved in this mechanism as well (Almeida *et al.*, 1989; Petraglia *et al.*, 1986). Norepinephrine initiates the preovulatory surge of gonadotropins by evoking the release of GnRH from the median eminence. IL-1 specifically blocks norepinephrine-stimulated GnRH and prostaglandin E_2 release from medial basal hypothalamic fragments (Rettori *et al.*, 1991).

10.3. Thyroid Hormones

This group includes thyroliberin [thyrotropin-releasing hormone (TRH)], thyrotropin [thyroid-stimulating hormone (TSH)], and of thyroid hormones, thyroxine (T_4) and triiodothyroxine (T_3). IL-1, TNF-α, and IFN-γ have an inhibitory effect on thyroid hormone secretion acting directly at the hypothalamic–pituitary level (Dubuis *et al.*, 1988). The literature, however, is not clear on the effect of IL-6. Thus, while IL-6 stimulates TSH secretion from anterior pituitary cells *in vitro* (Bernton *et al.*, 1987; Spangelo *et al.*, 1989), its intracerebral injection inhibits TSH release (Lyson *et al.*, 1991; Rettori *et al.*, 1987) and at the same time stimulates TRH release from medial basal hypothalamic explants (Lyson *et al.*, 1991).

Cytokines were also shown to exert a complex action on thyroid follicular cell growth. Furthermore, IL-1 stimulates growth of cells of the FRTL-5 thyroid cell line *in vitro* (Mine *et al.*, 1987) and of rat thyroid gland *in vivo* (Zerek-Melen *et al.*, 1993). However, IL-1 suppresses the proliferation of FRTL-5 cells induced by TSH or forskolin (Zeki *et al.*, 1991), and inhibition of TSH-induced growth of fetal thyroid cells in culture by IFN-γ was also observed (Huber and Davies, 1990). Moreover, TNF-α and interferons induce expression of class I and class II HLA antigens in thyrocytes (Nagataki and Eguchi, 1992).

10.4. Prolactin (PRL)

In addition to ACTH and GH, PRL is released in response to stress and intracerebroventricular injection of IL-1 also stimulates PRL secretion. Since PRL is mainly under the inhibitory control of hypothalamic dopamine, it was thought that dopamine is involved in the cytokine-induced release of PRL. Although IL-1, IL-6, and TNF-α have not been shown to have any effect on hypothalamic dopamine release, the observations cannot be interpreted as evidence against the possibility that hypothalamic dopamine is somehow involved in the mechanism of stress-induced PRL release (Yamaguchi *et al.*, 1991b).

IL-1, IL-6, TNF-α, and the interferons (α, β, and γ) all stimulate prolactin release from anterior pituitary cells (Yamaguchi *et al.*, 1991a,b; Schettini *et al.*, 1989). IL-6 release is stimulated from the anterior pituitary by IL-1 (Spangelo *et al.*, 1991a; Jones *et al.*, 1993), vasoactive intestinal peptide (Spangelo *et al.*, 1990), pituitary adenylate cyclase-activating polypeptide (PACAP), and calcitonin gene-related peptide (Tatsuno *et al.*, 1992). It appears that there are two separate systems by which IL-6 synthesis and release can be influenced, a cyclic AMP-dependent and a cyclic AMP-independent mechanism. This is supported by the following combination of findings: (1) activation of the adenylate cyclase–cyclic AMP system by forskolin, cholera toxin, or by the addition of dibutyryl cyclic AMP all stimulate IL-6 with prolonged incubation; (2) dexamethasone inhibits IL-6 secretin (Tatsuno *et al.*, 1992); (3) the 5′ promoter region of the IL-6 gene has cyclic AMP and glucocorticoid responsive elements (Kishimoto, 1989) which may very well be the sites of action on IL-6 synthesis by these agents; and (4) IL-1 has no effect on pituitary cyclic AMP levels (Spangelo *et al.*, 1991b).

In closing this section, it is important to note that the placental lactogens (PL) represent another hormone family closely related to PRL and these together with GH are critically important for the development and function of the immune system. Because of the pioneering investigations of Berczi and his associates in the past two decades, it is now clear that the growth and lactogenic hormones are critically required for the development and maintenance of immunocompetence (for recent reviews see Berczi, 1993, 1994; Berczi and Nagy, 1994).

10.5. Growth Hormone (GH)

Growth hormone secretion by the pituitary is mainly controlled by a balance of the stimulatory effect of growth hormone releasing hormone (GHRH) and the inhibitory effect of somatostatin. IL-1 specifically stimulates both the release of GHRH and somatostatin from rat hypothalamus (Honegger *et al.*, 1991) and increases somatostatin synthesis in the fetal hypothalamus (Scarborough, 1990). The predominant effect of IL-1 is on somatostatin release and this may result in an overall suppression of GH secretion (Huber and Davies, 1990). In the study by Honegger and co-workers, the hypothalamic site of action was not the medial basal hypothalamus or the median eminence, i.e., the hypothalamic areas most commonly involved in somatostatin release suggesting that this particular IL-1 effect is at a higher level of the hypothalamus. It may be added that GH release by IL-1 in the hypothalamus is mediated by a prostaglandin cyclooxygenase-dependent mechanism (Huber and Davies, 1990) similar to the earlier-described CRF release by IL-1 (Navarra *et al.*, 1991). Neither IL-6 nor TNF has an effect on GHRH or somatostatin release (Huber and Davies, 1990).

11. EXTRAHYPOTHALAMIC NEURAL STRUCTURES AND THE IMMUNE RESPONSE

In general, the immune response can basically be influenced in at least two ways: humoral (neuroendocrine) and through nerve connections (neural). Each of these pathways has afferent and efferent components.

The first pathway, i.e., the neuroendocrine pathway, employs mainly hormones and cytokines as its humoral effectors and the main structures are the hypothalamus, pituitary, and adrenals. The functioning of the neuroendocrine pathway with respect to both its component parts as well as its entirety is well understood and has been described above.

In sharp contrast, the functioning of the second pathway, i.e., the neural pathway operating through nerve connections, is only incompletely understood. Mainly, what is known is that the efferent and afferent nerve supply of lymphoid organs belongs primarily to the autonomic nervous system (Bulloch and Moore, 1981; Bulloch, 1985; Livnat *et al.*, 1985; Magni *et al.*, 1987; Romano *et al.*, 1991; Lorton *et al.*, 1991; Kendall and Alshawaf, 1991). Thus, lymphoid tissues are innervated by both sympathetic and parasympathetic fibers which interact with corresponding receptors on the lymphocytes (Strom *et al.*, 1974, 1981; Roszman and Brooks, 1985; Roszman *et al.*, 1985; Plaut, 1987; Rinner *et al.*, 1990). Also, nerve endings in the lymphoid organs (Magni *et al.*, 1987; Romano *et al.*, 1991; Kendall and Alshawaf, 1991) may be stimulated by cytokines released from immunocompetent cells so that the neurons serve in a sense as "immunoreceptors" (Weihe *et al.*, 1980, 1991) that feed on stimulation to secondary spinal neurons that transmit to the brain. This arrangement conjures up the image of the established organization of somatomotor or visceromotor reflexes, i.e., ascending and descending structures that are connected through the CNS influence or control the corresponding reflex (Petrovicky *et al.*, 1981; Petrovicky, 1989; Mogenson, 1990) and therefore could be considered as an "immune reflex arc" (Petrovicky *et al.*, 1994).

When viewed in this framework, the principal question that emerges is the identity of the anatomical substrate of the immune reflex arc, i.e., the nature of what is described in the literature as the "brain regulatory system for the immune response" (BRSIR).

In a series of experiments, Masek, Petrovicky, and associates (Masek *et al.*, 1983, 1992; Petrovicky *et al.*, 1981, 1994; Petrovicky, 1989) have undertaken to identify the anatomical structures that represent the BRSIR by using small electrolytic lesions placed in different areas of the nervous system and delayed skin hypersensitivity together with [^{3}H]thymidine uptake into DNA following injection of MDP. Lesions were placed from the spinal cord and through the brain stem to the cerebral cortex. The methodology and the results obtained in the studies are discussed in detail in Petrovicky *et al.* (1994). Here we only summarize the most important findings. It was found that the medial frontal cortex, the subnucleus basomedialis and centralis of the amygdala, the subnucleus medialis and dorsolateralis of the nucleus parabrachialis, the lateral reticular formation (nucleus paracellularis—mainly areas corresponding with aminergic groups), part of the raphe reticular formation (nucleus raphealis dorsalis and nuclear linearis, i.e., mainly areas corresponding with serotoninergic groups), and the spinal cord represent the main structures of the BRSIR. These are very important findings and one awaits their conceptual integration into the immune neuroendocrine circuitry with great expectations.

12. THE FUTURE

The immune–neuroendocrine circuitry represents an immensely complex, powerful, and wide-ranging charter of human physiologic and pathologic possibilities, which, among others, is working its way to the creation of a new immunology based on a vastly enlarged vision of immunologic potential in health and disease. The emergence of this new interdisciplinary field will require a critical reexamination of some of our basic current views on the pathophysiologic and immunopharmacologic realities surrounding immune manifestations in health and disease.

ACKNOWLEDGMENTS. This chapter is dedicated with gratitude to Doctors Judith Szentivanyi, David W. Talmage, Samuel C. Bukantz, David S. Pearlman, Charles E. Reed, Robert A. Townley, and Robert A. Good.

REFERENCES

Abe-Dohmae, S., Harada, N., Yamada, K., and Tanaka, R., 1993, Bcl-2 gene is highly expressed during neurogenesis in the central nervous system, *Biochem. Biophys. Res. Commun.* **191**:915.

Aggarwal, B. B., and Gutterman, J. U., 1992, *Leukemia Inhibitory Factor in Human Cytokines*, Blackwell, Oxford.

Akbar, A. N., Borthwick, N., Salmon, M., Gombert, W., Bofill, M., Shamsadeen, N., Pilling, D., Petts, S., Grundy, J. E., and Janossy, G., 1993a, The significance of low bcl-2 expression by CD45RO T-cells in normal individuals and patients with acute viral infections. The role of apoptosis in T-cell memory, *J. Exp. Med.* **178**:427.

Akbar, A. N., Salmon, M., Savill, J., and Janossy, G., 1993b, A possible role for bcl-2 in regulating T-cell memory—A "balancing act" between cell death and survival, *Immunol. Today* **14**:526.

Allaerts, W., Carmeliet, P., and Denef, C., 1990, New perspectives in the function of pituitary folliculostellate cells, *Mol. Cell. Endocrinol.* **71**:73.

Allsopp, T. E., Wyatt, S., Paterson, H. F., and Davies, A. M., 1993, The proto-oncogene bcl-2 can selectively rescue neurotrophic factor-dependent neurons from apoptosis, *Cell* **73**:295.

Almeida, O. F. X., Nikolarakis, K. E., and Sirinathsinghji, D. T. S., and Herz, A., 1989, Opioid mediated inhibition of sexual behavior and luteinizing hormone secretion by corticotrophin-releasing hormone, in: *Brain Opioid Systems in Reproduction* (R. G. Dyer and R. J. Bickness, eds.), Oxford University Press, London, pp. 223–233.

Aloisi, F., Rosa, S., Testa, U., Bonsi, P., Russo, G., Peschle, C., and Levi, G., 1994, Regulation of leukemia inhibitory factor synthesis in cultured human astrocytes, *J. Immunol.* **152**:5022.

Anegon, I., and Grolleau, D., 1991, Regulation of HILDA/LIF gene expression in activated human monocytic cells, *J. Immunol.* **147**:3973.

Arquint, M., Roder, J., Chia, L. S., Down, J., Wilkinson, D., Bayley, H., Braun, P., and Dunn, R., 1987, Molecular cloning and primary structure of myelin-associated glycoprotein, *Proc. Natl. Acad. Sci. USA* **84**:600.

Awatsuji, H., Furukawa, Y., Hirota, M., Murakami, Y., Nii, S., Furukawa, S., and Hayashi, K., 1993, Interleukin-4 and -5 as modulators of nerve growth factor synthesis/secretion in astrocytes, *Neurosci. Res.* **34**:539.

Bamber, B. A., Masters, B. A., Hoyle, G. W., Brinster, R. L., and Palmiter, K. D., 1994, Leukemia inhibitory factor induces neurotransmitter switching in transgenic mice, *Proc. Natl. Acad. Sci. USA* **91**:7839.

Barbin, G., Manthorpe, M., and Varon, S., 1984, Purification of the chick eye ciliary neuronotrophic factor, *J. Neurochem.* **43**:1468.

Barinaga, M., 1994, Neurotrophic factors enter the clinic, *Science* **264**:772.

Bazan, J. F., 1990, Structural design and molecular evolution of a cytokine receptor superfamily, *Proc. Natl. Acad. Sci. USA* **87**:6934.

Bazan, J. F., 1991, Neuropoietic cytokines in the hematopoietic fold, *Neuron* **7**:197.

Bekkers, J. M., and Stevens, C. F., 1990, Presynaptic mechanism for long-term potentiation in the hippocampus, *Nature* **346**:724.

Berczi, I., 1993, Neuroendocrine defense in endotoxin shock, *Acta Microbiol. Hung.* **40**:265.

Berczi, I., 1994, Role of the growth and lactogenic hormone family in immune function, *J. Neuroimmunol.* **1**:201.

Berczi, I., and Nagy, E., 1994, Neurohormonal control of cytokines during injury, in: *Brain Control of Responses in Trauma* (N. J. Rothwell and F. Berkenbosch, eds.), Cambridge University Press, London, pp. 32–107.

Berkemeier, L. R., Winslow, J. W., Kaplan, D. R., Nikolics, K., Goeddel, D. V., and Rosenthal, A., 1991, Neurotrophin-5: A novel neurotrophic factor that activates trkA and trkB, *Neuron* **7**:857.

Berkenbosch, F., Van Oers, J., del Rey, A., Tilders, F., and Besedovsky, H., 1987, Corticotropin-releasing factor producing neurons in the rat activated by interleukin-1, *Science* **238**:524.

Bernandini, R., Kamilaris, T. C., Calogero, A. E., Johnson, E. O., Gomez, M. T., Gold, P. W., and Chrousos, G. P., 1990, Interactions between tumor necrosis factor-α, hypothalamic corticotropin-releasing hormone and adrenocorticotropin secretion in the rat, *Endocrinology* **126**:2876.

Bernton, E. W., Beach, J. E., Holaday, J. W., Smallridge, R. C., and Fein, H. G., 1987, Release of multiple hormones by a direct action of interleukin-1 on pituitary cells, *Science* **238**:519.

Besedovsky, H. O., Sorkin, E., Felix, D., and Haas, H., 1977, Hypothalamic changes during the immune response, *Eur. J. Immunol.* **7**:325.

Bhatt, H., Brunet, L. J., and Stewart, C. L., 1991, Uterine expression of leukemia inhibitory factor coincides with the onset of blastocyst implantation, *Proc. Natl. Acad. Sci. USA* **88:**11408.

Birnbaumer, L., and Brown, A. M., 1990, G proteins and the mechanism of action of hormones, neurotransmitters, and autocrine and paracrine regulatory factors, *Am. Rev. Respir. Dis.* **141:**S106.

Bischoff, S. C., and Dahinden, C. A., 1992, Effect of nerve growth factor on the release of inflammatory mediators by mature human basophils, *Blood* **79:**2662.

Boise, L. H., Gonzalez-Garcia, M., Postema, C. E., Ding, L., Lindsten, T., Turka, L. A., Mao, X., Nunez, G., and Thompson, C. B., 1983, Bcl-X, a bcl-2 related gene that functions as a dominant regulator of apoptopic cell death, *Cell* **74:**597.

Bracci-Laudeiro, L., Aloe, L., Levi-Montalcini, R., Galeazzi, M., Schilter, D., Scully, J. L., and Otten, U., 1993, Increased levels of NGF in sera of systemic lupus erythematosus patients, *Neuroreport* **4:**563.

Bradshaw, R. A., Blundell, T. L., Lapatto, R., McDonald, N. Q., and Murray-Rust, J., 1993, Nerve growth factor revisited, *Trends Biochem. Sci.* **18:**48.

Breder, C. D., Dinarello, C. A., and Safer, C. B., 1988, Interleukin-1 immunoreactive innervations of the rat hypothalamus, *Science* **240:**321.

Bruce, A. G., Hoggatt, I. H., and Rose, T. M., 1992a, Oncostatin M is a differentiation factor for myeloid leukemia cells, *J. Immunol.* **149:**1271.

Bruce, A. G., Linsley, P. S., and Rose, T. M., 1992b, Oncostatin M, *Prog. Growth Factor Res.* **4:**157.

Brümmendorf, T., and Rathjen, F. G., 1994, Cell adhesion molecules 1: Immunoglobulin superfamily, *Protein Profile* **1:**9.

Bulloch, K., 1985, Neuroanatomy of lymphoid tissue: A review, in: *Neural Modulation of Immunity* (R. Guillemin, M. Cohn, and T. Melnechuk, eds.), Raven Press, New York, pp. 111–142.

Bulloch, K., and Moore, R. Y., 1981, Innervation of the thymus gland by brain stem and spinal cord in mouse and rat, *Am. J. Anat.* **162:**157.

Cai, J., Gill, P. S., Masood, P., Chandrasoma, P., Jung, B., Law, R. E., and Radka, S. F., 1994, Oncostatin M is an autocrine growth factor in Kaposi's sarcoma, *Am. J. Pathol.* **145:**74.

Cambronero, J. C., Rivas, F. J., Borrell, J., and Guaza, C., 1992, Interleukin-2 induces corticotropin-releasing hormone release from superfused rat hypothalami: Influence of glucocorticoids, *Endocrinology* **131:**677.

Carman-Krzan, M., Vige, X., and Wise, B. C., 1991, Regulation by interleukin-1 of nerve growth factor secretion and nerve growth factor mRNA expression in rat primary astroglial cultures, *J. Neurochem.* **56:**636.

Chao, M. V., 1992, Neurotrophin receptors: A window into neuronal differentiation, *Neuron* **9:**583.

Cheema, S. S., Richards, L., Murphy, M., and Bartlett, P. F., 1994a, Leukemia inhibitory factor prevents the death of axotomized sensory neurons in the dorsal root ganglia of the neonatal rat, *J. Neurosci. Res.* **37:**213.

Cheema, S. S., Richards, L., Murphy, M., and Bartlett, P. F., 1994b, Leukemia inhibitory factor rescues motoneurons from axotomy-induced cell death, *Neuroreport* **5:**989.

Chevalier, S., Praloran, V., Smith, C., MacGrogan, D., Ip, N. Y., Yancopoulos, G. D., Brochet, P., Pouplard, A., and Gascan, H., 1994, Expression and functionality of the trkA proto-oncogene product/NGF receptor in undifferentiated hematopoietic cells, *Blood* **83:**1479.

Cotzias, G. C., and Tang, L. C., 1977, Adenylate cyclase of brain reflects propensity for breast cancer in mice, *Science* **197:**1094.

Cunningham, B. A., Hemperley, J. J., Murray, B. A., Prediger, E. A., Brackenbury, R., and Edelman, G. M., 1987, Neural cell adhesion molecule: Structure, immunoglobulin-like domains, cell surface modulation, and alternative RNA splicing, *Science* **236:**799.

Davis, S., Aldrich, T. H., Valenzuela, D. M., Wong, V., Furth, M. E., Squinto, S. P., and Yancopoulos, G. D., 1991, The receptor for ciliary neurotrophic factor, *Science* **253:**59.

DeSimone, R., Alleva, E., Tirassa, P., and Aloe, L., 1990, Nerve growth factor released into the bloodstream following intraspecies fighting induces mast cell degranulation in adult male mice, *Brain Behav. Immun.* **4:**74.

Dougherty, P. M., and Dafny, N., 1987, Central opioid systems are differentially affected by products of the immune response, *Soc. Neurosci. Abstr.* **13:**1437.

Dubuis, J. M., Dayer, J. M., Siegnist-Kaiser, C. A., and Burger, A. G., 1988, Human recombinant interleukin-1β decreases plasma thyroid hormone and thyroid-stimulating hormone levels in rats, *Endocrinology* **123:**2175.

Dudai, Y., 1988, Neurogenetic dissection of learning and short-term memory in Drosophila, *Annu. Rev. Neurosci.* **11:**537.

Dunn, A. J., Powell, M. L., Moreshead, W. V., Gaskin, J. M., and Hall, N. R., 1987, Effects of Newcastle disease virus administration to mice on the metabolism of cerebral biogenic amines, plasma corticosterone and lymphocyte proliferation, *Brain, Behavior & Immunity* **1:**216–230.

Ebendal, T., 1992, Function and evolution in the NGF family and its receptors, *J. Neurosci. Res.* **32:**461.

Edelman, G. M., 1987, *Neural Darwinism*, Basic Books, New York.

Edelman, G. M., 1988, Morphoregulatory molecules, *Biochemistry* **27:**3534.

Edelman, G. M., 1989, Topobiology, *Sci. Am.* **260:**44.

Ehrhard, P. B., Erb, P., Graumann, U., and Otten, U., 1993a, Expression of nerve growth factor and nerve growth factor receptor tyrosine kinase Trk in activated CD4-positive T-cell clones, *Proc. Natl. Acad. Sci. USA* **90:**10984.

Ehrhard, P. B., Ganter, U., Bauer, J., and Otten, U., 1993b, Expression of functional trk protooncogene in human monocytes, *Proc. Natl. Acad. Sci. USA* **90:**5423.

Eremina, O. F., and Devoino, L. V., 1973, Production of humoral antibodies in rabbits following destruction of the nucleus of the midbrain raphe, *Byull, Eksp. Biol. Med.* **74:**258.

Evercooren, A. B., Kleinman, H. K., Ohno, S., Marangos, P., Schwartz, J. P., and DuBois-Dalq, M. E., 1982, Nerve growth factor, laminin and fibronectin promote neurite growth in human fetal sensory ganglia cultures, *J. Neurosci.* **8:**179.

Farrar, W. L., Kilian, P. L. Ruff, M. R., Hill, J. M., and Pert, C. B., 1987, Visualization and characterization of interleukin-1 receptors in brain, *J. Immunol.* **139:**459.

Filipp, G., and Szentivanyi, A., 1953, Frage der Organlokalisation der allergischen Reaktion, *Wien. Klin. Wochenschr.* **65:**620.

Filipp, G., and Szentivanyi, A., 1956, Experimentelle Data zur regulativen Rolle des Neuroendokriniums in experimenteller Anaphylaxie I. Relazioni e Communicazioni, *Rome Il Pansiero Scientifico* **229:**1.

Filipp, G., and Szentivanyi, A., 1957, Die Wirkung von Hypothalamuslasionen auf den anaphylaktischen Schock des Meerschweinchens, *Allerg. Asthmaforsch. Bd.* **1:**12

Filipp, G., and Szentivanyi, A., 1958, Anaphylaxis and the nervous system. Part III, *Ann. Allergy* **16:**306.

Filipp, G., and Szentivanyi, A., 1985, Anaphylaxis and the nervous system. Part III, in: *Foundations of Psychoneuroimmunology* (S. Locke, R. Ader, H. O. Besedovsky, N. R. Hall, G. Solomon, and T. Strom, eds.), Aldine Publishing, Hawthorne, NY, pp. 1–12.

Filipp, G., Szentivanyi, A., and Mess, B., 1952, Anaphylaxis and nervous system, *Acta Med. Hung. Tomus III, Fasciculus* **2:**163.

Fillion, M. P., Prudhomme, N., Haour, F., Fillion, G., Bonnet, M., Lespinats, G., Masek, K., Flegel, M., Corvaia, N., and Launay, J. M., 1989, Hypothetical role of the serotonergic system in neuroimmunomodulation: Preliminary molecular studies, in: *Interactions Among Central Nervous System, Neuroendocrine and Immune Systems* (J. W. Hadden, K. Masek, and G. Nistico, eds.), Pythagora Press, Rome, pp. 235–250.

Forger, N. G., Roberts, S. L., Wong, V., and Breedlove, S. M., 1993, Ciliary neurotrophic factor maintains motoneurons and their target muscles in developing rats, *J. Neurosci.* **13:**4720.

Friedman, H., Klein, T. W., and Szentivanyi, A., eds., 1981, *Immunomodulation by Bacteria and Their Products*, Plenum Press, New York.

Gearing, D. P., 1993, The leukemia inhibitory factor and its receptor, *Adv. Immunol.* **53:**31.

Gearing, D. P., and Cosman, D., 1991, Homology of the p40 subunit of natural killer cell stimulatory factor with the extracellular domain of the interleukin-6 receptor, *Cell* **66:**8.

Gearing, D. P., Thut, C. J., VandenBos, T., Gimpel, S. D., Delaney, P. B., King, J., Price, V., Cosman, D., and Beckmann, M. P., 1991, Leukemia inhibitory factor receptor is structurally related to the IL-6 signal transducer, gp130, *EMBO J.* **10:**2839.

Geschwind, N., 1983, Preface, in: *Mind and Immunity. Behavioral Immunology* (S. E. Locke and M. Hornig-Rohan, eds.), Institute for the Advancement of Health, New York, pp. 1–6.

Geschwind, N., and Galaburda, A. M., 1985, Cerebral lateralization: Biological mechanisms, associations, and pathology. Parts I–III, *Arch. Neurol.* **42:**428.

Gillett, N. A., Lowe, D., Lu, L., Chan, C., and Ferrara, N., 1993, Leukemia inhibitory factor expression in human carotid plaques: Possible mechanism for inhibition of large vessel endothelial regrowth, *Growth Factors* **9:**301.

Giovannini, M., Selleri, L., Hermanson, G. G., and Evans, G. A., 1993, Localization of the human oncostatin M gene (OSM) to chromosome 22q12, distal to the Ewing's sarcoma breakpoint, *Cytogenet. Cell Genet.* **62:**32.

Goodman, C. S., and Pearson, K. G., 1982, Neuronal development: Cellular approaches in invertebrates, *Neurosci. Res. Prog. Bull.* **20:**777.

Gough, N. M., 1992, Molecular genetics of leukemia inhibitory factor (LIF) and its receptor, *Growth Factors* **7:**175.

Graf, J., Iwamoto, Y., Sasaki, M., Martin, G. R., Kleinman, H. K., Robey, F. A., and Yamada, Y., 1987, Identification of an amino acid sequence in laminin mediating cell attachment, chemotaxis, and receptor binding, *Cell* **48:**989.

Graninger, W. B., 1992, Transcriptional overexpression of the proto-oncogene bcl-2 in patients with lupus erythematosus, *Wien. Klin. Wochenschr.* **104:**205.

Griffin, D. E., Levine, B., Tyor, W. R., Tucker, P. G., and Hardwick, J. M., 1994, Age-dependent susceptibility to fatal encephalitis: Alpha virus infection of neurons, *Arch. Virol. Suppl.* **9:**31.

Hadcock, J. R., Port, J. D., and Malbon, C. C., 1991, Cross-regulation between G-protein mediated pathways. Activation of the inhibitory pathway of adenylycyclase increases the expression of β_2-adrenergic receptors, *J. Biol. Chem.* **266:**11915.

Hadden, J. W., and Szentivanyi, A., eds., 1985, *The Pharmacology of the Reticuloendothelial System*, Plenum Press, New York.

Hagg, T., Quon, D., Higaki, J., and Varon, S., 1992, Ciliary neurotrophic factor prevents neuronal degeneration and promotes low affinity NGF receptor expression in the adult rat CNS, *Neuron* **8:**145.

Hall, A. K., and Rao, M. S., 1992, Cytokines and neurokines: Related ligands and related receptors, *Trends Neurosci.* **15:**35.

Hama, T., Kushima, Y., Miyamoto, M., Kubota, M., Takei, N., and Hatanaka, H., 1991, Interleukin-6 improves the survival of mesencephalic catecholaminergic and septal cholinergic neurons from postnatal, two-week-old rats in cultures, *Neuroscience* **40:**445.

He, X., and Rosenfeld, M. G., 1991, Mechanisms of complex transcriptional regulation: Implication for brain development, *Neuron* **7:**183.

Hirano, T., Matsuda, T., and Nakajima, K., 1994, Signal transduction through gp130 that is shared among the receptors for the interleukin-6 related cytokine subfamily, *Stem Cells* **12:**262.

Hockenbery, D. M., 1992, The bcl-2 oncogene and apoptosis, *Semin Immunol.* **4:**413.

Honegger, J., Spagnoli, A., D'Urso, R., Navarra, P., Tsagarkis, S., Besser, G. M., and Grossman, A. B., 1991, Interleukin-1β modulates the acute release of growth hormone-releasing hormone and somatostatin from rat hypothalamus in vitro, whereas tumor necrosis factor and interleukin-6 have no effect, *Endocrinology* **129:**1275.

Huber, G. K., and Davies, T. F., 1990, Human fetal thyroid cell growth in vitro: System characterization and cytokine inhibition, *Endocrinology* **126:**869.

Hughes, S. M., Lillien, L. E., Roff, M. C., Rohrer, H., and Sendtner, M., 1988, Ciliary neurotrophic factor induces type 2 astrocyte differentiation in culture, *Nature* **335:**70.

Ip, N. Y., Ibanez, C. F., Nye, S. H., McClain, J., Jones, P. F., Gies, D. R., Belluscio, L., LeBeau, M. M., Espinosa, R., III, and Squinto, S. P., 1992a, Mammalian neurotrophin-4: Structure, chromosomal localization, tissue distribution and receptor specificity, *Proc. Natl. Acad. Sci. USA* **89:**3060.

Ip, N. Y., Nye, S. H., Boulton, T. G., Davis, S., Taga, T., Li, Y., Birren, S. J., Yasukawa, K., Kishimoto, T., Anderson, D. J., Stahl, N., and Yancopoulos, G. D., 1992b, CNTF and LIF act on neuronal cells via shared signal pathway that involve the IL-6 signal transducing receptor component, gp130, *Cell* **69:**1121.

Iwane, M., Kitamura, Y., Kaisho, Y., Yoshimura, K., Shintani, A., Sasada, R., Nakagawa, S., Kawahara, K.,

Nakahama, K., and Kakimura, A., 1990, Production, purification and characterization of biologically active recombinant human nerve growth factor, *Biochem. Biophys. Res. Commun.* **171:**116.

Jeffery, E., Price, V., and Gearing, D. P., 1993, Close proximity of the genes for leukemia inhibitory factor and oncostatin M, *Cytokine* **5:**107.

Jessell, T. M., and Melton, D. A., 1992, Diffusible factors in vertebrate embryonic induction, *Cell* **68:**257.

Jones, K. R., and Reichardt, L. F., 1990, Molecular cloning of a human gene that is a member of the nerve growth factor family, *Proc. Natl. Acad. Sci. USA* **87:**8060.

Jones, T. H., and Kennedy, R. L., 1993, Cytokines and hypothalamic–pituitary function, *Cytokine* **5:**531–538.

Jones, T. H., Kennedy, R. L., Justice, S. K., and Price, A., 1993, Interleukin-1 stimulated the release of interleukin-6 from cultured human pituitary adenoma cells, *Acta Endocrinol.* **128:**405.

Kakihana, M., Kato, K., Fukumoto, H., Fujiwara, E., Iwane, M., and Suno, M., 1993, Detailed characterization of the biological activities of recombinant human nerve growth factor expressed in Chinese hamster ovary cells, *Mol. Chem. Neuropathol.* **18:**51.

Kallestad J. C., Shoyab, M., and Linsley, P. S., 1991, Disulfide bond arrangement and identification of regions required for functional activity of oncostatin M, *J. Biol. Chem.* **266:**8940.

Kalra, P. S., Figuentes, M., Sahu, A., and Kalra, S. P., 1990a, Endogeneous opioid peptides mediate the interleukin-1 induced inhibition of the release of luteinizing hormone (LH) releasing hormone and LH, *Endocrinology* **127:**2381.

Kalra, P. S., Sahu, A., and Kalra, S. P., 1990b, Interleukin-1 inhibits the ovarian steroid-induced luteinizing hormone surge and release of hypothalamic luteinizing hormone releasing hormone in rats, *Endocrinology* **126:**2145.

Karady, S., Selye, H., and Brownie, J. S. L., 1938, The influence of the alarm reaction on the development of anaphylactic shock, *J. Immunol.* **35:**335.

Kato, S., Negishi, K., Hayashi, Y., and Miki, N., 1983, Enhancement of neurite outgrowth and aspartate–glutamate uptake system in retinal explants cultured with chick gizzard extract, *J. Neurochem.* **40:**929.

Kato, S., Taniura, H., Taira, E., and Miki, N., 1992, Involvement of a receptor for neurite outgrowth factor (NOFR) in cerebellar neurogenesis, *Neurosci. Lett.* **140:**78.

Katsuura, G., Gottschall, P. E., Dahl, R. R., and Arimura, A., 1988, Adrenocorticotropin release induced by intracerebroventricular injection of recombinant human interleukin-1 in rats: Possible involvement of prostaglandin, *Endocrinology* **122:**1773–1779.

Katsuura, G., Arimura, A., Koves, K., and Gottschall, P. E., 1990, Involvement of organum vasculosum of lamina terminalis and preoptic area in interleukin-1beta induced ACTH release, *Am. J. Physiol.* **258:**E163–171.

Kendall, M. D., and Alshawaf, A. A., 1991, Innervation of the rat thymus gland, *Brain Behav. Immun.* **5:**9.

Kimata, H., Yoshida, A., Ishioka, C., Kusunoki, T., Hosoi, S., and Mikawa, H., 1991, Nerve growth factor specifically induces human IgG4 production, *Eur. J. Immunol.* **21:**137.

Kishimoto, T., 1989, The biology of interleukin-6, *Blood* **74:**1.

Klein, T. W., Specter, S., Friedman, H., and Szentivanyi, A., eds., 1983, *Biological Response Modifiers in Human Oncology and Immunology*, Plenum Press, New York.

Korneva, E. A., and Klimenko, V. M., 1976, Neuronale hypothalamusaktivitt und homoostatische rektionen, *Ergebn. Exp. Med.* **23:**373.

Korsching, S., 1993, The neurotrophic factor concept: A reexamination, *J. Neurosci.* **13:**2739.

Korsmeyer, S. J., 1992a, Bcl-2: An antidote to programmed cell death, *Cancer Surv.* **15:**105.

Korsmeyer, S. J., 1992b, Chromosomal translocations in lymphoid malignancies reveal novel proto-oncogenes, *Annu. Rev. Immunol.* **10:**785.

Kotzbauer, P. T., Lampe, P. A., Estus, S., Milbrandt, J., and Johnson, E. M., Jr., 1994, Postnatal development of survival responsiveness in rat sympathetic neurons to leukemia inhibitory factor and ciliary neurotrophic factor, *Neuron* **12:**763.

Krueger, J. M., Obal, F., Jr., Johannsen, L., Cady, A. B., and Toth, L., 1988, Endogenous slow-wave sleep substances: A review, in: *Current Trends in Slow-Wave Sleep Research* (C. Dugsovic and A. Wauquier, eds.), Raven Press, New York, pp. 97–112.

Krueger, J. M., Obal, F., Jr., Opp, M., Johannsen, L., Cady, A. B., and Toth, L., 1989, Immune response modifiers and sleep, in: *Interactions Among Central Nervous System, Neuroendocrine and Immune Systems* (J. W. Hadden, K. Masek, and G. Nistico, eds.), Pythagora Press, Rome, pp. 323–350.

Kurzrock, R., Estrov, Z., Wetzler, M., Gutterman, J. U., and Talpaz, M., 1991, LIF: Not just a leukemia inhibitory factor, *Endocrine Rev.* **12:**208.

Lam, A., Fuller, F., Miller, J., Kloss, J., Manthorpe, M., Varon, S., and Cordell, B., 1991, Sequence and structural organization of the human gene encoding ciliary neurotrophic factor, *Gene* **102:**271.

Lams, B. E., and Isacson, O., 1988, Loss of transmitter-associated enzyme staining following axotomy does not indicate death of brainstem cholinergic neurons, *Brain Res.* **475:**401.

Landis, S., 1990, Target regulation of neurotransmitter phenotype, *Trends Neurosci.* **13:**344.

Leary, A. G., Wong, G. G., Clark, S. C., Smith, A. G., and Ogawa, M., 1990, Leukemia inhibitory factor differentiation-inhibiting activity/human interleukin for DA cells augments proliferation of human hematopoietic stem cells, *Blood* **75:**1960.

LeDouarin, N., 1982, *The Neural Crest*, Cambridge University Press, London.

Lee, S. W., Tsou, A. P., Chan, H., Thomas, J., Petrie, K., Eugui, A. M., and Allison, A. C., 1988, Glucocorticoids selectively inhibit the transcription of interleukin-1β gene and decrease the stability of interleukin-1β mRNA, *Proc. Natl. Acad. Sci. USA* **85:**1204.

Leon, A., Buriani, A., DalToso, R., Fabris, M., Romanello, S., Aloe, L., and Levi-Montalcini, R., 1994, Mast cells synthesize, store, and release nerve growth factor, *Proc. Natl. Acad. Sci. USA* **91:**3739.

Levi-Montalcini, R., and Hamburger, V., 1951, Selective growth stimulating effects of mouse sarcoma on the sensory and sympathetic nervous system of the chick embryo, *J. Exp. Zool.* **116:**321.

Lin, L. F. H., Mismer, D., Lile, J. D., Armes, L. G., Butler, E. T., III, Vannice, J. L., and Collins, F., 1989, Purification, cloning, and expression of ciliary neurotrophic factor (CNTF), *Science* **246:**1023.

Livnat, S., Felten, S. Y., Carlson, S. L., Bellinger, D. L., and Felten, D. L., 1985, Involvement of peripheral and central catecholamine systems in neural immune interactions, *J. Neuroimmunol.* **10:**5.

Lochrie, M. A., and Simon, M. I., 1988, G protein multiplicity in eukaryotic signal transduction systems, *Biochemistry* **17:**4957.

Lorenzo, J. A., Jastrzebski, S. L., Kalinowski, J. F., Downie, E., and Korn, J. H., 1994, Tumor necrosis factor-alpha stimulates production of leukemia inhibitory factor in human dermal fibroblast cultures, *Clin. Immunol. Immunopathol.* **70:**260.

Lorton, D., Bellinger, D. L., Felten, S. Y., and Felten, D. L., 1991, Substance P innervation of spleen in rats: Nerve fibers associate with lymphocytes and macrophages in specific compartments of the spleen, *Brain Behav. Immun.* **5:**29.

Louis, J. C., Magal, E., Burnham, P., and Varon, S., 1993, Cooperative effectives of ciliary neurotrophic factor and norepinephrine on tyrosine hydroxylase expression in cultured rat locus coeruleus neurons, *Dev. Biol.* **155:**1.

Loze, M. T., Frana, L. W., Sharrow, S. O., Robb, R. J., and Rosenberg, S. A., 1985, In vivo administration of purified human interleukin-2. I. Half-life and immunological effects of the Jurkat cell line derived interleukin-2, *J. Immunol.* **134:**157.

Ludlam, W. H., Zang, Z., McCarson, K. E., Krause, J. E., Spray, D. C., and Kessler, J. A., 1994, mRNAs encoding muscarinic and substance P receptors in cultured sympathetic neurons are differentially regulated by LIF and CNTF, *Dev. Biol.* **164:**528.

Lyson, K., and McCann, S. M., 1991, The effect of interleukin-6 on pituitary hormone release in vivo and in vitro, *Neuroendocrinology* **54:**262.

Lyson, K., Milenkovic, L., and McCann, S. M., 1991, The stimulatory effect of interleukin-6 on corticotropin-releasing hormone and thyrotropin-releasing hormone release in vitro, *Neuroendocrinology* **4:**161.

McFadden, P. N., and Koshland, D. E., Jr., 1990a, Habituation in the single cell: Diminished secretion of norepinephrine with repetitive depolarization in PC12 cells, *Proc. Natl. Acad. Sci. USA* **87:**2031.

McFadden, P. N., and Koshland, D. E., Jr., 1990b, Parallel pathways for habituation in repetitively stimulated PC12 cells, *Neuron* **4:**615.

Magal, E., Burnham, P., and Varon, S., 1991a, Effect of ciliary neurotrophic factor on low affinity nerve growth factor receptor expression by cultured neurons from different rat brain regions, *J. Neurosci. Res.* **30:**560.

Magal, E., Burnham, P., and Varon, S., 1991b, Effects of ciliary neurotrophic factor on rat spinal cord neurons in vitro: Survival and expression of choline acetyltransferase and low-affinity nerve growth factor, *Dev. Brain Res.* **63:**141.

Magni, F., Bruschi, F., and Kasti, M., 1987, The afferent innervation of the thymus gland in the rat, *Brain Res.* **424:**379.

Malik, N., Kallestad, J. C., Gunderson, N. L., Austin, S. D., Neubauer, M. G., Ochs, V., Marquardt, H., Zarling, J. M., Shoyab, M., and Wei, C. M., 1989, Molecular cloning, sequence analysis and functional expression of a novel growth regulator, oncostatin M, *Mol. Cell. Biol.* **9:**2847.

Malinow, R., and Tsien, R. W., 1990, Presynaptic enhancement shown by whole-cell recordings of long-term potentiation in hippocampal slices, *Nature* **346:**177.

Manthorpe, M., Skaper, S. D., Williams, L. R., and Varon, S., 1986, Purification of adult rat sciatic nerve ciliary neurotrophic factor, *Brain Res.* **367:**282.

Markowska, A. L., Koliatsos, V. E., Breckler, S. J., Price, D. L., and Olton, D. S., 1994, Human nerve growth factor improves spatial memory in aged but not young rats, *J. Neurosci.* **14:**4815.

Marshall, J. S., Gauldie, J., Nielsen, L., and Bienenstock, J., 1993, Leukemia inhibitory factor production by rat mast cells, *Eur. J. Immunol.* **23:**2116.

Martinou, J. C., Martinou, I., and Kato, A. C., 1992, Cholinergic differentiation factor (CDF/LIF) promotes survival of isolated rat embryonic motoneurons in vitro, *Neuron* **8:**737.

Masek, K., Kadlecova, O., and Petrovicky, P., 1983, The effect of brain stem lesions on the immune response, in: *Advances in Immunopharmacology* (J. Hadden, ed.), Pergamon Press, Oxford, pp. 443–450.

Masek, K., Horak, P., Kadlec, O., and Flegel, M., 1989, The interactions between neuroendocrine and immune systems at the receptor level. The possible role of serotonergic system, in: *Interactions Among Central Nervous System, Neuroendocrine and Immune Systems* (J. W. Hadden, K. Masek, and G. Nistico, eds.), Pythagora Press, Rome, pp. 225–234.

Masek, K., Petrovicky, P., and Seifert, J., 1992, An introduction to the possible role of central nervous system structures in neuroendocrine immune systems interaction, *Int. J. Immunopharmacol.* **14:**317.

Mattoli, S., Miante, S., Calabro, F., Mezzetti, M., Fasoli, A., and Allegra, L., 1990, Bronchial epithelial cells exposed to isocyanates potentiate activation and proliferation of T cells, *Am. J. Physiol.* **259:**L320.

Mayer, M., Bhakoo, K., and Noble, M., 1994, Ciliary neurotrophic factor and leukemia inhibitory factor promote the generation, maturation and survival of oligodendrocytes in vitro, *Development* **120:**143.

Meakin, S. O., and Shooter, E. M., 1992, The nerve growth factor family of receptors, *Trends Neurosci.* **15:**323.

Metcalf, D., 1992, Leukemia inhibitory factor—A puzzling polyfunctional regulator, *Growth Factors* **7:**169.

Metcalf, D., Hilton, D., and Nicola, J. A., 1991, Leukemia inhibitory factor can potentiate murine megakaryocyte production in vitro, *Blood* **77:**2150.

Milner, R. J., Lai, C., Sutcliffe, J. G., and Bloom, F. E., 1989, Expression of immunoglobulin-like proteins in the nervous system: Properties of the neural protein 1B236/MAG, in: *Neuroimmune Networks: Physiology and Diseases* (E. J. Goetzl and N. H. Spector, eds.), Liss, New York, pp. 9–15.

Mine, M., Tramontano, D., Chin, W. W., and Ingbar, S. H., 1987, Interleukin-1 stimulates thyroid cell growth and increases the concentration of the c-myc proto-oncogene mRNA in thyroid follicular cells in culture, *Endocrinology* **120:**1212.

Missale, C., Boroni, F., Sigala, S., Zanellato, A., DalToso, R., Balsari, A., and Spano, P., 1994, Nerve growth factor directs differentiation of the bipotential cell line GH-3 into the mammotroph phenotype, *Endocrinology* **135:**290.

Miyajima, A., Kitamura, T., Harada, N., Yokota, N., and Arai, K., 1992, Cytokine receptors and signal transduction, *Annu. Rev. Immunol.* **10:**295.

Mogenson, G. J., 1990, Brain stem systems for the control of behavioral acts, in: *Brain Stem Mechanisms of Behavior* (E. Klemm and R. P. Vertes, eds.), Wiley, New York, pp. 171–198.

Morimoto, A., Murakami, N., Nakamori, T., Sakata, Y., and Watanabe, T., 1989, Possible involvement of porstaglandin E in development of ACTH response in rats induced by human recombinant interleukin-1, *J. Physiol.* **411:**245–256.

Morimoto, B. H., and Koshland, D. E., Jr., 1990a, Excitatory amino acid uptake and N-methyl-D-aspartate-mediated secretion in a neural cell line, *Proc. Natl. Acad. Sci. USA* **87**:3518.

Morimoto, B. H., and Koshland, D. E., Jr., 1990b, Induction and expression of long- and short-term neurosecretory potentiation in a neural cell line, *Neuron* **5**:875.

Morimoto, M., Morita, N., and Kawata, M., 1994, The effects of NGF and glucocorticoid on the cytological features of rat chromaffin cells in vitro, *Neuroreport* **5**:954.

Morris, G. M., Hadcock, J. R., and Malbon, C. C., 1991, Cross-regulation between G-protein-coupled receptors. Activation of β_2-adrenergic receptors increases α1-adrenergic receptor mRNA levels, *J. Biol. Chem.* **266**:2233.

Muller, Y., Duperray, F., Caruso, F., and Clos, J., 1994, Autocrine regulation of proliferation of cerebellar granule neurons by nerve growth factor, *J. Neurosci. Res.* **38**:41.

Murphy, M., Reid, K., Hilton, D. J., and Bartlett, P. F., 1991, Generation of sensory neurons is stimulated by leukemia inhibitory factor, *Proc. Natl. Acad. Sci. USA* **88**:3498.

Murphy, M., Reid, K., Brown, M. A., and Bartlett, P. F., 1993, Involvement of leukemia inhibitory factor and nerve growth factor in the development of dorsal root ganglion neurons, *Development* **117**:1173.

Nagataki, S., and Eguchi, K., 1992, Cytokines and immune regulation in thyroid autoimmunity, *Autoimmunity* **13**:27.

Naito, Y., Fukata, J., Tominaga, T., Nakai, Y., Tamai, S., Mori, K., and Imura, H., 1988, Interleukin-6 stimulates the secretion of adrenocorticotropic hormone in conscious, freely moving rats, *Biochem. Biophys. Res. Commun.* **155**:1459.

Naito, Y., Fukata, J., Tominaga, T., Masui, Y., Hirai, Y., Murakami, N., Tamai, S., Mori, K., and Imura, H., 1989, Adrenocorticotropic hormone releasing activities of interleukins in a homologous in vivo system, *Biochem. Biophys. Res. Commun.* **164**:1262.

Naito, Y., Fukata, J., Shindo, K., Ebisui, O., Murakami, N., Tominaga, T., Nakai, Y., Mori, K., Kasting, N. W., and Imura, H., 1991, Effects of interleukins on plasma arginine vasopressin and oxytocin levels in conscious, freely moving rats, *Biochem. Biophys. Res. Commun.* **179**:1189.

Navarra, P., Tsagarakis, S., Faria, M. S., Rees, L. H., Besser, G. M., and Grossman, A. B., 1991, Interleukin-1 and interleukin-6 stimulate the release of corticotropin-releasing hormone-YI from rat hypothalamus in vitro via the eicosanoid cyclooxygenase pathway, *Endocrinology* **128**:37.

Nikolarakis, K. E., Almeida, O. F. X., and Herz, A., 1986, Corticotropin-releasing factor (CRF) inhibits gonadotropin-releasing hormone release from superfused rat hypothalami in vitro, *Brain Res.* **377**:388.

Nishimoto, N., Ogata, A., Shima, Y., Tani, Y., Ogawa, H., Nakagawa, M., Sugiyama, H., Yoshizaki, K., and Kishimoto, T., 1994, Oncostatin M, leukemia inhibitory factor, and interleukin-6 induce proliferation of human plasmacytoma cells via the common signal transducer gp130, *J. Exp. Med.* **179**:1343.

Novack, D. V., and Korsmeyer, S. J., 1994, Bcl-2 protein expression during murine development, *Am. J. Pathol.* **145**:61.

Nunez, G., Hockenbery, D., McDonnel, T. J., Sorensen, C. M., and Korsmeyer, S. J., 1991, Bcl-2 maintains B-cell memory, *Nature* **353**:71.

Otten, U., Ehrhard, P., and Peck, R., 1989, Nerve growth factor induces growth and differentiation of human B lymphocytes, *Proc. Natl. Acad. Sci. USA* **86**:10059.

Panayotou, G., End, P., Aumailly, M., Timpl, R., and Engel, J., 1989, Domains of laminin with growth factor activity, *Cell* **56**:93.

Patterson, P. H., 1992, The emerging neuropoietic cytokine family: First CDF/LIF, CNTF and IL-6; next ONC, MGF, GCSF? *Curr. Opin. Neurobiol.* **2**:94.

Patterson, P. H., and Nawa, H., 1993, Neuronal differentiation factors/cytokines and synaptic plasticity, *Cell* **72**(Suppl.):123.

Petraglia, F., Vale, W., and Rivier, C., 1986, Opioids act centrally to modulate stress-induced decrease in luteinizing hormone in the rat, *Endocrinology* **119**:2445.

Petraglia, F., Sutton, S., Vale, W., and Plotsky, P., 1987, Corticotropin-releasing factor decreases plasma LH levels in female rats by inhibiting gonadotropin-releasing hormone release into hypophyseal-portal circulation, *Endocrinology* **120**:1083.

Petrovicky, P., 1989, Relationship between the central nervous and immune systems: A neuroanatomical aspect, in: *Interactions Among Central Nervous System, Neuroendocrine and Immune Systems* (J. W. Hadden, K. Masek, and G. Nistico, eds.), Pythagora Press, Rome, pp. 5–16.

Petrovicky, P., Kadlecova, O., and Masek, K., 1981, Mutual connections of the raphe system and the hypothalamus and their relationship to thermoregulation and fever, *Brain Res. Bull.* **7**:131.

Petrovicky, P., Masek, K., and Seifert, J., 1994, Brain regulatory system for the immune response: Immunopharmacology and morphology, *Neuroimmunomodulation* **1**:165.

Plaut, M., 1987, Lymphocyte hormone receptors, *Annu. Rev. Immunol.* **5**:261.

Qui, L., Bernd, P., and Fukada, K., 1994, Cholinergic neuronal differentiation factor (CDF)/leukemia inhibitory factor (LIF) binds to specific regions of the developing nervous system in vivo, *Dev. Biol.* **163**:518.

Rao, M. S., Tyrrell S., Landis, S. C., and Patterson, P. H., 1992, Effects of ciliary neurotrophic factor (CNTF) and depolarization on neuropeptide expression in cultured sympathetic neurons, *Dev. Biol.* **150**:281.

Rathjen, F. G., and Schachner, M., 1984, Immunocytological and biochemical characterization of a new neuronal cell surface component (LI antigen) which is involved in cell adhesions, *EMBO J.* **3**:1.

Rende, M., Muir, D., Ruoslahti, E., Hagg, T., Varon, S., and Manthorpe, M., 1992, Immunolocalization of ciliary neurotrophic factor in adult rat sciatic nerve, *GLIA* **5**:25.

Renoux, G., Biziere, K., Renoux, M., Bardos, P., and Degenne, D., 1987, Consequences of bilateral brain neocortical ablation on imuthiol-induced immunostimulation in mice, *Ann. N.Y. Acad. Sci.* **496**:346.

Rettori, V., Jurcovicova, J., and McCann, S. M., 1987, Central action of interleukin-1 in altering the release of TSH, growth hormone, and prolactin in the male rat, *J. Neurosci. Res.* **18**:179.

Rettori, V., Gimeno, M. F., Karara, A., Gonzalez, M. C., and McCann, S. M., 1991, Interleukin-1α inhibits prostaglandin E_2 release to suppress pulsatile release of luteinizing hormone but not follicle stimulating hormone, *Proc. Natl. Acad. Sci. USA* **88**:2763.

Rinner, I., Porta, S., and Schauenstein, K., 1990, Characterization of ^{3}H-N-methylscopolamine binding to intact rat thymocytes, *Endocrinol. Exp.* **24**:125.

Rivier, C., and Vale, W., 1989, In the rat interleukin-1 alpha acts at the level of the brain and the gonads to interfere with gonadotropin and sex steroid secretion, *Endocrinology* **124**:2105.

Rivier, C., and Vale, W., 1990, Cytokines act within the brain to inhibit luteinizing hormone secretion and ovulation in the rat, *Endocrinology* **127**:849.

Rivier, C., Chizonnite, R., and Vale, W., 1989, In the mouse the activation of the hypothalamic–pituitary–adrenal axis by a lipopolysaccharide (endotoxin) is mediated through interleukin-1, *Endocrinology* **125**:2800.

Robicsek, S., Szentivanyi, A., Calderon, E. G., Heim, O., Schultze, P., Wagner, H., Lockey, R. F., and Dwornik, J. J., 1992, Concentrated IL-1α derived from human T-lymphocytes binds to a specific single class surface receptor on human bronchial epithelial cells and induces the production of beta-adrenoceptor mRNA via an associated or separate receptor-linked signalling pathway, *J. Allergy Clin. Immunol.* **89**:212.

Romano, T. A., Felten, S. Y., Felten, D. L., and Olschowaka, J. A., 1991, Neuropeptide Y innervation of the rat spleen: Another potential immunomodulatory neuropeptide, *Brain Behav. Immun.* **5**:116.

Rose, T. M., and Bruce, A. G., 1991, Oncostatin M is a member of a cytokine family that includes leukemia inhibitory factor, granulocyte colony-stimulating factor and interleukin-6, *Proc. Natl. Acad. Sci. USA* **88**:8641.

Rosenthal, A., Goeddel, D. V., Nguyen, T., Lewis, M., Shih, A., Laramee, G. F., Nikolics, K., and Winslow, J. W., 1990, Primary structure and biological activity of a novel human neurotrophic factor, *Neuron.* **4**:767.

Roszman, T. L., and Brooks, W. H., 1985, Neural modulation of immune function, *J. Neuroimmunol.* **10**:59.

Roszman, T. L., Cross, R. J., Brooks, W. H., and Markesbery, W. R., 1985, Neuroimmunomodulation: Effect of neural lesions on cellular immunity, in: *Neural Modulation of Immunity* (R. Guillemin, M. Cohn, and T. Melnechnuk, eds.), Raven Press New York, pp. 95–110.

Rudge, J. S., Morrissey, D., Lindsay, R. M., and Pasnikowski, E., 1994, Regulation of ciliary neutrophic factor in cultured rat hippocampal astrocytes, *Eur. J. Neurosci.* **6**:218.

Saadat, S., Sendtner, M., and Rohrer, H., 1989, Ciliary neurotrophic factor induces cholinergic differentiation of rat sympathetic neurons in culture, *J. Cell Biol.* **108:**1807.

Sakamoto, Y., Kitamura, K., Yoshimura, K., Nishijima, T., and Uyemura, K., 1987, Complete amino acid sequence of PO protein in bovine peripheral nerve myelin, *J. Biol. Chem.* **262:**4208.

Salzer, J. L., and Colman, D. R., 1989, Mechanisms of cell adhesion in the nervous system: Role of the immunoglobulin gene superfamily, *Dev. Neurosci.* **11:**377.

Scarborough, D. E., 1990, Cytokine modulation of pituitary hormone secretion, *Ann. N.Y. Acad. Sci.* **594:**169.

Schechter, G., 1989, A good relationship: Sensitive, synchronized and synergistic, *Prog. Neuro-Endocrine Immunol.* **2:**35.

Schena, M., Larsson, L. G., Gottardi, D., Gaidano, G., Carlsson, M., Nilsson, K., and Caligaris-Cappio, F., 1992, Growth and differentiation-associated expression of bcl-2 in B-chronic lymphocytic leukemia cells, *Blood* **79:**2981.

Schena, M., Gottardi, D., Ghia, P., Larsson, L. G., Carlsson, M., and Nilsson, K., 1993, The role of bcl-2 in the pathogenesis of B chronic lymphocyte leukemia, *Leuk. Lymphoma* **11:**173.

Schettini, G., Landolfi, E., Grimaldi, M., Meucci, O., Postiglione, A., Florio, T., and Ventra, C., 1989, Interleukin-1β inhibition of TRH-stimulated prolactin secretion and phosphoinositide metabolism, *Biochem. Biophys. Res. Commun.* **165:**496.

Schwartz, M. E., Reiner, S., Heim, O., Abarca, C. M., and Szentivanyi, A., 1988, Further observations on the cellular and molecular mechanisms involved in the reciprocal histamine–catecholamine counter-regulatory interplay in relation to induction of histidine decarboxylase synthesis by interleukin-3 and granulocyte–macrophage colony stimulating factor, in: *Proceedings of XIII International Congress of Allergology and Clinical Immunology*, Mosby–Yearbook, St. Louis, p. 64.

Selye, H., 1936, A syndrome produced by diverse nocuous agents, *Nature* **138:**32.

Selye, H., 1943, Morphological changes in the fowl following chronic overdosage with various steroids, *J. Morphol.* **73:**401.

Selye, H., 1946, The general adaptation syndrome and the diseases of adaptation, *J. Clin. Endocrinol.* **6:**117.

Selye, H., 1949, Effect of ACTH and cortisone upon an "anaphylactoid reaction," *Can. Med. Assoc. J.* **61:**553.

Sendtner, M., Schmalbruch, H., Stockli, K. A., Carroll, P., Kreutzberg, G. W., and Thoenen, H., 1992, Ciliary neurotrophic factor prevents degeneration of motor neurons in mouse mutant progressive motor neuronopathy, *Nature* **358:**502.

Shapiro, L., Zhang, X. X., Rupp, R. G., Wolff, S. M., and Dinarello, C. A., 1993, Ciliary neurotrophic factor is an endogenous pyrogen, *Proc. Natl. Acad. Sci. USA* **90:**8614.

Snyder, D. S., and Unanne, E. R., 1982, Corticosteroids inhibit murine macrophage la expression and interleukin-1 production, *J. Immunol.* **129:**1803.

Spangelo, B. L., Judd, A. M., Isakson, P. C., and MacLeod, R. M., 1989, Interleukin-6 stimulated anterior pituitary hormone release in vitro, *Endocrinology* **125:**575.

Spangelo, B. L., Judd, A. M., MacLeod, R. M., and Goodman, D. W., 1990, Endotoxin-induced release of interleukin-6 from rat medial basal hypothalamus, *Endocrinology* **127:**1779.

Spangelo, B. L., Jarvis, W. D., Judd, A. M., and MacLeod, R. M., 1991a, Induction of interleukin-6 release by interleukin-1 in rat anterior pituitary cells in vitro: Evidence for an eicosanoid-dependent mechanism, *Endocrinology* **129:**2886.

Spangelo, B. J., Judd, A. M., Isakson, P. C., and MacLeod, R. M., 1991b, Interleukin-1 stimulates interleukin-6 release from rat anterior pituitary cells in vitro, *Endocrinology* **128:**2686.

Sporeno, E., Paonessa, G., Salvati, A. L., Graziani, R., Delmastro, P., Ciliberto, G., and Toniatti, C., 1994, Oncostatin M binds directly to gp 130 and behaves as interleukin-6 antagonist on a cell line expressing gp130 but lacking functional oncostatin M receptors, *J. Biol. Chem.* **269:**10991.

Srebro, Z., Spisak-Plonka, I., and Szirmai, E., 1974, Neurosecretion in mice during skin allograft rejection, *Agressologie* **15:**125.

Stockli, K. A., Lottspeich, F., Sendtner, M., Masiakowski, P., Carroll, P., Gotz, R., Lindholm, D., and Thoenen, H., 1989, Molecular cloning, expression and regional distribution of rat ciliary neurotrophic factor, *Nature* **342:**920.

Stockli, K. A., Lillien, L. F., Naher-Noe, M., Breitfeld, G., Hughes, R. A., Raff, M. C., Thoenen, H., and Sendtner, H., 1991, Regional distribution, developmental changes, and cellular localization of ciliary neurotrophic factor mRNA and protein in the rat brain, *J. Cell Biol.* **115:**447.

Strom, T. B., Syrokowski, A. T., Carpenter, C. B., and Merrill, J. B., 1974, Cholinergic augmentation of lymphocyte-mediated cytotoxicity: A study of the cholinergic receptor of cytotoxic T lymphocytes, *Proc. Natl. Acad. Sci. USA* **71:**1330.

Strom, T. B., Laane, M. A., and George, K., 1981, The parallel time-dependent, bimodal change in lymphocytic cholinergic binding activity and cholinergic influence upon lymphocyte-mediated cytotoxicity after lymphocyte activation, *J. Immunol.* **127:**705.

Suda, T., Tozawa, F., Ushiyama, T., Tomori, N., Sumitomo, T., Nakgami, Y., Yamada, M., Demura, H., and Shizume, K., 1989, Effects of protein kinase C related adrenocorticotropic secretagogues and interleukin-1 on proopiomelanocortin gene expression in rat anterior pituitary cells, *Endocrinology* **124:**1444.

Szeberenyi, J., and Erhardt, P., 1994, Cellular components of nerve growth factor signalling, *Biochim. Biophys. Acta* **1222:**187.

Szentendrei, T., Nakane, T., Lazarj-Wesley, E., Virmani, M., and Kunos, G., 1991, Regulation of beta-adrenergic receptor gene expression by interleukin-1, *Pharmacologist* **33:**225.

Szentivanyi, A., 1953, Allergie und Zentralnervensystem, *Acta Allergol.* **6:**27.

Szentivanyi, A., 1961, Hypothalamic influences on antibody formation and on bronchial responses to histamine, in: *Proceedings of the Fourth Aspen Conference on research in Emphysema and Asthma*, Aspen, CO, p. 78.

Szentivanyi, A., 1968, The beta-adrenergic theory of the atopic abnormality in bronchial asthma, *J. Allergy* **42:**203.

Szentivanyi, A., 1988a, The discovery of immune–neuroendocrine circuits and the concepts of prevailing immunologic thought that impeded the timely recognition of their role in immune-homeostasis, in: *Proceedings of the International Symposium on Interactions Between the Neuroendocrine and Immune Systems*, Pythagora Press, Rome, pp. 23–24.

Szentivanyi, A., 1988b, Plenary Lecture: Natural neuropeptides in the immunologic inflammation of the airways in asthma, in: *Proceedings of XIV World Congress of Natural Medicines*, Málaga, Spain.

Szentivanyi, A., 1989, The discovery of immune–neuroendocrine circuits in the fall of 1951, in: *Interactions Among Central Nervous System, Neuroendocrine and Immune Systems* (J. W. Hadden, G. Nistico, and K. Masek, eds.), Pythagora Press, Rome, pp. 1–5.

Szentivanyi, A., 1991, Beta-adrenergic subsensitivity in asthma and atopic dermatitis: A status report, *Acta Biomed. Hung. Am.* **1:**1.

Szentivanyi, A., 1993a, Adrenergic regulation, in: *Bronchial Asthma—Mechanisms and Therapeutics* (E. B. Weiss and M. Stein, eds.), Little, Brown, Boston, pp. 165–191.

Szentivanyi, A., 1993b, The immune–neuroendocrine circuitry and its relation to asthma, in: *Bronchial Asthma—Mechanisms and Therapeutics* (E. B. Weiss and M. Stein, eds.), Little, Brown, Boston, pp. 421–438.

Szentivanyi, A., and Filipp, G., 1956, Experimentelle Data zur regulativen Rolle des Neuroendokriniums in experimenteller Anaphylaxie. II. Relazionie e Communicazioni, *Rome Il Pansiero Scientifico* **237:**1.

Szentivanyi, A., and Filipp, G., 1958, Anaphylaxis and the nervous system. Part II, *Ann. Allergy* **16:**143.

Szentivanyi, A., and Filipp, G., 1962, *Propriètès Immuno-Chimiques et Physico-Chimiques des Anticorps*, Editions Mèdicales Flammarion, Paris.

Szentivanyi, A., and Fishel, C. W., 1965, Effect of bacterial products on responses to the allergic mediators, in: *Immunological Diseases* (M. Samter, ed.), Little, Brown, Boston, pp. 226–241.

Szentivanyi, A., and Fishel, C. W., 1966, Die Amin-Mediatorstoffe der allergischen Reaktion und die reaktionsfahiegheit ihrer Erfolgeszellen, in: *Pathogenese und Therapie allergischer Reaktionen* (G. Filipp and A. Szentivanyi, eds.), Ferdinand Enke Verlag, Stuttgart, pp. 588–683.

Szentivanyi, A., and Fitzpatrick, D. F., 1980, The altered reactivity of the effector cells to antigenic and pharmacological influences and its relation to cyclic nucleotides. II. Effector reactivities in the efferent loop of the immune response, in: *Pathomechanismus und Pathogenese Allergischer Reaktionen* (G. Filipp, ed.), Werk-Verlag Dr. Edmund Banachewski, Munich, pp. 511–580.

Szentivanyi, A., and Szekely, J., 1956, Effect of injury to, and electrical stimulation of hypothalamic areas on the anaphylactic and histamine shock of guinea pig, *Ann. Allergy* **14:**259.

Szentivanyi, A., and Szekely, J., 1957a, Uber den Effekt der Schadigung und der elektrischen Reizung der hypothalamischen Gegenden auf den anaphylaktischen und Histamin-Schock des Meerschweinchens, *Allerg. Asthmaforsch. Bd.* **1:**28.

Szentivanyi, A., and Szekely, J., 1957b, Wirkung der konstanten Reizung hypothalamischer Strukturen durch Tiefenelektroden auf den histaminbedingten und anaphylaktischen Schock des Meerschweinchens, *Acta Physiol. Hung. Suppl V* **11:**41.

Szentivanyi, A., and Szekely, J., 1958, Anaphylaxis and the nervous system. Part IV, *Ann. Allergy* **16:**389.

Szentivanyi, A., and Szentivanyi, J., 1982a, Immunomodulatory effects of central and peripheral autonomic mechanisms mediated by neuroeffector molecules, in: *Proceedings of International Symposium on Biological Response Modifiers in Clinical Oncology and Immunology*, Plenum Press, New York. p. 8.

Szentivanyi, A., and Szentivanyi, J., 1982b, The emergence of neuroendocrine disorders as a new group of autoimmune diseases, in: *Proceedings of Symposium on Clinical Laboratory Immunology*, Plenum Press, New York, p. 3.

Szentivanyi, A., and Szentivanyi, J., 1987, Immune–neuroendocrine circuits in antibiotic–bacterial interactions, in: *Proceedings of Third International Symposium on the Influence of Antibiotics on the Host–Parasite Relationship*, Springer-Verlag, Berlin, Abstr. 40.

Szentivanyi, A., and Szentivanyi, J., 1988, Antibiotic–bacterial interactions in relation to immune–neuroendocrine circuits, in: *Proceedings of XIII International Congress of Allergology and Clinical Immunology*, Mosby–Yearbook, St. Louis, Abstr. 986.

Szentivanyi, A., Filipp, G., and Legeza, I., 1952, Investigations on tobacco sensitivity, *Acta Med. Hung. Tomus III, Fasciculus* **2:**175.

Szentivanyi, A., Krzanowski, J. J., and Polson, J. B., 1978, The autonomic nervous system: Structure, function, and altered effector responses, in: *Allergy: Principles and Practice* (E. Middleton, C. E. Reed, and E. F. Ellis, eds.), Mosby, St. Louis, pp. 256–300.

Szentivanyi, A., Polson, J. B., and Krzanowski, J. J., 1980, The altered reactivity of the effector cells to antigenic and pharmacological influences and its relation to cyclic nucleotides. I. Effector reactivities in the efferent loop of the immune response, in: *Pathomechanismus und Pathogenese Allergischer Reaktionen* (G. Filipp, ed.), Werk-Verlag Dr. Edmund Banachewski, Munich, pp. 460–510.

Szentivanyi, A., Middleton, E., Williams, J. F., and Friedman, F., 1983, Effect of microbial agents on the immune network and associated pharmacologic reactivities, in: *Allergy: Principles and Practice* (E. Middleton, C. E. Reed, and E. F. Ellis, eds.), Mosby, St. Louis, pp. 211–236.

Szentivanyi, A., Maurer, P., and Janicki, B. W., eds., 1987a, *Antibodies: Structure, Synthesis, Function, and Immunologic Intervention in Disease*, Plenum Press, New York.

Szentivanyi, A., Reiner, S., Filipp, G., and Heim, O., 1987b, The influence of anterior hypothalamic lesions on the kinetic parameters of ^{125}I-VIP (vasoactive intestinal peptide) binding to murine mononuclear cells, in: *Proceedings of Workshop 12 on Mediators in Asthma, XII World Congress of Asthmology*, Editorial Garsi, Madrid, p. 41.

Szentivanyi, A., Haberman, K., Heim, O., Schultze, P., Filipp, G., and Reiner, S., 1988a, Hypothalamic and other central influences on antibiosis and host immunity, in: *Proceedings of the Fourth International Conference on Immunopharmacology*, Pergamon Press, Oxford, Abstr. 5101.

Szentivanyi, A., Krzanowski, J. J., and Polson, J. B., 1988b, The autonomic nervous system and altered effector responses, in: *Allergy: Principles and Practice* (E. Middleton, C. E. Reed, and E. F. Ellis, eds.), Mosby, St. Louis, pp. 461–493.

Szentivanyi, A., Reiner, S., Heim, O., Filipp, G., and Abarca, C. M., 1988c, The effect of 6-hydroxydopamine hydrobromide on endotoxin-induced adrenergic mechanisms, in: *Proceedings of Second International Meeting on Respiratory Allergy*, Pythagora Press, Rome, Abstr. 311.

Szentivanyi, A., Reiner, S., Heim, O., Filipp, G., and Abarca, C. M., 1988d, Some biochemical and cellular features of adrenergic mechanisms induced by bacterial lipopolysaccharide endotoxin in rats with or without chemical sympathetic ablation achieved by 6-hydroxydopamine hydrobromide (6-OHDA), in: *Proceedings of International Symposium on Endotoxin*, Jichi Medical School, Tochigi, Japan, Abstr. SV-8.

Szentivanyi, A., Szentivanyi, J., Haberman, K., and Heim, O., 1988e, Nonantibiotic properties of antibiotics in relationship to immune–neuroendocrine influences, *Clin. Pharmacol. Ther.* **43:**166.

Szentivanyi, A., Reiner, S., Heim, O., Filipp, G., and Abarca, C. M., 1989a, The effect of sympathetic ablation [6-hydroxydopamine hydrobromide (6-OHDA); axotomy] on endotoxin induced adrenergic mechanisms, *Pharmacologist* **31:**118.

Szentivanyi, A., Reiner, S., Schwartz, M. E., Heim, O., Szentivanyi, J., and Robicsek, S., 1989b, Restoration of normal beta adrenoceptor concentrations in A549 lung adenocarcinoma cells by leukocyte protein factors and recombinant interleukin-1α, *Cytokine* **1:**118.

Szentivanyi, A., Krzanowski, J. J., Polson, J. B., and Abarca, C. M., 1990, The pharmacology of microbial modulation in the induction and expression of immune reactivities. I. The pharmacologically active effector molecules of immunologic inflammation, immunity, and hypersensitivity, *Immunopharmacol. Rev.* **1:**159.

Szentivanyi, A., Calderon, E. G., Heim, O., Schultze, P., Wagner, H., Zority, J., Lockey, R. F., Dwornik, J. J., and Robicsek, S., 1992, Cell- and species-specific dissociation in the beta-adrenoceptor upregulating effects of IL-1α derived from lymphocyte conditioned medium and cortisol, *J. Allergy Clin. Immunol.* **89:**274.

Szentivanyi, J., Szentivanyi, A., Williams, J. F., and Friedman, H., 1986, Virus associated immune and pharmacologic mechanisms in disorders of respiratory and cutaneous atopy, in: *Viruses, Immunity and Immunodeficiency* (A. Szentivanyi and H. Friedman, eds.), Plenum Press, New York, pp. 211–244.

Szentivanyi, J., Szentivanyi, A., Schultze, P., Filipp, G., and Heim, O., 1988, Influences of hypothalamic and extrahypothalamic brain structures on the immunogenicity of antibiotic-pretreated bacteria, in: *Proceedings of Annual Meeting of the International Society for Interferon Research*, Japanese Society for Interferon Research, Kanagawa, p. 325.

Szentivanyi, J., Schultz, P., Heim, O., Abarca, C., and Szentivanyi, A., 1989a, Hypothalamic and other central influences on antibiotic modulated bacterial immunogenicity, *Pharmacologist* **31:**193.

Szentivanyi, J., Schultze, P., Heim, O., Reiner, S., Robicsek, S., Abarca, C., and Szentivanyi, A., 1989b, The effect of hypothalamic and extrahypothalamic nuclear groupings on the antibiotic modulated bacterial immunogenicity and production of IL-1, IFN and TNF, *Cytokine* **1:**364.

Szentivanyi, J., Szentivanyi, A., Schultze, P., Filipp, G., and Heim, O., 1989c, Changes in the immune parameters of antibiotic–bacterial interactions induced by hypothalamic and other electrolytic brain lesions produced through stereotaxically implanted depth electrodes, in: *The Influence of Antibiotics on the Host–Parasite Relationship* (G. Gillissen, W. Opferkuch, G. Peters and G. Pulverer, eds.), Springer-Verlag, Berlin, pp. 237–244.

Taga, T., Higi, M., Hirata, Y., Yamasaki, K., Yasukawa, K., Matsuda, T., Hirano, T., and Kishimoto, T., 1989, Interleukin-6 triggers the association of its receptor with a possible signal transducer, gp130, *Cell* **58:**573.

Taira, E., Takaha, N., and Miki, N., 1993, Extracellular matrix proteins with neurite promoting activity and their receptors, *Neurosci. Res.* **17:**1.

Talmage, D. W., 1988, Introduction to basic immunology, in: *Immunological Diseases* (M. Samter, ed.), Little, Brown, Boston, pp. 1–3.

Tanaka, H., Matsui, T., Agata, A., Tomura, M., Kubota, I., McFarland, K. C., Kohn, B., Lee, A., Phillips, H., and Shelton, D. L., 1991, Molecular cloning and expression of a novel adhesion molecule, *Neuron* **7:**535.

Taniura, H., Hayashi, Y., and Miki, N., 1991, Purification and characterization of an 82-KD membrane protein as a neurite outgrowth factor binding protein: Possible involvement of NOF binding protein in axonal outgrowth in developing retina, *J. Cell Biol.* **112:**313.

Tischler, A. S., Riseberg, J. C., Hardenbrook, M. A., and Cherington, V., 1993, Nerve growth factor is a potent inducer of proliferation and neuronal differentiation for adult rat chromaffin cells in vitro, *J. Neurosci.* **13:**1533.

Tokiwa, M. A., Gaspar, E. M., and Doering, L. C., 1994, CNTF is superior to NGF as a survival enhancement factor for adrenal medulla cells in vitro, *Neuroreport* **5**:549.

Tsuda, T., Wong, D., Dolovich, J., Bienenstock, J., Marshall, J., and Denburg, J. A., 1991, Synergistic effects of nerve growth factor and granulocyte macrophage colony stimulating factor on human basophilic cell differentiation, *Blood* **77**:971.

Uehara, A., Gottschall, P. E., Dahl, R. R., and Arimura, A., 1987, Interleukin-1 stimulates ACTH release by an indirect action which requires endogeneous corticotropin releasing factor, *Endocrinology* **121**:1580.

Ullrich, A., Gray, A., Berman, C., and Dull, T. J., 1983, Human beta-nerve growth factor gene sequence highly homologous to that of mouse, *Nature* **303**:821.

Vankele-Com, H., Carmeliet, P., Van Damme, J., Billiau, A., and Denef, C., 1990, Production of interleukin-6 by folliculo-stellate cells and hormone-secreting cells in perfused anterior pituitary cell aggregates, *Neuroendocrinology* **49**:102.

Van Vlasselaer, P., 1992, Leukemia inhibitory factor: A growth factor with pleiotropic effects on bone biology, *Prog. Growth Factor Res.* **4**:337.

Vekshina, N., and Magaeva, S. V., 1974, Changes in the serotonin concentration in the limbic structures of the brain during immunization, *Bull. Exp. Biol. Med.* **77**:625.

Villuendas, R., Piris, M. A., Orradre, J. L., Mollejo, M., Rodriguez, R., and Morente, M., 1991, Different bcl-2 protein expression in high-grade B-cell lymphomas derived from lymph node or mucosa-associated lymphoid tissue, *Am. J. Pathol.* **139**:989.

Weihe, E., Muller, S., Fink, T., and Zentel, H. J., 1980, Tachykinins, calcitonin gene-related peptide and neuropeptide Y in nerves of the mammalian thymus: Interactions with mast cells in autoimmune and sensory neuroimmunomodulation, *Neurosci. Lett.* **100**:77.

Weihe, E., Nohr, D., Michel, S., Muller, S., Zentel, H. J., Fink, T., and Krekel, J., 1991, Molecular anatomy of the neuroimmune connections, *Int. J. Neurosci.* **59**:1.

Whitnall, M. H., Perlstein, R. S., Mougey, E. H., and Neta, R., 1992, Effects of interleukin-1 on the stress-responsive and nonresponsive subtypes of corticotropin-releasing hormone neurosecretory axons, *Endocrinology* **131**:37.

Williams, A. F., and Barclay, A. N., 1988, The immunoglobulin superfamily—Domains for cell surface recognition, *Annu. Rev. Immunol.* **6**:381.

Willkinson, D. G., and Krumlauf, R., 1990, Molecular approaches to the segmentation of the hindbrain, *Trends Neurosci.* **13**:335.

Yamaguchi, M., Koike, K., Matsuzaki, N., Yoshimoto, Y., Taniguchi, T., Miyake, A., and Tanizawa, O., 1991a, The interferon family stimulates the secretions of prolactin and interleukin-6 by the pituitary gland in vitro, *J. Endocrinol. Invest.* **14**:457.

Yamaguchi, M., Koike, K., Yoshimoto, Y., Ikegami, H., Miyake, A., and Tanizawa, O., 1991b, Effect of TNF-alpha on prolactin secretion from rat anterior pituitary and dopamine release from the hypothalamus: Comparison with the effect of IL-1β, *Endocrinol. Jpn.* **38**:357.

Yamamori, T., 1992, Molecular mechanisms for generation of neural diversity and specificity: Roles of polypeptide factors in development of postmitotic neurons, *Neurosci. Res.* **12**:545.

Yamamori, T., and Sarai, A., 1992, Coevolution of cytokine receptor families in the immune and nervous systems, *Neurosci. Res.* **16**:235–236.

Yamamori, T., Fukada, K., Aebersold, R., Korsching, S., Fann, S. M., and Patterson, P. H., 1989, The cholinergic neuronal differentiation factor from heart cells is identical to leukemia inhibitory factor, *Science* **246**:1412.

Zarling, J. M., Shoyab, M., Marquardt, H., Hanson, M. B., Lioubin, M. N., and Todaro, G. J., 1986, Oncostatin M: A growth regulator produced by differentiated histiocytic lymphoma cells, *Proc. Natl. Acad. Sci. USA* **83**:9739.

Zeki, K., Azuma, H., Suzuki, H., Morimoto, I., and Eto, S., 1991, Effects of interleukin-1 on growth and adenosine 3′,5′-monophosphate generation of the rat thyroid cell line, FRTL-5 cells, *Acta Endocrinol.* **124**:60.

Zerek-Melen, G., Pawlikowski, M., Winczyk, K., Lachowica-Ochedalska, A., Legowska, A., Kwasny, H., Przybylski, J., and Szadowska, A., 1993, Effects of new somatostatin analogs on the cell proliferation of colonic crypts and colonic cancers in rats, *Neuropeptides* **25:**57.

Zhang, X. G., Gu, J.-J., Lu, Z.-Y., Kasukawa, K., Yancopoulos, G. D., Turner, K., Shoyab, M., Taga, T., Kishimoto, T., Bataille, R., and Klein, B., 1994, Ciliary neurotropic factor, interleukin-11, leukemia inhibitory factor and oncostatin M are growth factors for human myeloma cell lines using the interleukin-6 signal transducer gp130, *J. Exp. Med.* **179:**1337.

Zhong, L. T., Kane, D. J., and Bredesen, D. E., 1993, Bcl-2 blocks glutamate toxicity in neural cell lines, *Brain Res.* **19:**353.

INDEX